CLINICAL TRIALS

Monographs in Epidemiology and Biostatistics
edited by Abraham M. Lilienfeld

Monographs in Epidemiology and Biostatistics
Volume 8

CLINICAL TRIALS
Design, Conduct, and Analysis

Curtis L. Meinert, Ph.D.

Professor of Epidemiology and Biostatistics
School of Hygiene and Public Health
The Johns Hopkins University

In collaboration with
Susan Tonascia, M.Sc.

Research Associate
School of Hygiene and Public Health
The Johns Hopkins University

New York   Oxford
OXFORD UNIVERSITY PRESS
1986

Oxford University Press

Oxford   New York   Toronto
Delhi   Bombay   Calcutta   Madras   Karachi
Petaling Jaya   Singapore   Hong Kong   Tokyo
Nairobi   Dar es Salaam   Cape Town
Melbourne   Auckland

and associated companies in
Beirut   Berlin   Ibadan   Nicosia

Published by Oxford University Press, Inc.,
198 Madison Avenue, New York, New York 10016-4314

Oxford is a registered trademark of Oxford University Press

Library of Congress Cataloging-in-Publication Data

Meinert, Curtis L.
Clinical trials.

(Monographs in epidemiology and biostatistics; v. 8)
Bibliography: p.
Includes indexes.
1. Clinical trials.   I. Tonascia, Susan.   II. Title.
III. Series. [DNLM: 1. Clinical Trials. W1 M0567Lt v.8
/ QV 771 M514c]
R853.C55M45   1986   610'.72   85-11530
ISBN-13 978-0-19-503568-1
ISBN 0-19-503568-2

Printing (last digit):   19 18 17

Printed in the United States of America
on acid-free paper

To
Susie, Julie, Nancy, and Jill

my wife and daughters for their help,
encouragement, forbearance, and understanding

Preface

And further, by these, my son, be admonished: Of making many books there is no end; and much study is a weariness of the flesh.

Ecclesiastes 12:12

This book consists of seven parts:

Part I: Introduction and Current Status (7 chapters)
Part II: Design Principles and Practices (5 chapters)
Part III: Execution (4 chapters)
Part IV: Data Analysis and Interpretation (4 chapters)
Part V: Management and Administration (3 chapters)
Part VI: Reporting Procedures (3 chapters)
Part VII: Appendixes (9 in number)

It is intended as a general reference for practitioners of clinical trials. The main focus is on trials involving uncrossed treatments and a clinical event as the outcome measure. It is not concerned with trials designed to assess bioavailability or with trials involving crossover designs. However, this is not to say that it is of no value for researchers with such interests, since some of the design and operating principles and practices described herein extend to such trials as well. Parts of this book, such as the chapters concerned with sample size calculation, randomization, forms design, quality assurance, and reporting procedures, apply to most kinds of trials.

This book deals with single-center as well as multicenter trials, as defined in Chapter 4. No distinction is made between the two types in most of the chapters, because the design and operating practices are largely the same for both. There are only two chapters, 5 and 23, that deal exclusively with multicenter trials, and even they have some relevance to single-center trials.

Appendix A contains a glossary of terms and acronyms used in this book and serves as a starting point for a dictionary of terms for clinical trials in general. Appendix B contains operational information for 14 of the trials referenced. Tabulations based on the information contained in this appendix appear in various chapters of the book. Appendix I contains a combined bibliography of references cited in the various chapters and appendixes (except B and C). References in the combined bibliography have been arranged alphabetically by first author and then chronologically. The reference lists in Table B–3, Appendix B, for the studies sketched, are in chronological order. Journal abbreviations used in the reference listings throughout correspond to those used by the National Library of Medicine in *Index Medicus* and MEDLINE. The other five appendixes relate to specific chapters in the book.

The impetus for this book emerged from a long-standing involvement in clinical trials, beginning with the University Group Diabetes Program in 1961. The urge to develop a general text concerned with the design and conduct of clinical trials led to development of an initial draft in the spring of 1972. The emphasis in that and subsequent drafts during the next two years focused exclusively on a few large-scale multicenter trials. Work continued, but at a decelerating rate, until it came to a virtual halt by 1975, primarily because of other work commitments. The work lay dormant until late 1978 when, while still at the University of Maryland School of Medicine, I was persuaded to start anew by the late Abraham Lilienfeld. The revised outline involved 8 chapters. It gradually expanded to the current size.

Writing proceeded slowly until my move to the Department of Epidemiology of The Johns Hopkins University School of Hygiene and Public Health in late 1979, where I was faced with the challenge of developing a course on the design and conduct of clinical trials. That teaching effort and Susan Tonascia's participation in that activity helped me to organize my thoughts and to collect the materials needed for this book. I am indebted to her for her help.

Baltimore, Maryland C.L.M.
November 1985

Acknowledgments

I wish to begin by expressing my thanks to two individuals who stimulated and focused my interest in clinical trials. My sincere thanks to Jacob Bearman for his confidence in me when I had none and to Chris Klimt for his role in developing and promoting my career and for giving me the chance to learn about clinical trials by doing. I am indebted as well to the late Abraham Lilienfeld for his words of encouragement and editorial help during this writing effort.

One other individual, James Tonascia, deserves special thanks. I have benefited immensely from his teaching and counsel. His ideas and input are reflected in various places throughout this book. In fact, his notes, developed for an advanced course in epidemiology at Johns Hopkins, provided the starting point for much of what is contained in Chapter 9 and for some of Chapters 10 and 18 as well. In addition, he has spent hours reviewing various parts of this book, including all of Chapter 9 and parts of Chapter 10 and the Glossary.

Various others helped on specific parts of the book. I wish to thank each of them for their contribution. They include:

- Helen Abbey, for review of Chapter 9
- Barbara Andreassen, for help on Chapter 12 and art work on figures in the book
- Steven F. Bingham, for review of the VACSP #43 sketch in Appendix B
- Thomas Blaszkowski, for review of glossary terms and for referencing help concerning administration of government grants and contracts
- Robert Bradley, for referencing help on Chapter 7
- Paul L. Canner, for review of the Coronary Drug Project sketch in Appendix B and for information concerning procedures used in the CDP
- Jeffrey A. Cutler, for review of the Multiple Risk Factor Intervention Trial sketch in Appendix B
- Marie Diener, for help on Chapter 7
- Lloyd Fisher, for review of the Coronary Artery Surgery Study sketch in Appendix B and for information concerning procedures used in CASS
- Lawrence Friedman, for review of glossary terms and for review of the Aspirin Myocardial Infarction Study sketch in Appendix B
- Curt Furberg, for review of glossary terms
- Barbara S. Hawkins, for review of glossary terms, for review of the Macular Photocoagulation Study sketch in Appendix B, and for information concerning procedures used in the MPS
- C. Morton Hawkins, for review of the Hypertension Detection and Follow-Up Program sketch in Appendix B
- Charles Hennekens, for review of the Physicians' Health Study sketch in Appendix B
- Fred Heydrick, for critical review of and editorial help on Chapter 21
- Genell L. Knatterud, for review of the University Group Diabetes Program sketch in Appendix B and for information concerning procedures used in the UGDP, DRS, and ETDRS
- William F. Krol, for review of the Persantine Aspirin Reinfarction Study sketch in Appendix B and for information concerning procedures used in PARIS and AMIS
- John M. Lachin, for review of the National Cooperative Gallstone Study sketch and for information concerning procedures used in the NCGS
- John M. Long, for review of the Program on the Surgical Control of Hyperlipidemia sketch in Appendix B
- Maureen Maguire, for help on Chapter 9
- Medical librarians of the Johns Hopkins University, especially Katherine Branch and Karen Higgins, for referencing help throughout the book

- Lisa Mele, for help on Chapter 7
- Larry Moulton, for help on Chapter 9
- Ronald Prineas, for review of the Hypertension Prevention Trial sketch in Appendix B
- Michael Terrin, for help in carrying out the SMOG analysis on consent statements contained in Appendix E
- Robert Weiss, for review of the International Reflux Study in Children sketch in Appendix B

Thanks also go to Sheila Booker, Janet Hiller, Mary Hurt, Joan Jefferys, Jeanette Lautenschlager, Teresa Lee, Mark Van Natta, and Deborah Zeiler for help in producing this manuscript. Sheila Booker deserves a special note of thanks since it is she who did the bulk of the typing, always with great efficiency, accuracy, and good grace, even when working with copy in my worst hand that was almost impossible to decipher, even by me!

A thank you also to colleagues in the School of Hygiene and Public Health for their encouragement and for providing an environment and support structure conducive to a writing effort of this sort. And last I wish to express my gratitude to Jeffrey W. House and Joan Bossert, editors at Oxford University Press in New York. I am especially indebted to Joan Bossert for her exquisite editorial eye and ear and for her professionalism, patience, and persistence in dealing with a stubborn Midwesterner!

Contents

Tables and figures

Part I. Introduction and current status

Chapters in This Part

1. Introduction
2. Clinical trials: A state-of-the-art assessment
3. The activities of a clinical trial
4. Single center versus multicenter trials
5. Coordinating and other resource centers in multicenter trials
6. Cost and related issues
7. The impact of clinical trials on the practice of medicine

The seven chapters in this Part cover a number of background issues. The first provides a historical sketch of clinical trials and defines the class of trials considered in this book. Chapter 2 reviews the state of the art of clinical trials, as gleaned from published reports of clinical trials. Chapter 3 defines the stages of activities in a "typical" trial and discusses factors which influence these activities. Chapter 4 provides a definition of single and multicenter trials and discusses a number of issues related to these two classes of trials. Chapter 5 focuses on specialty centers of a multicenter trial with emphasis on coordinating centers. Chapter 6 summarizes available cost data on trials, as provided in the National Institutes of Health Inventory of Clinical Trials, and reviews factors that influence the cost of trials. The last chapter discusses factors that influence the way in which results from trials are viewed and used in everyday medical practice. The University Group Diabetes Program is used as a case study.

1. Introduction

Those who cannot remember the past are condemned to repeat it.

George Santayana

1.1 DEFINITION

A clinical trial is a planned experiment designed to assess the efficacy of a treatment in man by comparing the outcomes in a group of patients treated with the test treatment with those observed in a comparable group of patients receiving a control treatment, where patients in both groups are enrolled, treated, and followed over the same time period. The groups may be established through randomization or some other method of assignment. The outcome measure may be death, a nonfatal clinical event, or a laboratory test. The period of observation may be short or long depending on the outcome measure.

Under this definition, studies involving test and control-treated groups that are treated and followed over different time periods, such as studies involving a historical control group, do not qualify as a clinical trial. Also excluded are comparative studies involving animals other than man, or studies that are carried out in vitro using biological substances from man.

1.2 HISTORY OF CLINICAL TRIALS

The history of clinical trials has been traced by several persons, most notably by Bull (1959) and more recently by Lilienfeld (1982). Table 1-1 provides a summary of some of the historical events in the field of clinical trials.

The concepts involved in clinical trials are ancient. The Book of Daniel, verses 12 through 15, contains an account of a planned experiment with both baseline and follow-up observations.

Prove thy servants, I beseech thee, ten days; and let them give us pulse to eat, and water to drink. Then let our countenances be looked upon before thee, and the countenance of the children that eat of the portion of the King's meat: and as thou seest, deal with thy servants. So he consented to them in this matter, and proved them ten days. And at the end of ten days their countenances appeared fairer and fatter in flesh than all the children which did eat the portion of the King's meat (American Bible Society, 1816).

Avicenna, an Arabian physician and philosopher (980-1037), in his encyclopedic *Canon of Medicine*, set down seven rules to evaluate the effect of drugs on diseases. He suggested that a remedy should be used in its natural state, with uncomplicated disease, and should be observed in two "contrary types of disease." His *Canon* also suggested that the time of action and reproducibility of the treatment effect should be studied (Crombie, 1952).

Many of the early observations affecting choice of treatment were fortuitous and arose from natural consequences rather than planned experiments. The famous observation of the Renaissance surgeon, Ambroise Paré (1510-1590), during the battle to capture the castle of Villaine in 1537, is a case in point (Packard, 1921). Normal treatment procedure for battlefield injuries was to pour boiling oil over the wound. When Paré ran out of oil he found it necessary to resort to an alternative treatment consisting of a digestive made of egg yolks, oil of roses, and turpentine. Paré recognized the superiority of the treatment the next day.

I raised myself very early to visit them, when beyond my hope I found those to whom I had applied the digestive medica-

3

Table 1-1   Historical events in the development of clinical trials

Date	Author	Event
1747	Lind	Experiment with untreated control group (Lind, 1753)
1799	Haygarth	Use of sham procedure (Haygarth, 1800)
1800	Waterhouse	U.S.-based smallpox trial (Waterhouse, 1800, 1802)
1863	Gull	Use of placebo treatment (Sutton, 1865)
1923	Fisher	Application of randomization to experimentation (Fisher and MacKenzie, 1923)
1931	—	Special committee on clinical trials created by the Medical Research Council of Great Britain (Medical Research Council, 1931)
1931	Amberson	Random allocation of treatment to groups of patients (Amberson et al., 1931)
1937	—	Start of NIH grant support with creation of the National Cancer Institute (National Institutes of Health, 1981b)
1944	—	Publication of multicenter trial on treatment for common cold (Patulin Clinical Trials Committee, 1944)
1946	—	Promulgation of Nuremberg Code for Human Experimentation (Curran and Shapiro, 1970)
1962	Hill	Publication of book on clinical trials (Hill, 1962)
1962	Kefauver, Harris	Amendments to the Food, Drug and Cosmetic Act of 1938 (United States Congress, 1962)
1966	—	Publication of U.S. Public Health Service regulations leading to creation of Institutional Review Boards for research involving humans (Levine, 1981)
1967	Chalmers	Structure for separating the treatment monitoring and treatment administration process (Coronary Drug Project Research Group, 1973a)
1979	—	Establishment of Society for Clinical Trials (Society for Clinical Trials, Inc., 1980)
1980	—	First issue of *Controlled Clinical Trials*

ment, feeling but little pain, their wounds neither swollen nor inflamed, and having slept through the night. The others to whom I had applied the boiling oil were feverish with much pain and swelling about their wounds. Then I determined never again to burn thus so cruelly the poor wounded by arquebuses (Packard, 1921).

An indication that lemon juice was effective in preventing scurvy was the result of a fortuitous decision made by the East India Shipping Company in 1600. Only one of the company's four ships that sailed February 13, 1600, that of General James Lancaster, was supplied with lemon juice. Almost all of the sailors on board Lancaster's vessel remained free of scurvy, while most of the men on board the other three vessels fell victim to the disease. This led shipping company officials to conclude:

And the reason why the General's men stood better in health then [sic] the men of other ships, was this: he brought to sea with him certaine Bottles of the Juice of Limons, which hee gave to each one, as long as it would last, three spoonfuls every morning fasting: not suffering them to eate any thing after it till noone. This juice worketh much the better if the partie keepe, a short Dyet, and wholly refraine salt meate, which salt meate, and long being at the Sea is the only cause of the breeding of this Disease (Drummond and Wilbraham, 1940).

The first planned experiments were done without a formal comparison group. The results of the experiment, contrasted with previous experience, provided the basis for evaluation. The early smallpox experiments are a case in point. A study carried out by Lady Mary Wortley-Montague and Maitland in 1721 involved six inmates from Newgate prison, all assumed to have had no previous exposure to smallpox. The inmates were recruited through a policy, urged by Lady Wortley-Montague, in which King George I commuted the sentence of convicted felons if they agreed to inoculation. The prisoners were inoculated by engrafting smallpox matter from a patient with the natural disease onto both arms and the right leg. The fact that they remained free of smallpox was taken as evidence in favor of inoculation[1] (Creighton, 1894).

Jenner (1749–1823) described a series of experiments that involved 14 persons, or thereabouts, who had been vaccinated with cowpox (Baron, 1838). He later inoculated three of these people with smallpox and the others with cowpox. He subsequently wrote:

> *After the many fruitless attempts to give the Small-pox to those who had had the Cow-pox, it did not appear necessary, nor was it convenient to me, to inoculate the whole of those who had been the subjects of these late trials; yet I thought it right to see the effects of variolous matter on some of them, particularly William Summers, the first of these patients who had been infected with matter taken from the cow. He was therefore inoculated with variolous matter from a fresh pustule; but, as in the preceding Cases, the system did not feel the effects of it in the smallest degree (Jenner, 1798).*

Early experiments with anesthetics (ether and chloroform) in the 1840s by Long, Wells, Morton, and Simpson involved only a few patients and no control group (Duncum, 1947). The ability to render an individual unconscious and then to revive that individual was sufficient to establish the usefulness of anesthetics.

None of the early evaluations of penicillin involved controls. The dramatic recoveries achieved in treating infections, theretofore fatal, were by themselves sufficient to establish the efficacy of the treatment (Keefer et al., 1943).

One of the first experiments designed with a concurrently treated control group involved scurvy victims and was carried out by James Lind in 1747, while at sea on board the *Salisbury*. The study consisted of six different dietary regimens as described by Lind.

> *On the 20th of May 1747, I took twelve patients in the scurvy, on board the* Salisbury *at sea. Their cases were as similar as I could have them. They all in general had putrid gums, the spots and lassitude, with weakness of their knees. They lay together in one place, being a proper apartment for the sick in the fore-hold; and had one diet common to all, viz., watergruel sweetened*

with sugar in the morning; fresh mutton-broth often times for dinner; at other times puddings, boiled biscuit with sugar, etc.; and for supper, barley and raisins, rice and currants, sago and wine, or the like. Two of these were ordered each a quart of cyder a-day. Two others took twenty-five gutts of elixir vitriol *three times a-day, upon an empty stomach; using a gargle strongly acidulated with it for their mouths. Two others took two spoonfuls of vinegar three times a-day, upon an empty stomach; having their gruels and their other food well acidulated with it, as also the gargle for their mouth. Two of the worst patients, with the tendons in the ham rigid, (a symptom none of the rest had), were put under a course of sea-water. Of this they drank half a pint every day, and sometimes more or less as it operated, by way of gentle physic. Two others had each two oranges and one lemon given them every day. These they eat with greediness, at different times, upon an empty stomach. They continued but six days under this course, having consumed the quantity that could be spared. The two remaining patients, took the bigness of a nutmeg three times a-day, of an electuary recommended by an hospital surgeon, made of garlic, mustard-seed, rad raphan, balsam of Peru, and gum myrrh; using for common drink, barley-water well acidulated with tamarinds; by a decoction of which, with the addition of cremor tartar, they were gently purged three or four times during the course.*

Those receiving a daily ration of oranges and lemons fared best.

> *The consequence was, that the most sudden and visible good effects were perceived from the use of the oranges and lemons; one of those who had taken them, being at the end of six days fit for duty (Lind, 1753).*

Still, in spite of these findings, Lind and others clung to the notion that the best treatment involved placing patients stricken with scurvy in "pure dry air." The reluctance to accept oranges and lemons as treatment for the disease had to do, in part, with the relative expense of acquiring such fruits as opposed to the "dry air" treatment. It was 1795 before the British Navy supplied lemon juice for its ships at sea (Drummond and Wilbraham, 1940).

---

1. The results were not as convincing as first perceived. One of the six inmates was subsequently found to have had smallpox before inoculation and a second may have had the disease in childhood (Creighton, 1894).

The importance of a control treatment as a means of identifying placebo effects was recognized by Haygarth (1740–1827) in his 1799 study of Perkins' Tractors—metallic rods used to stroke the body of an ailing person (Haygarth, 1800). The rods were widely used at the time for a variety of conditions, including crippling rheumatism, pain in the joints, wounds, gout, pleurisy, and inflammatory tumors, as well as for "sedating violent cases of insanity." Haygarth used imitation tractors made of wood on five patients affected with chronic rheumatism.

Let their [the Tractors'] merit be impartially investigated, in order to support their fame, if it be well founded, or to correct the public opinion, if merely formed upon delusion. Such a trial may be accomplished in the most satisfactory manner, and ought to be performed without any prejudice. Prepare a pair of false, exactly to resemble the true Tractors. Let the secret be kept inviolable, not only from the patient, but every other person. Let the efficacy of both be impartially tried; beginning always with the false Tractors. The cases should be accurately stated, and the reports of the effects produced by the true and false Tractors be fully given, in the words of the patients. . . .

On the 7th of January, 1799, the wooden Tractors were employed. All the five patients, except one, assured us that their pain was relieved, . . .

The following day Haygarth used the metallic tractors on the same patients. He observed:

All the patients were in some measure, but not more relieved by the second application, except one, who received no benefit from the former operation, and who was not a proper subject for the experiment, having no existing pain, but only stiffness of her ankle (Haygarth, 1800).

Sir William Gull (1816–1890), in collaboration with Henry Sutton, demonstrated the importance of placebo treatment in assessing the natural variability of the course of disease and the possibility of spontaneous cure. They gave mint water to 44 rheumatic fever patients and, after close observation, concluded:

The cases show that too much importance has been attached to the use of medicines, especially those acute cases where the tendency to a natural cure is the greatest (Sutton, 1865).

Most of the early experiments involved arbitrary, nonsystematic schemes for assigning patients to treatment, such as that described by Lind. More systematic approaches were needed for trials in which patients were enrolled in a sequential fashion. Johannes Fibiger, in an evaluation of a therapeutic serum for the treatment of diphtheria patients, used a scheme in which "serum was injected into all those admitted on every other day" (Fibiger, 1898). Park and co-workers, in 1928, described a scheme involving use of an experimental treatment for lobar pneumonia on every other patient.

Patients were therefore taken alternatively for antibody treatment or control depending only on the order of their admission to the service. It was believed that with a sufficiently large series the distribution of cases by type would be equalized between the treated and the untreated group (Park et al., 1928).

The concept of randomization as a device for treatment assignment was introduced by Fisher while he was involved in agricultural experimentation (Box, 1980; Fisher and MacKenzie, 1923; Fisher, 1926, 1973). Amberson and his co-workers, in a study of sanocrysin in the treatment of pulmonary tuberculosis, were among the first to use the concept for treatment assignment in an actual clinical trial.

The 24 patients were then divided into two approximately comparable groups of 12 each. The cases were individually matched, one with another, in making this division. . . . Then, by a flip of the coin, one group became identified as group I (sanocrysin-treated) and the other as group II (control). The members of the separate groups were known only to the nurse in charge of the ward and to two of us. The patients themselves were not aware of any distinctions in the treatment administered (Amberson et al., 1931).

It was several years later before the process of randomization was used for assigning individual patients to treatment. Diehl and co-workers (1938) described a method of randomly assigning University of Minnesota student volunteers to treatment in a double-masked, placebo-controlled trial involving treatment of the common cold.

Great Britain, under the influence of men such as Sir Austin Bradford Hill, has been a leading force in the development of modern-day clinical trials. His book *Statistical Methods in Clinical and Preventive Medicine* (1962) represents an important milestone in the field of clinical trials.

The Medical Research Council of the United Kingdom recognized the need for clinical trials at least as early as 1930. An announcement in a 1931 issue of *Lancet* stated:

> The Medical Research Council announce that they have appointed a Therapeutic Trials Committee, as follows, to advise and assist them in arranging for properly controlled clinical tests of new products that seem likely, on experimental grounds, to have value in the treatment of disease. . . . The Therapeutic Trials Committee will be prepared to consider applications by commercial firms for the examination of new products, submitted with the available experimental evidence of their value, and appropriate clinical trials will be arranged in suitable cases (*Medical Research Council, 1931*).

The concept of multiple investigators from different sites, all following a common study protocol in the conduct of a clinical trial, did not emerge until the late 1930s and early 1940s. One of the first applications of this approach appeared in a 1944 publication of a trial to evaluate patulin for treatment of the common cold (Patulin Clinical Trials Committee, 1944).

A multicenter trial involving the use of streptomycin in patients with pulmonary tuberculosis was published in 1948 (Medical Research Council, 1948). One of the first multicenter trials in the United States involved assessment of the same drug (Mount and Ferebee 1952, 1953a, 1953b). The study was initiated about the same time as the British study but did not produce any published results until 1952—four years after the British publication.

The Veterans Administration (VA), in conjunction with the United States Armed Services, carried out a series of multicenter trials between 1945 and 1960 in an attempt to establish the efficacy of various chemotherapeutic agents in the treatment of tuberculosis (Tucker, 1960). The VA provided support for various other multicenter trials in the 1960s under a relatively informal funding structure. A more formal structure was created in 1972.

The United States poliomyelitis vaccine trials, started in the autumn of 1953, sponsored by the National Foundation for Infantile Paralysis and done in collaboration with the Public Health Service and state health departments, were multi-center (Francis et al., 1955). They are noteworthy because of their size. They involved tens of thousands of volunteers.

The creation of the National Cancer Institute in 1937 signaled the start of federally sponsored medical research in the United States and the creation of what ultimately has come to constitute the National Institutes of Health (National Institutes of Health, 1981b). The Institutes of this agency support by far the largest number of trials among all United States governmental agencies. The largest and most complex multicenter trials have been carried out by the National Heart, Lung, and Blood Institute (NHLBI). Some, such as the Multiple Risk Factor Intervention Trial (Multiple Risk Factor Intervention Trial Research Group, 1977) and the Hypertension Detection and Follow-Up Program (Hypertension Detection and Follow-Up Program Cooperative Group, 1979a), have involved thousands of patients and years of follow-up.

One of the first multicenter trials sponsored by the National Heart Institute (now the National Heart, Lung, and Blood Institute) was a trial involving the use of ACTH, cortisone, and aspirin as a treatment for rheumatic heart disease. The trial was initiated in 1951 and was carried out in conjunction with the Medical Research Council of Great Britain, the American Heart Association, and the Canadian Arthritis and Rheumatism Society (Rheumatic Fever Working Party, 1960).

Multicenter trials, focusing on the treatment of chronic noninfectious diseases, began to appear in the 1960s. One of the first examples in this category was the University Group Diabetes Program, started in 1960 and completed in 1974 (University Group Diabetes Program Research Group, 1970e, 1978).

The advent of multicenter clinical trials as a treatment evaluation tool has required collaboration among various disciplines. In addition to medical and biostatistical expertise, a typical large-scale multicenter trial requires close participation with various other specialists. This multidisciplinary approach has served to stimulate communication across disciplines, as evidenced by formation of the Society for Clinical Trials in 1979 and publication of *Controlled Clinical Trials* starting in 1980.

A major stimulus for the execution of clinical trials in the United States arose from language included in the 1962 Kefauver-Harris amendments to the United States Food, Drug and Cosmetic Act of 1938. The Act set forth a series of legal requirements which had to be satisfied be-fore a drug could be approved by the Food and Drug Administration—FDA (Colsky, 1963; Food and Drug Administration, 1963; Kelsey, 1963; United States Congress, 1962). A unique feature of the amendment was language spelling out the nature of scientific evidence required for a drug to be approved for human use—a specifi-cation heavily dependent on what are referred to in the act as "adequate and well-controlled in-vestigations."

The term "substantial evidence" means evi-dence consisting of adequate and well-controlled investigations, including clinical investigations, by experts qualified by sci-entific training and experience to evaluate the effectiveness of the drug involved, on the basis of which it could fairly and re-sponsibly be concluded by such experts that the drug will have the effect it purports or is represented to have under the conditions of its use prescribed, recommended, or sug-gested in the labeling or proposed labeling thereof (United States Congress, 1962).

Regulations published in the *Federal Register* (Food and Drug Administration, 1969a, 1969b, 1970a, 1970b) have set forth general design and execution standards for trials carried out as part of a FDA Investigational New Drug Applica-tion (INDA) and New Drug Application (NDA) processes. They were taken in large measure from testimony given by William Beaver in a court case involving the Pharmaceutical Manu-facturers Association versus Robert H. Finch, Secretary of Health, Education and Welfare, and Herbert L. Ley, Commissioner of Food and Drugs (Crout, 1982; United States District Court, 1969, 1970).

The Medical Device Amendments of 1976 have extended some of the testing requirements established for drugs to medical devices as well (United States Congress, 1976). Certain devices cannot be marketed without supporting evi-dence of safety and efficacy as obtained through controlled trials.

The importance of safe and effective treat-ments for major diseases has led Congress to earmark money for targeted areas of research. The Coronary Drug Project (CDP) is an early example of a trial funded via this route (Coro-nary Drug Project Research Group, 1973a). The emphasis on focused research has led to in-creased use of research contracts in place of grants by the NIH as funding vehicles for many

of the large-scale multicenter trials (see Chap-ters 5 and 21).

The long-term multicenter trial has created a new class of organizational and analysis prob-lems. A special task force convened by the Na-tional Heart Institute in 1967 outlined organiza-tion guidelines that have been used for many of the large-scale trials since then (Greenberg, 1967).[2] The analytic problems created by the need for periodic data analyses as the trial pro-ceeds have led to the development of organiza-tional structures that provide for a separation of the patient care and treatment evaluation func-tions. The structures, described in Chapter 23, emerged from concerns regarding the possibility of bias if study physicians are permitted access to study data during the course of the trial (Mei-nert, 1981). Chalmers was an early proponent of this separation of functions in the organization of the CDP.[3]

Cornfield played a major role in developing a philosophy that dealt with the problems of on-going analyses in long-term clinical trials (Green-house and Halperin, 1980; Seigel, 1982). His work on Bayesian analysis and on the use of the likelihood principle as an analytic tool served to de-emphasize the role of significance testing in data evaluation (Cornfield, 1969).

1.3   TERMINOLOGY CONVENTIONS

The language of clinical trials is confusing. Lan-guage conventions have not been established for characterizing the key design, organizational, and operational elements of trials (Meinert, 1980a). Appendix A provides a glossary of terms, abbreviations, and acronyms used in this book.

The term *patient* (see Glossary for the deriva-tion) will be used throughout to denote an indi-vidual enrolled in a trial. It will be used even though it may not always be appropriate, for example, as in trials that involve people without clinical disease. The term *test treatment* will de-note the treatment to be evaluated in the trial. The term *control treatment* will denote the treat-ment used for comparison with the test treat-

2. This report, according to William Zukel of the NHLBI (per-sonal communication, 1982), drew heavily on organizational expe-rience gained from earlier multicenter studies, most notably those done by the Committee on Lipoproteins (1956) and by the Rheu-matic Fever Working Party (1960).
3. A written communication from Thomas Chalmers to the Chair-man of the CDP Policy Board, Robert Wilkins, in 1967, led to the separation of these functions in the CDP.

Table 1-2 Frequency of selected terms in titles published in 1980*

	Titles under:			
Term used	MeSH of clinical trials		Other MeSH	
Titles containing the term *trial(s)*	502	(100)	191	(100)
Titles containing the term *trial(s)* plus:				
Clinical	201	(40)	41	(22)
Controlled	131	(26)	23	(12)
Double-blind	79	(16)	16	(8)
Random(ized)	74	(15)	13	(7)
Comparative	22	(4)	9	(5)
Field	15	(3)	4	(2)
Titles containing the term *trial(s)* and none of the above terms	99	(20)	103	(54)

*MEDLINE search, as of June 1982. Run restricted to nonreview articles in English appearing under the check tag *human*.

ment. For convenience, study designs will be discussed as if they involve a single test and control treatment, although certain trials may involve several test treatments. The term *study treatments* will denote the entire set of test and control treatments used in a trial.

The term *trial* is from the Anglo-French word *trier*, meaning to choose, sort, select, or try (Klein, 1971). Thomas Bayes (1702–1761), an English mathematician, made frequent use of the term in a nonmedical experimental sense in an essay on probability involving repeated drops of a billiard ball onto a surface to observe the position of its fall (Bayes, 1763). The use of the term in a medical context is not easy to trace. However, even a cursory search indicates it has been in use for some time. It appears in the writings of both Haygarth and Jenner around 1800. Its use today covers a wide variety of designs ranging from uncontrolled observations involving the first use of a treatment in man to a formal experiment, complete with a control treatment and randomization. The use of the term without modifiers implies nothing about the observational unit. It may be man or some other animal species—always man in this book.

Trial is frequently modified by the term *clinical* and/or one or more design terms (e.g., *randomized, placebo, controlled,* or *double-blind*). Table 1-2 provides an indication of modifier usage as seen in 1980 nonreview, publications in English appearing in the MEDLINE[4] data file.

The results presented are for articles appearing under the check tag *human*—a designation applied by indexers at the National Library of Medicine (NLM) to identify studies involving humans.[5] Tabulations presented in the first column of the table are based on a search of all the titles indexed under the medical subject heading (MeSH) *clinical trials* (1,949). Of the 502 articles containing the term *trials*, 40% also contained the term *clincial*. The term *trial* appeared without any of the modifiers listed in Table 1-2 in 20% of the titles (99 out of 502). It is worth noting that nearly three-fourths of the 1,949 articles screened did not contain the term *trial*. Other more nondescript terms such as *study* were used instead (see Chapter 2 and Coordinating Center Models Project Research Group, 1979e). Unfortunately, this pattern of use creates problems when an attempt is made to identify trials via title searching routines.

The results in the last column in Table 1-2 concern the use of the term *trial(s)* in articles appearing under MeSH headings other than *clinical trials*. A number of these may very well involve studies that are nonexperimental. Theoretically, this should be true for all articles not classified under the MeSH *clinical trials*. However, some of the articles identified appear to be germane to the field, as suggested by use of modifiers such as *clinical, controlled, double-blind, random,* or *randomized*.

4. Medical Literature Analysis Retrieval System On Line, a computer database of literature citations produced by the National Library of Medicine (Williams et al., 1979).

5. Most of the articles under the heading *clinical trials* appear under this tag. However, beginning in January 1981, the heading includes veterinary studies and hence contains studies where only the check tag *animal* is used.

1.4 FOCUS

This book will focus on the class of trials that involve:

- Man
- A fixed, nonsequential sample size design
- Random allocation of individual patients to treatment, as opposed to some larger randomization unit such as family, hospital ward, community, etc.
- An uncrossed treatment design (i.e., where the treatment design requires patients to receive either the test or control treatment, but not both)
- Concurrent enrollment, treatment, and follow-up of patients in the test and control treatment groups
- A clinical event, such as death or some other nonfatal event (e.g., a myocardial infarction, recurrence of cancer, loss of vision,

etc.), as the primary outcome measure for evaluating the test treatment

The fixed sample size design is by far the most commonly used design for the class of trials considered. Sequential designs (see Chapter 9 for further discussion) are not practical for comparing treatments in trials requiring long periods of follow-up for outcome assessment.

Emphasis will be on trials that require multiple clinics in order to enroll the required number of patients (see Appendix B for examples). The researcher who can cope with the challenges presented by such trials is in a good position to deal with less complicated trials carried out in a single clinic.

Many of the principles discussed herein have applicability beyond the setting outlined. This is true for several of the chapters, particularly those concerned with data collection (Chapter 12) and with organization and management practices (Chapters 22 and 23).

2. Clinical trials: A state-of-the-art assessment

One's knowledge of Science begins when he can measure what he is speaking about and express it in numbers.

Lord Nelson

2.1 EXISTING INVENTORIES

Various groups have assumed responsibility for developing and maintaining inventories of ongoing clinical trials. Some are organized according to disease; others relate to trials sponsored by a specific agency. An early example of the first type of inventory originated from the National Institute of Mental Health with the creation of the Biometric Laboratory Information Processing System (BLIPS) in the mid-1960s. The in-

ventory was created to provide information for ongoing trials of psychopharmacological agents in the United States and elsewhere (Levine et al., 1974). The National Cancer Institute (1983), via the International Cancer Research Data Bank, maintains a worldwide file of ongoing phase II and phase III cancer trials. The Veterans Administration (VA) maintains a list of trials carried out under its collaborative studies program (list available from the VA Central Office, 810 Vermont Avenue N.W., Washington, D.C.).

The Division of Research Grants of the National Institutes of Health (NIH) has maintained an inventory of NIH-sponsored trials for several years (National Institutes of Health, 1975, 1980). Responsible officials of institutes of the NIH involved in extramural or intramural research are asked to complete inventory sheets for all ongoing studies that they consider to satisfy the definition of a clinical trial, as specified in the inventory. The definition used is:

A scientific research activity undertaken to define prospectively the effect and value of prophylactic/diagnostic/therapeutic agents, devices, regimens, procedures, etc., applied to human subjects. It is essential that the study be prospective, and that intervention of some sort occur. The choice of number of cases or patients will depend on the hypothesis being tested, but must be sufficient to permit a definite result to be anticipated. Phase I, feasibility, or pilot studies are excluded.

This definition allows inclusion of trials with only one treatment group. One can only surmise that evaluation of the treatment is made against some hypothetical standard control treatment or through use of historical controls in such cases (see Chapter 1 and Glossary for definition of *clinical trial* as used in this book). The broad nature of the definition and the lack of surveillance by the Division of Research Grants in monitoring for differences in how the definition is applied allows for considerable variability in the reporting behavior of institutes contributing to the inventory. It is likely that some of the variation among institutes, within and across years, evident in tables in this chapter and in Chapters 5 and 6, is due to differences in reporting practices. Unfortunately, the inventory is not designed to provide data on the nature of the differences.

The number of trials reported for the 5-year period for which inventory data are available ranged from a low of 746 in 1977 to a high of 986 in 1979 (Table 2-1). The "typical" NIH trial, as reflected in the 1979 NIH Inventory,[1] involved between 30 and 300 patients (median sample size: 100) apportioned among the different treatment groups (Table 2-2). Most of the trials were classified as therapeutic (81%), as compared to

1. There have been no inventories since 1979, but one is planned for 1984 or 1985.

prophylactic (13%) and diagnostic (6%) (see Glossary for definitions). The majority (65%) were funded for a period of 3 years or longer.

Trials sponsored by the individual institutes vary in number and size (Table 2-3). The National Cancer Institute (NCI) sponsored by far

Table 2-1 Number of trials, median sample size, and percent randomized by fiscal year, as reported in NIH Inventories of Clinical Trials

Fiscal year	Total number of trials	Median sample size	Percent randomized
1975	755	127	62
1976	926	114	60
1977	746	125	62
1978	845	103	60
1979	986	100	60

Table 2-2 Design features of trials reported in the 1979 NIH Inventory of Clinical Trials

Design features	Number of trials	Percent
Number of treatment groups per trial		
1	258	26
2	438	44
≥3	290	29
Median number of treatment groups/trial: 1.48		
Sample size		
Median number of patients/trial	100	
Range (20th to 80th percentile)	30 to 300	
Number of patients/trial/treatment group*	68	
Range (20th to 80th percentile)	20 to 203	
Method of treatment allocation		
Random	589	60
Nonrandom	391	40
Method not reported	6	0
Type of trial		
Therapeutic	801	81
Prophylactic	126	13
Diagnostic	58	6
Anticipated length of trial		
≤1 year	19	2
1 year to ≤2 years	101	10
2 years to ≤3 years	223	23
>3 years	642	65
Total number of trials listed	986	100

*Calculated by dividing median number of patients per trial by the median number of treatment groups per trial.

Table 2-3 Number of trials, median sample size, and percent randomized, as reported in the 1979 NIH Inventory of Clinical Trials

Institute	Number of trials	Median sample size	Percent randomized
National Cancer Institute (NCI)	654	100	59
National Eye Institute (NEI)	26	200	85
National Heart, Lung, and Blood Institute (NHLBI)	20	850	100
National Institute of Allergy and Infectious Diseases (NIAID)	120	100	53
National Institute of Arthritis, Metabolism, and Digestive Diseases (NIAMDD)	67	70	60
National Institute of Child Health and Human Development (NICHD)	32	100	62
National Institute of Dental Research (NIDR)	26	663	65
National Institute of Neurological and Communicative Disorders and Stroke (NINCDS)	40	30	55
Total	985*	100	60

*One trial sponsored by the National Institute of General Medical Services not included.

the most trials (654 out of the 985 listed for 66% of all NIH trials). The National Heart, Lung, and Blood Institute (NHLBI) sponsored the largest trials (median sample size: 850). This variation in size is due, in part, to differences in the nature of the health problems addressed. The NCI plays a major role in developing and testing chemotherapeutic agents. Hence, many of their trials are of the phase I or II variety (see Glossary), involving relatively small numbers of patients. The NHLBI has concentrated on assessing the usefulness of various drugs and procedures in the primary or secondary prevention of heart disease. Their trials, of necessity, have had to involve large numbers of patients and long periods of follow-up because of low underlying event rates for the outcomes of interest.

2.2 TRIALS AS SEEN THROUGH THE PUBLISHED LITERATURE

An indication of the nature of completed trials can be obtained from a review of the published literature, as identified through *Index Medicus* or MEDLINE—the computerized version of *Index Medicus* (Beatty, 1979; Charen, 1977; Kenton and Scott, 1978; McCarn, 1980; Williams et al., 1979). The introduction in 1980 of a subject heading for *clinical trials* has made it possible to retrieve articles under this heading.[2] The

definition used by indexers at the National Library of Medicine—the agency responsible for entries into *Index Medicus* and MEDLINE—is:

Pre-planned usually controlled studies of the safety, efficacy, or optimum dosage schedule (if appropriate) of one or more diagnostic, therapeutic, or prophylactic drugs or technics in humans selected according to pre-determined criteria of eligibility and observed for pre-defined evidence of favorable and unfavorable effects (National Library of Medicine, 1980).

This definition, as with the one used by NIH, is designed to permit inclusion of studies with a wider number of design features, including some without a comparison group.

The heading included 2,409 citations bearing a 1980 publication date, as of an October 1981 MEDLINE search.[3] This number represents less than 1% of the total 1980 MEDLINE citations (Table 2-4). The 1,796 titles remaining after exclusion of review articles and foreign-language papers were ordered by date of entry into the MEDLINE file (approximately chronological by date of publication) and then sampled using a random start and a 1 in 10 sampling fraction. A total of 67 (37%) of the 180 papers selected were

2. Before 1980, trials were classified under the general heading *clinical research.*

3. This run included most of the 1980 publications. Evidence from previous years indicates that 95% of all entries for a given calendar year are indexed and entered into the system by October of the following year.

Table 2-4 1980 publications cited in MEDLINE as of October 1981

249,150	Total number of 1980 entries in MEDLINE
2,409	Number of 1980 titles under heading *clinical trials*
2,317	Number of 1980 titles remaining after exclusion of review articles
1,796	Number of 1980 titles remaining after the exclusion of review and foreign-language publications

Table 2-6 Number of journals represented in sample of 113 papers

Number of journals represented in sample of 113 papers	82
Number of journals with:	
1 of the 113 papers	65
2 of the 113 papers	9
3 or more of the 113 papers (see Table 2-7)	8

Source: Reference citation 321. Reprinted with permission of Elsevier Science Publishing Co., Inc., New York.

eliminated for reasons indicated in Table 2-5. The tabulations given in Tables 2-6 through 2-9 are based on the 113 remaining papers. Appendix C contains a list of all 180 papers (see also Meinert et al., 1984).

It would have been necessary to subscribe to no less than 82 different journals in order to have access to the 113 articles reviewed. Moreover, no combination of 4 or 5 journals accounted for a majority of the articles. Only 17 of the 82 journals contained 2 or more of the papers selected for review (Table 2-6). The 8 most frequently cited journals accounted for a little more than a quarter (27%) of the 113 articles (Table 2-7).

Each paper in the sample was classified as to major subject area (Table 2-8). General design characteristics of the trials represented in the sample are summarized in Table 2-9. The typical trial, as seen through published literature, is carried out in a single clinic and involves about 25 patients per treatment group followed over a relatively short time—usually less than 3 months.

Over 70% of the trials were classified as therapeutic (see Glossary for definition). The overwhelming proportion of trials involved drug treatments. Only 10 of the 113 studies involved some other form of treatment. Of the 10, 5 were surgical trials, 2 involved behavior modification, 2 involved a radiologic procedure, and 1 involved testing a medical device. Approximately a third (31%) of the trials used crossover designs (see Glossary).

The median length of follow-up was slightly over 2 months. There were only 12 trials that provided for a year or more of follow-up. Over two-thirds of the trials were reported to be double-masked; 80% of the reports indicated use of some random method for treatment assignment. Treatment assignment was classified in the nonrandom or unstated category if the paper contained an explicit statement indicating use of a nonrandom method or if there was no way to determine how assignments were made.

Fifteen of the trials (13%) were classified as multicenter. The remainder were classified as

Table 2-5 Literature selection process for papers appearing under heading *clinical trials*

Total number of English, nonreview, 1980 publications	1,796
Number of papers selected in sample	180
Number of papers excluded after initial review	67
No comparison group	15
Editorial or letter	17
Review or methodological paper	24
Other reasons*	11
Number reviewed	113

*Includes 1 paper that could not be located, 8 position or philosophical papers, and 2 others not classified as clinical trials under the definition used in this book (see Chapter 1 and Glossary).

Table 2-7 Journal of publication for 113 papers reviewed

Journal	Number of papers
Br Med J	6
Lancet	5
J Clin Pharmacol	4
Br J Clin Pharmacol	3
Br J Dis Chest	3
Cancer	3
J Int Med Res	3
S Afr Med J	3
All other journals (74)	83
Total number of papers in sample	113

Source: Reference citation 321. Reprinted with permission of Elsevier Science Publishing Co., Inc., New York.

Table 2-8   Subject matter of 113 papers reviewed

Subject	Number of papers
Cardiovascular	14
Gastrointestinal	14
Psycho-neurological	13
Cancer	10
Urinary system	8
Bone and joint	7
Dermatology	6
Dental	5
Respiratory	5
Allergy	4
Gynecologic	4
Ophthalmologic	3
Pain relief	3
Infectious disease	3
Other*	14
Total number of papers in sample	113

Source: Reference citation 321. Reprinted with permission of Elsevier Science Publishing Co., Inc., New York.

*Anesthesiology; ear, nose, and throat; diabetes; contraception; narcotics; diagnostic; trauma; drugs; and weight control.

single-center (89 studies) or could not be classified because of lack of information in the papers (9 studies). Slightly over half of the papers (53%) indicated a source of funding. Acknowledgment of a contribution of a supply item, such as drugs, was ignored in the classification, unless there was evidence that money was also provided.

Most trials presented results for a number of outcome measures (see Glossary). Many of the papers presented results for several different outcomes. It was impossible in nearly all those cases to identify the measure considered to be primary (see Glossary for definition). Most measures were of a nonclinical nature (e.g., usually laboratory or physiological measures). Only 3 trials used mortality as an outcome measure.

2.3   SMALL SAMPLE SIZE: A COMMON DESIGN FLAW

Only 2 of the 113 trials showed any evidence of a sample size calculation and they involved sequential designs. Of the others, 3 mentioned the statistical power (see Glossary) associated with the trial. The virtual disregard of power considerations is consistent with other literature reviews. None of the 83 gastrointestinal trials reviewed by Chalmers and co-workers (1978) included any discussion of power. Only 2 of the 93 papers from breast cancer trials reviewed by

Mosteller and co-workers (1980) contained a discussion of power. Power considerations are especially important in trials where investigators conclude in favor of the null hypothesis (Freiman and co-workers, 1978).

2.4   FUTURE NEEDS

The annals of medicine are filled with accounts of potions, drugs, devices, and the like, that have been heralded as great advances only to be shown as useless or even harmful later on. Bloodletting (venesection) has been used therapeutically as well as prophylactically from prehistoric times to the 1950s (Bryan, 1964; Holman, 1955; King, 1961). The death of George Washington was presumably associated with bloodletting (Donaldson and Donaldson, 1980; Knox, 1933). It fell from favor as a treatment for hypertension, not so much because of concerns regarding efficacy of the treatment, but rather, because of the advent of other modes of therapy. Holman, as late as 1955, after a review of medical texts in use at that time, wrote:

Bloodletting is still mentioned for control of arterial hypertension. . . . Hypertensive patients not in circulatory failure have often been observed to get symptomatic relief from venesection for varying periods of time. . . . If the early promise of Rauwolfia and similar recently introduced antihypertensive agents is fulfilled, this indication for venesection is apt to be supplanted also.

Perkins' tractors, introduced in 1795 and mentioned in Chapter 1, continued to be used long after Haygarth's study in 1800 showed them to be of no value (Elliott, 1913; Haygarth, 1800). Nathan Smith, the founder of the Yale Medical School, not only gave testimony to their efficacy but was reported to have sold them (Haggard, 1932).

Changes in treatment philosophy are slow to occur, especially if the new philosophy must replace an established one. Max Planck (1858–1947), a physicist, noted that:

A new scientific truth does not triumph by convincing its opponents and making them see the light, but rather because its opponents eventually die, and a new generation grows up that is familiar with it (Strauss, 1968).

The promotion and use of ineffective treatments is not simply a mistake of the past, as is

Table 2-9 Design characteristics of sample of 113 trials appearing in 1980 published literature

Design characteristic	Number of trials	Percent
Number of treatment groups		
2	70	62
3	24	21
≥4	19	17
Type of trial		
Therapeutic	81	72
Prophylactic	21	19
Diagnostic	2	2
Uncertain	9	8
Treatment design		
Drug trials	103	91
Uncrossed treatment	68	66
Crossed treatment	32	31
Treatment structure unclear	3	3
Other trials	10	9
Sample size		
≤20	19	17
21–49	36	32
50–99	21	19
100–299	20	18
≥300	15	13
Unstated	2	2
Median number: 52.5 (range 4 to 3,427)		
Median number per treatment group: 26.2 (range 2 to 1,714)		
Length of follow-up		
≤1 week	22	19
>1 week but ≤1 month	20	18
>1 month but ≤3 months	26	23
>3 months but ≤1 year	19	17
>1 year	12	11
Not stated	14	12
Median: 2.1 months (range <1 day to >2 years)		
Method of treatment assignment		
Random	90	80
Nonrandom or not stated	23	20
Level of treatment masking		
Double-masked	76	67
Single-masked	4	4
Unmasked	17	15
Not stated	16	14
Number of centers		
Single center*	98	87
Multicenter	15	13
Type of funding		
Public	24	21
Private	22	19
Public and private	14	12
Not stated	53	47

Source: Reference citation 321. Reprinted with permission of Elsevier Science Publishing Co., Inc., New York.

*This category includes 9 trials with inadequate information to make a classification.

evident from work of the Drug Efficacy Study Implementation, DESI (Food and Drug Administration, 1972b). Of the 3,185 prescription drugs reviewed by the FDA as of June 1982, 31% were classified as ineffective.[4]

The adoption of treatments as established forms of therapy without adequate testing applies to nondrug forms of therapy as well. Coronary artery bypass surgery was introduced in 1964 (DeBakey and Lawrie, 1978; Garrett et al., 1973). Since that time it has become one of the most common forms of surgery performed. Only recently have trials been mounted to evaluate the efficacy of the operation (Braunwald, 1977; Coronary Artery Surgery Research Group, 1981, 1983; European Coronary Surgery Study Group, 1982b; Murphy et al., 1977).

Coronary care units, regarded as standard treatment for patients with myocardial infarction since their introduction in 1962, have never been adequately evaluated (Day, 1965; Gordis et al., 1977). The few controlled trials that have been done raise doubts concerning widespread use of such units (Christiansen et al., 1971; Hill et al., 1977, 1978; Mather et al., 1971, 1976).

The development of electronic fetal monitoring (EFM) devices in the late 1960s has led to their widespread use in delivery rooms. Their use has been accompanied by a marked rise in cesarean section rates, without any apparent improvement in neonatal outcome (Haupt, 1982; Ott, 1981). All of the randomized trials reported to date have failed to show any benefit for the EFM devices tested (Haverkamp et al., 1976, 1979; Kelso et al., 1978; Renou et al., 1976). However, those results have not had any apparent effect on the use of the devices.

Demands from the public for access to new "miracle" drugs can also influence health care practices. Public clamor for Laetrile has led state legislators in 26 states to enact laws making the drug available to the public,[5] in spite of a skeptical medical profession and trials failing to indicate any merit for the treatment (Bross, 1982; Moertel et al., 1982; Relman, 1982). Lobbying by lay groups for a relaxation of proscriptions against the use of dimethyl sulfoxide (DMSO) has led to availability of the compound in 9 states[5] even though there are serious doubts regarding its usefulness (National Research Council, 1973).

The need for clinical trials is not limited to the medical profession. A case in point is the widespread and often indiscriminate use of diethylcarbamazine to protect dogs against heart worms. The risks associated with the chronic use of such medications, year in and year out for the life of a dog, may be greater than the risk from the heart worm itself, especially if the animal lives in a low infestation area and spends most of its time indoors.

The clinical trial has been termed the "indispensable ordeal" by Fredrickson (1968). Indeed it is, if we are to eliminate the uncertainty that stems from lack of data needed to evaluate the merit of many of our current treatment practices.

4. Personal communication with staff of the Office of the Division of Federal and State Relations, Food and Drug Administration, 1982.

5. Personal communication with staff of the Office of the Division of Federal and State Relations, Food and Drug Administration, 1982.

3. The activities of a clinical trial

Field trials are indispensable. They will continue to be an ordeal. They lack glamor, they strain our resources and patience, and they protract the moment of truth to excrutiating limits. Still, they are among the most challenging tests of our skills. I have no doubt that when the problem is well chosen, the study is appropriately designed, and that when all the populations concerned are made aware of the route and the goal, the reward can be commensurate with the effort. If, in major medical dilemmas, the alternative is to pay the cost of perpetual uncertainty, have we really any choice?

Donald Fredrickson (1968)

3.1 STAGES OF A CLINICAL TRIAL

A clinical trial progresses through a series of stages from beginning to end. The stages discussed in this book are outlined in Table 3–1, along with the event that is used to designate the end of one stage and the start of the next. The dates listed in the last column of the table are from the CDP (Coronary Drug Project Research Group, 1973a, 1976).

Appendix D provides a listing of activities by stage. The list is an adaptation of one developed as part of the Coordinating Center Models Project—CCMP (Coordinating Center Models Project Research Group, 1979d). It should be used only as a rough guide to activities in specific trials. It has been constructed assuming no overlap of activities from one stage to the next. In actual fact, as noted in Section 3.3.3, the overlap can be quite extensive.

3.2 DIVISION OF RESPONSIBILITIES

Any trial involving two or more investigators, whether done at a single center or multiple centers, must provide for a division of responsibilities. Some responsibilities, such as those related to patient care or to data analysis, require specialized skills associated with a particular discipline and may automatically be assumed by persons trained in that discipline. However, many of the required functions are not uniquely associated with a specific discipline and can be performed by any one of several individuals or groups in the trial. This fact was evident in the review of the data coordinating centers carried out as part of the CCMP. All centers had the responsibility for data intake and analysis, but they showed wide variation in the number of other general support functions performed. In some trials, the center had responsibility for virtually all support functions, whereas in others responsibilities were shared with or assumed by individuals or groups outside the center (McDill, 1979).

It is useful to list required activities and the individual or group expected to perform them.

Table 3-1 Stages of a clinical trial

Stage	Event marking end of stage	Illustration using CDP*
I. Initial design	Initiation of funding	March 1965
II. Protocol development	Initiation of patient recruitment	March 1966
III. Patient recruitment	Completion of patient recruitment	October 1969
IV. Treatment and follow-up	Initiation of patient close-out	May 1974
V. Patient close-out	Completion of patient close-out	August 1974
VI. Termination	Termination of funding for original trial	March 1979
VII. Post-trial follow-up (optional)	Termination of all follow-up	December 1983

*The CDP is considered to have started in 1961 with the first planning meeting. The initial funding for the trial was awarded in March of 1965.

This should be done early in the trial to avoid confusion as to who is doing what. These specifications are especially important in trials with multiple resource centers that have overlapping responsibilities (McDill, 1979). The specifications, once developed, should be reviewed and revised at intervals over the course of the trial to cover new responsibilities and to realign old ones.

3.3 COMMON IMPEDIMENTS TO THE ORDERLY PERFORMANCE OF ACTIVITIES

3.3.1 Separation of responsibilities in government-initiated trials

The responsibilities for planning and executing a trial rest with the investigators in the typical investigator-initiated trial. They design it, they propose the investigators to be involved in it, and they carry it out. The sponsor has only a peripheral role. The situation is different in a typical sponsor-initiated trial. In this case, the sponsor assumes major responsibility for design of the trial and for selection of the investigators to carry it out. The separation of the design and execution functions may lead to sponsor-investigator tensions that may impede progress in the trial if they are not addressed.

3.3.2 Structural deficiencies

In a survey of multicenter trials, Smith (1978) classified over half of the operational problems encountered as organizational or administrative in nature. Many of these organizational problems can be traced to ambiguities in decision-making processes for resolving key design and operational issues (e.g., when to stop patient recruitment, how long to continue patient follow-up, when to terminate a treatment because of adverse or beneficial effects). The ambiguities can cause different individuals or groups to view themselves as the "final authority" in resolving a particular issue and can cause delays and inefficiencies in the way activities are conducted.

3.3.3 Overlap of activities from stage to stage

The activities normally associated with a particular stage may continue into the next or subsequent stages. Experience during the patient recruitment stage may require re-evaluation of sample size and other criteria set down when the study was designed. New treatments may be added after the start of patient recruitment, for example, as in the UGDP (University Group Diabetes Program Research Group, 1970d).

Similarly, it is rare for patient recruitment to be completed by the time treatment and follow-up begin. In fact, it is not uncommon for all three of these processes to go on simultaneously in long-term trials. In addition, data analyses, while typically associated with the termination stage, may be necessary long before that point is reached for performance and treatment monitoring, as discussed in Chapters 16 and 20, respectively.

Overlap of activities from one stage to the next has staffing implications. A trial in which patients are still being recruited, while others are in various stages of follow-up or have already been separated from the study, requires more elaborate organization and staffing than one in which it is possible to complete one stage before the next one starts.

3.3.4 Inadequate time for planning, development, and implementation

The time schedule for a trial, as established in the design stage, often proves to be unrealistic. Among the ten Requests for Proposals (RFPs) reviewed in the CCMP, only six made any mention of a time period for planning and protocol development (Coordinating Center Models Project Research Group, 1979b). The start-up time (i.e., time from start of funding to the enrollment of the first patient) for the trials listed in Appendix B ranged from 2 months to 3 years. The average time was just over 1 year.

Unrealistically ambitious time schedules tend to exert pressure on investigators to initiate data collection before the necessary data forms and related documents have been fully developed and tested. Doing so can lead to a chronic crisis atmosphere in the data center as staff struggle to develop better data forms and intake procedures while trying to maintain existing procedures.

3.3.5 Inadequate funding

The level of activities in a trial should be compatible with available funding. It is a mistake to embark on a trial without adequate support. The effort proposed should be scaled to match available support. Further, funds should be equitably distributed across activities within the trial. Situations should be avoided where support for one aspect of the trial, such as data collection, is overfunded, while another, such as data intake and analysis, is underfunded. A successful trial requires balance in the amount of money available for all essential activities.

3.4 APPROACHES TO ENSURE ORDERLY TRANSITION OF ACTIVITIES

3.4.1 Phased initiation of data intake

It may be prudent to limit the number of patients to be enrolled at the outset, especially if a clinic has a large backlog of patients waiting to be enrolled. The limit may be lifted once a clinic has demonstrated proficiency in the data collection process and after the basic data forms and intake procedures have been shown to work.

One approach to phased data collection in trials with multiple clinics involves funding only a small number of clinics at the outset, with new clinics being added as the trial proceeds. This approach was used in the CDP. It started with five clinics. Additional clinics were added over a 2-year period to make up the total of 55 ultimately involved in the trial (Coronary Drug Project Research Group, 1973a).

A gradual progression to full-scale recruitment and data collection can be part of the study plan, even if all the participating clinics are identified from the outset. It may be wise in such cases to designate one or two clinics to serve as testing sites for the treatment protocol and data collection procedures before the others are brought into the study. This approach was used in the Multiple Risk Factor Intervention Trial (Sherwin et al., 1981). Another approach allows all clinics to begin recruitment at the same time, but at a reduced rate to start with. The Hypertension Prevention Trial—HPT (see Sketch 13, Appendix B) used this approach. Each of the 4 clinics in that trial was required to enroll a test cohort of 20 patients before it was allowed to start full-scale recruitment.

3.4.2 An adequate organizational structure

Coordination of activities in a trial requires a sound organizational structure. One of the first orders of business should be its development. A sound structure takes time to develop and to reach maturity. There should be adequate time for that maturation process before the start of patient intake. As a rule, the period of time required for this process is related to the size and complexity of the trial, and it may be longer for sponsor-initiated trials than for investigator-initiated trials. A well-designed investigator-initiated trial will include details on organization in the funding application. The period of time between submission of the application and initiation of funding (see Section 21.2.1 of Chapter 21) may provide investigators with opportunities to refine the structure proposed and may even allow it to reach a degree of functional maturity because of investigator interactions required in preparing and defending the funding request. Such opportunities do not exist in the typical sponsor-initiated trial because of the way centers are selected (see Section 21.3 of Chapter 21).

3.4.3 Opportunities for design modifications in sponsor-initiated trials

The separation of responsibilities discussed in Section 3.3.1 is an inherent feature of most sponsor-initiated trials, especially those initiated by the government via RFPs. The timetable for the trial should provide investigators with adequate opportunity to consider and accept the design tenets proposed before the start of data collection. This process begins before the proposal is submitted in the typical investigator-initiated trial, but cannot begin until after the centers are selected and funded in the typical government-initiated trial.

3.4.4 Certification as a management tool

Patient recruitment should not start until the clinics and data center have demonstrated that they are properly staffed and equipped to support this activity. Some trials, such as the National Cooperative Gallstone Study (see Sketch 5, Appendix B), have required clinics to carry a minimum number of patients through key study procedures before recruitment could begin. A formal certification of clinics was required in the HPT prior to the start of recruitment.

The certification process has been extended to individuals making key measurements in some trials (e.g., see Early Treatment of Diabetic Retinopathy Research Group, 1982; Knatterud, 1981; Rand and Knatterud, 1980). The personnel certification process is useful in that it provides a landmark that must be passed before a person is cleared for data collection in a trial.

3.4.5 Realistic timetables

The timetables for activities proposed in grant applications or RFPs for clinical trials should be based on realistic appraisals of times required to complete those activities. Unrealistically ambitious schedules may raise doubts regarding the feasibility of the study in the minds of those responsible for overseeing it, may lead to frustration among investigators in the trial, and may result in decisions to implement activities before the required procedures and support systems have been adequately tested and developed. The timetable constructed at the beginning of a trial should be reviewed and, when necessary, revised

as the trial proceeds if it is to retain its value as a management tool and performance monitoring standard over the course of the trial.

3.4.6 Ongoing planning and priority assessment

Planning and priority assessment are continuing needs in a trial. The leadership of the trial has a responsibility for implementing an active review process in order to make certain that work schedules and goals are compatible with the needs and resources of the trial. When they are not, priorities must be revised to reflect reality.

The leadership committee of the trial should take responsibility for setting priorities for data analyses when demands for them exceed resources available in the data center for carrying them out. The failure of the leadership committee to act in this capacity will leave staff in the data center open to criticisms if the priorities they set are not acceptable to everyone in the trial.

3.4.7 Minimal overlap of activities

The mix of activities under way at any one time influences the staffing needs of centers in the trial. The greater the heterogeneity of activities, the larger the staffing needs. The goal should be to minimize the number of activities under way at any one time. Pursuing this goal requires completion of patient recruitment in the shortest possible time. This means that all clinics in a multicenter trial should be prepared to continue patient enrollment until the study recruitment goal is met, even if some clinics exceed their goals while others fall short of theirs. For example, the CDP cut off patient enrollment at all clinics at the same time, even though it used a phased approach to clinic enrollment (see Section 3.4.1). Clinics that achieved their stated recruitment goal were asked to continue enrollment in order to reduce the time needed to achieve the study-wide recruitment goal of 8,300. Allowing each clinic to cut off recruitment when it achieves its prestated goal is inefficient for the data center, especially if there is wide variability among the clinics as to when the cutoff occurs. The data center will be required to maintain treatment allocation and baseline data intake procedures as long as recruitment continues in any clinic.

Similarly, the patient close-out process is most efficient when all patients are separated from the trial at the same time, regardless of when they were enrolled. The alternative is to separate each patient after a specified period of follow-up (e.g., 2 years). However, this approach is inefficient when patient recruitment has extended over a long period of time. See Chapter 15 for discussion.

4. Single-center versus multicenter trials

It is not the fault of our doctors that the medical service of the community, as at present provided for, is a murderous absurdity. . . . To give a surgeon a pecuniary interest in cutting off your leg, is enough to make one despair of political humanity. . . . And the more appalling the mutilation, the more the mutilator is paid. He who corrects the ingrowing toe-nail receives a few shillings; he who cuts your insides out receives hundreds of guineas, except when he does it to a poor person for practice.

George Bernard Shaw

4.1 DEFINITION

A center, in this book, is defined as any autonomous unit in a clinical trial that is involved in the collection, determination, classification, assessment, or analysis of data, or that provides logistical support for the trial. Included are clinical centers, data centers, coordinating centers, project offices, central laboratories, reading centers, quality control centers, and procurement and distribution centers. To qualify as a center, a unit must have a defined function to perform during one or more stages of a trial. In addition, it must be administratively distinct from other centers in the trial, and must be made up of two or more individuals who devote some portion of their time to the defined functions of the center.

A trial, to be considered as multicenter in this book, must involve:

- Two or more clinics
- A common treatment and data collection protocol
- A center to receive and process study data

All other trials will be considered single-center. This category includes:

- A single clinic, with or without satellite clinics (see Glossary) and with or without a center to receive and process study data or other resource centers (see Glossary)
- A trial involving multiple clinics, with or without satellite clinics, but not having a common study protocol, regardless of whether it has a center to receive and process study data
- A trial involving multiple clinics, with or without satellite clinics, that does not have a center to receive and process study data, even if clinics purport to follow a common study protocol
- A trial, such as the Physicians' Health Study (PHS), that does not involve any clinical centers, even if it has multiple resource centers

The four elements of the definition are necessary with the binary language structure used to characterize the physical structure of trials. However, the fact is that most trials are characterized by the first element in the category and, hence, they are discussed from this perspective throughout this book.

4.2 NATIONAL INSTITUTES OF HEALTH (NIH) COUNT OF SINGLE-CENTER AND MULTICENTER TRIALS

The 1979 NIH Inventory of Clinical Trials was the first inventory generated by that agency that distinguished between single-center and multicenter trials (National Institutes of Health, 1975, 1980). The institutes vary widely with regard to support for the two types of trials.[1] For example, all of the 26 trials supported by the National Institute of Dental Research were single-center, whereas all but 1 of the 20 trials sponsored by the National Heart, Lung, and Blood Institute were multicenter (Table 4-1). The differences are due, in part, to the nature of the evaluation

1. The definition of multicenter trials used by the NIH is less stringent than the one stated above. Trials in the Inventory were classified as multicenter without the requirement of a common protocol or the presence of a center to receive and process study data.

question faced by the various institutes (see Section 2.1).

Overall, the institutes of the NIH sponsor about as many multicenter trials, 476, as single-center trials, 510 (last line, Table 4-1). It is interesting, in view of this fact, to note the preponderance of single-center trials in published literature. Only 25% of the 306 gastrointestinal trials reviewed by Juhl and co-workers (1977) involved multiple clinics. Chalmers and co-workers (1972), in their review of cancer trials, identified only 49 as multicenter trials out of 252 reviewed. Only 15 of the 113 trials published in 1980 and reviewed for this book were multicenter by the definition used in this book (Table 4-3).

4.3 DESIGN CHARACTERISTICS OF SINGLE-CENTER VERSUS MULTICENTER TRIALS

Table 4-2 provides a summary of a few of the key design features of single-center trials versus multicenter trials for NIH-sponsored trials reported in the 1979 NIH Inventory (National Institutes of Health, 1980). Table 4-3 provides a corresponding summary for the 113 trials discussed in Chapter 2.

A major difference between multicenter and single-center trials, apparent in both tables, is

Table 4-1 NIH-sponsored single-center and multicenter trials by institute for fiscal year 1979

Sponsoring institute	Total number of trials	Single-center		Multicenter	
		Number	Percent	Number	Percent
National Cancer Institute (NCI)	654	261	39.9	393	60.1
National Eye Institute (NEI)	26	18	69.2	8	30.8
National Heart, Lung, and Blood Institute (NHLBI)	20	1	5.0	19	95.0
National Institute of Allergy and Infectious Disease (NIAID)	120	104	86.7	16	13.3
National Institute of Arthritis, Diabetes, and Digestive and Kidney Diseases (NIADDK)	67	42	62.7	25	37.3
National Institute of Child Health and Human Development (NICHD)	32	29	90.6	3	9.4
National Institute of Dental Research (NIDR)	26	26	100.0	0	0.0
National Institute of Neurological and Communicative Disorders and Stroke (NINCDS)	40	29	72.5	11	27.5
National Institute of General Medical Sciences (NIGMS)	1	0	0.0	1	100.0
Total	986	510	51.7	476	48.3

Table 4-2 Design features of NIH single-center and multicenter trials

	Single-center		Multicenter	
Feature	Number	Percent	Number	Percent
Total number of trials	510	100.0	476	100.0
Number of treatment groups/trial				
1	159	31.2	99	20.8
2	217	42.6	221	46.4
≥3	134	36.3	156	32.8
Median number	2		2	
Sample size				
Median number of patients/trial	60		166	
Range*	25 to 200		52 to 362	
Number of patients/trial/treatment group†	30		83	
Range*	12 to 100		26 to 181	
Method of treatment allocation				
Random	259	50.8	334	70.2
Nonrandom	251	49.2	142	29.8
Type of trial				
Therapeutic	369	72.5	432	90.8
Prophylactic	90	17.7	36	7.6
Diagnostic	50	9.8	8	1.7
Anticipated length of funding				
>1 year ≤ 2 years	10	2.0	9	1.9
>2 years ≤ 3 years	51	10.0	50	10.5
	129	25.3	94	19.7
	319	62.7	323	67.9

*20th to 80th percentile.
†Calculated by dividing median number of patients per trial by the median number of treatment groups per trial.

sample size. The typical multicenter trial has more patients than does the typical single-center trial. This difference is most apparent for the 113 papers reviewed in Chapter 2. The median number of patients enrolled per trial was 283 for the 15 multicenter trials, which contrasts with 40 for the 98 single-center trials (Table 4–3).

4.4 THE PROS AND CONS OF SINGLE-CENTER VERSUS MULTICENTER TRIALS

Certain features of single-center trials make them appealing. They are generally easier to mount and carry out than their multicenter counterparts. The fact that all study personnel are located in the same institution in most single-center trials obviates the need for and expense of maintaining communications and decision-making structures needed for execution of most multicenter trials. In addition, the physical proxim-

ity of study personnel may make it possible for them to work more efficiently and to achieve a higher degree of uniformity in the procedures they perform than might be expected in a multicenter trial. Further, the fact that all patients enrolled in the trial come from the same area in the typical single-center trial should produce a more homogeneous study population than might be expected of a population made up of patients from different clinics.

The main weaknesses of the single-center trial are sample size and resource limitations. One center and a few investigators will find it difficult to recruit and follow the numbers of patients needed. Compromises will have to be made in order to bring the number of patients required for study into line with reality while still providing adequate type I and II error (see Glossary) protection. The original trial, planned to focus on a single clinical event as the outcome, may have to be converted to one involving composite

Table 4-3   Design features of single-center and multicenter trials, as reflected in a 1980 sample of clinical trial publications*

Feature	Single-center		Multicenter	
	Number	Percent	Number	Percent
Total number of trials	98†	100.0	15	100.0
Number of treatment groups/trial				
2	62	63.3	8	53.3
≥3	36	36.7	7	46.6
Median number		2		2
Sample size				
Median number of patients/trial (enrolled)		40		283
Median number of patients/trial (used in analysis)		34		217
Method of treatment allocation				
Random	77	78.6	13	86.7
Nonrandom	21	21.4	2	13.3
Type of trial				
Therapeutic	66	67.3	15	100.0
Prophylactic	21	21.4	0	0.0
Diagnostic	2	2.0	0	0.0
Unable to classify	9	9.2	0	0.0
Anticipated length of follow-up				
≤1 week	20	20.4	2	13.3
>1 week ≤1 month	20	20.4	0	0.0
>1 month ≤3 months	21	21.4	5	33.3
>3 months ≤1 year	15	15.3	4	26.7
>1 year	9	9.2	3	20.0
Not stated	13	13.3	1	6.7

*See Chapter 2 and Appendix C for description.

†Includes 9 trials that could not be classified because of the lack of information in the published reports. They are assumed to have been from single-center trials for purposes of this analysis.

events or a surrogate outcome (see Glossary) simply as a means of arriving at a feasible sample size.

Often, the only way to preserve the clinical relevance of a trial and desired levels of error protection is to have multiple clinics enroll, treat, and follow patients under a common study protocol (Meinert, 1981). All other things being equal, a treatment effect may be more difficult to detect in a multicenter trial than in a single-center trial. However, the effects that are detected are likely to be more convincing than those found in a single, highly homogeneous population.

The physical separation of personnel involved in a multicenter trial requires a more systematic approach to documentation of the methods and procedures used than is typically the case in a single-center trial. This is largely because of the amount of money involved and the conse-quences of a botched performance. Further, economies of scale make it possible to establish dedicated resource centers, staffed with trained personnel, to perform essential functions, such as quality control, performance monitoring, and data analysis. Centers of this type are beyond the means of most single-center trials.

One feature of a multicenter trial, sometimes considered a disadvantage, has to do with the nature of the organizational structure required to link centers into a functioning whole. These structures (see Chapter 23), while cumbersome, provide an essential framework for discussion and decision making and for ensuring adherence to established procedures in the trials they support. The physical separation of personnel in a multi-center trial underscores the need for discussion to resolve differences in treatment and data collection philosophies. Those differences may exist in a single-center setting as well, but may never be identified in the absence of a formal organizational and management structure for the trial.

The typical study population of a multicenter trial will be more heterogeneous than its single-center counterpart. The increased variability is both a virtue and a curse. There is no doubt that it makes it more difficult to detect treatment differences. Indeed, the more heterogeneous the population, the larger the sample size required to detect a given difference. However, at the same time, a heterogeneous population provides added opportunities for subgroup analyses, such as those done in conjunction with the dextrothyroxine treatment in the CDP (Coronary Drug Project Research Group, 1972). It also provides a broader basis for generalizations than is the case with highly homogeneous populations. In addition, the fact that each clinic represents a quasi-independent replication of the study design makes it possible to examine the consistency of treatment results across clinics. Considerations of this sort were important in the University Group Diabetes Program (UGDP). The fact that none of the 12 clinics produced results favoring the tolbutamide treatment added to investigator concerns regarding the usefulness of the treatment (University Group Diabetes Program Research Group, 1970e).

4.5 INITIATION OF SINGLE-CENTER VERSUS MULTICENTER TRIALS

The mechanisms available for initiation and funding a trial are the same for both types of trials (see Chapter 21). The initiative may arise from interested investigators or from the sponsoring agency. The mode of support (grant or contract) will depend on the method of initiation and on funding practices of the sponsor.

A comparison of the characteristics of trials by mode of initiation and mode of support is hampered by the lack of information needed to make such comparisons. The only database available comes from the NIH Inventory of Clinical Trials, and then only with regard to mode of support. There are marked differences among the institutes with respect to mode of support. Most (88%) of the multicenter trials sponsored by the National Cancer Institute in fiscal year 1979 were grant supported, as opposed to 34% of the multicenter trials funded by the other institutes (Table 4-4). The differences are due to the size of the trials undertaken and operational and philosophical differences among the institutes in the way trials are managed.

The information given in Table 4-4 provides a few clues with regard to the mode of initiation. Trials supported by grants are more likely to have arisen from investigator initiative than those supported by contracts. However, there are exceptions, as discussed in Chapter 21.

4.6 INVESTIGATOR INCENTIVES FOR SINGLE-CENTER VERSUS MULTICENTER TRIALS

The multicenter trial is an important research tool. More, not fewer, are needed to address a variety of treatment questions. It is ironic in view of this fact that present-day reward and incentive systems tend to favor single-center over multicenter trials. One reason has to do with the ef-

Table 4-4   Funding mode for NIH extramural trials in fiscal year 1979

Type of trial	Funding mode							
	Grant		Contract		Mixed*		All modes	
	Number	Percent	Number	Percent	Number	Percent	Number	Percent
NCI								
Single-center	75	46.9	82	51.2	3	1.9	160	100.0
Multicenter	340	88.3	38	9.9	7	1.8	385	100.0
All other institutes								
Single-center	153	76.5	47	23.5	0	0.0	200	100.0
Multicenter	24	33.8	46	64.8	1	1.4	71	100.0
Total	592	72.5	213	26.1	11	1.3	816	100.0

*Includes trials supported by grant and contract funds as well as trials with an intramural component.

forts involved in mounting and carrying out a multicenter trial. It is much easier and less time consuming to design and carry out a short-term trial in a single clinic than it is to mount and execute one extending over a period of years and involving multiple clinics. Most investigators lack the time and wherewithal to initiate such trials. And even if they do have the resolve to carry such efforts forward, they may not have the support needed to cover developmental costs for the work. The demise of NIH planning grants has virtually precluded the acquisition of government funds for planning multicenter trials. As a result, responsibility for initiative rests in the hands of senior investigators with other sources of support and in the hands of sponsoring agencies.

Another reason for the prominence of single-center trials is that promotions in most academic institutions are based, in large measure, on the originality, number, and quality of papers produced by those considered for promotion. As a result, an investigator who carries out a number of short-term, single-center trials and who uses them to produce a series of papers as sole or senior author is more likely to be promoted than one who works on a few long-term multicenter trials and who produces relatively few papers, even if of high quality. The prospects for promotion may be further diminished if the papers produced are written under a corporate masthead (see Remington, 1979, and see also Chapter 24 for a discussion of authorship policies).

4.7 TIMING OF SINGLE-CENTER VERSUS MULTICENTER TRIALS

Many investigations of a new or existing treatment modality begin with uncontrolled observational studies, followed by small-scale clinical trials. Only after the results of these trials begin to appear in print, and especially if they are inconclusive or conflicting, is the need for larger trials recognized. Even then, sponsors and the review groups that advise them will be reluctant to commit the money required for a multicenter trial if they think answers can be obtained with less effort and money.

Some evaluation questions are slow to progress beyond the stage of uncontrolled studies— some never progress beyond that point. Others may be considered only in the context of multicenter trials from the outset. A case in point is risk factor reduction for cardiovascular disease. There is no realistic way to address this issue, except via large-scale trials, such as MRFIT (Multiple Risk Factor Intervention Trial Research Group, 1982).

Three general conditions should be satisfied before a multicenter trial is considered. First, there should be evidence that multiple clinics are needed to meet the sample size requirements of the trial. A single-center trial may suffice if the sample size requirement is modest. Second, there should be an identifiable group of clinical investigators who are willing and able to follow a common treatment and data collection proto-

Table 4-5 NIH expenditures for trials in fiscal year 1979 by type of trial

Type of trial	Trials		Amount (millions of dollars)		Median patient cost per year*
	Number	Percent	Dollars	Percent	
Single-center	510	51.7	35.0	25.7	$587
Multicenter	476	48.3	101.1	74.2	$523
Total	986	100.0	136.2	100.0	$574

*The dollar cost per patient per year for a given trial was derived by dividing the total projected expenditures for that trial by the product of the number of patients to be enrolled (projected) and years of support (projected) required for execution of the trial. The median dollar cost per patient per year for a given type of trial was determined by ranking the resulting figures for individual trials from lowest to highest and then locating the dollar value corresponding to the 50th percentile point in the resulting distribution (median value).

col. Third, there should be an identifiable set of clinics with adequate support staff and facilities to carry out the trial.

4.8 COST OF SINGLE-CENTER VERSUS MULTICENTER TRIALS

The only database available for a comparative analysis of cost is that provided via the 1979 NIH Inventory of Clinical Trials.[2] The total dollar cost for multicenter trials was nearly three times that for single center trials in 1979 (101.1 million versus 35.0 million). However, this figure is misleading in that it is not adjusted for the differences in sample size noted in Table 4–2 for the two types of trials. This has been done in Table 4–5 using median cost per patient per year of study. When viewed in this way, the cost is actually less than for single-center trials—a noteworthy fact in view of oft-expressed concerns regarding the cost of multicenter trials.

2. See footnote 1, page 12.

5. Coordinating and other resource centers in multicenter trials

Technical skills, like fire, can be an admirable servant and a dangerous master.

A. Bradford Hill (1971)

5.1 INTRODUCTION

A resource center is any center involved in a trial, other than a clinical center, that is in charge of performing a specific set of functions concerned with the design, conduct, or analysis of the trial. Resource centers include (see Glossary for definitions):

- Data centers
- Data coordinating centers
- Treatment coordinating centers
- Coordinating centers
- Project offices
- Central laboratories
- Reading centers
- Quality control centers
- Procurement and distribution centers

This chapter focuses on coordinating centers because of their key role in the typical multicenter trial. The coordinating center, or data coordinating center when there are separate coordinating centers for data collection and treatment, will be among the first to be funded and the last to cease operations when the trial is completed. It may, in fact, operate after the trial is terminated if post-trial follow-up (see Glossary) is required.

All 14 trials sketched in Appendix B included either a coordinating center or data coordinating center. No other resource center was common to all the trials (Table 5-1).

5.2 COORDINATING CENTERS

As noted in the previous chapter, a multicenter trial is defined herein to include a center that is

Table 5-1 Type of resource center represented in the 14 trials sketched in Appendix B*

Type of center	Number of trials with center†
Coordinating center‡	14
Project office	13
Reading center	12
Central laboratory	11
Procurement and distribution center	6
Quality control center	2

*All of the trials were classified as multicenter except one, the Physicians' Health Study (PHS).

†Several trials had multiple laboratories and/or reading centers. See item 10, Table B-4, Appendix B for specifics.

‡Three of the trials had both a data and treatment coordinating center.

responsible for receiving, editing, processing, analyzing, and storing data generated in the trial. In fact, some studies may use multiple centers to perform this function. The most common approach when this is the case, is to establish regional data centers, with each of the centers performing identical functions. Such structures, while relatively uncommon for studies done in one country, may be necessary in international studies, especially when different languages are involved. Both the International Reflux Study in Children, IRSC (see Sketch 14, Appendix B), and the International Mexiletine Placebo Antiarrhythmic Coronary Trial, IMPACT (Alamercery et al., 1982) had separate data coordinating centers to service United States and European based clinics.

The data center (or centers), at least in the larger multicenter trials, will typically have a number of coordination responsibilities. This book makes a distinction between two types of coordinating functions—those related to data collection and those related to treatment. A *data coordinating center* is defined as one that, in addition to responsibilities for receiving, editing, processing, analyzing, and storing data generated in a trial, has responsibilities for coordinating the data generation activities of the clinics and for implementing and maintaining quality assurance procedures related to the data generation process. Responsibilities for coordinating the administration of treatments in the trial and for surveillance of clinic activities are vested in a second center—a *treatment coordinating center.*

The unmodified term *coordinating center* will be used to designate a center that fulfills both the data and treatment coordination functions.

Use of the term *coordinating center* outside this book does not always conform to these conventions. For example, the facility designated as the coordinating center in the National Cooperative Gallstone Study (NCGS) was responsible for treatment coordination and for dispersal of funds to the other participating centers, but had no data coordinating responsibilities. The center with those responsibilities in the NCGS was referred to as the Biostatistical Center (National Cooperative Gallstone Study Group, 1981a).

5.2.1 General activities

The general activities of the coordinating center by stage of the trial are summarized in Table 5-2 (see also Appendix D). The list is adapted from one developed in the Coordinating Center Models Project, CCMP (Coordinating Center Models Project Research Group, 1979a, 1979d). The activities listed for the first stage—the initial design stage—and some of those for the second stage—the protocol development stage—may be assumed by the sponsor in sponsor-initiated trials.

No one center will necessarily have responsibilities for all the functions listed, especially if there are separate centers for treatment and data coordination. A review of coordinating centers for the trials included in the CCMP revealed important differences in their duties, partly because of the differences in the roles assumed by other units in the trial, most notably the project office and the office of the study chairman (McDill, 1979).

One of the major responsibilities of the coordinating center relates to preparation and distribution of key study documents, such as the manual of operations and data collection forms. In addition, the center typically serves as the repository for completed data forms (except for studies with distributed data entry systems), minutes of study meetings, progress reports, performance monitoring reports, and treatment effects monitoring reports.

5.2.2 Location

The coordinating center, under ideal circumstances, will be administratively and physically distinct from the sponsor and from all other cen-

Table 5-2   Coordinating center activities by stage of trial, with emphasis on data coordination activities

Initial design stage

- Calculate required sample size
- Outline data collection schedule, quality control procedures, data analysis plans, and data intake and editing procedures
- Develop organizational structure of the trial
- Prepare funding proposal for coordinating center
- Coordinate preparation of the funding application

Protocol development stage

- Develop treatment allocation procedures
- Develop computer programs and related procedures for receiving, processing, editing, and analyzing study data
- Design and test data forms
- Develop interface for data transmission from clinics and other resource centers to coordinating center
- Train clinic personnel in required data collection procedures
- Implement clinic and personnel certification procedures
- Distribute study data forms and related materials
- Develop manuals needed in the trial, including the treatment protocol, clinic manual of operations, coordinating center manual of operations, etc.
- Provide a repository for official records of the study, including minutes of meetings, manuals of operation, etc.
- Serve as the funding center for a trial operated under a consortium agreement, unless this function is fulfilled by some other center
- Serve as the payment center for general study needs, such as study insurance, and other specialized procedures not provided for in the grants or contracts of other participating centers

Patient recruitment stage

- Administer treatment allocations, including checks for breakdowns in the assignment process
- Assume leadership role in outlining study needs for quality assurance
- Implement editing procedures to detect data deficiencies
- Develop performance monitoring procedures and prepare data reports to summarize performance of participating clinics
- Develop treatment monitoring and reporting procedures to detect evidence of adverse or beneficial treatment effects
- Respond to requests for analyses from within the study structure
- Site visit participating clinics
- Prepare study progress reports for submission to sponsor

- Prepare, in conjunction with the study leadership, renewal or supplemental funding requests
- Update study manuals

Treatment and follow-up stage

- Prepare periodic data reports for safety monitoring committee
- Prepare periodic reports on performance of clinical and resource centers
- Carry out periodic training sessions to maintain high level of proficiency at clinics in treatment and data collection procedures
- Evaluate data processing procedures and modify as necessary
- Develop and test data collection forms for close-out stage
- Prepare summary of study results for presentation to participating investigators for use in close-out stage
- Assume responsibility for location of patients lost to follow-up
- Take initiative for reviewing study priorities and for proposing changes in the organizational or operating structure of the trial
- Assume major role in writing paper on design and methods

Patient close-out stage

- Monitor for adherence to agreed-upon patient close-out procedures
- Develop plans for final data editing
- Design and test computer programs needed for final data analysis
- Develop plans for final disposition of study data
- Coordinate logistics of patient disengagement from treatment
- Assume key role in writing papers summarizing results of the trial
- Develop plans for disengagement of clinical centers from the trial

Termination stage

- Perform final data edit and undertake final analysis of data according to plans outlined by study leadership
- Implement study plans for disposition of study records
- Assume leadership role in paper writing activities
- Undertake extra measures to locate patients lost to follow-up
- Supervise collection and disposal of unused study medications
- Distribute draft manuscripts and published papers to participating centers
- Serve as funding center for activities in the trial after termination of support for clinics

Table 5-2 Coordinating center activities by stage of trial, with emphasis on data coordination activities (*continued*)

Post-trial follow-up stage (optional)
- Compile a list of patients eligible for post-trial follow-up
- Implement procedures to locate patients whose current whereabouts are unknown
- Coordinate mailings, telephone calls, or clinic visits required for post-trial follow-up

- Update existing data files with data collected during post-trial follow-up
- Assume leadership role in drafting and distributing any manuscript using post-trial follow-up results
- Store, under adequate security, names of study patients and other identifying information for future follow-up

ters in the trial. This separation insulates the center from the direct administrative control of the sponsor, and helps it to establish and maintain balanced working relationships with all other centers in the trial. This balance may be difficult to achieve if the center is part of the sponsoring agency or if it is physically or fiscally a part of one of the clinics in the trial.

Twelve of the 14 trials sketched in Appendix B had coordinating or data coordinating centers located in academic institutions. This setting has pluses and minuses. A prestigious teaching institution, especially one with a recognized degree program in biostatistics, epidemiology, or related fields, provides a pool of bright and energetic people to meet the programming and data analysis needs of the center. In addition, the opportunity to teach and to interact with other faculty may help the center attract and retain senior professional personnel.

The minuses stem from the internal bureaucracy of any large academic institution. Most of the coordinating centers reviewed in the CCMP (all except one of ten centers reviewed were located in academic institutions) complained of difficulties in recruiting intermediate-level personnel because of pay and promotional restrictions imposed by their respective institutions. Several had difficulty in purchasing computing hardware for their own needs because of policies aimed at discouraging dedicated facilities.

The real or perceived lack of administrative flexibility of such settings, coupled with small business set-asides for government-funded studies (United States Congress, 1981), has given impetus to coordinating centers located in private (profit or nonprofit) business firms. The Persantine Aspirin Reinfarction Study (PARIS) coordinating center, located at the Maryland Medical Research Institute, is a case in point (Persantine Aspirin Reinfarction Study Research Group, 1980a). The main advantage of this setting is the administrative flexibility it provides for personnel hiring and pay practices and for acquisition of needed computing hardware and software. The main disadvantage stems from the lack of stability of any operation devoted to a specialized set of activities. That lack may make it difficult to recruit and retain needed personnel.

5.2.3 Staffing

Ten of the 14 trials sketched in Appendix B had coordinating centers headed by persons with a doctorate in biostatistics. Three centers were headed by persons with M.D. degrees; and one was headed by a person with a master's degree in applied mathematics.

All coordinating centers require expertise in the areas of biostatistics and computer programming. Ideally, the staff should include someone trained in medicine who is knowledgeable in the disease under treatment as well. When this is not possible, the director of the center should establish a working relationship with appropriate medical personnel located outside the center. The relationship may be established via collaboration with a medical department in the director's parent institution or nearby medical facility, or via relations with one of the clinics in the trial.

The CCMP has provided summary staffing data for seven of the coordinating centers reviewed in that project (Hawkins, 1979). A detailed staffing profile for the Coronary Drug Project (CDP) coordinating center is provided in Table 5-3 (see also Meinert et al., 1983). The figures in the table were based on data contained in annual budget requests of the CDP coordinating center to the National Heart, Lung, and Blood Institute (NHLBI).

The total number of full-time equivalents (FTEs) rose from 7 in the first year to a high of 36 in the tenth year (column 3 of Table 5-3). Programmers and master's-level statisticians accounted for about one-quarter of the staff during the 13-year period covered in the table

Table 5-3   Percent of full-time equivalents by category of personnel and year of study for the CDP Coordinating Center

Year of study*	Stage	Total FTEs	Percent of full-time equivalents (FTEs)			
			MD or PhD in statistics	MSc in statistics	Data coords, key punch, coders	Support personnel†
1st	Protocol dev.	6.8	27.0	29.2	29.2	14.6
2nd	Recruitment	14.8	32.4	20.3	27.0	20.3
3rd	Recruitment	19.0	20.1	31.5	31.5	16.8
4th	Recruitment	24.3	19.8	28.8	32.9	18.5
5th	Follow-up	24.8	17.3	24.2	32.3	26.2
6th	Follow-up	26.4	18.6	22.7	26.5	32.2
7th	Follow-up	27.3	17.6	22.0	25.6	34.8
8th	Follow-up	30.3	15.8	26.4	23.1	34.6
9th	Follow-up	29.5	16.3	23.7	24.4	35.6
10th	Close-out	35.7	12.3	23.8	23.8	40.1
11th	Termination	22.6	14.2	24.8	23.5	37.6
12th	Termination	17.2	18.6	27.9	19.2	34.3
13th	Termination	11.5	21.7	25.2	17.4	35.7

Source: Reference citation 320. Reprinted with permission of Elsevier Science Publishing Co., Inc., New York.

*The study started in April 1965. Patient recruitment began near the end of the first year (March 1966) and was completed during the fourth year of the study (October 1969). Close-out of follow-up occurred in 1974 during the first half of the tenth year. The main activity thereafter had to do with analyses for paper-writing activities.

†Administrative, secretarial, and clerical personnel. Also includes a graphic artist.

(column 5). Data processing activities were concentrated on systems development and programming for data intake and editing during the early part of the trial. Reductions in these activities as the study progressed were offset by increased demands for data analyses.

Data coordinators, key-punch operators, and coders accounted for one-quarter to one-third of all coordinating center personnel through the eleventh year (column 6 of Table 5-3). The drop in years 12 and 13 resulted from reductions in data intake and keying operations following completion of patient close-out.

Secretarial, clerical, and administrative staff constituted the largest personnel category starting with the sixth year. Growth of this category from 15% in the first year to more than 40% of the FTEs in the tenth year was a reflection of an increasing workload associated with manuscript production and maintenance of various reading and quality control procedures in the study.

5.2.4   Equipment

The equipment listed in Table 5-4 represents items that are likely to be needed in a "typical" coordinating center operation. The list does not include general office furniture and equipment, such as desks, chairs, typewriters, and dictating and transcribing equipment. These are assumed to be part of any office setting.

The approach a coordinating center takes to data entry and processing may be dictated in large measure by the equipment that exists at the institution housing the center and the data processing philosophy held by key people in that institution. The factors that should be considered in choosing between a dedicated or centralized approach to computing are discussed in Chapter 17.

5.2.5   Relative cost

Table 5-5 provides data on the relative cost of five coordinating centers reviewed in the CCMP (Meinert, 1979a). The percentage annual cost of the individual centers, relative to the total cost of the trials for that year, ranged from 5.1 to 51.7 in the first year and from 7.3 to 16.8 for the other years covered in the table.

Figure 5-1 is based on data from the CDP (Meinert et al., 1983). As in Table 5-5, the values reported represent the proportionate cost of the coordinating center, expressed as a percentage of the total direct cost of the study. The majority of the expenditures during the first year occurred in connection with equipment purchases

Table 5-4 General equipment requirements of coordinating centers

- Computing facilities* for storing, editing, and analyzing study data
- CRT work stations for use by programming and data processing staff
- RJE station with high-speed printer
- Dedicated minicomputer for data storage and simple analyses
- Computer-controlled graphics equipment
- Electronic calculator*
- Data entry equipment* (e.g., key punches, key-to-tape units, key-to-diskette units)
- Word processing equipment*
- Photocopying equipment*
- Collation and report binding equipment
- Telecopier (for transmitting and receiving special documents)
- Mailing equipment (postage meter, scale, etc.)
- Filing cabinets with locks*
- Microfilming equipment and viewers
- Fireproof, environment-controlled storage vaults for data tapes and other essential study documents

*Essential items.

and work in developing data forms and manuals for the study. Expenditures in the clinics were modest until the start of patient recruitment in the second year. Support for clinics terminated during the eleventh year. Only the coordinating center was supported beyond that time. The gradual increase in proportionate costs starting with the third year and continuing through the tenth year is a reflection of increased demands for analyses related to treatment and performance monitoring and for paper writing, superimposed on continuing demands for maintenance of established data collection, intake, and editing procedures.

There are no accepted rules of thumb for determining the correct allocation of funds for the coordinating center, relative to other centers in the trial. The amount will depend on the nature and complexity of the data collection, editing, and analysis procedures needed, and on the total number of clinical centers in the trial. The relative costs, all other things being equal, will fall as the number of clinics increases, since many of the developmental, programming, and analysis costs incurred by the coordinating center are independent of the number of clinics. Part of the drop in relative cost, shown in Figure 5-1, is due to the addition of new clinics during the first two years of the CDP. There were only five clinics funded during the first year. Twenty-three additional clinics were funded early in the second year. The last complement of 27 clinics was added near the end of the second year.

The funds available for the coordinating center must be in line with the demands placed on it. Experienced investigators and sponsors will review the overall allocation of funds at intervals over the course of the trial and will reallocate funds among centers if there are gross imbalances. The way in which this is done depends on the funding vehicle. It is relatively easy to do with either a consortium approach to funding or with contracts, but not when each center has its own grant (see Chapter 21).

Table 5-5 Relative cost of coordinating centers for five trials* reviewed in the Coordinating Center Models Project

Year of trial	Number of trials†	Percent of total study cost		
		Lowest	*Median*	*Highest*
1	5	5.1	9.0	51.7
2	5	7.3	9.7	16.8
3	5	8.6	10.1	14.0
4	4	9.7	10.1	13.6
5	4	9.8	11.2	13.6
6	3	10.7	11.4	16.1

*Aspirin Myocardial Infarction Study (AMIS), Coronary Drug Project (CDP), Hypertension Detection and Follow-Up Program (HDFP), Lipid Research Clinics, Coronary Primary Prevention Trial (LRC-CPPT), and Multiple Risk Factor Intervention Trial (MRFIT).
†AMIS reported data through the third year. MRFIT reported data through the fifth year.

Figure 5-1   Percentage cost of the CDP Coordinating Center, relative to total direct study cost.*

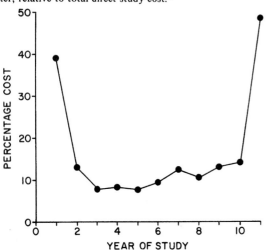

*Based on direct cost expenditure data from the NHLBI, excluding costs for the central laboratory and drug distribution center. Total costs for all the centers combined ranged from $3.3 to $4.3 million during the third through the tenth year of the study. Figures for the first two years and the eleventh year were $0.5, $1.3, and $0.9 million, respectively.

Source: Reference citation 320. Reprinted with permission of Elsevier Science Publishing Co., Inc., New York.

5.2.6   Internal allocation of funds

The allocation of funds within the coordinating center is as important as the allocation of funds among centers. The amount of support available for personnel must be balanced against that available for equipment, computing, and other support services.

The internal allocation of funds, as reflected by annual budget requests submitted to the sponsoring agency for several different centers, is given in Table 5-6 (Meinert, 1979a). Table 5-7 provides a detailed look at the allocation of funds within the CDP coordinating center (Meinert, 1983). Ideally, the results in both tables should be based on after-the-fact expenditure data, but reliable data of this sort are almost impossible to obtain.

The typical coordinating center, as reflected by the median values recorded in Table 5-6, budgeted somewhere between 50 and 60% of its direct cost funds to personnel and about 20% to computing. The latter category includes funds for rental of data processing equipment, as well as time charges for computer use and for software rentals or purchases.

Funds requested for travel ranged from 3 to 6% of the annual budget. They were used to cover travel for center staff to attend study committee meetings, meetings of the entire investigative group, visits to participating centers, and scientific meetings. The "All other categories" in Tables 5-6 and 5-7 contain cost items needed to support general activities in the trials and include funds for items such as study publications, study insurance, and consultant fees and related expenses.

5.3   CENTRAL LABORATORIES

An issue in any trial that requires laboratory determinations is where those determinations are to be made. In this regard it is important to

Table 5-6   Budget allocation for coordinating centers by category and year of study. Results for centers from AMIS, CDP, CAST, HDFP, LRC-CPPT, and MRFIT

Year of study	Number of centers	*Median percent of direct costs devoted to:*			
		Personnel	Computing†	Travel	All other categories
1	6	50	19	6	25
2	6	62	19	6	13
3	6	60	16	4	20
4	6	61	18	3	18
5	5*	60	18	4	18
6	4*	60	16	4	20

*Budget data were available for all six centers only through the first four years at the time the table was prepared. AMIS did not yield data for years 5 and 6. CASS did not yield data for year 6. Also, one center did not provide a personnel budget for year 5. Hence, the median value for personnel for that year is based on results from only four centers. All other entries for that year are based on five studies.

†Includes funds for computer time, as well as for purchase or rental of data entry equipment and for computing hardware and software.

Table 5-7 Budget allocation of the CDP Coordinating Center, by category and year of study

Year study	Stage	CC funds requested (direct costs)	Percent of direct costs devoted to:			
			Personnel	Computing*	Travel	All other categories
1st	Protocol dev.	$188,111	29.0	55.7	2.1	13.2
2nd	Recruitment	196,103	75.7	8.9	4.1	11.3
3rd	Recruitment	279,749	73.0	12.2	2.9	11.9
4th	Recruitment	316,384	65.6	22.4	2.5	9.5
5th	Follow-up	372,242	68.1	22.1	2.4	7.4
6th	Follow-up	403,991	67.6	17.6	2.2	12.6
7th	Follow-up	507,745	75.1	15.4	2.1	7.4
8th	Follow-up	432,996	73.7	12.1	1.8	12.4
9th	Follow-up	569,170	72.5	16.9	1.9	8.7
10th	Close-out	595,756	73.8	17.1	1.8	7.3
11th	Termination	498,494	67.8	20.6	2.2	9.4
12th	Termination	396,023	64.2	24.7	2.5	8.6
13th	Termination	339,736	60.2	25.3	2.4	12.1

Source: Reference citation 320. Reprinted with permission of Elsevier Science Publishing Co., Inc., New York.
*Includes funds for computer time as well as for purchase or rental of data entry equipment and for computer hardware and software.

distinguish between determinations required for routine patient care and those needed for treatment comparisons. The former set of determinations may be performed locally and need not even be part of the central data file. The latter set of determinations may be done locally or in a central laboratory and should be part of the central data file.

All but three of the trials listed in Appendix B relied on central laboratories for making certain determinations. However, many of those same trials also relied on local laboratories for other determinations.

It will be necessary to rely on local determinations where it is impractical to use a central laboratory or where rapid feedback is required (e.g., in determining patient eligibility or in making treatment decisions that depend on laboratory values). Even if this is done, however, the determinations may be repeated at a central laboratory in order to provide results that are free of laboratory variation. In such cases, investigators must decide which set of determinations are to be used for assessment of patient eligibility and for treatment decisions.

The general factors to be considered in deciding whether to use a central laboratory at all are outlined in Table 5-8. The costs and logistical difficulties of establishing and operating a central laboratory must be balanced against need. Valid treatment comparisons can be made with results obtained from local laboratories as long

Table 5-8 Central versus local laboratories in multicenter trials

Local laboratory needed or permissible when:

- Specimens cannot be preserved for shipment to a central laboratory
- Determinations are needed quickly for the acute management of patients
- Higher level of precision possible through use of a central laboratory not essential to the trial
- All participating clinics have laboratories that perform the required determinations
- Individual laboratories are all certified by the same agency and are part of an ongoing standardization and quality assurance program
- Local laboratories agree to participate in standardization and monitoring efforts required by the study
- Senior personnel of each local laboratory are sensitive to the specific needs of the study and are willing to make adjustments in their procedures
- Risks of treatment feedback bias (i.e., where the laboratory reading obtained is influenced by knowledge of a patient's treatment) is minimal, e.g., as in double-masked trials

Central laboratory needed or desired when:

- Required determinations cannot be performed at the local laboratory
- Required level of standardization is not feasible with individual laboratories
- Separation of laboratory and clinics is needed to restrict flow of laboratory results back to clinics
- Laboratory measure is subject to wide variability from laboratory to laboratory

as the treatment allocations are balanced by clinic.

The fact that the central laboratory is remote from the clinics has advantages and disadvantages. The location adds to the cost and logistical difficulties involved in transport of the specimens. However, it also helps to ensure that the required masks are maintained (e.g., that the determinations are performed by personnel with no knowledge of patient treatments).

5.4 READING CENTERS

A reading center is a facility designed to provide the technical skills needed to read and code materials or records collected in the trial. The readings should be made by individuals who have no knowledge of the treatment assignment to ensure separation of the treatment and reading processes. They may involve extracting information from ECGs, fundus photographs of the eye, angiograms of the vascular structure of the heart, cholecystograms, chest x-rays, liver biopsies, food records, death certificates, or autopsy material. Of the 14 trials sketched in Appendix B, 12 had one or more such centers.

The conditions under which a centralized approach to reading is advantageous are outlined in Table 5–9. They are in large measure similar to those discussed for central laboratories.

The way in which central readings for eligibility assessments are to be used poses problems when they do not agree with local readings, if local readings are used for decisions on enrollment and randomization. Decisions must be made in such cases as to the disposition of patients where there are disagreements. Patients should be retained if the disagreements are minor. Procedures that allow investigators to exclude patients after randomization must be administered by personnel masked to treatment assignment and treatment results (see questions 38b, 39, and 50, Chapter 19).

The number of independent readings per record is a design question that should be resolved before any records are read. It is common to require two independent readings, with or without subsequent adjudication of disagreements. Duplicate readings offer a more precise basis for treatment comparisons than is possible with a single reading. However, valid comparisons can be made with just one reading per record, so long as the readings are independent of treatment assignment.

Table 5–9 Conditions under which centralized readings may be required

- Reading procedures are complex and require special skills or training
- High degree of uniformity and standardization is required in the readings, especially for determining eligibility for the trial and for key items of follow-up information
- Large volumes of records are to be read
- Separation of the reading and treatment process is desired

5.5 PROJECT OFFICES

The project office, as defined in this book, is located at the sponsoring agency and is designed to serve as an interface between the sponsor and the investigative group involved in the trial. The main functions assumed by staff in the project office are to:

- Represent the interests of the sponsor in the design and operation of the trial
- Perform coordinating functions assigned by the leadership committee of the study
- Perform special functions assumed or assigned to the office by the sponsor or investigative group
- Serve as members of the key leadership committees of the study
- Carry out special analyses and tabulations

The National Institutes of Health (NIH) has used different terms to designate the office fulfilling these functions. It is usually designated as the project office but may have other names, such as medical liaison office or program office. The role of the project office will be related to the perceived importance of the trial by the sponsoring agency and the size of its financial investment. Generally, the greater the investment, the greater the involvement of the project office. Its role will also be influenced by the responsibilities of the sponsor in initiating the project. It will tend to have a more pronounced role in sponsor-initiated trials than in investigator-initiated trials.

There should be a well-defined division of responsibilities between the project office and the coordinating center. Failure to specify a division can lead to friction between the office and the center. Any division is workable so long as the principals involved understand and accept it.

The role assumed by the project officer is influenced by his or her personality. A strong, assertive person will automatically have an active role in the trial. The project officer's role is also heavily influenced by the personalities of others in the trial. The opportunity for an active role will be encouraged by a weak study leadership structure and discouraged by a strong one.

5.6 OTHER RESOURCE CENTERS

Several trials sketched in Appendix B included a drug procurement and distribution center. The VA Cooperative Studies Program has a general facility located in Albuquerque, New Mexico, that fulfills this function for all its drug trials (Hagans, 1974; Veterans Administration Cooperative Studies Program, 1982).

PARIS had a quality control center. Its duties are outlined in one of the publications from that study (Persantine Aspirin Reinfarction Study Research Group, 1980a; see also Sketch 8, Appendix B). One of the prime functions of the center was to check on the accuracy of the data entry and analysis procedures carried out by the coordinating center. It also played a role in the development of new data analysis procedures for the trial.

The HPT (Sketch 13, Appendix B) includes a treatment coordinating center. One of its duties is to compile materials used in counseling study patients to make the required diet changes.

6. Cost and related issues

A man may do research for the fun of doing it but he cannot expect to be supported for the fun of doing it.

J. Howard Brown

6.1 GOVERNMENT EXPENDITURES FOR CLINICAL TRIALS

Table 6-1 gives a count of trials for the various institutes of the NIH by fiscal year (National Institutes of Health, 1975, 1980). The number of trials reported ranged from a low of 746 in fiscal year (FY) 1977 to a high of 986 in FY 1979. Table 6-2 gives the NIH expenditures for clinical trials as a percentage of total NIH appropriations. The dollar figures given for total appropriations are from an NIH fact book (National Institutes of Health, 1981a). Expenditures for clinical trials represented from 4.1 to 5.3% of total appropriations over the 5-year period covered in the table. (See Section 2.1 for notes on how the inventories were compiled.)

Table 6-3 gives expenditures by institute and fiscal year for clinical trials as a percentage of total NIH expenditures. The relative distribution of expenditures among institutes has remained fairly constant over the 5-year period covered. The National Heart, Lung, and Blood Institute (NHLBI) has had the largest expenditures for trials, even though the number of trials (Table 6-1) is small relative to some of the other institutes. This Institute plus the Cancer Institute accounted for over three-fourths of all expenditures for trials in the 5-year period covered. (See Section 2.1 for comments on differences in the type of trials undertaken by the two institutes.)

The total projected expenditures[1] for clinical trials are shown in Table 6-4 by FY. Results in the table are given as a percentage of the total projected expenditures for all institutes combined. The percentage distribution for FY 1979 expenditures (Table 6-3) was about the same as for FY 1979 projected expenditures (Table 6-4). This was not true for FY 1975 through FY 1978. Some of the change was due to the length of trials sponsored by the NHLBI and NCI. The average length of NCI trials listed in the 1975 Inventory was 2.47 years, contrasted with 2.74 years in the 1979 Inventory. The corresponding figures for NHLBI trials were 3.58 and 2.85, respectively.

---

1. Previous expenditures plus projected future expenditures for trials counted in Table 6-1.

Table 6-1   Number of NIH-sponsored trials, by institute and fiscal year

Institute	Fiscal year (FY)				
	1975	*1976*	*1977*	*1978*	*1979*
Cancer (NCI)	405	522	418	515	654
Eye (NEI)	20	21	22	28	26
Allergy and Infectious Diseases (NIAID)	109	141	93	99	120
Arthritis, Diabetes, and Digestive and Kidney Diseases (NIADDK)	49	50	49	51	67
Child Health and Human Development (NICHD)	41	52	53	39	32
Dental Research (NIDR)	44	34	36	37	26
General Medical Services (NIGMS)	2	0	0	1	1
Neurological and Communicative Diseases and Stroke (NINCDS)	59	73	51	55	40
Heart, Lung, and Blood (NHLBI)	26	26	24	20	20
All NIH	755	926*	746	845	986

*Includes 7 trials done in the NIH Clinical Center.

Table 6-5 provides total projected expenditures per patient-year of study for FY 1979 trials. This figure, for a given trial, was derived by dividing the total projected expenditures for that trial by the product of the projected sample size and the number of years the trial was expected to run. This calculation was made for each trial listed in the Inventory. The resulting values were ranked from lowest to highest. The value falling at the 50th percentile constituted the median projected expenditure per patient-year of study. The mean projected expenditure per patient-year was calculated by dividing the total projected expenditures for all trials by the sum of products derived by multiplying the projected sample size and expected duration of the individual trials.

Note that both the median and mean are underestimates of the actual per patient-year expenditures since they are derived under the assumptions that the full complement of patients, as given by the projected sample size, is enrolled as soon as the trial is funded and that it remains under follow-up to the end of funding for the study. Neither assumption is likely to be true. However, more refined calculations were not possible with the data provided.

The median expenditure per patient-year for FY 1979 trials was $574 and ranged from a low of $70 to a high of $1,657. The mean expenditure was $273 and ranged from $31 to $889. (See Chapter 4 and Meinert, 1982, for discussion of expenditures for single-center versus multicenter trials.)

Table 6-5 also provides sample size data. The median sample size of all 986 trials was 100 (range 30 to 850). The mean was 670 (range 99 to 2,589).

Table 6-6 provides expenditure data[2] from 1970 through 1981 for Veterans Administration

2. From the Veterans Administration Cooperative Studies Program, VA Central Office, Washington, D.C., 1981.

Table 6-2   NIH expenditures for clinical trials as a percentage of total NIH appropriations

		Fiscal year (FY)				
		1975	*1976*	*1977*	*1978*	*1979*
A.	Total NIH appropriations (millions $)	$2,093	$2,302	$2,544	$2,843	$3,190
B.	NIH expenditures* for clinical trials (millions $)	$88	$121	$105	$122	$136
C.	Percent of total (i.e., B ÷ A × 100)	4.2	5.3	4.1	4.3	4.3

*Excludes general support provided to the Division of Research Resources of the NIH and to the NIH Clinical Center.

Table 6-3   Percent distribution of total NIH expenditures for clinical trials, by institute and fiscal year

Institute	Fiscal year (FY)				
	1975	1976	1977	1978	1979
Cancer (NCI)	30.2	34.7	35.9	31.9	34.8
Eye (NEI)	3.5	3.9	4.4	5.3	6.3
Allergy and Infectious Diseases (NIAID)	3.5	4.1	2.8	3.1	4.8
Arthritis, Diabetes, and Digestive and Kidney Diseases (NIADDK)	3.8	6.4	6.1	6.6	6.1
Child Health and Human Development (NICHD)	4.4	5.0	4.3	3.1	3.1
Dental Research (NIDR)	2.0	1.3	2.7	2.5	1.3
General Medical Services (NIGMS)	0.1	0.0	0.0	0.2	0.2
Neurological and Communicative Diseases and Stroke (NINCDS)	3.9	2.4	2.6	2.5	2.0
Heart, Lung, and Blood (NHLBI)	48.6	42.1	41.1	44.9	41.5
All NIH	100.0	100.0	100.0	100.0	100.0
Total NIH expenditures for clinical trials (millions $)	$87.8	$120.6*	$105.3	$122.3	$136.2

*Includes expenditures for 7 trials done in the NIH Clinical Center.

(VA) sponsored multicenter trials. The support for such trials represented a little over 3% of the total VA research and development (R and D) budget in 1970, contrasted with slightly over 7% in 1981. The portion of VA research funds awarded to individual centers to conduct single-center trials was not available.

6.2   WHO SHOULD FINANCE CLINICAL TRIALS?

Clearly, the federal government via the NIH, VA, or other agencies can provide only a fraction of the support needed to carry out clinical trials. In fact, there is concern that the present level of

Table 6-4   Percent distribution of total NIH projected expenditures* for clinical trials, by institute and fiscal year

Institute	Fiscal year (FY)				
	1975	1976	1977	1978	1979
Cancer (NCI)	20.6	23.2	22.9	24.2	37.0
Eye (NEI)	3.1	3.3	7.4	7.7	6.8
Allergy and Infectious Diseases (NIAID)	2.0	2.9	2.2	2.2	2.5
Arthritis, Diabetes, and Digestive and Kidney Diseases (NIADDK)	5.4	6.2	5.8	6.0	5.4
Child Health and Human Development (NICHD)	3.0	3.8	3.3	2.9	2.1
Dental Research (NIDR)	1.8	1.6	1.6	1.7	1.0
General Medical Services (NIGMS)	0.0	0.0	0.0	0.0	0.0
Neurological and Communicative Disorders and Stroke (NINCDS)	2.8	3.1	2.3	2.5	1.3
Heart, Lung, and Blood (NHLBI)	61.4	55.9	54.5	52.7	43.8
All NIH	100.0	100.0	100.0	100.0	100.0
Total projected expenditures for clinical trials (millions $)	$641.8	$739.3†	$848.6	$848.4	$1,083.0

*Includes expenditures through the indicated fiscal year plus projected future expenditures (see Table 6-1 for count).
†Includes expenditures for 7 trials done in the NIH Clinical Center.

Table 6-5   Mean and median projected expenditures* per patient-year of study for trials listed in the 1979 Inventory

Institute	Number of trials	Sample size		Projected expenditure per patient-year	
		Mean	Median	Mean	Median
Cancer (NCI)	654	269	100	$237	$ 603
Eye (NEI)	26	482	200	$706	$ 350
Allergy and Infectious Diseases (NIAID)	120	1,373	100	$ 31	$ 302
Arthritis, Diabetes, and Digestive and Kidney Diseases (NIADDK)	67	180	70	$674	$1,036
Child Health and Human Development (NICHD)	32	473	100	$383	$ 483
Dental Research (NIDR)	26	943	663	$ 55	$ 70
Neurological and Communicative Disorders and Stroke (NINCDS)	40	99	30	$889	$1,155
Heart, Lung, and Blood (NHLBI)	20	2,589	850	$873	$1,657
All NIH	986†	670	100	$273	$ 574

*Includes expenditures through FY 1979 plus projected future expenditures.

†Includes 1 trial sponsored by the National Institute of General Medical Sciences.

government funding is already too high and that the support is siphoning funds from other more basic areas of research.

In an ideal world, the drug and device industry would underwrite the costs for establishing both the efficacy and long-term safety of proprietary products. Government support would be limited primarily to commercial products that offer manufacturers little or no opportunity for profits. Health insurance carriers, such as Blue Cross and Blue Shield, as well as Medicare and Medicaid, would support trials designed to evaluate specific health care procedures, as well as trials aimed at assessing the cost effectiveness of different methods of health care delivery.

We are still a long way from the ideal. Drugs such as the hypoglycemic agents have been marketed without any evidence of long-term safety or efficacy in relation to the prime reason for their continued use—reduction of morbidity and premature death associated with diabetes. Most of the data on the long-term safety and efficacy of proprietary drugs used for chronic conditions, such as diabetes and heart disease, have been assembled at government expense.

Health insurance carriers and their clients, instead of encouraging trials, have payment policies that discourage them. The general proscription against payments for "experimental" procedures in most health insurance plans leads to the paradox in which coverage may be denied when a procedure is being tested as part of a clinical trial but not when that same procedure is used by practitioners outside the context of any trial.

The drug prescribing practices of the medical profession have an effect on the testing and licensing practices of the drug industry. It is clear that physicians prescribe drugs for purposes

Table 6-6   VA expenditures for multicenter clinical trials, by fiscal year

Fiscal year	Total R and D budget*	Multicenter clinical trials*	Cost as percent of total R and D budget
1970	$ 58.1	$1.8	3.1
1971	$ 60.9	$1.8	3.0
1972	$ 69.1	$1.8	2.6
1973	$ 78.6	$2.4	3.1
1974	$ 81.8	$4.3	5.3
1975	$ 95.4	$5.4	5.7
1976†	$101.6	$5.9	5.8
1977	$109.6	$5.8	5.3
1978	$118.0	$6.3	5.3
1979	$126.3	$8.5	6.7
1980	$137.7	$9.0	6.5
1981	$137.5	$9.7	7.1

*In millions of dollars.

†Adjusted for switch in starting date for fiscal year from July 1 to October 1.

other than the approved indications (Committee on Drugs, 1978; Erickson et al., 1980; Mundy et al., 1974). The sales spurt following approval of cimetidine (Tagamet®) in 1977 for use with duodenal ulcer and Zollinger-Ellison syndrome is a case in point. The spurt was due in large measure to use of the drug for unapproved indications. A total of 2,840 patients were identified as having received cimetidine in two Baltimore area hospitals from July 1978 to January 1979 (Cocco and Cocco, 1981). Among this number, only 604 (21%) had established diagnoses for the two approved indications. A survey by Schade and Donaldson (1981) involved 200 consecutive patients admitted to the Yale University Hospital and the West Haven Veterans Administration Medical Center (100 patients from each of the two institutions) who received a prescription for cimetidine. Only 15 of the patients (7.5%) were given the drug for an approved indication. The authors concluded that:

> *Our findings strongly suggest that physicians now prescribe cimetidine for remarkably diverse purposes, most of which have not been validated.*

Why should a drug company undertake the expense of testing an established drug for a new indication if it is already being used for that indication?

The Food and Drug Administration (FDA) approval process for a drug to be used with a chronic condition, such as elevated blood glucose or lipid levels, requires the manufacturer to show only that the proposed drug is safe and effective (e.g., in the case of a hypoglycemic agent, that it lowers blood glucose levels). Evidence of effectiveness in reducing morbidity or mortality associated with the condition is not required. Others, outside the drug industry, via government funded trials such as the UGDP and CDP, have had to gather the evidence (see Coronary Drug Project Research Group, 1973a; University Group Diabetes Program Research Group, 1970d).

Even the patent law that protects proprietary drugs may serve to reduce incentives for industry-sponsored long-term trials. Protection is limited to a 17-year period. Proprietary products can be marketed by other manufacturers under their own trade names once the period of protection expires. The period for protected sales will be less, sometimes much less, than the 17 years after deducting time needed by the manufacturer to test the drug and obtain approval from the FDA for marketing the drug.

There are proposals before the United States Congress to extend the period of protection, but they have not yet been acted upon. The recent legislation involving so-called orphan drugs is an example of the importance of the legislative process in facilitating the development of drugs—in this case for rare diseases that offer little opportunity for industry profit (Finkel, 1982).

Mechanisms need to be developed that will facilitate the mixture of public and private funds for conduct of worthwhile trials. Drug firms do provide limited support for some government-sponsored trials, via drugs, devices, and other materials they supply free of charge. However, they will be reluctant to provide massive financial aid unless the leadership of the study is responsive to their needs in the FDA approval process. A prototype organizational structure is required. In fact, many of the necessary organizational principles have already been developed. For example, the organizational guidelines for ensuring a separation of functions in PARIS (Persantine Aspirin Reinfarction Study Research Group, 1980a) were similar to those used in AMIS (Aspirin Myocardial Infarction Study Research Group, 1980a). The latter trial was government funded; the former was privately funded.

Private health insurance companies and their clients must be encouraged to take a more positive approach toward the support of worthwhile trials. Investments of this sort could pay dividends in reduced costs for health care insurance in the future, if coverage for new procedures was denied until or unless they were shown to be of benefit via properly designed and executed trials. The NIH, even with greatly expanded resources, cannot be expected to bear the full burden of these costs and still provide needed support for basic research. Other resources are required if the momentum developed in the 1970s for planned evaluations is to be continued into the eighties and beyond.

Expenditures for health care have increased at an average rate of nearly 12% per year during the last two decades, as contrasted with 8.6% for the gross national product for the same period (Weichert, 1981). Expenditures totaled $247 billion in 1980 with $20 billion for Medicaid and $28 billion for Medicare in FY 1979 (Department of Health and Human Services, 1982a). Expenditures for trials aimed at evaluation of designated health care procedures are minuscule in comparison. There is need for a more realistic balance. Creation of a fund pegged at just 1% of the U.S. expenditure for health care would have yielded an evaluation budget of nearly $2.5 billion in 1980. Contrast that with the $136 million expenditure in FY 1979 for NIH-sponsored clinical trials (Table 6-2).

6.3. FACTORS THAT INFLUENCE THE COST OF A TRIAL

6.3.1 Design

A trial, especially when carefully designed and executed, can be a costly undertaking. The need for cost efficiency is obvious, particularly in an era of shrinking budgets and skyrocketing costs. Factors influencing cost include:

- Patient eligibility criteria
- Number of patients required for study
- Time required to develop the study protocol and data collection forms
- Outcome variable to be used to measure success of the treatments
- Number of clinics and speciality resource centers required for the trial
- Treatment procedures to be used
- Ease of patient identification and enrollment
- Complexity and frequency of data collection
- Length of follow-up
- Frequency of follow-up contacts and examinations
- Time required for final data analysis
- Time required to close out the study

The frequency of patient contacts and the amount of data collected per contact is a major cost determinant. A trial requiring treatment administration over an extended time period and an outcome measure that can be observed only via regular clinic visits will require a more elaborate follow-up examination schedule than one involving a short period of treatment and death or some other easily diagnosed event as the outcome measure. The Physicians' Health Study— PHS (Sketch 1, Appendix B) is an example of a long-term drug trial not involving any direct patient contact. Patients—in this case physicians—are recruited via mail. Those who agree to participate receive their assigned medication (daily doses of aspirin, aspirin and beta-carotene, or placebo) in the mail. Follow-up for mortality is done via the National Death Index (National

Center for Health Statistics, 1981) or via patients' families.

No-contact designs, such as that used in the PHS, can be considered only under special circumstances. General conditions required include use of:

- A reliable, easily observed outcome measure
- Treatments that have few side effects or complications
- Entry criteria that are not dependent on clinical assessments
- A literate, reasonably sophisticated study population

6.3.2 Planning

Starting a trial with an ill-conceived research plan or inadequately tested data forms can result in a waste of money. Serious design mistakes may make it necessary to abort the trial. Even if such drastic action is not needed, modifications to the data collection procedures after the trial is under way can be costly to implement, especially when the formats of data that have already been collected must be changed to render them compatible with revised formats. A cost element that is often underestimated is that of data processing and analysis. Underfunding this activity can seriously hamper the entire data collection process (see Chapter 5 for a discussion of data center costs).

It is not uncommon for long-term trials to cost more than originally anticipated. This can be illustrated with trials sponsored by the NHLBI, although the problem is not unique by any means to this Institute. Among the NHLBI trials appearing in both the 1975 and 1979 NIH inventories of clinical trials, only one reported a lower projected cost in 1979 than in 1975. The projected total expenditures given in 1979 were more than double the figures given in 1975 for three of the trials. Some of the changes undoubtedly were due to failure to anticipate inflationary trends over the 5-year period. However, most of the increases were too large to be explained by inflation.

One reason for increased costs has to do with shortfalls in patient recruitment and the actions taken to make up for the shorfalls via more intensive recruitment efforts and extensions of the periods of follow-up. A paper published by investigators in the Cooperative Studies Program of the Veterans Administration reviewed the recruitment performance of seven multicenter trials supported by that program (Collins et al., 1980). One trial was terminated due to recruitment problems. None of the other six trials were able to complete recruitment within the time frame originally proposed. All six required extensions for patient recruitment or had to settle for fewer patients than originally planned. Even with extensions, none of the trials achieved the original sample size goal.

6.3.3 Multipurpose studies

It is not unusual for a trial to be designed to satisfy a number of secondary objectives in addition to the primary one. A common one relates to the description of the natural history of the disease under treatment in long-term trials, such as the CDP (Coronary Drug Project Research Group, 1973a). The addition of secondary objectives can add to the cost of the trial. The increase will be smallest for objectives that can be pursued with data needed for the primary objective as well, and largest when added data are needed. The decision as to whether to pursue secondary objectives should depend on the scientific importance of those objectives, the suitability of the trial as a vehicle for pursuing them, the chances of successfully achieving them, and the costs associated with their pursuit.

6.3.4 Ancillary studies

The trial, especially in a large multicenter trial, may provide investigators with opportunities for a number of ancillary studies (see Glossary for definition). Some may involve added patients, whereas others may simply require special analyses of existing data. However, as with pursuit of secondary objectives, they can add to the cost and complexity of the trial. Priorities should be given to those studies that are needed to understand the action of the treatments under study and to those concerning methodological issues of direct importance to the trial. No study should be undertaken that jeopardizes pursuit of the primary objective.

6.3.5 Equating the data collection needs of the trial with those for patient care

The data required to satisfy the research aims of the trial may be different from those needed for patient care. Failure to distinguish data needed for this latter purpose from those needed for the

trial can lead to the collection of superfluous information that is a burden to collect and to process.

6.3.6 Undisciplined data collection philosophy

The data collection schedule for the trial should be kept as simple as possible. Strong leadership is required to ensure the development of a focused data collection philosophy and related set of data forms. Without this leadership, the data collection scheme can be a hodgepodge of peripherally related data items designed to cater to the special interests of specific investigators in the trial.

6.4 COST CONTROL PROCEDURES

6.4.1 General cost control procedures

Cost control is the combined responsibility of the sponsor and study investigators. There is no substitute for a cost-conscious investigatorship. Some of the more obvious extravagances to be avoided are:

- Use of costly state-of-the-art technology when less sophisticated technology will suffice
- Unnecessary travel at study expense
- Use of study funds for lavish office furnishings or for activities not related to the trial
- Overstaffing

"Cost saving" measures to be avoided include:

- Submission of an unrealistically low budget request in the hope of improving the prospects for funding
- Undue reliance on existing staff paid from other sources to perform essential functions in the trial
- Cutbacks on financial support for data analysis in order to increase support for data collection activities
- Reduction of the sample size requirement for the trial by switching from a single event to a composite of events or to a laboratory measure as the outcome measure
- Changing the sample size calculation so as to bring it in line with the number of patients available for study
- Sponsor-imposed travel restrictions in a multicenter trial that limit the ability of investigators to interact and function as a cohesive unit

6.4.2 Method of funding

The funding structure for the trial will in itself provide some cost controls. Ceilings placed on expenditures when awards are made, as with most NIH grant awards, encourage the conservation of funds, provided unused funds accrued in one year can be carried over for use in the next year. Awards with cost-reimbursement features, as with some NIH contracts, generally include provisions for periodic cost reviews by the sponsor over the life of the award (see Chapter 21 for additional discussion).

The differences between grant and contract methods of funding are most apparent in the budgeting process. An investigator is required to submit a budget for the specified number of years before the start of the trial with a fixed cost multiyear grant. Budgeting is done with the realization that the funds requested may be reduced if the budget is perceived as excessive by reviewers of the proposal. Approved applications that are funded are supported up to, but not above, the approved ceiling figures set when awards are made. An investigator who has done a poor job in anticipating costs for the trial will have to cut back on activities planned or seek supplemental funds to make up for deficits.

The budget preparation process is different for cost-reimbursement contracts. Costs can exceed the original budget and still be recovered. However, reliance on the cost-reimbursement mode of funding can pose dilemmas for investigators when preparing their initial budget requests in conjunction with Request for Proposals (RFP). Submission of a realistic budget that includes support for activities deemed necessary by the investigator but not mentioned in the RFP may cause the response to be viewed as noncompetitive. Realization of this fact may tempt him to adopt a more "pragmatic" approach to the budgeting process (i.e., by preparing a budget which he believes to be in the competitive range, even if he considers it to be too small), since the costs for "unanticipated" but justifiable activities can be recovered later as part of the cost-reimbursement process.

Funding is tied to the actual level of activities in the cost-reimbursement approach. This is more difficult to do with fixed-cost awards. One method of funding that combines features of the two approaches, at least for clinics, involves awarding a designated amount for fixed costs, plus a variable sum that depends on numbers of patients enrolled and followed. However, a word of warning is in order. Capitation forms of payment can lead to questionable practices if clinic personnel are tempted to cut corners in order to ensure an adequate flow of patients to maintain a desired level of funding.

6.4.3 Cost reviews

The investigator cannot develop or maintain a cost-conscious attitude without periodic reviews of activities and their associated costs. Such reviews are especially important in trials involving two or more primary work components, such as in CASS (Coronary Artery Surgery Study Research Group, 1981). That study required a separation of the coordinating center costs for the trial and registry components of the study. The separation was used as a management tool to make certain that data intake and analysis priorities were met for both components.

6.4.4 Periodic priority assessments

The usual approach is to add new data collection and quality control procedures as they are needed over the course of the trial, without much thought regarding their importance in meeting the main objectives of the trial (Meinert, 1977). Periodic revisions and prunings performed by the leadership of the trial are necessary if the procedures are to remain lean and efficient.

6.4.5 Review and funding for ancillary studies

The study leadership should develop an internal review process for proposed ancillary studies (see Glossary). Only those studies that do not interfere with patient recruitment, data collection, or other essential activities in the trial, should be approved. Studies that are too costly to undertake without additional funding should be reviewed subject to acquisition of funding.

Ancillary studies, by definition, are designed to address questions that are of secondary or peripheral importance to the main objectives of the trial. However, since they are done by investigators involved in the trial and are often carried out on subgroups of study patients, they can add to both the cost and the complexity of the trial. They may even compromise the ability of the investigators to pursue the main aims of the trial. Part of the purpose of the review process is to make certain that this does not happen and to ensure that the investigations do not siphon away resources needed for the trial itself. Small amounts of support, particularly in the form of study staff, may be derived from the trial. Undertakings requiring added staff should be funded and operated independently of the trial.

6.4.6   Justification of data items

The data collection requirements of the trial should be limited to those that are directly related to the aims of the trial and should not be confused with other needs, such as those required for patient care or for ancillary studies. Every item that appears on the data forms should be required for pursuit of one of the aims of the trial. Items that cannot be justified in this manner should not be made part of the official data set of the trial.

6.4.7   Use of low-technology procedures

The cost of a trial will be influenced by the level of technology needed for the procedure used in the trial. Insistence on high-technology procedures can result in a significant increase in expenses, especially if special equipment must be purchased and skilled personnel hired to operate it. State-of-the-art instrumentation is generally not essential to the success of most trials.

6.5   NEED FOR BETTER COST DATA

Reliable data on the costs of trials are difficult to obtain. Expenditure records maintained by the NIH are too crude to permit anything more than a rough analysis of cost (Meinert, 1979a). Cost comparisons across governmental agencies, such as the NIH and VA, are further complicated by differences in funding and accounting practices. For example, NIH-sponsored trials typically include salary support for senior as well as essential support staff, whereas personnel costs in VA-sponsored trials are generally limited to those needed for essential support staff. Comparisons between countries are even more difficult to make. For example, studies done in the United Kingdom always appear to be less expensive than in the United States because of fundamental differences in the way health care procedures are paid for in the two countries.

Reliable cost data for industry-sponsored trials are even more difficult to obtain. A for-profit business firm is not eager to provide detailed research expenditure data for review by the general public or competing firms.

Nevertheless, designers of trials need to have a better understanding of the way in which costs accumulate and how they are influenced by factors under the designers' control, especially in relation to the types and amounts of data collected. This understanding can only be achieved through the collection of detailed cost data related to specific data collection and analysis activities in a variety of trials.

7. Impact of clinical trials on the practice of medicine

A new scientific truth does not triumph by convincing its opponents and making them see the light, but rather because its opponents eventually die, and a new generation grows up that is familiar with it.

Max Planck

7.1 INTRODUCTION

There is need for a better understanding of the way trials influence the practice of medicine. What is their role in establishing new treatments or in discrediting old ones? When can they be expected to play a role and when not? Does the design or the way in which a trial is executed influence the way it is perceived—in the medical community and by the lay public? Answers to questions of this kind could promote the design of better, more potent, trials in the future. (See references 59 and 366 for additional discussion.)

7.2 FACTORS INFLUENCING TREATMENT ACCEPTANCE

7.2.1 Prior opinion and previous experience with a treatment

A treatment that has been around for a long time, even if trials have shown it to be of no value, will fade from favor more slowly than one still in its infancy. Chalmers has noted the continued use of bed rest in the treatment of acute viral hepatitis after several trials, all of which have failed to indicate any merit for the treatment. Similarly, ulcer patients continue to be placed on "sippy" diets, even though trials have failed to show the value of such diets (Chalmers, 1974).

The time to do a trial is before the treatment is accepted as standard practice. It will be difficult to mount one once that has happened. For example, it would be quite difficult to mount trials now to evaluate the efficacy of coronary care units (CCU) in the treatment of acute myocardial infarction (MI) victims. The units are presumed to be of value. Assigning patients to a CCU or regular hospital care at random might well be regarded as a questionable practice in today's climate.

7.2.2 Clinical relevance of the outcome measure

All other things being equal, a trial with death or some other serious morbid event as the outcome should receive more attention than one involving less relevant outcomes. It is distressing, in this context, to note the number of trials that rely on nonclinical measures, such as a laboratory test, to evaluate a treatment (see Chapter 2).

7.2.3 Degree to which test treatment simulates real-world treatment

Ideally, the test treatment should be used in the exact same manner as in the real world. However, this is not always possible. The need for uniformity in the treatment process makes it necessary to impose conditions on usage not ordinarily encountered in real life. For example, drugs may have to be given in a single fixed dose in double-masked trials, even though they are not used this way in practice.

7.2.4 Consistency of findings with previous results

The judgment regarding the virtues of a treatment should be based on a digest of all pertinent data—not only the last report. Survey papers, such as those produced by Chalmers and co-workers (1972, 1977), represent examples of efforts aimed at amalgamating information from several trials to assess the merits of a treatment.

It is desirable to have several replications of a trial before reaching a conclusion regarding a treatment. Unfortunately, the world is usually not so obliging. The high cost of some trials, such as the Multiple Risk Factor Intervention Trial (in excess of $100 million), makes it impractical to consider replication. Replication in other cases may be ruled out on ethical grounds. For example, it would be impossible to replicate

the Veterans Administration (VA) studies on frank hypertensives. No physician would be prepared to have such patients assigned to a piacebo treatment (Veterans Administration Cooperative Study Group on Antihypertensive Agents, 1967, 1970).

7.2.5 Direction of results

The direction of the trial results will influence the way in which they are received. It is easier to accept a positive finding than a negative one, especially if the finding pertains to an "established" treatment. Physicians are trained to be more comfortable giving a treatment than withholding one. Patients as well usually find it more consoling to receive a treatment than to be denied one.

7.2.6 Importance of the treatment

The interest generated by a particular trial will be influenced by the number of persons in the medical community who regard the treatment as useful. The attention accorded the UGDP findings was much greater than that for the Coronary Drug Project (CDP). Undoubtedly, the difference was due in part to the fact that the treatments used in the UGDP were established modes of therapy for the mild, noninsulin dependent diabetic, whereas this was not the case for the drugs used in the CDP for patients with a prior MI.

7.2.7 Cost and payment schedule

The cost of the treatment and the opportunity for covering those costs from third-party sources, such as insurance carriers, will play a role in treatment "acceptance." Use of dialysis for end-stage renal disease is a case in point. The big spurt in use of the treatment came with enactment of legislation in 1972 that provided payment for the procedure from Social Security funds. The number of people on dialysis in the United States jumped from 2,400 in 1970 to nearly 27,000 by 1977 and to over 44,000 by 1979 (Burton and Hirschman, 1979a, 1979b).

7.2.8 Treatment facilities and resources

The opportunities for administering a treatment will be limited by the nature of staff and support facilities needed for its administration. Liver transplantation is a case in point. The utility of the treatment is limited by organ availability, the number of trained transplant teams, and available support facilities.

7.2.9 Design and operating features of the trial

Ideally, the weight given to a result should be determined by an unbiased, objective evaluation of the strengths and weaknesses of the trial. In fact, the evaluation may be done carelessly and from a preconceived point of view. Design or operating features regarded as major weaknesses in one trial may be overlooked or ignored in another, depending on the direction of the results. Evidence of such double standards can be seen from a comparison of the criticisms directed at the UGDP study of tolbutamide with those directed at studies done by Keen and by Paasikivi (Keen and Jarrett, 1970; Keen, 1971; Paasikivi, 1970). The UGDP results were negative, whereas the other two were considered to be positive.

7.2.10 Study population

The degree to which the study population approximates a real-life mix of patients may influence the way results are received. A clinician's perception that patients treated in the trial were markedly different from those he treats may lead him to downplay or completely reject the results.

7.2.11 Method of presentation

Treatment acceptance can be influenced by the way in which results are presented. Negative attitudes that develop in the medical community because of the mode of presentation may cause its members to reject the findings for emotional reasons. There is some evidence that this happened with the UGDP. The tolbutamide findings were presented at a national meeting of the American Diabetes Association (ADA) in June 1970. The paper containing the results first appeared 5 months after the presentation, and then only in a speciality journal with limited circulation (University Group Diabetes Program Research Group, 1970e). The press coverage following the presentation resulted in a deluge of inquiries to practicing diabetologists around the country regarding the treatment. Many of them resented having to deal with the questions before the results were published.

The potential for ill will is not limited to trials with negative findings, as may be seen in the Macular Photocoagulation Study (MPS) with presentation of results for treatment of senile macular degeneration (Macular Photocoagulation Study Group, 1982, 1984). The study avoided the UGDP publication lag by mailing a preprint of the manuscript to all practicing ophthalmologists in the U.S. The National Eye Institute scheduled a press conference a few days after the mailing and just before the manuscript appeared in print. The national TV coverage of the results took many treating ophthalmologists by surprise, particularly those who had not yet received the paper or who had not read it. The public relations problem might have been avoided if there had not been a press conference, but public awareness of the results was considered to be essential because of the need for patients to recognize the symptoms of senile macular degeneration so as to obtain early diagnosis and treatment.

7.2.12 Counterforces

There may be a number of counterforces working against the acceptance of a finding. Such forces can be expected to emerge whenever results run contrary to established dogma, and especially when major financial considerations are involved. A medical specialist whose practice depends on the treatment being questioned will be much more reluctant to accept negative findings than positive findings. The Committee for the Care of the Diabetic was formed by a group of diabetologists largely as a means of counteracting the UGDP findings and the proposed Food and Drug Administration (FDA) labeling changes for the oral hypoglycemic agents (see Section 7.4).

The drug company whose product is threatened by the study can be expected to question the findings and to express doubts regarding the study. These expressions may take the form of prepared press releases indicating that the trial should not be regarded as definitive and making the universal call for further research. Upjohn, the manufacturer of Orinase® (tolbutamide), as well as other manufacturers of hypoglycemic agents, sent "Dear Doctor" letters to practicing diabetologists warning of the need for caution when interpreting the findings of the UGDP (see Knox, 1971, and Mintz, 1970b for references to the letters). Consultants were hired by Upjohn to critique the study and to speak at meetings where the findings were discussed. Company sales personnel were provided with "informational material" for answering questions concerning the study. The material summarized criticisms of the study and reminded physicians of other work supportive of the treatment.

Another force with interests allied to the pharmaceutical firms is that associated with the so-called "throw-away" medical journals.[1] Such publications rely heavily on advertising from drug manufacturers for their income (Chalmers, 1982a; Warner et al., 1978). The editorial policy of publications such as the *Medical Tribune* and the *Hospital Tribune* was negative, if not downright hostile, toward the UGDP, while carrying ads for hypoglycemic agents.

7.3   IMPACT ASSESSMENT

Changes in health care practices occur gradually and for a variety of reasons. Methods used to relate such changes to specific events, such as the publication of results from a particular trial, are at best approximate. It is always dangerous to associate any change involving complex behaviors with any single event. A case in point is the growing emphasis on the diagnosis and treatment of hypertension. Unquestionably, the emphasis stems, at least in part, from trials supporting the value of antihypertensive treatment. But it is also due to massive efforts by the federal government and the medical profession to alert the public to the dangers of hypertension. Communities throughout the nation have carried out screening programs to identify hypertensives. The National High Blood Pressure Education Program, founded in 1972 and sponsored by the National Heart, Lung, and Blood Institute (NHLBI), has been aimed at educating members of the public and the medical community to the importance of blood pressure control (National Heart, Lung, and Blood Institute, 1973; Szklo, 1980). Physician visits during which at least one antihypertensive drug was prescribed increased by about a third from 1968 to 1978 (from data provided in the National Disease and Therapeutic Index, IMS America Ltd.,[2] Ambler, Pennsylvania). There was a 27% decrease in mortality rates for coronary heart disease over the same time interval (Working Group on Arteriosclerosis, 1981).

In the light of such evidence, it is tempting to attribute the decline to more aggressive treatment resulting from trials and educational programs. However, those who do so ignore the fact that mortality due to cardiovascular disease was already on the decline before the first VA hypertension trials started and before widespread public awareness of the dangers of hypertension.

Prescription and sales data can be used to provide gross indications of changes in treatment patterns. Data from IMS are used in Section 7.4 to chart changes in the use of oral hypoglycemic agents from 1964 forward.

Other indications of change may be obtained from other data sources, such as the Professional Services Review Organization (PSRO) or from the Commission on Professional and Hospital Activities (CPHA). The Commission is based in Ann Arbor, Michigan, and maintains a variety of usage statistics for member hospitals. Payment data maintained by private health insurance carriers and by Medicare and Medicaid also can be helpful in tracing treatment patterns.

More direct measures of change can be obtained from special surveys, such as the one done by Stross and Harlan (1979) designed to assess the awareness of primary-care physicians regarding results from the Diabetic Retinopathy Study—DRS (done about 18 months after the DRS results were published). Only 28% (38 out of 137) of the family physicians and 46% of the internists surveyed (42 out of 91) were aware of the results. A similar approach was used to assess the level of physician familiarity with results from the Hypertension Detection and Follow-Up Program—HDFP (Stross and Harlan, 1981). Survey techniques also were used in a contract issued by the NHLBI to assess physician knowledge of findings from the CDP and Aspirin Myocardial Infarction Study—AMIS (Market Facts, Inc., 1982).

7.4   THE UNIVERSITY GROUP DIABETES PROGRAM: A CASE STUDY

The UGDP was started in 1960, enrolled its first patient in 1961, completed data collection in 1975, and published its final report in 1982. Citations 464 through 470, 472, 473, 475, and 476 (Appendix I) refer to a series of original publications that detail the design, methods, and results of the study. Citations 83, 95, 161, 173, 183–188, 192–194, 261, 386, 409, 413, 419, 459, 460, and 471, relate to the controversy that developed starting in mid-1970 with a UGDP data presentation that questioned the value of tolbutamide for use in diabetics. Table 7–1 provides a chro-

---

1. So termed because they are distributed to practicing physicians free of charge.

2. IMS is a private firm that specializes in the compilation of drug utilization data for sale to various business firms and agencies.

Table 7-1 Chronology of events associated with the UGDP

Year	Month, day	Event
1959	June	First planning meeting of UGDP investigators (467)*
1960	September	Initiation of grant support for the coordinating center and first 7 clinics (467)
1961	February	Enrollment of first patient (467)
1962	September	Addition of phenformin to the study and recruitment of 5 additional clinics (467)
1966	February	Completion of patient recruitment (467, 468)
1969	June 6	UGDP investigators vote to discontinue tolbutamide treatment (468 and UGDP meeting minutes)
1970	May 20	Tolbutamide results on Dow Jones ticker tape (327)
1970	May 21, 22	*Wall Street Journal, Washington Post,* and *New York Times* articles on tolbutamide results (280, 326, 408)
1970	June 14	Tolbutamide results presented at American Diabetes Association meeting, St. Louis (464, 465, 466)
1970	October	Food and Drug Administration (FDA) distributes bulletin supporting findings (179)
1970	November	Tolbutamide results published (468)
1970	November	Committee for the Care of Diabetics (CCD) formed (183)†
1971	April	Feinstein criticism of UGDP published (161)
1971	May 16	UGDP investigators vote to discontinue phenformin treatment in UGDP (470, 472, and UGDP meeting minutes)
1971	June	FDA outlines labeling changes for sulfonylureas (180)
1971	August 9	UGDP preliminary report on phenformin published (470)
1971	September 14	Associate Director of National Institutes of Health (NIH) asks president of International Biometrics Society to appoint a committee to review UGDP (83)
1971	September 20	Schor criticism of UGDP published (409)
1971	September 20	Cornfield defense of UGDP published (95)
1971	October 7	CCD petitions commissioner of the FDA to rescind proposed label change (183 and actual petition)
1972	May	FDA reaffirms position on proposed labeling change (181)
1972	June 5	FDA commissioner denies October 1971 request to rescind proposed label change (183)
1972	July 13	CCD requests evidentiary hearing before FDA commissioner on proposed labeling changes (183)
1972	August 3	Commissioner of FDA denies CCD request for evidentiary hearing (451)
1972	August 11	CCD argues to have the FDA enjoined from implementing labeling change before the United States District Court for the District of Massachusetts (451)
1972	August 30	Request to have the FDA enjoined from making labeling change denied by Judge Campbell of the United States District Court for the District of Massachusetts (183, 451)
1972	August	Biometrics Society Committee starts review of UGDP and other related studies (83)
1972	September	Seltzer criticism of UGDP published (419)
1972	October 17	Second motion for injunction against label change filed by CCD in the United States District Court for the District of Massachusetts (451)
1972	October	Response to Seltzer critique published (471)
1972	November 3	Temporary injunction order granted by Judge Murray of the United States District Court for the District of Massachusetts (451)
1972	November 7	Preliminary injunction against proposed label change granted by United States District Court for the District of Massachusetts (183)

Table 7-1   Chronology of events associated with the UGDP (*continued*)

Year	Month, day	Event
1973	July 31	Preliminary injunction vacated by Judge Coffin of United States Court of Appeals for the First Circuit. Case sent back to FDA for further deliberations (183, 451)
1973	October	FDA hearing on labeling of oral agents (183)
1974	February	FDA circulates proposed labeling revision (183)
1974	March–April	FDA holds meeting on proposed label change, then postpones action on change until report of Biometrics Committee (183)
1974	September 18, 19, 20	Testimony taken concerning use of oral hypoglycemic agents before the United States Senate Select Committee on Small Business, Monopoly Subcommittee (459)
1975	January 31	Added testimony concerning use of oral hypoglycemic agents before the United States Senate Select Committee on Small Business, Monopoly Subcommittee (460)
1975	February 10	Report of the Biometrics Committee published (83)
1975	February	UGDP final report on phenformin published (472)
1975	July 9, 10	Added testimony concerning use of oral hypoglycemic agents before the United States Senate Select Committee on Small Business, Monopoly Subcommittee (460)
1975	August	Termination of patient follow-up in UGDP (476)
1975	September 30	CCD files suit against David Mathews, Secretary of Health, Education and Welfare, et al., for access to UGDP raw data under the Freedom of Information Act (FOIA) in the United States District Court for the District of Columbia (452)
1975	October 14	Ciba-Geigy files suit against David Mathews, Secretary of Health, Education and Welfare, et al., for access to UGDP raw data under the FOIA in the United States District Court for the Southern District of New York (457)
1975	December	FDA announces intent to audit UGDP results (461)
1976	February 5	United States District Court for the District of Columbia rules UGDP raw data not subject to FOIA (453)
1976	February 25	CCD files appeal of February 5 decision in United States Court of Appeals for the District of Columbia Circuit (461)
1976	September	FDA audit of UGDP begins
1976	October	FDA Endocrinology and Metabolism Advisory Committee recommends removal of phenformin from market (184)
1977	March 8	United States District Court for the Southern District of New York rejects Ciba-Geigy request for UGDP raw data (458)
1977	April 22	Health Research Group (HRG) of Washington, D.C., petitions Secretary of HEW to suspend phenformin from market under imminent hazard provision of law (185)
1977	May 6	FDA begins formal proceedings to remove phenformin from market (185)
1977	May 13	FDA holds public hearing on petition of HRG (185)
1977	July 25	Secretary of HEW announces decision to suspend New Drug Applications (NDAs) for phenformin in 90 days (185)
1977	August	CCD requests that United States District Court for the District of Columbia issue an injunction against HEW order to suspend NDAs for phenformin†
1977	October 21	CCD request to United States District Court for the District of Columbia for injunction against HEW order to suspend NDAs for phenformin denied†
1977	October 23	NDAs for phenformin suspended by Secretary of HEW under imminent hazard provision of law (187)
1977	December	UGDP announces release of data listings for individual patients (474)

Table 7-1 Chronology of events associated with the UGDP (*continued*)

Year	Month, day	Event
1978	January	Appeal of October 21, 1977, court ruling filed by CCD in United States Court of Appeals for the District of Columbia Circuit
1978	July 7	Preliminary report on insulin findings published (474)
1978	July 11	Judges Leventhal and MacKinnon of the United States Court of Appeals for the District of Columbia Circuit rule that public does not have right to UGDP raw data under the FOIA. Judge Bazelon dissents (450, 461)
1978	July 25	CCD petitions United States Court of Appeal for the District of Columbia Circuit for rehearing on July 11 ruling (461)
1978	October 17	Petition for rehearing at the United States Court of Appeals for the District of Columbia Circuit denied (461)
1978	November 14	Results of FDA audit of UGDP announced (188)
1978	November 15	Commissioner of FDA orders phenformin withdrawn from market (462)
1979	January 15	CCD petitions the United States Supreme Court for writ of certiorari to the United States Court of Appeals for the District of Columbia Circuit (461)
1979	April 10	Appeal of October 21, 1977, ruling denied†
1979	May 14	Writ of certiorari granted
1979	October 31	UGDP case of Forsham et al., versus Harris et al., argued before the United States Supreme Court (462)
1980	March 3	United States Supreme Court holds that HEW need not produce UGDP raw data in 6 to 2 decision (462)
1982	April	Expiration of NIH grant support for UGDP
1982	November	Final report on insulin results published (476)
1982	November	UGDP deposits patient listings plus other information at the National Technical Information Service for public access (476, 477, 478)
1984	March 16	Revised label for sulfonylurea class of drugs released (192, 193, 194)

*Numbers in parentheses refer to citations in the Combined Bibliography (Appendix I).

†Personal communications with Robert F. Bradley, Joslin Diabetes Center, Boston, who was the first chairman of the CCD.

nology of UGDP related events (see also Appendix B for a sketch of the UGDP).

Table 7-2 provides a listing of the main criticisms of the study as offered by others and comments on their validity by the author (one of the investigators in the trial). Most of the attention has focused on the tolbutamide results because they were the first released and because of the popularity of the drug. Table 7-2 reflects this focus.

The news media carried a number of articles on the tolbutamide results, beginning with a report on May 20 appearing on the Dow Jones tickertape.[3] One article in particular, suggesting

that the drug caused as many as 8,000 deaths per year,[4] created a good deal of patient anxiety and physician hostility toward the study even before the results were presented in June. (Incidentally, the number had escalated from 10,000 to 15,000 without benefit of any new data in news reports a few years later, e.g., as in the *Philadelphia Inquirer*, January 28, 1975.)

The controversy and resulting doubts about the study led to two independent audits of it. The first was undertaken by a blue-ribbon committee appointed by the International Biometrics Society and was published in 1975 (see citation 83). The second was carried out by the FDA and appeared in November, 1978 (see citation 188). Neither audit found any basis to reject the conclusions of the study.

3. The report was prepared from information in an abstract of a paper submitted to the American Diabetes Association (ADA) for presentation at its June meeting. Study investigators were surprised by the publicity before the meeting. They were not aware that it was the practice of the ADA to make the program, and abstracts contained therein, available to the press in advance of its annual meeting.

4. The article appeared in *The Washington Post* on May 22, 1970, and in several other papers around the country over the next several days.

Table 7-2   Criticisms of the UGDP and comments pertaining to them

Criticism	Comment
• The study was not designed to detect differences in mortality (Schor, 1971).	• The main aim of the trial was to detect differences in nonfatal vascular complications of diabetes (UGDP Research Group, 1970d). However, this focus in no way precludes comparisons for mortality differences. In fact, it is not possible to interpret results for nonfatal events in the absence of data on fatal events.
• The observed mortality difference was small and not statistically significant (Feinstein, 1971; Kilo et al., 1980).	• It is unethical to continue a trial, especially one involving an elective treatment, to produce unequivocal evidence of harm.
• The baseline differences in the composition of the study groups are large enough to account for excess mortality in the tolbutamide treatment group (Feinstein, 1971; Kilo et al., 1980; Schor, 1971; Seltzer, 1972).	• The tolbutamide-placebo mortality difference remains after adjustment for important baseline characteristics (Cornfield, 1971).
• The tolbutamide-treated group had a higher concentration of baseline cardiovascular risk factors than any of the other treatment groups (Feinstein, 1971; Kilo et al., 1980; Schor, 1971; Seltzer, 1972).	• Differences in the distribution of baseline characteristics, including CV risk factors, is within the range of chance. Further, the mortality excess is as great for the subgroup of patients who were free of CV risk factors as for those who were not. Finally, simultaneous adjustment for major CV baseline risk factors did not eliminate the excess (UGDP Research Group, 1970e; Cornfield, 1971).
• The treatment groups included patients who did not meet study eligibility criteria (Feinstein, 1971; Schor, 1971).	• Correct. However, the number of such cases was small and not differential by treatment group. Further, analyses in which ineligible patients were removed did not effect the tolbutamide-placebo mortality difference (UGDP Research Group, 1970d).
• Data from patients who received little or none of the assigned study medication should have been removed from analysis (Kilo et al., 1980; Seltzer, 1972).	• The initial analysis included all patients to avoid the introduction of selection biases. This analysis approach tends to underestimate the true effect. Analyses in which noncompliant patients were not counted enhanced, rather than diminished, the mortality difference (UGDP Research Group, 1970d).
• The data analysis should have been restricted to patients with good blood glucose control (Kilo et al., 1980).	• The analysis philosophy for this variable was the same as for drug compliance. The removal of patients using a variable influenced by treatment has a good chance of rendering the treatment groups noncomparable with regard to important baseline characteristics. In any case, analyses by level of blood glucose control did not account for the mortality difference (UGDP Research Group, 1971a).
• The study failed to collect relevant clinical data (Feinstein, 1971; Seltzer, 1972).	• The criticism is unjustified. The study collected data on a number of variables needed for assessing the occurrence of various kinds of peripheral vascular events. It is always possible to identify some variable that should have been observed with the perspective of hindsight. The criticism lacks credibility, in general and especially in this case, because of the nature of the result observed. It is hard to envision other clinical observations that would offset mortality, an outcome difficult to reverse!
• There were changes in the ECG coding procedures midway in the course of the study (Schor, 1971; Seltzer, 1972).	• Correct. However, the changes were made before investigators had noted any real difference in mortality and were, in any case, made without regard to observed treatment results (Cornfield, 1971).
• The patients did not receive enough medication for effective control of blood glucose levels (Seltzer, 1972).	• A higher percent of tolbutamide-treated patients had blood glucose values in the range indicative of good control than did the placebo-treated pa-

Table 7-2 Criticisms of the UGDP and comments pertaining to them (*continued*)

Criticism	Comment
	tients. The percentage of patients judged to have fair or good control, based on blood glucose determinations done over the course of the study, was 74 in the tolbutamide-treated group versus 59 in the placebo-treated group (UGDP Research Group, 1971a, 1976).
• The excess mortality can be accounted for by differences in the smoking behavior of the treatment group (source unknown).	• The argument is not plausible. While it is true that the study did not collect baseline smoking histories, there is no reason to believe the distribution of this characteristic would be so skewed so as to account for the excess (Cornfield, 1971). The study did in fact make an effort to rectify this oversight around 1972 with the collection of retrospective smoking histories. There were no major differences among the treatment groups with regard to smoking. However, the results were never published because of obvious questions involved in constructing baseline smoking histories long after patients were enrolled and then with the use of surrogate respondents for deceased patients. The oversight is understandable in view of the time the trial was designed. Cigarette smoking, while recognized at that time as a risk factor for cancer, was not widely recognized as a risk factor for coronary heart disease.
• The observed mortality difference can be accounted for by differences in the composition of the treatment group for unobserved baseline characteristics (Feinstein, 1971; Schor, 1971).	• This criticism can be raised for any trial. However, it lacks validity since there is no reason to assume treatment groups in a randomized trial are any less comparable for unobserved characteristics than for observed characteristics. And even if differences do exist, they will not have any effect on observed treatment differences unless the variables in question are important predictors of outcome.
• The majority of deaths were concentrated in a few clinics (Feinstein, 1971; Seltzer, 1972).	• Differences in the number of deaths by clinic are to be expected in any multicenter trial. However, they are irrelevant to comparisons by treatment groups in the UGDP, since the number of patients assigned to treatment groups was balanced by clinic (UGDP Research Group, 1970d, 1970e).
• The study included patients who did not meet the "usual" criteria for diabetes (Seltzer, 1972).	• There are a variety of criteria used for diagnosing diabetes, all of which are based, in part or totally, on the glucose tolerance test. The sum of the fasting one, two, and three hour glucose tolerance test values used in the UGDP represented an attempt to make efficient use of all the information provided by the test (UGDP Research Group, 1970d).
• The patients received a fixed dose of tolbutamide. The usual practice is to vary dosage, depending on need (Feinstein, 1971; Schor, 1971; Seltzer, 1972).	• Most patients in the real world receive the dosage used in the study (UGDP Research Group, 1972).
• The randomization schedules were not followed (Schor, 1971).	• The Biometrics Committee reviewed the randomization procedure and found no evidence of any breakdown in the assignment process (Committee for the Assessment of Biometric Aspects of Controlled Trials of Hypoglycemic Agents, 1975).
• There were "numerous" coding errors made at the coordinating center in transcription of data into computer readable formats (Feinstein, 1971).	• There is no evidence of any problem in this regard. The few errors noted in audits performed by the Biometrics Committee and FDA audit team were of no consequence in the findings of the trial (Committee for Assessment of Biometric Aspects of Controlled Trials of Hypoglycemic Agents, 1975, Food and Drug Administration, 1978).

Table 7-2   Criticisms of the UGDP and comments pertaining to them (*continued*)

Criticism	Comment
• There were coding and classification discrepancies in the assembled data (Kolata, 1979).	• The coding and classification error rate was in fact low and the errors that did occur were not differential by treatment group. There were no errors in the classification of patients by treatment assignment or by vital status. Hence, the argument does not provide a valid explanation of the mortality differences observed (Committee for the Assessment of Biometric Aspects of Controlled Trials of Hypoglycemic Agents, 1975; Food and Drug Administration, 1978; Prout et al., 1979).
• The cause of death information was not accurate (Feinstein, 1971; Schor, 1971; Seltzer, 1972).	• Independent review of individual death records by the FDA audit team revealed only three classification discrepancies, only one of which affected the tolbutamide-placebo comparison (Food and Drug Administration, 1978). However, in any case, the main analyses in the study and the conclusions drawn from them relate to overall mortality.
• The study does not prove tolbutamide is harmful (Feinstein, 1971; Schor, 1971; Seltzer, 1972).	• Correct. It would be unethical to continue a trial to establish the toxicity of an elective treatment. Toxicity is not needed to terminate an elective treatment (UGDP Research Group, 1970d).

The FDA started work on a revised label insert for tolbutamide shortly after the results were presented in 1970. The revised label warned of potential cardiovascular complications associated with prolonged use of the drug (Food and Drug Administration, 1972a). Doubts regarding the validity of the study and concerns regarding the implications of the proposed label change led to the formation of the Committee for the Care of the Diabetic (CCD). The committee was made up of practicing diabetologists from around the country (first headed by Robert F. Bradley of the Joslin Clinic and subsequently by Peter H. Forsham of the University of California). This committee, with legal counsel, obtained a court order on November 7, 1972 staying the use of the revised label[5] (Food and Drug Administration, 1975).

A side issue of importance to the field of clinical trials—and other research fields as well for that matter—had to do with public access to UGDP raw data. Records generated by the study and housed at the UGDP Coordinating Center in Baltimore were requested on behalf of the CCD under the Freedom of Information Act—FOIA (Morris et al., 1981; Stallones, 1982; Watson, 1981; see also Chapter 24). The request was denied by the United States District Court for the District of Columbia on February 5, 1976 (see citation 453). The decision was ultimately upheld by the United States Supreme Court in a six-to-two decision issued March 3, 1980 (see citation 462).

In spite of the controversy—or more likely because of it—the study appears to have had an effect on the treatment practices of diabetologists. It has caused both friends and foes of the study alike to re-examine the underlying rationale for treatment of the noninsulin-dependent diabetic and to consider dietary rather than pharmacological treatment of such patients (Beeson et al., 1979; West, 1980).

Sales data compiled by IMS from the National Prescription Audit[6] show a drop in the use of the oral hypoglycemic agents beginning with 1974. The estimated total number of prescrip-

5. The revised label had actually been prepared and distributed to manufacturers for use when the restraining order was issued. It contained a special warning concerning the possibility of an increased risk of cardiovascular death with the use of sulfonylurea oral hypoglycemic agents and referred specifically to the UGDP results. The label was finally revised in 1984 to include the special warning and a synopsis of the UGDP results (see citations 192, 193, and 194).

6. The National Prescription Audit is based on a nationwide sample of pharmacies that supply monthly data to IMS on the number of new and refill prescriptions issued per month. Reporting procedures were changed in 1981 and again in 1982. As a result, data obtained after the changes are difficult to compare with those obtained before the change. Therefore, they are not presented herein.

tions (new as well as refills) for all hypoglycemic oral agents in the United States has declined from a high of 21 million in 1973 to 13.6 million in 1980 (Figure 7-1, Part A). The largest decrease occurred for the sulfonylurea, tolbutamide (Figure 7-1, Part B). However, it is worth noting that the decrease began before publication of the UGDP results and that it was accompanied by increases in sales of chlorpropamide and tolazamide, also members of the family of sulfonylurea compounds.

The decline of phenformin sales, beginning with 1973, was the result of a general concern in the medical community related to isolated cases of lactic acidosis and of a negative report from the UGDP on the treatment. The drug was for all intents and purposes removed from the market in 1977 through special powers vested in the Secretary of Health, Education and Welfare (see citations 184, 185, and 187).

The de-emphasis on the oral hypoglycemic agents is reflected by advertising, as seen in the *Journal of the American Medical Association* (see Table 7-3). The only product advertised in 1979 was Pfizer's Diabinese®. In addition, advertising for the oral hypoglycemic agents represented 4.6% of the total advertising space in the journal in 1969, compared with 2.3% in 1979 (total advertising space estimated from a 25% sample of the 52 issues of the Journal published in the two time periods).

The National Therapeutic Index provides a more direct measure of physician prescribing habits. Data in this Index (IMS America, Ltd.,

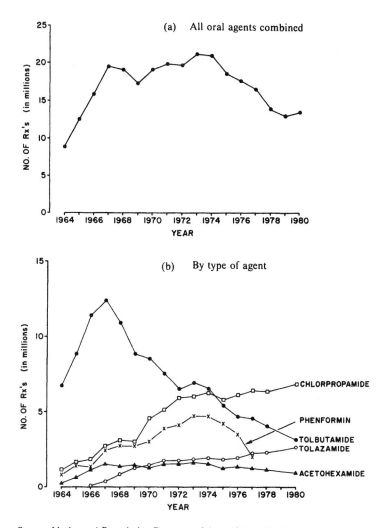

Figure 7-1 Estimated total number of hypoglycemic prescriptions (new and refill) for the U.S.

Source: Market and Prescription Data, copyright © 1964–1980, IMS America, Ltd., Ambler, Pa. (reference citation 244).

Table 7-3 Advertising for oral hypoglycemic agents in the *Journal of the American Medical Association* for 1969 and 1979

	1969		1979	
Drug	*Number of pages*	*Percent*	*Number of pages*	*Percent*
DBI®	2	1	0	0
Diabinese®	0	0	36	100
Dymelor®	11	8	0	0
Orinase®	49	36	0	0
Tolinase®	74	54	0	0
Total for hypoglycemic agents	136	100	36	100
Total number of advertising pages	2953		1597	

1977) are obtained from participating physicians. According to data in the Index, the number of physician visits of diabetics that resulted in a prescription of an oral hypoglycemic agent declined from 56% in 1969 to 36% by 1976, while the number of visits involving insulin prescriptions increased from 29% to 34% (Table 7-4). The apparent increase in use of insulin is reflected in Figure 7-2 as well. The figure suggests an increasing use of insulin relative to the oral agents. However, this conclusion is valid only if it is reasonable to assume that participating pharmacies in the National Prescription Audit have not changed their reporting habits with regard to insulin.[7]

Data from the CPHA indicate a similar trend for patient discharge data from U.S. short-term,

7. Technically, insulin is not a prescription drug, although it is usually issued by prescription and, hence, reported in the Audit.

nonfederal, general hospitals (Figure 7-3). A survey of 14 large teaching hospitals in 1969 and again in 1971 showed less reliance on oral agents and a sharper drop in their use than noted for general hospitals (Commission on Professional and Hospital Activities, 1972, 1976). The percentages of patients receiving a prescription for an oral hypoglycemic agent on discharge dropped from 33% in 1969 to 24% in 1971 for the 14 teaching hospitals, as contrasted with a drop from 38% to 34% for general hospitals. There was only a slight increase in the use of insulin for the time period in the teaching hospitals (63% in 1969 and 64% in 1971), as compared with a somewhat larger increase in the general hospitals (61% in 1969 and 64% in 1971).

The UGDP cost about $8.5 million to carry out. That cost is minuscule when contrasted with the amount of money spent on prescriptions for oral hypoglycemic agents (Table 7-5). The esti-

Table 7-4 Percentage of patient-physician visits for diabetics by type of prescription issued

Type of Rx given	*1969*	*1970*	*1973*	*Oct. 1974 through Sept. 1975*	*Oct. 1975 through Sept. 1976*
No drug Rx	16	19	24	26	28
Drug Rx	84	81	76	74	72
Oral hypoglycemics	56	52	45	41	36
Sulfonylureas	49	45	37	34	30
Phenformin	10	11	12	10	8
Insulin	29	28	29	31	34
Total	100	100	100	100	100

Source: Market and Prescription Data, copyright © 1964–1980, IMS America, Ltd., Ambler, Pa. (reference citation 244).

Figure 7-2 Estimated number of insulin prescriptions (new and refill) and ratio of oral hypoglycemic Rx's to insulin Rx's for the U.S.

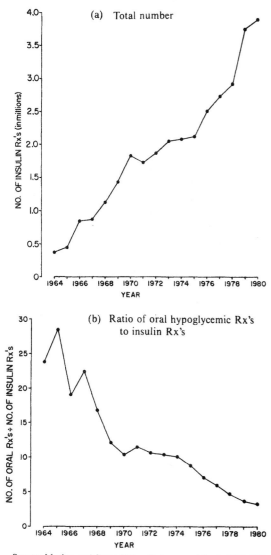

Table 7-5 Estimated U.S. wholesale dollar cost for oral hypoglycemic prescriptions

	Estimated* wholesale dollar cost (in millions)		
Year	*Phenformin*	*Tolbutamide*	*All oral agents*
1964	2.3	22.4	28.9
1965	3.9	28.2	38.6
1966	3.5	35.1	47.2
1967	7.1	38.1	58.0
1968	7.9	35.3	58.9
1969	8.4	28.7	54.5
1970	10.5	29.0	62.1
1971	14.0	24.7	65.0
1972	15.2	21.8	65.8
1973	26.7	34.8	104.8
1974	28.3	34.1	112.0
1975	26.7	31.2	109.3
1976	25.2	28.4	114.9
1977	17.1†	31.8	119.8
1978	†	30.9	109.8
1979	†	26.4	110.5

Source: Market and Prescription Data, copyright © 1964–1980, IMS America, Ltd., Ambler, Pa. (reference citation 244).

*Method of estimation changed in 1973. The large increase from 1972 to 1973 is an artifact of that change.

†NDAs for drug suspended in 1977; ordered off the market in 1978.

Figure 7-3 Type of hypoglycemic prescription on discharge from general hospitals for diabetes as a percentage of total diabetic discharges.

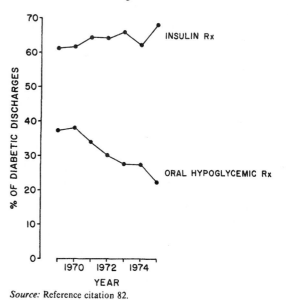

Source: Reference citation 82.

Source: Market and Prescription Data, copyright © 1964–1980, IMS America, Ltd., Ambler, Pa. (reference citation 244).

mated wholesale cost of the 21 million prescriptions for oral hypoglycemic agents written in 1973 (Figure 7-1) was $105 million. This translates into an average cost of $10 per prescription, assuming retail cost is twice wholesale cost. The drop in 1980 to 13.5 million oral hypoglycemic prescriptions represents a "savings" of $75 million—about nine times the cost of the study.

7.5   WAYS TO INCREASE THE IMPACT OF CLINICAL TRIALS

One obvious way to increase the impact of clinical trials is through improvements in their design and conduct. Continued proliferation of trials that have inadequate sample sizes, that involve clinically irrelevant outcome measures, and that are poorly executed cannot help having an adverse effect on the way clinical trials are viewed by the public.

The pharmaceutical industry needs to be encouraged to develop better structures for their trials. There needs to be a clearer separation of those responsible for execution of the trial from the sponsoring firm. The collection and analysis of data by firms with a proprietary interest in the product being tested is automatically open to question. Both industry and the public would ultimately benefit from trials that are above reproach.

There must also be efforts made to educate the public on the importance of clinical trials as an evaluation tool. The public must be taught to have a realistic appreciation of the strengths and weaknesses of the tool. Research societies, such as the Society for Clinical Trials and others, have a responsibility to assume leadership roles in this education process.

Investigators carrying out trials have, in effect, a public trust. They must take pains to avoid even the appearance of conflict of interest in the collection, analysis, or interpretation of results. A public trust cannot be established and maintained without high standards of integrity on the part of everyone involved in trials.

Editors of journals can help by establishing more stringent review criteria to make certain that the results of trials that are published have been generated and analyzed using sound methods. They should reject papers from trials with inadequate design features or standards of execution. Imposition of higher editorial standards would ultimately serve to elevate the design and execution standards of future trials.

Finally, as mentioned at the beginning of this chapter, there is a need for a better understanding of the way in which clinical trials influence the practice of medicine.

Part II. Design principles and practices

Chapters in This Part

The five chapters of this Part are intended to outline the primary principles and procedures to be followed in designing a trial. Chapter 8 discusses the general principles underlying selection of the study treatment, the choice of the outcome measure, and the roles of randomization and masking in data collection. Chapter 9 discusses the role of sample size and power estimates in planning a trial and details the methods for making such calculations in trials involving fixed sample size designs. Chapter 10 is devoted to a discussion of the principles and practices to be followed in administering the randomization schedule. Chapter 11 details the items that must be addressed in developing the study plan and treatment protocol for the trial. Chapter 12 outlines factors that influence the data collection schedule and contains suggestions concerning the design and content of data forms.

8. Essential design features of a controlled clinical trial

> On being asked to talk on the principles of research, my first thought was to arise after the chairman's introduction, to say, "Be careful," and to sit down.
>
> Jerome Cornfield (1959)

8.1 INTRODUCTION

The first question in any clinical trial is whether it is appropriate to mount the trial at all. Timing is of prime importance. The trial cannot proceed in the face of widespread doubts regarding its ethical base. Investigators must be satisfied that it is proper to expose patients to either the test or the control treatment. The ethical window for a trial may be quite narrow. Use of an agent in any trial setting may be deemed unethical if the agent is regarded as "too" experimental, yet that same agent may be accepted by the medical profession a short time later as the standard of treatment—without the benefit of any experimental evidence.

Ideally, the best time to start a trial is with the introduction of a treatment, before preconceived notions regarding its merit develop. Chalmers has argued for randomized trials the moment a new treatment is introduced (Chalmers, 1975, 1982b). This approach, while laudable, is not without problems. The rush to start may lead to a series of uncoordinated, small-scale efforts, none of which is adequate to answer the question of interest. Randomization of patients should not be started until there is a defined treatment protocol and a support organization to monitor the trial for evidence of adverse or beneficial treatment effects. The time involved in developing a common study protocol, writing and testing the necessary data forms, obtaining required support staff, and establishing the structure needed for proper data intake and analysis, not to mention the time needed to fund the trial, makes it difficult to start randomization with the first use of a treatment.

Once the question of timing has been resolved, the next set of issues involves basic design questions. Any controlled clinical trial requires specification of:

- A test and control treatment
- An outcome measure for evaluating the study treatments
- A bias-free method for assigning patients to the study treatments

Considerations in arriving at each of these specifications are discussed in the sections that follow.

8.2 CHOICE OF THE TEST AND CONTROL TREATMENTS

The choice of the test and control treatments is key. The general requirements to be satisfied are outlined in Table 8–1. The test treatment must be different from the control treatment; otherwise there is no point to the trial. Further, both treatments must be justifiable on medical grounds in order to allow investigators to assign patients to either treatment.

The choice of the test treatment is straightforward in settings where there is only one viable alternative to the control treatment, or where there are practical reasons for concentrating on a particular treatment (e.g., in an industry-sponsored trial done to satisfy Food and Drug Administration requirements for licensure of a particular drug). It is not when a number of

Table 8-1 Requirements for the test and control treatments

- They must be distinguishable from one another
- They must be medically justifiable
- There must be an ethical base for use of either treatment
- Use of the treatments must be compatible with the health care needs of study patients
- Either treatment must be acceptable to study patients and to physicians administering them
- There must be a reasonable doubt regarding the efficacy of the test treatment
- There should be reason to believe that the benefits will outweigh the risks of treatment
- The method of treatment administration must be compatible with the design needs of the trial (e.g., method of administration must be the same for all the treatments in a double-masked trial) and should be as similar to real-world use as practical

---

alternatives exist. This was the situation faced by investigators designing the University Group Diabetes Program (UGDP). They had to choose from among several different types of hypoglycemic agents (University Group Diabetes Program Research Group, 1970d). The same was true for planners of the Coronary Drug Project (CDP) in choosing among various lipid-lowering drugs (Coronary Drug Project Research Group, 1973a).

The choice of the control treatment has implications for the size of the treatment difference that can be expected. The largest difference can be expected when the control treatment is inactive. However, this design is only feasible when it is ethical to allow patients assigned to the control treatment to remain untreated (except for use of a placebo or sham treatment). The more effective the control treatment, the more difficult it will be to establish the superiority of the test treatment.

The choice of the control treatment will be dictated by current medical practice. The usual control in a surgery trial is the best available medical therapy. Some surgery trials have used sham operations as controls (Cobb et al., 1959; Dimond et al., 1960; Perry et al., 1964). However, their use has been curtailed in recent years for ethical reasons. The control treatment in a drug trial will be a standard form of drug therapy, a placebo, or no treatment at all, depending on the nature of the disease.

Treatment cannot be withheld from control patients if it is unethical to do so. Some form of medical care must be provided if a patient has a condition that requires treatment. The nature of the treatment chosen can cause a dilemma for investigators, especially when the test treatment is a refinement of the standard treatment. Investigators in the Hypertension Detection and Follow-Up Program (HDFP) had to face this problem. It was recognized that it would be unethical to identify hypertensive patients and then leave them untreated. It was also recognized that clinic personnel could not be expected to adopt two standards of care—an aggressive approach to blood pressure control for patients assigned to stepped-care and a laissez-faire approach to patients assigned to regular care. The dilemma was resolved by referring patients assigned to the control treatment back to their private physicians for treatment (Hypertension Detection and Follow-Up Program Cooperative Group, 1979b).

Some trials may involve more than one control treatment. The UGDP included both a placebo and fixed-dose insulin treatment group. The placebo treatment was used primarily for comparison with the tolbutamide and phenformin treatments, whereas both the fixed-dose insulin and placebo treatments were useful in evaluating the insulin variable treatment (University Group Diabetes Program Research Group, 1970e, 1971b, 1978, 1982).

8.3 PRINCIPLES IN THE SELECTION OF THE OUTCOME MEASURE

The outcome measure used for treatment comparisons will be a clinical event (e.g., death, myocardial infarction, significant loss of vision, recurrence of a disease) or a surrogate outcome measure (e.g., a score on a psychological test, blood pressure change, serum lipid level). The focus in this book is on trials using a clinical event as the outcome measure.

Table 8-2 provides a list of desired characteristics for the primary outcome measure. The measure should be specified when the trial is planned, before the start of data collection. Otherwise the value of the trial may be compromised, especially if there is reason to believe that data collected during the trial were used to select the measure.

The rate of occurrence of the outcome event will affect the power of the study and the length of time it is required to run (see Chapter 9). Trials involving a laboratory measure or some other surrogate outcome usually involve fewer

Table 8–2 Desired characteristics of the primary outcome measure

- Easy to diagnose or observe
- Free of measurement or ascertainment errors
- Capable of being observed independent of treatment assignment
- Clinically relevant
- Chosen before the start of data collection

patients and take less time to complete than those using death or some other nonfatal clinical event as the outcome, but these economies are achieved at the expense of medical relevancy. The implications of a trial with a clinical event as the outcome will, as a rule, be easier to understand than one in which clinical relevance must be inferred by relying on the presumed relationship of a surrogate outcome and the clinical condition of interest.

It is not uncommon for trials to provide data on a number of secondary outcome measures as well. This is almost always the case in a trial in which mortality serves as the primary outcome. For example, the CDP collected data on the occurrence of myocardial infarctions and a series of other nonfatal events in addition to data on deaths (Coronary Drug Project Research Group, 1973a).

Investigators may design the trial to detect a specified treatment difference using a combination of events. Use of composite events will increase the expected event rates and hence may reduce the required size of the trial (see Chapter 9). However, the practice is ill advised because of the potential for confusion when interpreting results based on composite measures.

8.4 PRINCIPLES OF ESTABLISHING COMPARABLE STUDY GROUPS

The baseline characteristics of the test- and control-treated groups must be more or less similar in order to provide a valid basis for comparison. This need was recognized by Lind in his famous scurvy experiment. He wrote:

On the 20th of May 1747, I took twelve patients in the scurvy, on board the Salisbury *at sea. Their cases were as similar as I could have them. They all in general had putrid gums, the spots and lassitude, with weakness of their knees. They lay together*

in one place, being a proper apartment for the sick in the fore-hold; and had one diet common to all. . . . (Lind, 1753)

The ideal experimental model for comparing two treatments is one in which the baseline characteristics of the two study groups are identical in all aspects. This requires a homogeneous group of patients who are arbitrarily assigned to the test and control treatments. An alternative design involves enrolling pairs of patients into the trial, with each pair matched on all important baseline characteristics, and where one member of the pair is assigned to the test treatment and the other to the control treatment. However, matching is not practical. The number of patients that must be screened to find suitable matches is usually unacceptably large, to say nothing of the time required to achieve even a modest recruitment goal.

Usually the focus is on the recruitment of patients one by one, with no attempt to match. The comparability of the study groups for a few key baseline characteristics may be assured by first classifying patients into subgroups defined by those characteristics, and then assigning members of each subgroup to the test or control treatment in the same proportion as for all other subgroups. However, this approach, referred to as stratification and discussed in Chapter 10, at best can control the distribution of only a few variables.

The need for comparability can be partially satisfied by appropriate patient selection. The eligibility and exclusion criteria in most trials are designed to reduce the variability of the study populations by placing restrictions on the type of patients that may be enrolled. However, the desire for patient homogeneity and the resultant improvement in study precision must be balanced against reduced opportunities for generalizations when a highly homogeneous population is studied.

Once an eligible patient has agreed to be enrolled, it is imperative that the treatment assignment be made free of influence from both the patient and clinic personnel so as to avoid selection biases in the way study groups are formed. The general conditions that should be satisfied in order to have a sound allocation scheme are outlined in Table 8–3.

Any system in which the study physician has access to a patient's treatment assignment before enrollment is open to suspicion and violates the first requirement listed in Table 8–3. This is the main problem with allocation procedures based on characteristics associated with patients, such as birth dates or Social Security numbers. Odd-even schemes, for example, in which patients seen on odd-numbered days receive one treatment and those seen on even-numbered days receive the other treatment, are unsatisfactory for the same reason. (See Wright et al., 1954, for example.) Schemes of this sort are open to challenge and are almost always impossible to defend.

Systematic schemes in which every other patient is assigned to the test treatment violate the second requirement listed in Table 8-3. Even random allocation schemes can violate this requirement if the assignments are balanced at intervals known to clinic personnel (e.g., after every second allocation in a study involving only two study treatments). Several of the papers reviewed in Chapter 2 described or alluded to systematic nonrandom allocation schemes that appeared not to meet the second requirement (e.g., deAlmeida et al., 1980; Marks et al., 1980; Milman et al., 1980; Scott et al., 1980). However, there was not sufficient information in most of the papers to make a reliable judgment as to the soundness of the allocation process.

The third requirement, that the sequence of assignments be reproducible, is violated by any scheme that does not generate the same sequence of assignments when replicated. Coin flips are unsatisfactory for this reason, among others.

Schemes in which individual assignments are contained in sealed envelopes at the clinics are preferable to schemes described above. However, they are subject to manipulation as well if they fail to satisfy the first requirement listed in Table 8-3 (see Carleton et al., 1960, for exam-

Table 8-3   Requirements of a sound treatment allocation scheme

- Assignment remains masked to the patient, physician, and all other clinic personnel until it is needed for initiation of treatment
- Future assignments cannot be predicted from past assignments
- The order of allocations is reproducible
- Methods for generation and administration of the schedule are documented
- The process used for generation has known mathematical properties
- The process provides a clear audit trail
- Departures from the established sequence of assignments can be detected

ple). Precautions must be taken to make certain that the envelopes are used in the order provided and that their contents remain unknown to clinic personnel until they are used.

The assignment process should have known mathematical properties. A major shortcoming of most informal methods of assignment, such as the odd-even scheme described above, is the absence of a mathematical base. It should also provide a clear audit trail and should be constructed and administered in such a way that departures from the established procedure can be detected.

The accepted standard for creating treatment groups is randomization. Unfortunately, there is still a good deal of misunderstanding regarding the reasons for randomizing. While the process does provide a basis for certain types of statistical analyses (Pitman, 1937), it is far more useful as a method of making bias-free treatment assignments. The term *random* is often misused in medical circles by investigators who equate haphazard and random processes (as in referring to a random blood sugar determination when really meaning a haphazard one, or in characterizing a group of arbitrarily selected individuals as a random sample). It should be reserved in research settings for processes that satisfy the definition stated in the Glossary.

Chapter 10 provides a discussion of methods for administering the treatment allocation schedule. It also contains a discussion of issues to be considered when the randomization schedule is constructed, including those related to stratification and blocking.

8.5   PRINCIPLES OF MASKING AND BIAS CONTROL

The aim of any trial should be to collect data that are free of bias, especially treatment-related bias (see Glossary for definition). The latter type of bias is of particular concern since it has the potential for obscuring a treatment difference or creating the impression that one exists when in fact it does not. The usual procedure used to protect against treatment-related bias is masking.

The term *masked*,[1] when used throughout this book, refers to a condition in which the treat-

---

1. Used in this book instead of *blinded* because it is regarded as a more apt description of the process involved. Further, use of the latter term, as in double-blinded trial, leads to confusion in some settings, such as in vision trials where the outcome measure is blindness.

ment assignment, or some other item of information, is withheld from some individual or group of individuals in the study as a means of improving the objectivity of the treatment, data collection, reporting, or analysis processes. It is conventional to refer to trials as unblinded, single-blinded, or double-blinded (unmasked, single-masked, or double-masked in this book). The terms serve as decriptors of the method of treatment administration. For example, a double-masked trial is one in which neither the patient nor the physician responsible for treatment is informed of the patient's treatment assignment; a single-masked trial is one in which the patient is not informed of the treatment assignment but the treating physician is, and an unmasked trial is one in which both the patient and the physician are informed of the treatment assignment. Technically, the term *single-masked* may be used to characterize a trial in which *either* the patient or physician is unaware of the treatment assignment; however, it usually refers to designs in which the patient is masked and the physician is not.

The logistics of masking are not simple. They are discussed in Chapter 10 in relation to bottling and dispensing drugs, and briefly in Chapter 19 in relation to data collection.

Among the randomized trials listed in the 1979 NIH Inventory of Clinical Trials (see Chapter 2), the majority were unmasked (388 out of 589, or 66%). Another 12% were single-masked, and 22% were double-masked. These results stand in marked contrast to published reports, as summarized in Chapter 2. Of the 113 trials reviewed, 76 (67%) were reported to be double-masked.

Reports of trials that are single- or double-masked should contain information on the effectiveness of the mask. The information is useful in assessing the possibility of bias in the study. However, only a few groups have addressed this issue (e.g., Beta Blocker Heart Attack Trial Research Group, 1981; Howard et al., 1981).

Treatment-specific side effects can reduce the effectiveness of the masking. This was the case with the estrogen treatments in the CDP. A total of 61% of patients assigned to the high dose of estrogen and 45% of patients assigned to the low dose of estrogen complained of decreased libido, as contrasted with only 1.5% of the placebo-treated patients (Coronary Drug Project Research Group, 1970a).

The principle of masking is general and applies whenever it is practical to withhold infor-

mation that, if known, may influence the way in which data are collected or how the treatments are adminstered. Table 8-4 lists suggested masking guidelines. Masked data collection is especially important in trials involving outcome measures that are subject to measurement or ascertainment errors.

A double-masked trial, as defined above, is characterized by masked data collection. However, even single-masked or unmasked trials may be designed so that data collection is done in a masked fashion via structures in which treatment information is withheld from personnel responsible for data collection. The structures require one set of personnel to administer the study treatments and another to collect the data needed for assessing the study treatments.

Laboratory tests should be performed, recorded, and reported by personnel who are masked to treatment assignment, regardless of the level of treatment masking in the rest of the trial. The only exceptions are cases in which treatment assignment is needed to determine the tests to be performed. Likewise, records such as ECGs, fundus photographs, and x-rays should be read by individuals who are masked to treatment assignment. The same is true of personnel responsible for coding or classifying outcome events.

Ideally, all keying, editing, and data analysis activities in the data center should be performed by personnel who are masked. This standard is not easy to achieve because of the obvious prac-

Table 8-4 Masking guidelines

- Use a treatment allocation scheme that meets the masking criteria listed in Table 8-3 (i.e., the treatment assignment for a patient cannot be determined in advance of enrollment)

- Administer treatments with the highest level of masking feasible (e.g., double-masked if possible; single-masked if double masking is impossible; unmasked only if any level of masking is out of the question)

- Require, when possible, that essential data collection, measurement, reading, and classification procedures on individual patients be made by persons who have no knowledge of treatment assignment or course of treatment

- Require, when possible, that outcome measurements that are subject to interpretation errors (e.g., measurements requiring a subjective evaluation) be made by personnel who are masked to treatment assignment

- Do not require masked treatment administration if doing so requires study patients to assume measurable risks in order to achieve or maintain the masking

tical problems involved in maintaining the mask. However, it is important when it cannot be achieved to make certain that decisions regarding the way in which data are keyed or used for analysis purposes are made without regard to treatment assignment or observed treatment differences.

The principle of masking has been extended to treatment monitoring committees as well. Treatment monitoring reports presented in the Diabetic Retinopathy Study (DRS) were masked with regard to treatment group, even though the trial itself was unmasked. However, in this case the masking was subsequently abandoned because of the logistical difficulties involved in producing the monitoring reports and because of its limited usefulness (Knatterud, 1977).

9. Sample size and power estimates

A difference to be a difference must make a difference.

Source unknown

9.1 SEQUENTIAL VERSUS FIXED SAMPLE SIZE DESIGNS

This chapter deals with sample size and power estimates for fixed sample size designs. All of the trials sketched in Appendix B are of this type. Strictly speaking, a fixed sample size design is one in which the investigator specifies the required sample size before starting the trial. The specification may be based on a formal sample size calculation or on practical considerations related to cost, patient availability, or other factors. The investigator then proceeds to enroll the number of patients specified, unless there are extenuating circumstances to the contrary (e.g., the specified number cannot be recruited as planned or recruitment has to be stopped because of adverse or beneficial treatment effects). In practice, the sample size may not be set until after the trial is started or may never be formally set in some cases. In other cases, it may be merely implied by other conditions, such as the amount of time allowed for patient recruitment.

The approach is quite different with sequential designs. A classical open sequential design provides for continued patient enrollment until the observed test-control treatment difference exceeds a predefined boundary value (see Figure 9–1). The simplest application of this design is the enrollment of patients in pairs. One member of each pair is assigned to the test treatment and the other member is assigned to the control treatment. The decision as to whether to enroll the next pair of patients is based on outcomes observed for patients already enrolled. The pair of patients is enrolled if the cumulative test-control difference for all previously enrolled pairs of patients is still within the defined boundaries. The pair is not enrolled if one of the two boundaries is exceeded.

The expected sample size, given a specified type I and II error level, is smaller for a sequential design than for its fixed sample size counterpart (Armitage, 1975). However, the number of patients required in any given replication can exceed the number required with a fixed sample size design. In fact, there is a chance, albeit infinitesimally small, that the treatment difference will remain within the defined boundaries no matter how many pairs of patients are en-

Figure 9-1   Schematic illustration of boundaries for open sequential design.

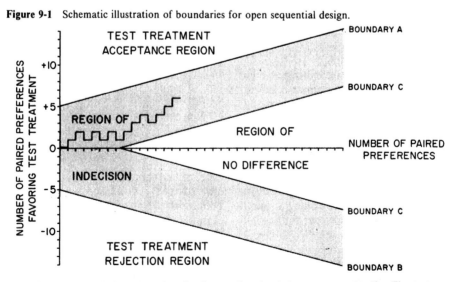

Note: Trial continues until observed number of preferences (ignoring ties) crosses a boundary line. The test treatment is considered superior to the control treatment if boundary line A is crossed, inferior to the control treatment if boundary B is crossed, and equal to the control treatment if boundary C is crossed. The C boundary lines are deleted in trials designed to continue until the test treatment is declared superior or inferior to the control treatment.

rolled. This possibility is eliminated by imposing a limit on the number of patients that may be enrolled, as illustrated in Figure 9-2. Closed sequential designs (so named because of the limit imposed on the number of patients that may be enrolled) are preferred to open sequential designs in most medical settings because they allow the investigator to stop the trial if the study treatments appear to be of about equal value.

The initial work on open sequential designs was done by Wald (1947). The closed modifications come from work by Bross (1952) and Armitage (1957). A book by Armitage (1975) focuses on applications of closed designs to medical trials. (See Grant, 1962, and Snell and Armitage, 1957, for examples of the two types of sequential designs).

There are sequential aspects to any trial, even if done using a fixed sample size design. Patients in both types of designs are typically enrolled over time. The temporal nature of the enrollment process leads to a gradual accumulation of outcome data for use in making treatment comparisons. As noted above, a new comparison is made after each pair of patients is enrolled in the classical sequential design. The results of the comparison are used to decide whether to stop patient enrollment. The decision-making process is more complicated in the typical fixed sample design, at least for the class of trials discussed in this book. An investigator must not only decide

whether it is appropriate to continue patient enrollment up to the limit set, but also whether it is appropriate to continue the trial after enrollment is completed. He should stop the trial once it becomes clear that the test treatment is superior or inferior to the control treatment, regardless of whether patients are still being enrolled (see Chapter 20 for further discussion).

The use of sequential designs is limited to situations in which outcome assessment can be made shortly after patients are enrolled in the trial. They are not practical where long periods of follow-up are required to accumulate sufficient outcome data to make reliable treatment comparisons. The usual approach in such cases is to use a fixed sample size design. This approach, as discussed herein, utilizes a frequentist analysis philosophy—a philosophy based on work of Neyman and Pearson (1966) and one that is widely used in biostatistics for analysis of medical research. Other analysis philosophies include those built on the likelihood principle and on Bayes' theorem. Plackett (1966) has reviewed all three philosophies. The frequentist approach is reviewed by Armitage (1963) and by Armitage and co-workers (1969). The likelihood approach is reviewed by Anscombe (1963). The Bayesian approach is reviewed by Colton (1963) and Cornfield (1966a).

Sample size and power estimates for fixed sample size designs are discussed by a number of

Figure 9-2 Schematic illustration of boundaries for closed sequential design.

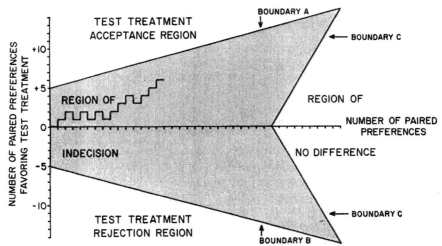

Note: Trial continues until observed number of preferences (ignoring ties) crosses a boundary line. The test treatment is considered superior to the control treatment if boundary line A is crossed, inferior to the control treatment if boundary line B is crossed, and equal to the control treatment if boundary line C is crossed.

authors, including Cochran and Cox (1957), Cox and Hinkley (1974), Fleiss (1981), Lachin (1981), Schlesselman (1982), and Snedecor and Cochran (1967). Readers may refer to these references or to other basic statistics texts for details not covered in this chapter.

9.2 SAMPLE SIZE AND POWER CALCULATIONS AS PLANNING GUIDES

It is unwise to undertake a fixed sample size trial without a calculation to determine the number of patients required or the power available with a specified sample size. With a sample size calculation, the investigator sets out to determine the number of patients required to detect a designated treatment difference with specified levels of type I and II error protection. With a power (see Glossary) calculation, the investigator determines the power associated with a specified treatment difference, given a specified sample size. Either one of these calculations, may lead to subsequent design modifications. The modifications may include expansion from a single center to multiple centers to increase the number of patients available for study, changes in the patient admission criteria to make recruitment easier, or abandonment of the trial.

The archives of clinical trials are cluttered with inconsequential trials. Such trials are, in one sense, unethical in that they require patients to accept the risks of treatment, however small, without any chance of benefit to them or future patients. Small-scale preliminary investigations may be justified when part of a larger plan, but not as an end in their own right.

The absence of a planned approach to study design is evident from a review of the published literature, as discussed in Chapter 2. Few of the trials cited there show any evidence of having involved sample size or power calculations (see also Freiman et al., 1978, and Mosteller et al., 1980).

The design documents prepared when the trial is planned should indicate the recruitment goal for the trial and how it was determined. If the goal was the result of a sample size calculation, the details of that calculation should be provided. If it was set by practical considerations, such as cost or the presumed availability of patients, it should be accompanied by appropriate calculations to indicate the power that can be expected with the proposed number of patients.

In either case, the calculations, such as shown in Tables 9-1 and 9-2, should indicate how the trial is affected if the control event rate used in the sample size calculation proves to be wrong, or how power changes as a function of sample size.

The main thrust of the discussion in this chapter relates to the use of sample size and power estimates in planning the trial. However, as noted in Section 9.7, the same methods are used for sample size adjustments during the trial or for posterior power calculations at the end of the trial.

9.3 SPECIFICATIONS FOR SAMPLE SIZE CALCULATIONS

A determination of the required sample size cannot be undertaken until the basic design features of the trial, such as outlined in Table 9–3, have been set. It may take months and a good deal of interaction between investigators, especially between the physicians and biostatisticians, to reach agreement on the specifications.

The subsections that follow detail the considerations that go into setting the specifications and provide discussion of the ways in which they influence sample size requirements. Most of the same points pertain to power calculations as well.

9.3.1 Number of treatment groups

The considerations involved in reaching a decision on the type and number of study treatments have been discussed in Chapter 8. The sample size formulations presented in Section 9.4 are for the case of a trial involving one test and one control treatment. However, they can be used for trials with any number of test treatments, so

Table 9-1 Illustration of a sample size presentation, $\alpha = 0.01$ (two-tailed), $\beta = 0.05$, and $\lambda = 1$

Control event rate, P_c	$\Delta_R = \dfrac{P_c - P_t}{P_c}$		
	0.125	0.250	0.375
0.10	19,373	4,549	1,888
0.15	12,246	2,886	1,202
0.20	8,682	2,055	859
0.30	5,119	1,223	516

Table 9-2 Illustration of a power presentation, given a sample size of 800 per treatment group, $\alpha = 0.01$ (two-tailed), and $\lambda = 1$

Control event rate, P_c	$\Delta_R = \dfrac{P_c - P_t}{P_c}$		
	0.125	*0.250*	*0.375*
0.10	0.043	0.209	0.574
0.15	0.067	0.359	0.812
0.20	0.099	0.525	0.935
0.30	0.181	0.800	0.996

long as investigators plan to allocate the same number of patients to each of the test treatments. The total sample size, N, for a trial with one control treatment and uniform allocation among the r test treatments is:

$$N = rn_t + n_c \qquad (9.1)$$

where

r = number of test treatments

n_t = sample size required for each of the r test treatments

and

n_c = sample size for the control treatment

For the purposes of calculation it is necessary to specify the test-control allocation ratio,

$$\lambda = n_t/n_c \qquad (9.2)$$

Table 9-3 Design specifications affecting sample size considerations

- Number of treatment groups to be studied
- Outcome measure
- Anticipated length of patient follow-up
- Alternative treatment hypothesis
- Detectable treatment difference
- Desired type I and II error protection
- Allocation ratio
- Anticipated rate of loss to follow-up
- Anticipated treatment noncompliance rate
- Anticipated treatment lag time
- Degree of stratification for baseline risk factors
- Level of type I and II error adjustment for multiple comparisons
- Level of type I and II error adjustment for multiple looks
- Level of type I and II error adjustment for multiple outcomes

It is simply the number of patients to be assigned to a test treatment divided by the number to be assigned to the control treatment. This quantity is fixed by the study investigators and is generally the same for each of the r test treatments in the trial (see Section 9.3.7 for factors determining the choice of λ).

The usual approach is to calculate the sample size requirement for n_t using the formulas given in Section 9.4 and then to derive the value of n_c from Equation 9.2 by noting that $n_c = n_t/\lambda$. For example, given $r = 3$, $\lambda = 0.5$, and a calculated value of 50 for n_t yields an n_c of $50/0.5 = 100$. The total sample size is 250, as derived from Equation 9.1.

The sample size is not given by Equation 9.1 if the trial involves more than one control treatment. The simplest approach in this case is to use just one of the control treatments for the sample size calculation—ideally the one that provides the best basis for assessing the test treatments. The value for n_c, as derived from Equation 9.2, would be used for each control treatment and the total sample size would be $N = rn_t + sn_c$, where s is the number of control treatment groups. An alternative approach, if a minimal level of type II error protection is desired for comparisons of a test treatment with any one of the control treatments, involves making a sample size calculation for each of the different control treatments and then using the largest value of N obtained to plan the trial.

9.3.2 Outcome measure[1]

Sample size and power formulations are given in this chapter for binary as well as continuous outcome measures. However, the main emphasis is on binary outcomes (see Glossary) because of the class of trials considered in this book, as outlined in Chapter 1. Trials with binary outcomes are characterized by data collection schemes in which patients may be classified at any point after enrollment as either having or not yet having experienced the event of interest. The event may be a desired or undesired outcome depending on the trial and patients selected for study. It will be desired (positive) in trials in which patients are watched for disappearance or amelioration of some medical condition. It will be undesired (negative) when they are watched for the occurrence of death or some

---

1. See Chapter 8 for additional discussion of factors influencing the choice of the primary outcome measure.

morbid event. All discussion and calculations in this chapter are for negative events.

For the purposes of sample size or power calculations, the investigator may decide to alter the form of the outcome measure when the underlying measure is polychotomous or continuous. The choice should be dictated by the anticipated analysis requirements at the end of the trial. The calculations should be made using the unaltered underlying measure if the aim of the trial is to assess distributional changes in the measure over the time course of the trial. They should be made using a binary event measure, constructed from a dichotomization of the underlying measure, if observed values of the measure, at or above a specified level, take on special medical or operational significance (e.g., as in the case with blood pressures over a defined level used to diagnose hypertension and signal the need to initiate treatment).

The decision as to whether to design the trial to detect a mean change in some continuous measure or a difference in some event rate can have major implications on how the trial is perceived when it is finished. It is one thing to conclude that there is a significant difference in mean diastolic blood pressure between the study treatment groups, and quite another to conclude there is a significant difference in the rate of development of hypertension in the two groups. The latter statement has far greater clinical relevance than the former.

9.3.3   Follow-up period

Sample size and power calculations require specification of the follow-up period. Generally, the longer the period, the higher the accumulated event rate and the smaller the required sample size for a given type I and II error level.

The specification used for planning purposes may be modified as the trial proceeds. For example, the follow-up period may be extended to compensate for a shortfall in patient recruitment or for a lower-than-anticipated control event rate. Or it may have to be curtailed because of funding or other problems.

9.3.4   Alternative treatment hypothesis

The calculations in this chapter are always made under the null hypothesis of no treatment effect versus a specified alternative. The alternative will be constructed to cover treatment effects of

a specified size that are either beneficial or adverse (two-sided alternative), or that are only beneficial (one-sided alternative). The decision as to whether to use a one- or two-sided alternative depends on the clinical importance of a positive versus a negative treatment effect and how much is known about the safety of the test treatment when the trial is planned.

Trials of the sort considered in this book are done to establish the efficacy of a treatment, not toxicity. This fact argues for use of a one-sided alternative in the calculation, even though practice seems to favor use of two-sided alternatives. The reason has to do with the amount of prior evidence investigators have regarding treatment safety. They may prefer a two-sided alternative simply as a means of documenting their own uncertainty regarding the potential merits of the test treatment. A side benefit of the practice is that it leads to a larger sample size than the same α and β using a one-sided test. The increased sample size represents a hedge against unanticipated losses, such as those due to lack of compliance to the treatment protocol during the trial.

9.3.5   Detectable treatment difference

The experimenter is required to specify the minimum treatment difference he wishes to detect under the alternative hypothesis. The larger the difference the smaller the required sample size.

The difference chosen should be realistic. A 50% reduction in the test treatment event rate, while of unquestioned clinical relevance if achieved, is unlikely in real life. Only miracle treatments produce reductions of this size and there are few such treatments around and even fewer that require discovery via a clinical trial. Generally, the gains with most new treatments are much more modest. Certainly a reduction in the event rate does not have to be enormous to be important. Small reductions, in the range of 5 to 10%, can have major public health implications if they apply to death or some other serious nonfatal event associated with a common disease.

9.3.5.1   Binary outcome measures

Specification of the difference, in this case, requires the experimenter to designate a value for both P_c and P_t, or for P_c and the percentage reduction in P_c to be achieved with the test treatment, where

P_c = anticipated event rate for the control-treated group

and

P_t = anticipated event rate for the test-treated group

The minimal detectable difference expressed in absolute terms is:

$$\Delta_A = P_c - P_t \qquad (9.3)$$

Expressed in relative terms, it is:

$$\Delta_R = \frac{P_c - P_t}{P_c} \qquad (9.4)$$

Although either form is acceptable, many investigators prefer to express the difference in relative terms using Δ_R, even though sample size and power formulas are conventionally expressed in terms of Δ_A. Equation 9.5 can be used to convert from a relative to an absolute difference.

$$\Delta_A = P_c \, \Delta_R \qquad (9.5)$$

Ideally, the value chosen for P_c should be derived from follow-up studies of patients similar to those to be enrolled in the trial and who received treatment similar to that planned for the control-treated group. Unfortunately, follow-up data such as these are usually not available. Hence, the experimenter may have to rely on an educated guess for P_c. The value chosen may turn out to be higher or lower than the one actually observed in the trial. Selection of a value for P_c that is lower than the one subsequently observed means the trial was larger than it needed to be to detect a given relative difference—not a serious problem unless the underestimation resulted in a significant increase in the cost and time needed to carry out the trial. (The reverse is true if $P_c + P_t < 1$ and the experimenter is interested in detecting a prespecified absolute difference.) A more serious and common problem stems from overestimation of P_c. The sample size estimate in such cases will be smaller than needed to achieve the required error protection. Overestimation can occur even in instances in which investigators have reasonably reliable information for determining P_c, as in the Coronary Drug Project (CDP). The P_c (5-year mortality rate) used for sample size calculations was 30 per 100 population. The observed rate was only 21 per 100 population (Coronary Drug Project Research Group, 1975).

The tendency to overestimate P_c arises, at least in part, from the failure or inability of the study planners to predict the impact of the proposed patient eligibility criteria on subsequent observed event rates. The exclusion of seriously ill patients from enrollment may well yield a population with a better than expected prognosis.

9.3.5.2 Continuous outcome measures

The difference to be detected in this case is expressed as a function of means, as discussed in Section 9.4.2. The variance estimate[2] required, like the value of P_c used for binary outcomes, should be based on actual data if at all possible. It is wise to explore the effect of a range of variance estimates on sample size if there is no reliable way of estimating variance before the start of the trial.

9.3.6 Error protection

The choice of α and β (probabilities of type I and II error, respectively, see Glossary for definition) is arbitrary. The first instinct of an inexperienced investigator is to want a trial that precludes any possibility of either type of error—a lofty goal since an infinite number of patients is required to achieve it!

The choice of α and β should depend on the medical and practical consequences of the two kinds of errors. Relatively high error rates (e.g., $\alpha = 0.10$ and $\beta = 0.2$) may be acceptable for preliminary trials that are likely to be replicated, whereas lower rates (e.g., $\alpha = 0.01$ and $\beta = 0.05$) should be used if replication is unlikely.

The consequences of both a type I and II error must be considered. For example, one might choose:

$\alpha = \beta$ if both the test and control treatments are new, about equal in cost, and there are good reasons to consider them both relatively safe

$\alpha > \beta$ if there is no established control treatment and the test treatment is relatively inexpensive, easy to apply and is not known to have any serious side effects

$\alpha < \beta$ if the control treatment is already widely used and is known to be reasonably safe and effective, whereas the test treatment is new, costly, and produces serious side effects

2. The need for an independent variance estimate is avoided for binary outcomes. The variance in such cases is a function of the specified event rates.

The most common approach is to set $\alpha < \beta$. However, this is only reasonable if the consequences of a type II error are considered to be less than those of a type I error.

9.3.7 Choice of allocation ratio

The allocation ratio is ordinarily under the control of the experimenter and is set before patient enrollment is started, except with some forms of adaptive allocation (see Chapter 10). All of the trials sketched in Appendix B involved preset allocation ratios, except one (see item 20.a of Table B–4 in Appendix B). A uniform allocation scheme, in which the probability of assignment to one treatment group is the same as for all other treatment groups, is generally preferred (used in 11 of the 14 trials sketched in Appendix B; see item 20.e of Table B–4). Nonuniform methods of allocation are used when there is a need to concentrate more patients in certain treatment groups to satisfy secondary aims of the trial or to provide increased precision for certain of the treatment comparisons. Investigators in the Persantine Aspirin Reinfarction Study (PARIS) decided to allocate twice as many patients to the aspirin and to the aspirin-persantine treatment groups than to the placebo treatment group. They made this choice because they considered comparison of the aspirin and aspirin-persantine treatment groups more important than comparison of either of these treatment groups with the placebo treatment group (Persantine Aspirin Reinfarction Study Research Group, 1980b).

The CDP allocated 2.5 times as many patients to the placebo treatment as to any one of the five test treatments (Coronary Drug Project Research Group, 1973a).[3] The allocation ratio was chosen to minimize the variance for the five test-control comparisons of 5-year mortality. A somewhat lower ratio would have been derived using an approach developed by Dunnett (1955). His method assumes the experimenter wishes to construct confidence intervals about each test-control outcome difference at the end of the trial, such that the risk of a type I error for all comparisons combined is α. This error probability condition is satisfied if $\sqrt{r}$ patients are assigned to the control treatment for every patient assigned to any one of the r test treatments used in

the trial. The CDP would have required an allocation ratio of 2.24 instead of the one used with this method of calculation.

9.3.8 Losses to follow-up

Losses to follow-up are concentrated in dropouts (throughout this book, patients enrolled in the trial who are no longer able or willing to return to the clinic for regular follow-up examinations) who can no longer be followed for the event of interest. A patient who drops out is automatically lost to outcome follow-up unless the event used for outcome assessment can be reliably observed and reported outside the clinic setting.

The loss to follow-up rate used in the sample size calculation is estimated by the experimenter. As with other variables, such as P_c, the value used should be based on relevant experience, if at all possible. The value chosen may be zero or very small in cases in which it is possible to continue follow-up of patients for the outcome of interest even if they refuse to return to the clinic for regular follow-up examinations (e.g., as with patients under follow-up for mortality or some other event that can be reliably observed and recorded outside the clinic setting). It may have to be set quite high if long periods of clinic surveillance are required for outcome measurement.

Clearly, any loss of outcome data, regardless of how it occurs, will reduce the statistical precision of the trial, and may introduce bias as well if the losses are differential by treatment group. Hence, the sample size estimate, as given by formulas in Section 9.4, must be increased to compensate for the anticipated loss. This is normally done by multiplying the sample size by the quantity, $1/(1 - d)$, where d is the anticipated loss rate. For example, a d of $10/100$ would mean that for every 100 patients enrolled, 10 could not be classified as to presence or absence of the outcome of interest because of the lack of follow-up data. It would require multiplying the calculated sample size by a factor of $1/0.9 = 1.11$ to compensate for the losses.

9.3.9 Losses due to treatment noncompliance

The sample size must be increased to compensate for loss of precision due to treatment non-

---

3. The actual ratio, as derived by methods described in the 1973 CDP publication, was 2.45. It was rounded up to 2.5 to simplify construction of the allocation schedules needed in the trial.

compliance as well. Treatment compliance is rarely an all-or-none phenomenon. The level of compliance achieved may range from low to high, depending on the patient. Perfect compliance may be difficult, if not impossible, to achieve, especially in drug trials where the patient is required to take the assigned medication over long periods of time.

There are two aspects to the determination of compliance. One has to do with the amount of exposure the patient has to the assigned treatment, and the other has to do with the amount of exposure to the other study treatments. Underexposure to the assigned treatment may arise from:

- Patient unwillingness to accept the assigned treatment
- Physician unwillingness to administer it
- Patient or physician unwillingness to use the full treatment dosage

Overexposure to the assigned treatment may arise from:

- A mistake by the study physician or patient in the assigned treatment (e.g., as in the case in which a patient takes twice as many pills as required)
- Administration of the same treatment outside the study clinic by the patient's private physician
- Patient self-treatment with medications obtained outside the study clinic (e.g., as with a patient in a myocardial infarction trial who is assigned to aspirin therapy and who takes his medication but who uses his own supply of aspirin for headaches and other ailments as needed)

Exposure to one of the other study treatments may arise in various ways. Examples include:

- A patient who takes a drug outside the trial that is similar to one of the test treatments (e.g., as with a patient assigned to the control treatment in an aspirin trial who uses an over-the-counter cold remedy containing aspirin)
- A patient who demands and receives, midway in the course of the trial, another study treatment in place of, or in addition to, the assigned treatment
- A physician who unwittingly switches a patient from the assigned treatment to another study treatment through a mix-up in prescriptions

- A physician who elects, for medical reasons, to administer another study treatment to a patient in the trial, in addition to, or in place of, the patient's assigned treatment

Any departure from the study treatment protocol, regardless of the nature of the departure, reduces the chances of finding a treatment difference. For example, a patient assigned to the test treatment who refuses the treatment may, in effect, expose himself to the control treatment (e.g., as in the case where the control treatment involves no treatment at all). This reduces the chance of finding a treatment difference, even if the adherence of patients actually assigned to the control treatment is excellent. Conversely, so does the exposure of control-treated patients to the test treatment (e.g., as in a coronary bypass surgery trial where a sizable number of the control-treated patients receive bypass surgery), even if the compliance of patients assigned to the test treatment is excellent.

Loss of precision due to noncompliance is not necessarily related to patient follow-up status. Dropouts, to be sure, automatically become noncompliant if the treatments to which they were assigned are stopped when they drop out. However, as noted above, patients who do not drop out can become noncompliant as well. Further, being a dropout does not necessarily imply a state of noncompliance if the treatment process, as specified by the study protocol, was completed before dropout and the patient is not exposed to any of the study treatments after dropout.

The loss of precision due to noncompliance is compensated for in the same way as losses to follow-up, as discussed in Section 9.3.8. The value for d will be based on the amount of noncompliance anticipated and its role in reducing the precision of the trial. Trials with losses from follow-up and noncompliance will require a composite multiplier to account for both kinds of losses. For example, the CDP used a combined d of 0.30. In actual fact, the losses were due almost exclusively to noncompliance, since it was possible to follow virtually every patient for mortality—the primary outcome measure.

9.3.10 Treatment lag time

Most calculations are made as if there is no treatment lag (i.e., the full effect of the treatment is realized as soon as it is applied). That convention is followed in this chapter. The approach is reasonable with some forms of treatment (e.g., most types of surgery and certain drug treatments), but not for others (e.g., with a drug given to dissolve atherosclerotic plaques). The decision of investigators in the Anturane Reinfarction Trial to ignore deaths that occurred within seven days after the initiation of treatment was based on a presumed treatment lag for Anturane (Anturane Reinfarction Trial Research Group, 1978, 1980; Temple and Pledger, 1980). One reason for ignoring lag times has to do with the mathematical difficulties involved in taking account of them in sample size calculations. Further, there is often no reliable way to estimate lag times.

The impact of lag time on sample size is illustrated below for a trial involving 5 years of follow-up for each patient enrolled, one test and one control treatment, $\lambda = 1$, $P_c = 0.30$, $\Delta_R = 0.30$, $\alpha = 0.01$ (one-tailed), $\beta = 0.05$, and $d = 0$. The sample sizes recorded are derived from tables developed by Halperin and co-workers (1968). The required sample size, given the above specifications, is 1,474 if the full effect of the treatment is realized as soon as it is administered. It is about twice this size if it takes 2.5 years for the treatment to reach full effectiveness and nearly 20 times as large if the lag time is 10 years.

Lag time	Sample size: $n_t + n_c$	Sample size ratio*
0	1,474	1.00
2 months	1,530	1.04
6 months	1,656	1.12
1 year	1,870	1.27
2 years	2,444	1.66
2.5 years	2,828	1.92
3 years	3,266	2.22
4 years	4,492	3.05
5 years	6,536	4.43
7.5 years	12,136	8.23
10 years	29,428	19.96

*Ratio of sample size for indicated lag time relative to size for 0 lag time.

9.3.11   Stratification for control of baseline risk factors

The sample size is influenced by the amount of stratification done to control for baseline varia-

tion. The issues involved in selection of stratification variables are discussed in Chapter 10. Technically, the sample size calculation should take account of the stratification planned. However, in actuality, most calculations are made ignoring stratification. Doing so can lead to an overestimate of the required sample size if the variables used for stratification represent important risk factors and if the calculated sample size is small (see Section 10.3.2 of Chapter 10).

9.3.12   Degree of type I and II error protection for multiple comparisons

The experimenter must also decide whether the error protection specified is to be for a single treatment comparison or for multiple treatment comparisons (see Glossary and Section 20.4 of Chapter 20). Section 9.3.7 alludes to methods of sample size calculation in which the investigator is interested in r test-control treatment comparisons. However, the need for making multiple comparisons is not limited to such cases. It can be just as great when $r = 1$ (i.e., where the trial involves only two treatment groups) if the investigator wishes to design the trial to provide a specified level of error protection for treatment comparisons within designated subgroups of patients. One approach in this setting is to calculate sample size estimates for each subgroup of interest. A drawback with it is that it leads to a series of recruitment quotas—one for each subgroup (see Section 14.1 of Chapter 14). An alternative and generally preferable approach is to ignore subgroups in making the sample size calculation and then to estimate the power provided for subgroups of interest. The total sample size may be increased (e.g., by making a new calculation using smaller values for α and β) if the power is considered to be inadequate for one or more of the subgroups of interest.

9.3.13   Degree of type I and II error protection for multiple looks for safety monitoring

The experimenter may plan to look at outcome data at various time points over the course of the trial in conjunction with the safety monitoring process (see Glossary and Chapter 20). Carrying out multiple looks will alter the type I and type II error levels (see Dupont, 1983a). Ideally, sample size should be estimated with the need for safety monitoring in mind from the outset. However, calculations are routinely made ignoring the need, in part because of difficulties in making the necessary adjustments. This practice is followed here. However, designers of trials should recognize that the error protection provided in such cases will be less than the levels used in making the calculations.

9.3.14 Degree of type I and II error protection for multiple outcomes

A trial, even though planned to focus on a primary outcome, will generate data for a number of secondary outcomes as well (see Glossary for definitions of primary and secondary outcome measures). The usual approach is to base the sample size calculations on the primary outcome of interest and to accept whatever power that calculation yields for the comparisons involving secondary outcome measures.

The only compensation made may be in the choice of α and β. The investigator may choose smaller values than normally used as a means of increasing the precision for the primary as well as secondary comparisons. He may be forced to make calculations for each outcome and then to use the largest size for planning the trial if he is unwilling to designate any of the measures as primary.

9.4 SAMPLE SIZE FORMULAS

Table 9–4 provides a summary of the calculations discussed in this Section and Section 9.5. Tables 9–5 and 9–6 are included for use in making sample size and power calculations. Other more extensive tables of the two functions may be found in many texts on statistics.

The method of analysis implied in the sample size calculation should be identical to that used when the results of the trial are analyzed. However, this is not always possible, as already noted with regard to the need for safety monitoring and the use of secondary outcomes in the analysis process. Technically, there are as many methods of sample size calculation as there are methods of data analysis. The methods presented in this Section are the most common ones.

The methods presented assume that the primary comparison will entail a simple comparison of proportions constructed at the end of the trial (or after a specified period of patient follow-up). Strictly speaking, they are not appropriate if the treatment groups are to be compared using life-table methods. The log rank test is the test of choice in such cases (Gail, 1985). It will yield smaller sample sizes than are obtained with the tests covered herein (i.e., it is more efficient). The difference is small for trials involving rapid patient accrual and low event

Table 9–4 Sample size and power calculation summary for Sections 9.4 and 9.5

Test	Sample size	Power	Assumptions	Applicability
A. Binary outcome measure				
Fisher's exact test	See Section 9.4.1.1	See Section 9.5.1.1	Independent observations	Applicable over entire event rate range from 0 to 1
Chi-square approximation	Eqs 9.6, 9.7	Eqs 9.16, 9.17	Independent observations	P_c and $P_t \geq 0.2$ but ≤ 0.8; $n_c P_c$, $n_c Q_c$, $n_t P_t$, and $n_t Q_t$ all ≥ 15
Inverse sine transform approximation	Eqs 9.8, 9.9	Eqs 9.18, 9.19	Independent observations	P_c and $P_t \geq 0.05$ but ≤ 0.95; $n_c P_c$, $n_c Q_c$, $n_t P_t$, and $n_t Q_t$ all ≥ 15
Poisson approximation	Eqs 9.10, 9.11	Eqs 9.20, 9.21	Independent observations	Low event rates (e.g., P_c and $P_t \leq 0.05$; $n_c P_c$, and $n_t P_t$ ≥ 10)
B. Continuous outcome measure				
Normal approximation for 2 independent means	Eqs 9.12, 9.13	Eqs 9.22, 9.23	Independent observations Common variance Normality	n_c and $n_t \geq 30$
Normal approximation for mean change	Eqs 9.14, 9.15	Eqs 9.24, 9.25	Independent observations between patients Common variance Normality	n_c and $n_t \geq 30$

Table 9-5 Z values for $N(0, 1)$ distribution for selected error levels

Error level	One-tailed	Two-tailed
0.500	0.000	0.674
0.400	0.253	0.842
0.300	0.524	1.036
0.200	0.842	1.282
0.100	1.282	1.645
0.050	1.645	1.960
0.025	1.960	2.248
0.010	2.326	2.576
0.005	2.576	2.813

rates. It is largest for trials involving slow accrual and high event rates.

Most of the formulations in this chapter are for one-tailed tests. However, they may be used for two-tailed tests by using $\alpha/2$ wherever α appears in the formulas cited. Strictly speaking this substitution should be used only when the allocation ratio, λ, equals 1, since there are disagreements among statisticians as to the validity of the substitution when $\lambda \neq 1$. However, the common practice is to use the substitution even if $\lambda \neq 1$.

9.4.1 Binary outcome measures

9.4.1.1 Fisher's exact test

Fisher's exact test is the test of choice for comparing simple counts or proportions based on binary data (Gart, 1971). The test, unlike others considered in this section, works for samples of

Table 9-6 Values of $\Phi(A)$, the proportion of area of a $N(0, 1)$ distribution point lying to the left of a designated point A, for selected values of A

A	$\Phi(A)$	A	$\Phi(A)$
−3.00	0.0013	3.00	0.9987
−2.50	0.0062	2.50	0.9938
−2.00	0.0228	2.00	0.9772
−1.50	0.0668	1.50	0.9332
−1.00	0.1587	1.00	0.8413
−0.75	0.2266	0.75	0.7734
−0.50	0.3085	0.50	0.6915
−0.40	0.3446	0.40	0.6554
−0.30	0.3821	0.30	0.6179
−0.20	0.4207	0.20	0.5793
−0.10	0.4602	0.10	0.5398
0.00	0.5000	0.00	0.5000

any size. It yields an exact *p*-value for the observed difference and, hence, the name.

Closed form sample size formulas for the test are not available. Required sample sizes must be read from tables (Casagrande et al. 1978; Gail and Gart, 1973; Haseman, 1978) or calculated using computer programs.

9.4.1.2 Chi-square approximation

The standard 2×2 chi-square test (without continuity correction) can be used in place of Fisher's exact text if there are 15 or more patients represented in each of the 4 cells of the table (i.e., there are at least 15 patients in each of the 2 treatment groups who have experienced the event and at least 15 others in each of the 2 treatment groups who have not). This rule is somewhat more stringent than the one proposed by Cochran (1954). He proposed a total sample size of 40 and a cell frequency of ≥ 5. Indications are that, even under these border conditions, the test provides a good approximation to the exact test.

The test can be used for sample size estimation if the event rates in both treatment groups are at or between 0.2 and 0.8 and provided the resulting estimates satisfy the above cell conditions. Fisher's exact test or one of the other tests discussed in this section should be used if the conditions are not satisfied. The formulas for uniform and nonuniform allocation, derived from the 2×2 chi-square test, are as follows:

Uniform allocation $(\lambda = 1)$

$$n_c = \left(Z_\alpha \sqrt{2\bar{P}\bar{Q}} + Z_\beta \sqrt{P_c Q_c + P_t Q_t} \right)^2 / \Delta_A^2 \qquad (9.6)$$

$$n_t = n_c$$
$$N = (r + 1)n_c$$

Nonuniform allocation $(\lambda \neq 1)$

$$n_c = \left(Z_\alpha \sqrt{\bar{P}\bar{Q}(\lambda + 1)/\lambda} + Z_\beta \sqrt{P_c Q_c + P_t Q_t/\lambda} \right)^2 / \Delta_A^2 \qquad (9.7)$$

$$n_t = \lambda n_c$$
$$N = rn_t + n_c$$

where

$\lambda = n_t/n_c$, the ratio of the number of patients assigned to a test-treated group to the number assigned to the control-treated group

n_c = required sample size for the control-treated group

n_t = required sample size for one of the test-treated groups

N = total sample size required in all groups combined

α = type 1 error probability

β = type II error probability

Z_α = point on the abscissa of a $N(0,1)$ curve (i.e., a normal distribution with mean 0 and variance 1) to the right of which is found $100(\alpha)\%$ of the total area under that curve

Z_β = point on the abscissa of a $N(0,1)$ distribution to the right of which is found $100(\beta)\%$ of the total area under that curve

P_c = assumed event rate (expressed as a proportion) for the outcome of interest in the control-treated group

P_t = assumed event rate (expressed as a proportion) for the outcome of interest in the test-treated group

$Q_c = 1 - P_c$

$Q_t = 1 - P_t$

$\bar{P} = (P_c + \lambda P_t)/(1 + \lambda)$, a weighted average of the 2 event rates

$\bar{Q} = 1 - \bar{P}$

$\Delta_A = P_c - P_t$

9.4.1.3 *Inverse sine transform approximation*

The inverse sine transform (denoted by $\sin^{-1}$ and expressed in radians) is also used as an approximation to Fisher's exact test (Cochran and Cox, 1957). It has the virtue of providing a good approximation to the exact test over a wider range of P values than is the case with the ordinary 2×2 chi-square test—0.05 to 0.95 compared with 0.2 to 0.8—given the same cell size conditions as specified in Section 9.4.1.2.

Uniform allocation ($\lambda = 1$)

$$n_c = \frac{(Z_\alpha + Z_\beta)^2}{2\left(\sin^{-1}\sqrt{P_c} - \sin^{-1}\sqrt{P_t}\right)^2} \quad (9.8)$$

$n_t = n_c$
$N = (r+1)n_c$

Nonuniform allocation ($\lambda \neq 1$)

$$n_c = \frac{(Z_\alpha + Z_\beta)^2 (\lambda + 1)/\lambda}{4\left(\sin^{-1}\sqrt{P_c} - \sin^{-1}\sqrt{P_t}\right)^2} \quad (9.9)$$

$n_t = \lambda n_c$
$N = rn_t + nc$

The definitions for P_c, P_t, Z_α, Z_β, and λ are the same as for Equations 9.6 and 9.7.

9.4.1.4 *Poisson approximation*

The Poisson approximation can be used for comparison of proportions that lie below the lower limit (i.e., 0.05) specified for the inverse sine transform, provided $n_c P_c$ and $n_t P_t$ are both ≥ 10 (Gail, 1974). The same approximation may be used for P values lying above the upper limit (i.e., 0.95) for the transform by using a complementary event (i.e., by using $1 - P_c$ and $1 - P_t$ in place of P_c and P_t in the formula).

Uniform allocation ($\lambda = 1$)

$$n_c = \frac{(Z_\alpha + Z_\beta)^2 (P_c + P_t)}{(P_c - P_t)^2} \quad (9.10)$$

$n_t = n_c$
$N = (r + 1)n_c$

Nonuniform allocation ($\lambda \neq 1$)

$$n_c = \frac{(Z_\alpha + Z_\beta)^2 (P_c + P_t/\lambda)}{(P_c - P_t)^2} \quad (9.11)$$

$n_t = \lambda n_c$
$N = rn_t + n_c$

9.4.2 Continuous outcome measures

The methods described above may be used for trials involving a continuous outcome measure if the investigator plans to base the primary analysis on a comparison of proportions using a binary categorization of the measure. He should use the methods described in this section if the primary outcome is continuous or near continuous. Conversion of continuous data to binary form for analysis purposes is unwise unless a binary categorization is considered to provide the most relevant treatment of the data. Any categorization reduces the amount of information provided by the data and, if used as a basis for sample size calculations, can be expected to yield an overestimate of the required sample size.

Equations 9.12 and 9.13 are derived using a statistical test for comparison of means observed after a specified period of follow-up. Equations 9.14 and 9.15 are derived using a statistical test for mean change from baseline to some specified period of follow-up. Both sets of equations are based on the normal approximation to the *t*-statistic. The approximation underestimates sample size if the estimated number of patients per treatment group is <30. Other formulations, such as those discussed by Lachin (1981) and Cochran and Cox (1957), can be used in such cases.

9.4.2.1   *Normal approximation for two independent means*

Uniform allocation ($\lambda = 1$)

$$n_c = \frac{2(Z_\alpha + Z_\beta)^2 \, \sigma^2}{(\mu_c - \mu_t)^2} \qquad (9.12)$$

$$n_t = n_c$$
$$N = (r + 1)n_c$$

Nonuniform allocation ($\lambda \neq 1$)

$$n_c = \frac{(Z_\alpha + Z_\beta)^2 \, \sigma^2 \, (\lambda + 1)/\lambda}{(\mu_c - \mu_t)^2} \qquad (9.13)$$

$$n_t = \lambda n_c$$
$$N = r n_t + n_c$$

where

μ_c = true mean of the outcome measure for control-treated patients

μ_t = true mean of the outcome measure for test-treated patients

σ^2 = variance of the outcome measure for a single individual (assumed to be the same for all patients in both treatment groups)

and where observed expressions of the outcome measure are assumed to be independent of one another and to be normally distributed. See Section 9.4.1.2 for notation.

9.4.2.2   *Normal approximation for mean changes from baseline*

Uniform allocation ($\lambda = 1$)

$$n_c = \frac{2(Z_\alpha + Z_\beta)^2 \sigma_d^2}{(\mu_{dc} - \mu_{dt})^2} \qquad (9.14)$$

$$n_t = n_c$$
$$N = (r + 1)n_c$$

Nonuniform allocation ($\lambda \neq 1$)

$$n_c = \frac{(Z_\alpha + Z_\beta)^2 \sigma_d^2 \, (\lambda + 1)/\lambda}{(\mu_{dc} - \mu_{dt})^2} \qquad (9.15)$$

$$n_t = \lambda n_c$$
$$N = r n_t + n_c$$

where

$\mu_{dc} = \mu_{1c} - \mu_{0c}$ is the true value of the difference in the outcome measure at follow-up and baseline for the control treatment

$\mu_{dt} = \mu_{1t} - \mu_{0t}$ is the corresponding value for the test treatment

μ_{0c} = true baseline mean (observed just before the initiation of treatment) for the outcome measure for patients assigned to the control treatment

μ_{1c} = true follow-up mean (observed after a specified period of follow-up) for the outcome measure for patients assigned to the control treatment

μ_{0t} and μ_{1t} are the corresponding means for patients assigned to the test treatment

$\sigma_d^2 = 2(1 - \rho)\sigma^2$

σ^2 = variance of the outcome measure on a single individual (assumed to be the same for all patients in both treatment groups) at either baseline or follow-up

ρ = correlation coefficient between baseline and follow-up outcome measures on a single individual

and where the baseline and follow-up measurements made on different patients are assumed to be independent of one another and normally distributed.

9.5   POWER FORMULAS

Sometimes the number of patients available for study is fixed by practical considerations. In these cases it is useful to calculate the power that can be expected with the available sample size.

The power functions for the chi-square approximation and inverse sine transforms are discussed by Lachin (1981). The formulations for the Poisson approximation are based on work by Gail (1974). The power function for Fisher's exact test involves a complicated summation formula that is not practical for routine use.

All of the power formulations given involve use of normal approximations in which

$$\text{Power} = 1 - \beta = 1 - \Phi(A)$$
where

$\Phi(A)$ = proportion of area of a $N(0,1)$ distribution that is to the left of a point A

All other notation is as defined in Section 9.4.

9.5.1   **Binary outcome measures**

9.5.1.1   *Fisher's exact test*

Power estimates must be computed or read from tables of the power functions (Casagrande et al., 1978).

9.5.1.2   *Chi-square approximation*

Uniform allocation ($\lambda = 1$)

Power $= 1 - \Phi \, (A)$

where

$$A = \frac{Z_\alpha \, \sqrt{2\bar{P}\bar{Q}/n_c} - |P_c - P_t|}{\sqrt{(P_c Q_c + P_t Q_t)/n_c}} \qquad (9.16)$$

Nonuniform allocation ($\lambda \neq 1$)

Power $= 1 - \Phi \, (A)$

where

$$A = \frac{Z_\alpha \, \sqrt{\bar{P}\bar{Q}/n_c + \bar{P}\bar{Q}/n_t} - |P_c - P_t|}{\sqrt{P_c Q_c/n_c + P_t Q_t/n_t}} \qquad (9.17)$$

9.5.1.3 Inverse sine transform approximation

Uniform allocation ($\lambda = 1$)

Power $= 1 - \Phi \, (A)$

where

$$A = Z_\alpha - \frac{2|\sin^{-1} \sqrt{P_c} - \sin^{-1} \sqrt{P_t}|}{\sqrt{2/n_c}} \qquad (9.18)$$

Nonuniform allocation ($\lambda \neq 1$)

Power $= 1 - \Phi \, (A)$

where

$$A = Z_\alpha - \frac{2|\sin^{-1} \sqrt{P_c} - \sin^{-1} \sqrt{P_t}|}{\sqrt{1/n_c + 1/n_t}} \qquad (9.19)$$

9.5.1.4 Poisson approximation

Uniform allocation ($\lambda = 1$)

Power $= 1 - \Phi \, (A)$

where

$$A = Z_\alpha - \frac{|P_c - P_t|}{\sqrt{(P_c + P_t)/n_c}} \qquad (9.20)$$

Nonuniform allocation ($\lambda \neq 1$)

Power $= 1 - \Phi \, (A)$

where

$$A = Z_\alpha - \frac{|P_c - P_t|}{\sqrt{(P_c + P_t/\lambda)/n_c}} \qquad (9.21)$$

9.5.2 Continuous outcome measures

9.5.2.1 Normal approximation for comparison of two independent means

Uniform allocation ($\lambda = 1$)

Power $= 1 - \Phi \, (A)$

where

$$A = Z_\alpha - \frac{|\mu_c - \mu_t|}{\sqrt{2\sigma^2/n_c}} \qquad (9.22)$$

Nonuniform allocation ($\lambda \neq 1$)

Power $= 1 - \Phi \, (A)$

where

$$A = Z_\alpha - \frac{|\mu_c - \mu_t|}{\sqrt{(n_t + n_c)\sigma^2/(n_t n_c)}} \qquad (9.23)$$

9.5.2.2 Normal approximation for mean changes from baseline

Uniform allocation ($\lambda = 1$)

Power $= 1 - \Phi \, (A)$

where

$$A = Z_\alpha - \frac{|\mu_{dc} - \mu_{dt}|}{\sqrt{2\sigma_d^2/n_c}} \qquad (9.24)$$

Nonuniform allocation ($\lambda \neq 1$)

Power $= 1 - \Phi \, (A)$

where

$$A = Z_\alpha - \frac{|\mu_{dc} - \mu_{dt}|}{\sqrt{(n_t + n_c)\sigma_d^2/(n_t n_c)}} \qquad (9.25)$$

9.6 SAMPLE SIZE AND POWER CALCULATION ILLUSTRATIONS

The examples that follow are designed to illustrate sample size and power calculations using the formulas provided in Sections 9.4 and 9.5. Values reported for n_c in illustrations 1 through 5 were rounded up to the next higher integer regardless of the size of the decimal fractions yielded by n_c in the calculations.

9.6.1 Illustration 1: Sample size calculation using chi-square and inverse sine transform approximation

a. Design specifications

- Number of treatment groups (see Section 9.3.1): 2 (i.e., one control and one test treatment)
- Outcome measure (see Section 9.3.2): death
- Follow-up period (see Section 9.3.3): 5 years
- Alternative treatment hypothesis (see Section 9.3.4): one-sided
- Detectable treatment difference in binary outcome (see Section 9.3.5):

$P_c = 0.40$ (5-year control treatment mortality rate)

$\Delta_A = P_c - P_t = 0.10$

- Error protection (see Section 9.3.6): $\alpha = 0.05$, $\beta = 0.05$
- Allocation ratio (see Section 9.3.7): 1:1 (i.e., $\lambda = 1$, equal numbers in test and control groups)
- Losses to follow-up (see Section 9.3.8): 0%
- Losses due to dropouts and noncompliance (see Section 9.3.9): 20%
- Treatment lag time (see Section 9.3.10): 0

b. Method of calculation

Equations 9.6 and 9.8

c. Results

Chi-square approximation (Equation 9.6, Section 9.4.1.2)

$$n_c = \left(1.645\sqrt{2(0.35)(0.65)}\right.$$
$$\left. + 1.645\sqrt{0.40\cdot0.60+0.30\cdot0.70}\right)^2/0.10^2$$
$$= 490$$

$n_c = (1/0.8) \times 490 = 613$ (adjusted for 20% loss)

$n_t = 613$

$N = n_c + n_t = 1226$

Inverse sine approximation (Equation 9.8, Section 9.4.1.3)

$$n_c = \frac{(1.645 + 1.645)^2}{2\left(\sin^{-1}\sqrt{0.40} - \sin^{-1}\sqrt{0.30}\right)^2}$$

$n_c = 491$

$n_c = (1/0.8) \times 491 = 614$ (adjusted for 20% loss)

$n_t = 614$

$N = n_c + n_t = 1228$

9.6.2   Illustration 2: Sample size calculation using Poisson approximation

a. Design specifications

Same as for Illustration 1 except:

- Detectable treatment difference (see Section 9.3.5)

  $P_c = 0.04$

  $\Delta_A = P_c - P_t = 0.016$

b. Method of calculation

Equation 9.10, Section 9.4.1.4

c. Results

$$n_c = \frac{(1.645 + 1.645)^2 (0.040 + 0.024)}{(0.040 - 0.024)^2}$$

$n_c = 2707$

$n_c = (1/0.8) \times 2707 = 3384$ (adjusted for 20% loss)

$N = 3384 + 3384 = 6768$

9.6.3   Illustration 3: Sample size calculation using Coronary Drug Project design specifications

a. Design specifications (Coronary Drug Project Research Group, 1973a)

- Number of treatment groups (see Section 9.3.1): 6 (i.e., 1 control and 5 test treatments)
- Outcome measure (see Section 9.3.2): death
- Follow-up period (see Section 9.3.3): minimum of 5 years
- Alternative treatment hypothesis in binary outcome (see Section 9.3.5): one-sided
- Detectable treatment difference in binary outcome (see Section 9.3.4):

  $P_c = 0.30$ (5-year control treatment mortality rate)

  $\Delta_R = \dfrac{P_c - P_t}{P_c} = 0.25$

- Error protection (see Section 9.3.6): $\alpha = 0.01$, $\beta = 0.05$
- Allocation ratio (see Section 9.3.7): 1:1:1:1:1:2.5 (i.e., $\lambda = 1/2.5$, for a control group that is 2.5 times as large as any of the five treatment groups)
- Losses to follow-up (see Section 9.3.9): 0%
- Losses due to dropouts and noncompliance (see Section 9.3.9): 30% after 5 years of follow-up
- Treatment lag time (see Section 9.3.10): 0

b. Method of calculation

Equation 9.7, Section 9.4.1.2

c. Results

$$n_c = \{2.326[0.279\cdot0.721\cdot(0.400+1)/0.400]^{\frac{1}{2}}$$
$$+1.645[0.300\cdot0.700+0.225\cdot0.775/$$
$$0.400]^{\frac{1}{2}}\}^2/0.075^2$$

$n_c = 1906$

$n_t = (1/2.5) \times 1906 = 762$

$n_c = (1/0.7) \times 1906 = 2723$ (adjusted for 30% loss)

$n_t = (1/0.7) \times 762 = 1089$ (adjusted for 30% loss)

$N = 5n_t + n_c = 5(1089) + 2723 = 8168$

The calculations shown above yield results quite similar to those in the Coronary Drug Project using a different method. The total number of patients derived via that method, after adjustment for losses, was $5(1117) + 2793 = 8378$.

9.6.4 Illustration 4: Sample size calculation for blood pressure change

a. Design specifications

- Number of treatment groups (see Section 9.3.1): 2 (i.e., 1 control and 1 test treatment)
- Outcome measure (see Section 9.3.2): blood pressure change after 3 years of treatment
- Follow-up period (see Section 9.3.3): 3 years
- Alternative treatment hypothesis in mean change from baseline (see Section 9.3.4): two-sided
- Detectable treatment difference in continuous outcome measure (see Section 9.3.5):

  $\Delta_A = \mu_{dc} - \mu_{dt} = 4 \; mm \; Hg$ (expected difference in mean change from baseline)

  $\sigma^2 = 100 \; (mm \; Hg)^2$ (variance of a single blood-pressure measurement)

  $\rho = 0.3$ (correlation between a baseline blood-pressure measure and the measure after 3 years of follow-up, both taken on the same individual)

  $\sigma_d^2 = 2(1 - \rho)\sigma^2 = 2(0.70)100 \; (mm \; Hg)^2 = 140 \; (mm \; Hg)^2$
- Error protection (see Section 9.3.6): $\alpha = 0.05$, $\beta = 0.05$
- Allocation ratio (see Section 9.3.7): 1:1 (i.e., $\lambda = 1$)
- Losses to follow-up due to dropouts and noncompliance (see Sections 9.3.8 and 9.3.9): 30%
- Treatment lag time (see Section 9.3.10): 0

b. Method of calculation

Equation 9.14, Section 9.4.2.2

c. Results

$$n_c = \frac{2(1.960 + 1.645)^2 (140 \; mm \; Hg)^2}{(4 \; mm \; Hg)^2}$$

$n_c = 228$

$n_c = (1/0.7) \times 228 = 326$ (adjusted for 30% loss)

$n_t = 326$

$N = 326 + 326 = 652$

9.6.5 Illustration 5: Sample size calculation using Fisher's exact test

a. Design specifications

- Number of treatment groups (see Section 9.3.1): 2 (i.e., 1 control and 1 test treatment)
- Outcome measure (see Section 9.3.2): death
- Follow-up period (see Section 9.3.3): 2 years
- Alternative treatment hypothesis in binary outcome (see Section 9.3.4): one-sided
- Detectable treatment difference in binary outcome (see Section 9.3.5):

  $P_c = 0.5$

  $P_t = 0.1$

  $\Delta_A = 0.4$
- Error protection (see Section 9.3.6): $\alpha = 0.05$, $\beta = 0.10$
- Allocation ratio (see Section 9.3.7): 1:1 (i.e., $\lambda = 1$, equal numbers in the test and control groups)
- Losses to follow-up (see Section 9.3.8): 0%
- Losses due to dropouts and noncompliance (see Section 9.3.9): 0%
- Treatment lag time (see Section 9.3.10):0

b. Method of calculation

Use tables produced by Haseman (1978) or Casagrande and co-workers (1978) and compare the result with that obtained using the chi-square and inverse sine transform approximation.

c. Results

$N = 50$ (25 in each group) from sample size tables in Haseman (1978) or Casagrande et al. (1978)

$N = 42$ (21 in each group) chi-square approximation (Equation 9.6, Section 9.4.1.2)

$N = 40$ (20 in each group) from inverse sine transform approximation (Equation 9.8, Section 9.4.1.3)

Note that $n_t p_t = 4$ is below the limit specified for use with the chi-square and inverse sine transform approximations and that they underestimate the required sample size.

9.6.6   Illustration 6: Power calculation based on chi-square and inverse sine transform approximation

a. Design specifications

- Number of treatment groups (see Section 9.3.1): 2 (i.e., 1 control and 1 test treatment)
- Outcome measure (see Section 9.3.2): death
- Follow-up period (see Section 9.3.3): 5 years
- Alternative treatment hypothesis (see Section 9.3.4): two-sided
- Detectable treatment difference in binary outcome measure (see Section 9.3.5):
  $P_c = 0.40$
  $P_t = 0.30$
  $\Delta_A = P_c - P_t = 0.4 - 0.3 = 0.1$
- Error protection (see Section 9.3.6): $\alpha = 0.05$, β to be determined
- Allocation ratio (see Section 9.3.7): 2:1 (i.e., $\lambda = 2$, twice as many patients in the test-treated group as in the control-treated group), with:
  $n_c = 300$
  $n_t = 600$
  $N = n_t + n_c = 900$
- Losses to follow-up (see Section 9.3.9): 0%
- Losses due to dropouts and noncompliance (see Section 9.3.9): 0%
- Treatment lag time (see Section 9.3.10): 0

b. Method of calculation

Equations 9.17 and 9.19

c. Results

Chi-square approximation:

$$A = [1.960(0.333 \cdot 0.667)(1/300 + 1/600)^{\frac{1}{2}} - |0.400 - 0.300|]/[0.400 \cdot 0.600/300 + 0.300 \cdot 0.700/600]^{\frac{1}{2}}$$
$$= -1.0242$$
Power $= 1 - \Phi(-1.0242) = 1 - 0.15 = 0.85$

Inverse sine transform approximation:

$$A = 1.96 - \frac{2|\sin^{-1}\sqrt{0.40} - \sin^{-1}\sqrt{0.30}|}{\sqrt{1/300 + 1/600}}$$
$$= -1.012$$
Power $= 1 - \Phi(-1.012) = 1 - 0.16 = 0.84$

9.6.7   Illustration 7: Power for design specifications given in Illustration 2 for 1500 patients per treatment group

a. Design specification

As given in Illustration 2 except:

- β to be determined for indicated sample size
- n_c and $n_t = 1500$ (effective sample size, i.e., after reduction for 20% loss due to dropout and noncompliance)

b. Method of calculation

Equation 9.20

c. Results

$$A = 1.645 - |0.040 - 0.024|/[(0.040 + 0.024)/1500]^{\frac{1}{2}}$$
$$= -0.8045$$
Power $= 1 - \Phi(-0.8045) = 1 - 0.21 = 0.79$

9.6.8   Illustration 8: Power for design specifications given in Illustration 4 for 150 patients per treatment group

a. Design specification

As given in illustration 4 except:

- β to be determined for indicated sample size
- n_c and $n_t = 150$ (effective sample size, i.e., after reduction for 30% loss due to dropout and noncompliance)

b. Method of calculation

Equation 9.24

c. Results

$$A = 1.96 - \frac{4 \text{ mm Hg}}{\sqrt{2(140 \text{ mm Hg}^2)/150}}$$
$$= -0.9677$$
Power $= 1 - \Phi(-0.9677) = 1 - 0.17 = 0.83$

9.7   POSTERIOR SAMPLE SIZE AND POWER ASSESSMENTS

The calculations made when the trial is planned will provide the recruitment goal. However, the goal may have to be changed during the trial.

For example, it may have to be raised if the observed event rate for the control-treated group during the early stages of recruitment is lower than expected or there is more loss of precision due to noncompliance and dropout than originally envisioned. The period of follow-up may have to be extended as well. Extension of follow-up may be the only option available if recruitment has been completed when the shortfall in desired error protection is first recognized.

There are occasions where an overestimate of P_c in the planning stage may be offset by lower than expected dropout and noncompliance rates during the trial. For example, this was the case in the CDP. The actual five-year mortality in the placebo-treated group was lower than expected, but so were the dropout and noncompliance rates (Coronary Drug Project Research Group, 1973a, 1975).

Power calculations should be made at the end of the trial using the observed sample size and actual losses due to noncompliance and dropouts. Such calculations should be a part of any finished report where the observed treatment effect is small and the authors, therefore, conclude in favor of the null hypothesis of no difference among treatment groups. The calculations, as noted by Freiman and co-workers (1978), are useful to readers when trying to decide whether or not to accept the author's conclusion. A reader may be inclined to accept the conclusion if the estimated power of the study was large enough to detect an important difference, but not otherwise (see also Mosteller et al., 1980).

10. Randomization and the mechanics of treatment masking

Chance favours only those who know how to court her.

Charles Nicolle

10.1 INTRODUCTION

A valid trial requires a method for assigning patients to a test or control treatment that is free of selection bias. The best method for ensuring bias-free selection is via a bona fide randomization scheme as discussed in Section 8.4 of Chapter 8. Nonrandom methods may be used, but they all suffer from defects that can be avoided with randomization. Hence, randomization is the only method of assignment discussed in this chapter.

Two general designs exist for randomization of patients to treatment: adaptive randomization and fixed randomization. With fixed randomization schemes, the assignment probabilities remain fixed over the course of the trial. In adaptive randomization schemes (also referred to as dynamic randomization, but not in this book) assignment probabilities for the treatments change as a function of the distribution of previous assignments, observed baseline characteristics, or observed outcomes.

The emphasis in this chapter is on fixed randomization. Only a brief overview of adaptive randomization is provided (Section 10.2). Fixed randomization is easier to manage than adaptive randomization. Assignment schedules can be generated before the start of patient recruitment. This is not possible with most adaptive schemes. Assignment must be generated as needed. Further, the generation process is usually complicated enough so that it has to be done on a computer to keep track of previous assignments and any other data used in the adaptation process. All of the trials listed in Appendix B, except one—the National Cooperative Gallstone Study—used fixed allocation schemes. None of the 113 reports of trials reviewed in Chapter 2 gave any indication of having used adaptive randomization. However, this count may be somewhat deceptive in that many of the reports lacked the details needed to reach a definitive judgment regarding the method of treatment assignment used.

10.2 ADAPTIVE RANDOMIZATION

There are three general types of adaptive randomization:

- Those in which the assignment probabilities are modified as a function of observed departures from the desired allocation ratio (number adaptive)
- Those in which the assignment probabilities are modified as a function of differences in the observed distribution of baseline characteristics among the treatment groups (baseline adaptive)
- Those in which the assignment probabilities are modified as a function of observed outcomes in the treatment groups (outcome adaptive)

The biased coin randomization procedure, proposed by Efron (1971), is an example of a number adaptive scheme. It is an alternative to blocking in a fixed randomization design (see Section 10.3.3). Patients are assigned to the treatment groups with preset probabilities so long as the difference in the number of patients assigned to the treatment groups remains within a specified range. The probability of assignment to a test treatment is increased or decreased, relative to that for the control treatment, when the range is exceeded.

Baseline adaptive randomization is designed to make certain that the treatment groups are balanced with regard to important baseline characteristics that may affect the outcome measure. In this approach, the assignment probabilities are a function of observed differences in the baseline composition of patients already enrolled (Begg and Iglewicz, 1980; Freedman and White, 1976; Friedman et al., 1982; Pocock, 1983; Pocock and Simon, 1975; Simon, 1977). The main advantage of the technique is the opportunity it provides for balancing the composition of treatment groups on several different baseline characteristics without stratification (see Section 10.3.2). The main disadvantage is in its administrative complexities. The technique cannot be managed without a computer.

The play-the-winner scheme, proposed by Zelen (1969), is an example of outcome adaptive randomization. The simplest version is one involving only one test and one control treatment, where the first patient enrolled has the same probability of being assigned to either treatment, and thereafter the assignment received by each patient is a function of the outcome observed and the treatment assignment of the preceding patient. The assignment will be the same as for the preceding patient if the outcome observed for that patient was favorable. The assignment will be to the other treatment if the outcome was unfavorable. Hence, the name, play-the-winner.

The main difficulty with the scheme, at least with simple versions such as the one described, is that it allows an investigator to predict the next assignment, thereby introducing the possibility of bias into the patient selection process. A second limitation is the need to determine the outcome for the last patient enrolled before the next one can be enrolled.

The play-the-winner algorithm has been modified to incorporate outcome information from multiple patients (Wei and Durham, 1978). This modification eliminates dependence on the last outcome observed and therefore makes it more difficult for an investigator to predict the next assignment. However, even modified in this way, the scheme has limited utility. The ability to identify a "winning" treatment and to have that knowledge influence treatment assignments during the patient recruitment process is minimal in most trials requiring long-term follow-up for outcome assessment.

10.3   FIXED RANDOMIZATION

Fixed randomization schemes require specification of the:

- Allocation ratio
- Allocation strata
- Block size

The considerations involved in making these specifications are outlined in the subsections that follow.

10.3.1   Allocation ratio

The number of allocations made to any one of the study treatments is a function of the assignment probabilities—assumed to be set in advance of patient recruitment and to be held fixed over the course of recruitment in fixed allocation schemes. The only changes that occur are due to major design modifications, such as occurred in the University Group Diabetes Program (UGDP) with the addition of a fifth treatment (phenformin) some 18 months after the start of patient recruitment (University Group Diabetes Program, 1970d).

The allocation of patients to the study treatments can be uniform or nonuniform. A design will be characterized as uniform if the assignment probabilities for the t test treatments and control treatment are equal, i.e.,

$$P_1 = P_2 = \cdots = P_i = \cdots = P_{t+1} \quad (10.1)$$

where

$P_i, i = 1, \cdots, t$, denote assignment probabilities for the t test treatments

and

P_{t+1} denotes the assignment probability for the control treatment

and where

$$\sum_{i=1}^{t+1} P_i = 1$$

It will be characterized as nonuniform if there is at least one probability value in Equation 10.1 that differs from the other values in the equation.

The entire allocation scheme for the trial can be expressed as a ratio of $t + 1$ numbers,

$$r_1 : r_2 : \cdots : r_i : \cdots : r_{t+1}$$

where r_i is the expected number of assignments to the ith test treatment and where all values of r are expressed as integers, reduced so as to have no multiplier in common other than 1 (e.g., an allocation ratio involving 1 assignment to the test treatment for every 2 assignments to the control treatment would be expressed as a ratio of 1:2). Expressed this way,

$$\sum_{i=1}^{t+1} r_i = B \quad (10.2)$$

where B is the minimum block size (see Glossary and Section 10.3.3). For example, the minimum block size in a 2-treatment trial with an allocation ratio of 1:1 is 2. It is 4 if the allocation ratio is 1:3. It is 5 for a 3-treatment trial with an allocation ratio of 2:2:1.

All $t + 1$ values of r are equal to 1 in uniform fixed allocation designs. At least one value of r will be greater than 1 in nonuniform fixed allocation designs.

The most common allocation design is one involving uniform allocation. All of the trials sketched in Appendix B, except three, were of this type (see line 20e, Table B-4, Appendix B). Uniform allocation should be used, except where there are valid reasons to allocate a disproportionately larger number of patients to one treatment than to another. The reasons may have to do with the cost of one treatment versus another, the way of administering one versus another, or the presumed safety or efficacy of one versus another (see Persantine Aspirin Reinfarction Trial Research Group, 1980a, for example of nonuniform allocation). Other reasons relate to statistical considerations, as discussed in Section 9.3.12, where the study involves multiple test treatments, each of which is to be contrasted with the same control treatment. A third set of reasons relate to secondary research aims that are best pursued via use of nonuniform allocation. One of the reasons why the Coronary Drug Project (CDP) enrolled more patients in the placebo-treated group than in any of the test-treated groups had to do with a secondary aim (Coronary Drug Project Research Group, 1973a).

10.3.2 Stratification

Stratification[1] during patient enrollment involves the placement of patients into defined strata for randomization. It is done to reduce or eliminate variation in the outcome measure due to the stratification variable(s) (see Table 10-1 for points concerning stratification during randomization). A variable is said to be controlled when patients are assigned to treatment in such a way so as to ensure that it has the same distribution in all treatment groups. Separate allocation schedules are required for the various levels or states assumed by the variables to be controlled. Allocations to each stratum are made using the same allocation ratio as for all other strata. A scheme requiring control of sex would require a separate allocation stratum for males and for females. A scheme requiring control of sex and age, the latter classified at three levels (e.g., <45, 45 through 55, and >55), would require six (i.e., $2 \cdot 3$) allocation strata, one for each age level and sex combination. In general terms, s stratification variables with l_i levels for the ith variable will produce a total of $l_1 \cdot l_2 \cdots l_i \cdots l_{s-1} \cdot l_s$ allocation strata.

The term *stratification*, as used throughout this chapter, refers to a process that takes place in conjunction with randomization, and that is based on data collected prior to randomization. Stratification that is done in conjunction with data analyses, as discussed in Chapter 18, is referred to as post-stratification. Both forms of stratification may be used in the same trial, but not on the same variable.

The main arguments for stratification involve a combination of philosophic and statistical considerations. Ideally, the goal in any trial is to carry out the comparison of the study treatments in groups of patients that are identical with regard to all entry characteristics that influence the outcome measure. The best way to achieve the goal is via matching for all variables of concern. However, it is impractical for reasons discussed in Chapter 8. The best that can be done is to stratify the study groups on a few variables and then to randomize within those strata.

Clearly, there is a practical limit to the number of variables that can be realistically controlled via stratification. The number of strata

1. Not to be confused with poststratification (see Glossary).

Table 10-1 Stratification considerations for randomization

- Only variables that are observed and recorded before randomization may be used for stratification in the treatment assignment process.

- Increased statistical efficiency resulting from stratification is minimal for trials involving ≥50 patients per treatment group.

- It is impractical to control for more than a few sources of variation via stratification at the time of randomization (i.e., generally no more than two or three).

- Use of a large number of allocation strata may allow for fairly large chance departures from the desired allocation ratio if there are only a small number of patients per stratum.

- Any gain in statistical efficiency resulting from stratification using a given variable will be a function of the relationship of that variable to the outcome measure. The gain will be small to nil if the relationship is weak or nonexistent. It will be greatest for variables that are highly predictive of outcome.

- Stratification on any patient characteristic complicates the randomization process; it may prolong the time needed to clear a patient for enrollment if stratification depends on readings or determinations made outside the clinic.

- Variables used for stratification should be easy to observe and reasonably free of measurement error.

- Variables that are subject to major sources of error due to differing interpretations should not be used for stratification. They are of limited use for variance control and the errors made may open the study to criticism when the results are published.

- It is unreasonable to expect that all important sources of baseline variation can be controlled via stratification during randomization. Analysis procedures involving post-stratification and multiple regression will be required to adjust treatment comparisons for baseline differences not controlled via stratification.

- Use of any stratification scheme that involves calculations or complicated interpretations should be avoided, especially in self-administered randomization schemes where the calculations or interpretations are not checked before treatment assignments are issued.

- Clinic should be used for stratification in multicenter trials. This form of stratification will control for differences in the study population due to environmental, social, demographic, and other factors related to clinic.

quickly reaches unmanageable limits when a number of different variables are used. As a result, the choice of variables must be judicious and by definition must be limited to variables that are independent of the treatment assignment. In addition, the choice should be limited to variables that are not subject to large observational or recording errors so as to minimize classification errors made in the stratification process.

The gain in statistical precision from stratification is inconsequential once the number of patients per treatment group reaches 50 or more. The greatest gains are for small trials involving 20 or fewer patients per treatment group (Grizzle, 1982; Meier, 1981).

Clinical trial researchers are divided over the wisdom of stratification at the time of randomization. Those in favor of the process presume that even if it does not increase statistical precision it is unlikely to reduce it. Therefore, why not stratify? Those who question use of the process argue that the statistical gain, at best, is likely to be small. This fact, coupled with the practical complexities involved in administering the process, serve as the main arguments against stratified randomization (see Brown, 1980, for pro arguments; Meier, 1981, and Peto and co-workers, 1976, for con arguments). The diversity of opinion is reflected in the trials sketched in Appendix B. Six of the trials did not stratify on any patient characteristic. The other eight used sex, age at entry, and/or some indicator of disease state for stratification (see item 20.b, Table B–4, Appendix B).

The goal in stratification is to reduce the variance associated with treatment comparisons through control of variables that affect outcome. Clearly, there will be no reduction, and hence no gain in statistical precision, if the variables are unrelated to outcome. The more restrictive the patient selection criteria, the less the need for any stratification. The relationship of a variable (e.g., age) to an outcome (e.g., death), even if quite striking when assessed over a broad range of unselected patients, may be modest over the range represented by patients enrolled into the trial.

The CDP provides graphic evidence of the futility of identifying factors that predict mortality, the outcome of interest in that study and several of the others sketched in Appendix B. A multiple linear regression model, using 40 different baseline characteristics as predictors for mortality, accounted for only 10.6% of the observed variance associated with mortality (Coronary Drug Project Research Group, 1974). Risk group, defined by number and severity of previous myocardial infarctions and the only variable used for stratification other than clinic, had little predictive value. It ranked 26 in the list of 40 variables in terms of predictive value. The five most important predictors, in order of impor-

tance using a stepwise regression procedure, were: ECG ST segment depression, cardiomegaly (as read from chest x-rays), New York Heart Association functional class, ventricular conduction defects (as read from ECGs), and history of use of diuretics. They accounted for over two-thirds of the total variance explained by the model.

Stratification using patient characteristics should not be undertaken lightly. It will complicate the randomization process since assignments cannot be made until all data needed for stratification are in hand. This may delay, sometimes by weeks, the enrollment of a patient if needed data come from laboratory determinations or readings made outside the clinic. Variables that require a series of complex and error-prone classifications in order to be converted into values suitable for use in stratification should be avoided. The same is true for variables requiring subjective interpretations. A high error rate in the classification of patients by strata can negate the effect of stratification and may open the study to criticism when the results are published.

Clinic is a natural stratification variable in multicenter trials. All of the 13 multicenter trials sketched in Appendix B (see item 20.b, Table B–4) used this form of stratification. The cautions expressed above with regard to use of patient characteristics for stratification do not apply to clinic. Use of separate allocation schedules by clinic, with each schedule having the same allocation ratio, ensures comparability of the treatment groups with regard to the mix of patients coming from the various clinics in the trial. This assurance is important since clinic populations can differ widely with regard to a host of characteristics, even if the study has fairly rigid entry criteria. Patients will come from different geographic areas and, hence, will have different environmental exposures and perhaps demographic characteristics as well. Further, there may be subtle differences in treatment patterns from clinic to clinic, even if the study has a well-defined treatment plan. In addition, there are practical reasons for the stratification, especially in masked drug trials in which clinics receive the drugs they are to use in coded bottles from a central supply point. It is much easier for the supplier to estimate the drug needs of individual clinics if the allocation ratio is fixed across clinics than when it is not.

Clinic variation in outcome event rates can be seen from inspection of the UGDP results. The number of deaths recorded ranged from a high of 23 out of the 90 patients enrolled in the Cincinnati clinic to a low of 1 out of the 87 patients enrolled in the Baltimore clinic when the first results from the trial were published (University Group Diabetes Program Research Group, 1970e). Four of the 12 clinics accounted for a little over 70% of all deaths reported. Critics of the study cited clinic variation in mortality as one of the explanations for the tolbutamide results (see Chapter 7). However, in doing so they failed to recognize that the variation was unlikely to be treatment-related because of the stratification by clinic in the randomization process.

Normally, the question of who treats within a clinic is ignored in the randomization process. None of the trials sketched in Appendix B controlled for this source of variation. Physician-to-physician variation in treatment practice may be small in masked drug trials, but may not be in unmasked trials, especially those involving surgical procedures. It may be appropriate in such cases to control for anticipated variation by stratifying on treating physician.

Statistical considerations are only one reason for stratification. It is sometimes done simply as a ploy to protect the study from criticism when it is finished. Indeed, it is easier to answer criticisms concerning the comparability of the study groups if the criticisms focus on variables that have been stratified. However, defensive stratification can backfire if the variables selected are viewed by critics as "inappropriate" or if they are able to make cogent arguments suggesting that other "more important" variables were left uncontrolled.

Stratification is also used to control for a variable known or suspected to interact with treatment (see Glossary for definition of treatment interaction). Stratification of this sort should be considered for any variable that, depending on its level, has the potential of ameliorating or enhancing a treatment effect. The experimenter, via stratification, is able to compare treatment effects across strata and thereby estimate the size of the interaction effect. In actual fact, however, most interactions, unless they are pronounced, are difficult to detect. The typical trial, because of its small size, provides little statistical power for their detection.

Extreme cases of interactions in which the treatment has a positive effect when the interacting variable assumes one state and the opposite effect when it assumes another state should not be controlled via stratification. They should be dealt with by constructing more restrictive selection criteria so only patients who react positively to the treatment are enrolled.

10.3.3 Block size

The investigator must decide whether to constrain the randomization process so as to ensure balance in the number of allocations made to the various treatment groups in a stratum at various points over the course of patient enrollment. Unconstrained randomization may lead to imbalances in the baseline characteristics of the treatment groups if there are, quite by chance, long unbroken runs of assignments to the same treatment and if the type of patients enrolled changes over time. Table 10-2 lists considerations involved in blocking.

The desired allocation ratio in a stratum could be achieved with a single blocking constraint if the exact number of patients to be enrolled in the stratum were known in advance. However, this approach is not recommended. First, there are few situations in which it is practical to recruit to a set limit within a stratum. Hence, failure to achieve the desired recruitment goal could mean that the study closes far from the desired allocation ratio. Second, the approach may allow too much room for variation around

Table 10-2 Blocking considerations

Blocking should be considered if:

- Patient enrollment is likely to continue over an extended period of time, or if the demographic or clinical characteristics of the study population can be expected to change over the course of enrollment
- There are practical or statistical reasons why it is important to satisfy the specified allocation ratio at various points during the enrollment process

Block size considerations:

- The smallest possible block size is the sum of integers defined by the allocation ratio (see Equation 10.2)
- The block sizes used for construction of an allocation schedule should not be divulged until it is appropriate to do so—and never before patient enrollment is completed
- The larger the block, the greater the chance of departure from the specified allocation ratio
- Variable block sizes are preferable to fixed blocks, especially in unmasked trials
- Use of a large number of allocation strata may lead to a large departure from the specified allocation ratio, unless small block sizes are used within each stratum

the desired allocation ratio over the course of patient enrollment. For example, the constraint in a trial involving two treatments, a 1:1 allocation ratio, and a single block of 100 patients does not take effect until 50 assignments have been made to one of the two treatment groups. Hence, in theory it is possible that the results of the trial could be completely confounded with time of enrollment if the first 50 patients are assigned to the same treatment. A third reason has to do with the need for interim analyses over the course of the trial, as discussed in Chapter 20. These analyses are easier to interpret if large departures from the desired allocation ratio have been avoided. Certainly, blocking is recommended any time recruitment extends over a long period of time.

The usual approach to blocking in fixed allocation schemes is to use a sequence of blocks of the same size or of differing sizes, each of which is constructed using the same allocation ratio. All of the 14 trials sketched in Appendix B, except two—the National Cooperative Gallstone Study (NCGS) and the Veterans Administration Cooperative Studies Program Number 43 (VACSP No. 43)—used this approach.

The blocking arrangement used should not be revealed to clinic personnel until it is appropriate to do so (after patient recruitment is completed in unmasked trials and after the trial is completed in double-masked trials). Further, the scheme used should be designed to minimize the chance of clinic personnel discovering the blocking scheme. Discovery of the scheme can lead to selection biases if the information is used to predict future assignments and if the predictions influence decisions on enrollment. The probability of making correct predictions is highest with simple blocking schemes involving small blocks of uniform size. For example, it is 0.5 in designs involving two treatment groups and an unmasked treatment assignment scheme using blocks of size two. The chance of discovering the blocking pattern is minimal with large blocks, even if blocks of uniform size are used, especially if treatments are administered in double-masked fashion as in the CDP (see Section 10.5 and Coronary Drug Project Research Group, 1973a).

The preferred approach, particularly in unmasked trials, involves a mix of different block sizes with the order specified. One arrangement is to have the blocks filled in order according to size. This arrangement may be considered if blocks of several different sizes are used and if

the largest block represents a sizable fraction of the total numbers of assignments anticipated in a stratum. The arrangement reduces the amount of variation around the specified allocation ratio as recruitment proceeds—a desirable feature if the designers wish to have an observed allocation ratio that is near the specified one when recruitment is finished. An alternative approach involves a random order of blocks according to size. It is preferred to the ordering described above when only two or three different block sizes are used and when each stratum contains several blocks of each size. The random ordering eliminates any chance of clinic personnel discovering the blocking pattern.

The usefulness of blocking can be reduced by the use of too many allocation strata. There can be large departures from the desired allocation ratio if none of the blocks in the individual strata are filled by the time patient recruitment is completed. Use of small block sizes will help guard against this problem, but their use may increase the chances of predicting future assignments, as discussed above.

10.4. CONSTRUCTION OF THE RANDOMIZATION SCHEDULE

The randomization schedule can be constructed once the design specifications outlined in Section 10.3 have been set. Construction may be done using output from:

- A published list of random numbers, e.g., as provided by The Rand Corporation (1955)
- Published random permutations of a set of numbers, e.g., those appearing in Cochran and Cox (1957) and Fisher and Yates (1963)
- A computer-based pseudo-random number generator

Methods such as coin flipping, where the order of assignment cannot be replicated, are unacceptable (see Chapter 8).

Most computer statistical packages include pseudo-random number[2] generators. They may be used for construction of the allocation schedule, but with some caution. Output from some of the generators involves serial correlations (e.g., see Hauck, 1982). While the defect is not of great concern in the allocation process, it is best to use

---

2. So termed because the numbers they generate are not the result of a random process, but have properties similar to those generated via a random process.

a generator that has been tested for the defect and found to be free of it.

An algorithm is needed to translate output obtained from the randomizing device into treatment assignments. The translation is straightforward for schemes based on tables of random permutations, as in Illustration 1 in Section 10.8.1. It is more complicated for schemes using output from tables of random numbers or from pseudo-random number generators. The method described in Table 10–3 is based on an algorithm proposed by Moses and Oakford (1963) and can be implemented using the worksheet displayed in Table 10–4. Use of the algorithm is illustrated in Table 10–5 for a random sequence of numbers selected from Table 10–6.

10.5 MECHANICS OF MASKING TREATMENT ASSIGNMENTS

Masked administration of treatment (see Chapter 8 for discussion of the rationale for masking) is feasible only in cases in which it is possible to administer all study treatments in an identical fashion and in which clinic personnel do not need to know the identity of the treatment being administered in order to care for the patient receiving it. Most applications of masked treat-

Table 10-3 Moses-Oakford assignment algorithm for block of size k

Step	Illustration (see Table 10–5)
1. Specify number of treatment groups, $t + 1$.	$t + 1 = 4$
2. Specify treatment allocation ratio, $r_1{:}r_2{:}\cdots{:}r_i{:}\cdots r_{t+1}$ such that $$\sum_{i=1}^{t+1} r_i = B \text{ (see Equation 10.2)}.$$	$r_1 = 1$ $r_2 = 1$ $r_3 = 1$ $r_4 = 1$ $B = 4$
3. Specify block size k such that it is $\geq B$ and is divisable by B.	$k = 8$
4. Specify treatment symbols or codes.	C = Control
5. Set down an arbitrary sequence of treatment symbols in column 2 of worksheet (Table 10–4), such that the allocation ratio specified in step 2 is satisfied.	T1 = Test treatment 1 T2 = Test treatment 2 T3 = Test treatment 3
6. Generate a random number,* N_1, such that it is ≥ 1 but $\leq k$; record value in column 5, line k, of worksheet.	$N_1 = 1$, record on line 8, col. 5
7. Take treatment symbol on line N_1, column 2, and record on line k, column 4.	C, from line 1, col. 2, record on line 8, col. 4
8. Cross out symbol on line N_1, column 2. Record symbol given on line k, column 2, on line N_1, column 3 (skip if $N_1 = k$).	Cross out C, line 1, col. 2, add T3 to line 1, col. 3
9. Generate a new random number N_2 such that it is ≥ 1 but $\leq k - 1$ and record in column 5, line $k - 1$.	$N_2 = 4$, record on line 7, col. 5
10. Take treatment symbol on line N_2, column 2 or from column 3, if any appear in column 3, record on line $k - 1$, column 4.	T1 from line 4, col. 2, record on line 7, col. 4
11. Cross out the symbol appearing in columns 2 or 3, line N_2. Record symbol given on line $k - 1$, columns 2 or 3 on line N_2, column 3 (skip if $N_2 = k - 1$).	Cross out T1, line 4, col. 2, add T3 to line 4, col. 3
12. Repeat steps 9, 10, and 11 reducing the upper limit of permissible random numbers by 1 for each repetition** until all but the last assignment has been made.	As outlined above
13. Complete the scheme by recording in column 4 the unused treatment symbol appearing on line 1, columns 2 or 3.	Take T3 from line 1, col. 3, record on line 1, col. 4

*Numbers are drawn from page 17 of The Rand Corporation's 1 million random digits (1955), as reproduced in Table 10-6.

**The algorithm is written to allow the user to work from the bottom up on the worksheet illustrated in Table 10-4. It can be written to allow use of the sheet from the top down but this arrangement complicates keeping track of the permissible range for the next random number to be selected. With the methods as outlined, the limit for the next number to be selected is given by the line number of the next line on the sheet to be filled.

Table 10-4 Moses-Oakford treatment assignment worksheet for block of size k

			Random numbers*
Block size	~~~ codes		Page Column Row
_____		Start ____ ____ ____
Allocation ratio		End ____ ____ ____
_____		Source: _____

(1)	(2)	(3)	(4)	(5)
		Treatment assignments		
Order of assignment	Initial	Replacements	Final	Random number
1	___	_____	___	___
2	___	_____	___	___
3	___	_____	___	___
4	___	_____	___	___
5	___	_____	___	___
6	___	_____	___	___
7	___	_____	___	___
8	___	_____	___	___
⋮	⋮	⋮	⋮	⋮
$k-2$	___	_____	___	___
$k-1$	___	_____	___	___
k	___	_____	___	___

*Reading rule:

ment administration arise in the context of drug trials. Masking is accomplished by bottling, packaging, labeling, and dispensing the test and control drug in an identical fashion. Tablets may have to be formulated using a taste-masking substance, such as quassin as in the CDP Aspirin Study (Coronary Drug Project Research Group, 1976), to obscure telltale tastes. Another alternative is to use an enteric coating on the tablets, provided the coating does not reduce the bioavailability of the drug. Generally, masking the identity of a drug is easier to accomplish if the drug is contained in capsules than if it is contained in tablets. The capsules help to obscure taste differences that may be present when tablets are used.

There can be subtle differences in sheen, color, or texture of tablets as well. For example, there was a slight difference in the sheen of tolbuta-mide tablets as contrasted with the corresponding placebo tablets in the UGDP. However, the difference was apparent only in indirect light, and then only in side-by-side comparisons of the two kinds of tablets. Such differences are avoided with opaque capsules.

Trials involving multiple test treatments should be designed with the goal of using a single placebo unless it is not possible or practical to do so. The goal cannot be achieved if the study medications are dispensed in different forms, as in the case of the UGDP. Two kinds of placebo pills were required, one to match tolbutamide tablets and the other to match phenformin capsules.

Use of a common placebo imposes the same pill schedule on all patients, regardless of treatment assignment. For example, the CDP required all patients to take nine capsules per day in order to deliver the required dosage of nicotinic acid. Several of the medications could have been delivered via a smaller number of capsules (Coronary Drug Project Research Group, 1973a). However, this would have required a different placebo for those drugs.

The way in which medications are bottled and labeled is important. There is no value in going to great lengths to develop matching tablets or capsules if the test and control medications arrive at the clinic in different sized or colored bottles. The differences do not have to be great to destroy the mask. Subtle variations in the way the bottles are capped or labeled may be enough to do the job. The best approach is to have all medications bottled and labeled at the same facility, under tightly controlled conditions. The VA Cooperative Studies Program has established a central pharmacy to supply its trials with needed study medications (Hagans, 1974). Various other trials, such as the CDP, have contracted with a single facility

to supply drugs to the study clinics (Coronary Drug Project Research Group, 1973a).

In a typical drug trial, clinics will dispense drugs by bottle number. The treatment assignment issued by the data center will indicate the bottle number to be used. The simplest bottle numbering scheme is one in which all bottles containing a given drug bear the same number or letter designation. The trouble with such schemes is that all patients on a drug are unmasked as soon as any one patient on the drug is unmasked. Use of a unique bottle number for every patient in a clinic avoids this problem, but such schemes complicate the logistics of supplying clinics with needed drugs. A compromise between these two extremes was used in the CDP. Each clinic was supplied with sets of bottles, labeled from 1 through 30, as discussed in Illustration 7 of Section 10.8.7. This meant that clinics had somewhere between 5 and 8 patients on the same bottle number by the time recruitment was finished.

Table 10-5 Illustration of Moses-Oakford algorithm

Block size	Treatment codes		Random numbers*		
				Page	Column	Row
———	C = Control		Start	17	27	16
Allocation ratio	T1 = Test trt 1					
	T2 = Test trt 2		End	17	27	24
1:1:1:1	T3 = Test trt 3		Source: Rand Corp. (1955)			

(1)	(2)	(3)	(4)	(5)
Order of assignment within block	Initial	Treatment assignments Replacements	Final	Random number
1	C	T3, T3	T3	—
2	C	T2, T2	T2	2
3	T1	T3	T3	1
4	T1	T3	T1	3
5	T2	———	T2	2
6	T2	———	C	2
7	T3	———	T1	4
8	T3	———	C	1

* Reading rule:

Read down to the end of column and from left to right. Ignore 0's and numbers in excess of number of lines remaining to be filled.

Table 10-6   First 25 lines of page 17 of The Rand Corporation's 1 million random digits

Row number	Column number									
	5	10	15	20	25	30	35	40	45	50
	00397	56753	53158	71872	68153	09298	20961	49656	33407	95683
	14328	44708	72952	27048	67887	28741	46752	88177	95894	40086
	88534	87112	68614	83073	88794	96799	67588	75049	84603	83140
	97347	87316	73087	77135	71883	98643	03808	08848	14133	60447
5	01366	72976	01868	51667	63279	60040	88264	79152	03474	61366
	20523	21584	93712	83654	89761	90154	96345	37539	32556	74254
	70603	97122	44978	78028	08943	13778	11080	34271	68266	85372
	48410	94516	15427	75323	71685	70774	50342	33771	03678	42321
	69788	41758	55004	30992	17402	63523	42328	87171	24751	15084
10	33884	83655	88345	69602	52606	57886	18034	03381	75796	35901
	77480	28683	68324	66035	07223	14926	16128	13645	90370	31949
	11057	98849	29499	21565	30786	83292	92392	37104	36899	49906
	79368	43710	80365	88735	75275	21664	57965	19002	00301	12658
	94385	01717	96191	50404	80166	93965	24688	27839	10812	31715
15	92127	42588	93307	80834	11317	26583	25769	98227	14887	58462
	29148	68662	26872	72927	79021	51622	29521	33355	45701	45996
	33782	93424	16530	96086	17329	74020	11501	46660	05583	22277
	77653	55430	84644	00448	86828	58855	67451	95264	67386	82424
	52611	60012	88620	72894	94716	22262	99813	69592	63464	33163
20	91857	47904	22209	78590	68615	52952	31441	41313	18550	72685
	68825	04795	53971	14592	39634	23682	76630	02731	81481	86542
	23727	54291	56045	61635	32186	90355	73416	63532	24340	18886
	84832	30654	48543	18339	65024	91197	64624	74648	09660	27897
	49771	11123	08732	49393	12911	72416	17834	18878	62754	85072
25	23727	56577	51257	83291	12329	16203	91681	68138	79959	43609

Source: Reference citation 387. Reprinted with permission of The Rand Corporation (New York: The Free Press, 1955). Copyright © 1955 and 1983 by The Rand Corporation.

However, it also meant that they could get by with a much smaller inventory of drugs than would have been required with individually numbered bottles.

Most prepackaged medications in masked trials will be supplied to clinics with a two-part label, as illustrated in Figure 10–1. One part of the label will be affixed to the package and dispensed with it. It should bear the name of the study, the bottle or container number, instructions for taking the medication, and the name of the physician or clinic responsible for dispensing the medication. The other part of the label is loosely affixed to the container. Its prime purpose is to indicate container contents, either on the face of the label (for single-masked trials), or by breaking a seal (for double-masked trials). It is required for interstate shipment of drugs under federal law; it is illegal to ship drugs across state lines without it. It is detached when the medication is dispensed and is ordinarily retained at the clinic to allow clinic personnel to unmask a medication in an emergency.

10.6   DOCUMENTATION OF THE RANDOMIZATION SCHEME

There should be a written description of the scheme used to generate the allocation schedule. It should be written when the randomization schedule is produced and should be checked for clarity and accuracy before it is filed for future reference. Table 10–7 provides an outline of the items to be covered in the writeup. The details should be sufficient to allow a person from outside the study to reproduce the schedule with the information provided.

The documentation may be needed to defend the study years after the completion of randomization. The UGDP serves as a case in point. The Committee for the Assessment of Biometric Aspects of Controlled Trials of Hypoglycemic

Part A: Attached portion of bottle label

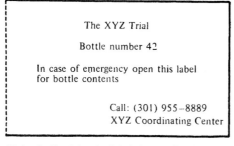

```
The XYZ Trial

Bottle number 42

R_x: Take one capsule each morning

For: Harry L. Green

Date: 3-7-85          John Smith, M.D.
                      Phone: 555-1701
```

Part B: Detachable portion of bottle label

```
The XYZ Trial

Bottle number 42

In case of emergency open this label
for bottle contents

                    Call: (301) 955-8889
                    XYZ Coordinating Center
```

Figure 10-1 Stylized bottle label for medications dispensed in the XYZ trial.

Agents (1975), appointed to review the study about 8 years after the completion of patient enrollment, was especially interested in the randomization process used.

10.7 ADMINISTRATION OF THE RANDOMIZATION PROCESS

An allocation scheme, no matter how carefully constructed, will be useless as a means of protecting against patient selection bias if it is not followed. Departures from the schedule to accommodate the desire of a patient or his physician, no matter how well motivated, are never justified. They can invalidate the results of the entire trial if they are numerous and if there are reasons to believe they are treatment related. A carefully executed trial will include various safeguards to make certain the assignment schedule is followed, as listed in Table 10-8.

The preferred system is one in which allocations are issued from a central point on a per-patient basis. The main advantage with such systems, as opposed to systems with no central control (e.g., as in systems with envelopes placed in the clinic to be used in the order provided), lies in the audit trail provided and the oppor-

Table 10-7 Items that should be included in the written documentation of the allocation scheme

A. For procedures using published lists of random numbers

- Reference citation to the published numbers
- Section of the table or list used (indicate enough detail to allow regeneration of the schedule)
- Reading instructions indicating the order in which numbers are read, including a description of any modular arithmetic used to convert numbers outside the usable range to usable values
- Specifications of the construction process, such as those listed for illustrations in Section 10.8
- Worksheets or computer program used to generate the assignment list
- Copy of the assignment list

B. For procedures using computer based pseudo-random number generators

- Reference citation to the pseudo-random number generator
- Program listing of the pseudo-random number generator
- Seed used to start the generation process
- First and last numbers generated with the seed
- Specifications for the construction process, such as those listed for illustrations in Section 10.8
- Computer programs used to generate the assignment list
- Copy of the assignment list

tunity to proscribe release of an assignment until a patient has been shown to be eligible for enrollment via the data provided, the required baseline data have been collected, and his consent to participate has been obtained. The CDP used a

Table 10-8 Safeguards for administration of treatment allocation schedules

- Avoid the use of any assignment scheme that has a high degree of predictability (e.g., use of small blocks as discussed in Section 10.3.3)
- Keep each treatment assignment masked to the patient, physician, and person issuing the assignment until the patient has been accepted into the study and is ready to start treatment
- Vest responsibility for issuing assignments in an individual or group located outside the clinic
- Withhold disclosure of an assignment until the patient is judged eligible for enrollment, has given his consent to be enrolled, and all essential baseline data have been obtained
- Make certain that the assignment process establishes a clear audit trail that indicates who requested the assignment and when it was issued

centrally administered mail-based assignment scheme (Coronary Drug Project Research Group, 1973a). The Coronary Artery Surgery Study (CASS) used a centrally administered telephone-based assignment scheme (Coronary Artery Surgery Study Research Group, 1981). Either scheme is preferable to one that is self-administered. Such systems are subject to the abuses noted in Section 8.4.

Table 10-9 contains a facsimile of an allocation schedule from the CDP, as used in the Coordinating Center for making assignments. The allocation process required the clinic to initiate the request. This was done by sending the forms completed for a patient's two prerandomization visits to the Coordinating Center. An állocation was not released by the Center if essential items of information were missing from the forms, if an eligibility stop condition (see Section 12.5.8) had been checked, or if the clinic did not indicate

that a signed consent had been obtained from the patient indicating his willingness to be enrolled into the trial.

Once all essential conditions were met, a treatment assignment form was prepared (Part A, Table 10–10). The bottle assignment recorded on the form was taken from the first topmost empty line of the allocation schedule for the clinic and stratum to which the patient belonged (the third line in the sample schedule in Table 10–9). The ID number and the name of the patient were entered on the line. After entry of the required data on the treatment assignment form, it was placed in an opaque envelope (Part B, Table 10–10), which was then sealed and placed in a larger envelope for mailing to the clinic. The inner envelope was retained in sealed condition at the clinic until the patient returned for his final baseline examination and was judged ready to start treatment. A patient was not considered enrolled

Table 10-9   Sample CDP treatment allocation schedule

Order of assignment within block	Bottle number to be assigned	Bottle contents	Patient ID number		Patient name or name code	
1	29	CPIB	(56-001	)	(JAMEI	)
2	14	NICA	(56-002	)	(ASJON	)
3	26	PLBO	(	)	(	)
4	2	ESG2	(	)	(	)
5	27	ESG1	(	)	(	)
6	19	NICA	(	)	(	)
7	15	DT4	(	)	(	)
8	16	CPIB	(	)	(	)
9	13	PLBO	(	)	(	)
10	25	PLBO	(	)	(	)
11	10	ESG1	(	)	(	)
12	4	ESG2	(	)	(	)
13	24	PLBO	(	)	(	)
14	23	PLBO	(	)	(	)
15	9	DT4	(	)	(	)
16	30	ESG2	(	)	(	)
17	17	DT4	(	)	(	)
18	20	DT4	(	)	(	)
19	11	PLBO	(	)	(	)
20	6	CPIB	(	)	(	)
21	5	PLBO	(	)	(	)
22	28	ESG1	(	)	(	)
23	22	CPIB	(	)	(	)
24	18	ESG1	(	)	(	)
25	7	ESG2	(	)	(	)
26	8	NICA	(	)	(	)
27	1	PLBO	(	)	(	)
28	12	PLBO	(	)	(	)
29	21	PLBO	(	)	(	)
30	3	NICA	(	)	(	)

Source: Reference citation 104. Adapted with permission of the American Heart Association, Inc., Dallas, Texas.

in the trial until the clinic opened the treatment allocation envelope. Once this was done, the patient was counted as a member of the treatment group to which he had been assigned. Assignments issued for patients who failed to return for their last baseline visit, or who withdrew their consent at that visit, were not counted, provided they were returned to the Coordinating Center in sealed condition. The ID numbers and names of such patients were deleted from the allocation schedule on receipt of the sealed envelopes at the Coordinating Center. The assign-

ments in question were not reissued. The small amount of imbalance introduced in this way was not considered serious enough to justify the effort involved in reissuing the assignments.

The allocation schedule used by personnel in the CDP Coordinating Center revealed the contents of the bottles assigned (see Table 10-9). The presence of this information violates one of the masking safeguards listed in Table 10-8. However, there is no evidence that this information had any effect on the assignment process.

The mail system described was made possible

Table 10-10 Sample CDP allocation form and envelope

Part A. CDP treatment allocation form

We have received your request for a treatment allocation for

Mr. _____

whose identifying number is   _____

This person should receive medication from bottles identified by the following number:

```
    _____
   |           |
   |           |
   |           |
   |_____|
```

The sealed tear off portion of the label on each bottle should be removed prior to dispensing. The patient's name, treating physician, date and prescription number should be recorded on the tear off portion of the label prior to filing with the patient's prescription record.

The treatment should be initiated at initial Visit 3 and should be administered on the following schedule:

   1   capsule three times a day after meals from initial visit 3 through initial visit 4.

   2   capsules three times a day after meals from initial visit 4 through initial visit 5.

   3   capsules three times a day after meals after initial visit 5 throughout the remainder of the study on the above named person unless clinically contraindicated

NOTE: If the date on which the treatment allocation envelope has been opened is more than four months after the date of initial Visit 1 (which, as indicated on Form 01, is _____), this allocation must be returned unused to the CDP Coordinating Center and this patient must start anew with initial Visit 1.

Date of Allocation _____

                                                  CDP Coordinating Center
                                                Baltimore, Maryland 21201

Part B: Treatment allocation envelope

CORONARY DRUG PROJECT

Treatment Allocation for

Mr. _____   I.D. No. _____

DO NOT OPEN until instructed to do so in Form 02 (at Initial Visit 3).

If not opened within four months following the date of Initial Visit 1, this envelope should be returned to the CDP Coordinating Center.

Source: Coronary Drug Project Research Group.

because of the time separation between initiation of the request and treatment—generally about a month. Telephone assignments were allowed only when there was not adequate time to complete the mail circuit and then only if Coordinating Center personnel were satisfied that the patient in question was eligible for enrollment, that the clinic had completed the necessary forms, and that they had obtained his consent for enrollment.

The scheme described above cannot be used in cases where clinic personnel have to have the assignment as soon as the patient agrees to enroll. A system for making telephone allocations, such as used in CASS, has to be used in such cases, unless the study is willing to rely on a noncentral self-administered scheme (not recommended). The procedure in CASS required Coordinating Center personnel to carry out a series of telephone-administered checks with the requesting party before an assignment could be released. They included:

- Checks for eligibility
- Checks on the disease classification (needed for proper stratification)
- Checks to determine if the patient had signed the study consent statement and had indi-

cated his willingness to accept either surgical or medical treatment.
- Checks to make certain a date for surgery had been set (for use if the patient was assigned to surgery)

CASS Coordinating Center personnel responsible for issuing assignments were masked with regard to assignments until the telephone interview was completed. This was done to protect against premature disclosure of assignments during the interview process.

The telephone assignment process used in CASS could be managed during the normal working hours of the Coordinating Center. This may not be possible in studies involving clinics scattered across a large number of time zones. Extended hours of phone coverage will be needed in such cases. Twenty-four-hour phone coverage will be needed when the trial involves emergency treatments that must be initiated as soon as possible.

The advent of low-cost, stand-alone minicomputers makes it possible to control the assignment process without any contact with the coordinating center, as in the Hypertension Prevention Trial (HPT). A clinic in that study initiated a request for assignment via an on-site computer (IBM S/23 DataMaster). The assignment was released via the computer, but only if the data forms entered by the clinic met the edit tests necessary for assignment.

Many trials, especially single-center trials, which cannot arrange for a centrally administered allocation scheme, must rely on self-administered schemes managed at the clinic. The usual approach in such cases is to place the assignments in sealed envelopes arranged in a predetermined order with personnel instructed to use the envelopes in order of arrangement, as indicated by numbers appearing on the faces of the envelopes. Strict ground rules should be established to indicate when envelopes are to be opened and to ensure that patients are counted in the trial once this has happened. Persons authorized to draw an allocation envelope should be required to check the prerandomization data form for missing data and for exclusion conditions before the envelope is opened. Documents completed in the allocation process should identify the patient for whom the assignment was intended and the time the envelope was opened. The time information is important when checks are made to determine if envelopes are used in the order indicated.

There is, of course, no method of allocation that is completely foolproof. It is important for this reason to perform periodic checks for breakdowns in the assignment process, regardless of how it is administered. It is dangerous to assume that the rules for allocation, no matter how explicitly outlined, will always be followed. The checking that is carried out should be performed by an individual or group of individuals not directly involved in the assignment process. For example, such checks in CASS were made by an external review team during visits to the CASS Coordinating Center. A similar function can be performed by the statistician or some other individual in the case of small-scale single-center trials using self-administered allocation schemes.

10.8 ILLUSTRATIONS

The illustrations in this section are designed to acquaint the reader with various techniques for constructing allocation schedules. The first 5 illustrations are for unmasked trials. Illustrations 6 and 7 are for masked trials. Illustration 1 involves use of random permutations of a set of numbers for constructing the randomization schedule. All of the remaining illustrations, except Illustration 5, involve use of random number tables. Illustra-

tion 5 involves use of a pseudo-random number generator.

10.8.1 Illustration 1: Restricted randomization using a table of random permutations

a. Specifications

- Treatment groups: 3
- Allocation ratio: $1:1:2$
- Blocking constraints:
  - Number of blocks: 3
  - Block sizes: $k_1 = 12$, $k_2 = 4$, $k_3 = 4$
- Treatment masking: None
- Stratification variables: None
- Random permutation source: Cochran and Cox (1957). See Table 10–11.

b. Approach

Step 1 Establish treatment notation. Let:
T1 denote test treatment 1
T2 denote test treatment 2
C denote control treatment

Step 2 Establish treatment coding rule. Assign:
C for integers 1 through $k/2$
T1 for integers $1 + (k/2)$ through $3k/4$
T2 for integers $1 + (3k/4)$ through k

Step 3 Select a random start in table of random permutations. Set 7, Table 10–11, in this example.

Step 4 Establish reading rules. Read from left to right, i.e., use set 7 for first block, set 8 for second block, and set 9 for third block. Skip numbers in a permutation set that exceed the indicated block size.

Step 5 Record the assignment sequence. See third column of Table 10–12.

c. Comment

Note that the allocation ratio of $1:1:2$ is satisfied in each of the three blocks.

10.8.2. Illustration 2: Unblocked allocations using a table of random numbers

a. Specifications

- Treatment groups: 2
- Allocation ratio: $1:1$
- Blocking constraints: None

Table 10-11   Reproduction of 20 sets of random permutations of first 16 integers, from page 584 of Cochran and Cox (1957)

Permutation set																				
1	*2*	*3*	*4*	*5*	*6*	*7*	*8*	*9*	*10*	*11*	*12*	*13*	*14*	*15*	*16*	*17*	*18*	*19*	*20*
9	16	15	12	2	11	4	16	11	10	2	5	5	14	11	2	14	13	16	6
11	3	2	6	15	13	10	1	4	13	11	8	16	16	4	3	5	15	5	15
14	14	8	16	11	15	5	14	14	11	1	14	15	15	13	5	7	11	11	16
4	13	1	3	5	7	6	2	16	1	14	9	14	3	3	1	6	16	6	10
6	6	10	7	13	10	16	7	2	12	6	12	6	13	8	9	15	9	1	11
2	10	14	9	12	3	3	10	5	6	5	16	12	10	15	10	11	4	9	8
5	15	11	14	10	4	14	13	6	4	12	4	11	5	10	14	16	5	7	9
16	5	13	10	3	9	12	6	3	7	3	7	3	11	14	7	3	14	4	12
8	12	7	11	7	8	13	15	13	9	4	3	8	1	12	6	9	8	15	14
1	8	3	2	1	5	15	9	9	3	10	11	13	8	5	13	12	3	3	5
13	9	9	1	6	2	11	3	8	8	15	1	7	9	7	8	8	6	2	3
15	1	5	5	9	6	9	4	10	5	8	13	10	7	9	15	2	10	8	4
7	4	12	13	16	1	2	11	12	2	16	15	2	4	2	11	1	7	13	1
10	2	4	15	4	16	1	12	7	15	9	10	9	12	16	4	13	2	10	13
3	7	6	8	8	14	7	5	1	14	13	2	4	2	1	16	4	1	12	7
12	11	16	4	14	12	8	8	15	16	7	6	1	6	6	12	10	12	14	2

Source: Reprinted with permission of John Wiley & Sons, Inc., New York (copyright © 1957).

Table 10-12   Allocations for Illustration 1

Order of assignment		Value from Table 10-11*	Treatment assignment
1	⎤	4	C
2		10	T2
3		5	C
4		6	C
5		3	C
6	⎱Block 1	12	T2
7		11	T2
8		9	T1
9		2	C
10		1	C
11		7	T1
12	⎦	8	T1
13	⎤	1	C
14	⎱Block 2	2	C
15		3	T1
16	⎦	4	T2
17	⎤	4	T2
18	⎱Block 3	2	C
19		3	T1
20	⎦	1	C

*Starting point: Permutation set number 7, Table 10-11.

- Treatment masking: None
- Stratification variables: None
- Random number source: Rand Corporation (1955)

b.   Approach

Step 1   Establish treatment codes. Let:
C   denote control treatment
T   denote test treatment

Step 2   Select an arbitrary starting point from table of random numbers. Suggested method:

i. Arbitrarily open book to some page and place the point of a pencil on the page without looking. Use the three digits to immediate right and nearest the point to designate the starting page (17 in example).

ii. Repeat the process described in step i to select a starting column (22 in example) and row (3 in example) for the page selected (page 17 in the example, see Table 10-6).

Step 3   Define order in which numbers are to be used. Read from left to right and down by row, beginning at the point designated in Step 2. Use single integers.

Step 4 Establish correspondence between numbers selected and treatment assignments. For this illustration use odd integers (1, 3, 5, 7, 9) to designate assignment to the control treatment (C) and even integers (0, 2, 4, 6, 8) to designate assignment to the test treatment (T).

Step 5 Record the treatment assignment sequence (see third column of Table 10–13).

c. Comment

Note that the sequence for the first 20 assignments provided 9 T assignments and 11 C assignments for an observed allocation ratio of 1:1.2 instead of the desired ratio of 1:1.

10.8.3 Illustration 3: Blocked allocations using the Moses-Oakford algorithm and a table of random numbers

a. Specifications

Same as for Illustration 2 except:

- Blocking constraints:
  - Number of blocks: 4
  - Block sizes: $k_1 = 10$, $k_2 = 4$, $k_3 = 2$, $k_4 = 4$

b. Approach

Step 1 Same as for Illustration 2.

Step 2 Starting point: row 9, column 42, Table 10–6.

Step 3 Reading instructions: Left to right to end of row, then down, row by row. Use pairs of integers as long as the remaining block size is ≥10. Skip 00 and pairs of integers that exceed remaining block size. Use single integers once the remaining block size is ≤9. Ignore 0. (*Note:* Most numbers exceeding the remaining block size could be converted to the usable range through subtraction of an appropriate multiplier of the remaining block size if desired. For example, the number 53 converts to 9 by subtracting 44 if the remaining block size is 11. However, such arithmetic is tedious and subject to error if done by hand and therefore is not done in this example.)

Step 4 Set down an arbitrary order of treatments, as shown in column 2, Table 10–14.

Step 5 Establish the final order of treatment assignment (column 4, Table 10–14) using the Moses-Oakford algorithm (Table 10–3).

c. Comment

The table below gives the location of the first and last numbers used from Table 10–6 for each of the four blocks.

Table 10-13 Allocations for Illustration 2

Order of assignment	Random number*	Treatment assignment
1	8	T
2	7	C
3	9	C
4	4	T
5	9	C
6	6	T
7	7	C
8	9	C
9	9	C
10	6	T
11	7	C
12	5	C
13	8	T
14	8	T
15	7	C
16	5	C
17	0	T
18	4	T
19	9	C
20	8	T

*Starting point: Row 3, Column 22, Table 10–6.

Block number	First number		Last number	
	Column	Row	Column	Row
1	42	9	22	10
2	31	10	40	10
3	50	10	50	10
4	3	11	14	11

10.8.4 Illustration 4: Stratified and blocked allocations using the Moses-Oakford algorithm and a table of random numbers

a. Specifications

- Treatment groups: 3
- Allocation ratio: 1:1:5
- Blocking constraints: Blocks of sizes 7 or 14 arranged in random sequence

Table 10-14 Allocations for Illustration 3

No. of blocks	Treatment codes		Random numbers*		
_4_			Page	Column	Row
Block sizes	C = Control				
_10, 4, 2, 4_	T = Test		Start _17_	_42_	_9_
Allocation ratio			End _17_	_14_	_11_
_1:1_			Source: _Rand Corp. (1955)_		

(1a)	(1)	(2)	(3)	(4)	(5)
	Order of assignment within block	Treatment assignments			
Order of assignment		Initial	Replacements	Final	Random number
1	_1_	_C_	_____	_C_	___
2	_2_	~~C~~	_T_	_T_	_2_
3	_3_	~~C~~	~~T,C,C,~~T	_T_	_2_
4	_4_	~~T~~	~~C,~~T	_C_	_3_
5	_5_	_C_	_____	_C_	_3_
6	_6_	_T_	_____	_C_	_4_
7	_7_	_C_	_____	_T_	_3_
8	_8_	~~C~~	_T_	_C_	_3_
9	_9_	_C_	_____	_T_	_4_
10	_10_	_T_	_____	_T_	_08_
11	_1_	~~C~~	~~C,~~T	_T_	___
12	_2_	_T_	_____	_T_	_1_
13	_3_	_C_	_____	_C_	_3_
14	_4_	_T_	_____	_C_	_1_
15	_1_	~~C~~	_T_	_T_	___
16	_2_	_T_	_____	_C_	_1_
17	_1_	_C_	_____	_C_	___
18	_2_	~~T~~	_C_	_C_	_2_
19	_3_	_C_	_____	_T_	_2_
20	_4_	_T_	_____	_T_	_4_

Blocks: rows 1–10 Blk 1; rows 11–14 Blk 2; rows 15–16 Blk 3; rows 17–20 Blk 4.

* Reading rule:

See Illustration 3 (Section 10.8.4) for reading instructions. Note also that the last two assignments in block 4 could be made without drawing any number since the two remaining assignments must be to the control treatment in order to satisfy the allocation ratio.

- Treatment masking: None
- Stratification variables: 1 (2 levels)
- Random number source: Rand Corporation (1955)

Step 1 Establish treatment codes (shown in Table 10–15)

Step 2 Starting point: row 10, column 6, Table 10–6.

Step 3 Reading rule: Read left to right using pairs of integers until remaining number of assignments to be made is ≤9, then use single integers. Ignore 00 and 0.

Step 4 Set down an arbitrary order of treatments, as shown in column 2, Table 10–15.

Step 5 Establish the final order of treatments (column 4, Table 10–15) using the Moses-Oakford algorithm (Table 10–3).

c. Comment

This problem requires construction of an allocation schedule for enrollment of an unspecified number of patients per stratum (See Chapter 14 for discussion of difficulties with designs involving recruitment quotas). One approach would be to develop 2 schedules, each one with enough allocations to meet the recruitment goal of the trial. However, this is wasteful since half of the assignments would remain unused. A more effi-

Table 10–15 Allocations for Illustration 4

Block number: 3
Block size: 14
Allocation ratio: 1:1:5

Treatment Codes:
C = Control
T1 = Test trt 1
T2 = Test trt 2

Random numbers*
	Page	Column	Row
Start	17	11	10
End	17	33	11

Source: Rand. Corp. (1955)

Patient ID number	(1a) Order of assignment	(1) Order of assignment within stratum	(2) Initial	(3) Replacements	(4) Final	(5) Random number
—	—	1	C	T1,C,C,C	C	—
—	—	2	C	T2,T1,C,C,C	C	1
—	—	3	C	T2, C	C	1
—	—	4	C	C	C	2
—	—	5	C		C	4
—	—	6	C		T1	1
—	—	7	C	C	T2	3
—	—	8	C		C	2
—	—	9	C		T1	2
—	—	10	C		C	07
—	—	11	T1		T2	02
—	—	12	T1		C	01
—	—	13	T2		C	03
—	—	14	T2		C	02

* Reading rule: See Illustration 4 for reading instructions (Section 10.8.4).

cient approach is to generate sets of worksheets arranged in the order generated as dictated by the random sequence of block sizes used (in this example, 7, 7, 14, 7, 14, etc.; see Table 10–15 for third block of size 14). They are then used in order, as needed, depending on enrollment patterns in the 2 strata. The first worksheet of block size 7 is used to make assignments for patients in the stratum represented by the first patient enrolled into the trial. For example, if the stratification variable is sex and the first patient enrolled is female, then the first worksheet is used for the first 7 females enrolled. The second sheet is not used until the eighth patient enters the same stratum, or until a patient enters who qualifies for the second stratum, in this example, a male. The stratum number is not placed on the sheet until it is used. The lines in the column labeled *Patient ID number* would be filled in as the individual assignments are issued. The numbers written in column 1a would depend on the number of sheets already used for allocations to the stratum in question. For example, they would run from 1 through 14 if there had been no previous assignments in the stratum, and from 8 through 21 if a block of size 7 had already been filled for the stratum.

10.8.5   Illustration 5: Sample allocation schedule for the Macular Photocoagulation Study using pseudo-random numbers

a. Specifications

- Treatment groups: 2
- Allocation ratio: 1:1
- Blocking constraints: Blocks of sizes 6 or 8 in random sequence
- Treatment masking: None
- Stratification variables: 2 (clinic and type of eye disease, three different types)

- Random number source: Computer based pseudo-random number generator

b. Approach

Step 1   Establish treatment codes. Let:
C   denote control treatment
T   denote test treatment

Step 2   Select a block size, 6 or 8, by some random or pseudo-random process (size 6 in this Illustration).

Step 3   Arrange treatment codes in arbitrary order (column 2, Table 10–16).

Step 4   Generate a sequence of 5-digit pseudo-random numbers and record in the order generated (column 3, Table 10–16).

Step 5   Link the treatment code (column 2, Table 10–16) and pseudo-random number (column 3, Table 10–16).

Step 6   Order the pseudo-random numbers with associated treatment codes (column 4, Table 10–16).

Step 7   Repeat steps 2 through 6 as necessary to generate the desired number of assignments.

c. Comment

Sheets should be used in the order needed, as discussed in Illustration 4.

10.8.6   Illustration 6: Double-masked allocation schedule using the Moses-Oakford algorithm and a table of random numbers

a. Specifications

- Treatment groups: 3
- Allocation ratio: 2:2:3

Table 10-16   Sample allocation schedule from the Macular Photocoagulation Study for Illustration 5

(1) Order of assignment in block	*(2)* Initial assignment	*(3)* Pseudo-random number	*(4)* Ordered pseudo-random number with treatment code	*(5)* Final assignment from column 4
1	T	26391	(T) 07631	T
2	C	29126	(C) 10645	C
3	T	07631	(C) 22846	C
4	C	22846	(T) 26391	T
5	T	30856	(C) 29126	C
6	C	10645	(T) 30856	T

- Blocking constraints: Uniform block size of 14
- Treatment masking: Double-masked
- Stratification variables: 1 (2 levels)
- Random number source: Rand Corporation (1955)

b. Approach

The first step is to denote the bottle numbers to be used. The designation in this Illustration was made by arbitrarily selecting a random permutation of the first 16 integers (set 12, Table 10–11). The first 6 values of size 14 or less in the permutation are used to denote bottles containing the control drug, the next 4 numbers are used to designate bottles containing test drug 1 and the last 4 numbers are used to denote bottles containing test drug 2. The bottle codes and associated treatment are recorded in column 2, Table 10–17, and then rearranged as described for Illustrations 3 and 4 to yield the bottle sequence indicated in column 6. The sheet provided is for 1 block in the scheme.

c. Comment

Note that each bottle number appears only once in Table 10–17. Subsequent blocks will contain different orderings of the same bottle numbers.

Table 10-17 Allocation schedule for double-masked drug trial described in Illustration 6

Block size: *14*

Allocation ratio: *2:2:3*

Treatment codes:
C: Bottle Nos. 4, 5, 8, 9, 12, 14
T1: Bottle Nos. 1, 3, 7, 11
T2: Bottle Nos. 2, 6, 10, 13

Random numbers*

	Page	Column	Row
Start	*17*	*21*	*7*
End	*17*	*19*	*8*

Source: _____

(1)	(2)	(3)	(4)	(5)	(6)
Order of assignment within block	Initial	Replacements	Final	Random number	Bottle number
1	*C-4*	*T1-1, T2-6*	*T2-6*	—	*6*
2	*C-5*	*T2-10*	*T2-10*	*2*	*10*
3	*C-8*	*T2-10*	*C-5*	*2*	*5*
4	*C-9*	*T1-11*	*T1-11*	*4*	*11*
5	*C-12*	*T2-6*	*T1-1*	*1*	*1*
6	*C-14*	_____	*C-14*	*6*	*14*
7	*T1-1*	_____	*C-4*	*1*	*4*
8	*T1-3*	*T2-13, T2-6*	*C-12*	*5*	*12*
9	*T1-7*	*T1-11*	*C-9*	*4*	*9*
10	*T1-11*	_____	*T1-7*	*09*	*7*
11	*T2-2*	*T2-10*	*C-8*	*03*	*8*
12	*T2-6*	_____	*T2-13*	*08*	*13*
13	*T2-10*	_____	*T2-2*	*11*	*2*
14	*T2-13*	_____	*T1-3*	*08*	*3*

* Reading rule:
Read numbers from left to right and down, row by row. Use pairs of numbers as long as the remaining block size is >10. Skip 00's and pairs of numbers which exceed the remaining block size. Use single integer once the remaining block size is ≤9. Skip 0's.

10.8.7   Illustration 7: Sample CDP double-masked allocation schedule

a. Specifications

- Number of assignments: 8,341
- Clinics: 53
- Treatment groups: 6
- Allocation ratio: 2:2:2:2:2:5
- Blocking constraints: Uniform block size of 15
- Treatment masking: Double-masked
- Stratification variables: 2 (clinic and risk group, two levels per clinic, to yield a total of $53 \times 2 = 106$ allocation strata)
- Random number source: Rand Corporation (1955)

b. Approach

The allocation procedure is described in a CDP publication (Coronary Drug Project Research Group, 1973a). Treatment assignments were identified by a 2-digit bottle number as shown in Table 10–9. The same bottle numbers were used in all clinics. Hence, all bottles bearing a particular number always contained the same medication, regardless of clinic.

c. Comment

Note that each bottle number appears once and only once in the 30 assignments listed in Table 10–9 and that both blocks in the table satisfy the allocation ratio (i.e., contain 2 assignments to each test treatment and 5 assignments to the placebo treatment).

11. The study plan

The way to improve a treatment is to eliminate controls.

Hugo Muench

11.1 INTRODUCTION

The basic elements of the plan for any trial will be set long before the first patient is enrolled. The nature of the test treatment and outcome measure will be specified in the funding proposal. Specifics having to do with execution of the study plan may not be addressed until the trial has been funded. The period of time between initiation of funding and enrollment of the first patient is one requiring intense effort to develop and test procedures needed for the trial. However, the planning and testing process does not end there. In fact, it is likely to continue over much of the course of the trial, particularly in long-term trials involving extended periods of patient recruitment or follow-up. The goal in such settings of maintaining the study plan unchanged once the first patient has been enrolled, while laudable, is not always practical.

The term *study plan* used in a broad sense refers to the design of the trial and all the organi-

zational and operational details needed to carry it out. In this sense, various other chapters, in addition to this one, relate to the study plan, starting with the two previous chapters and including most of those that follow.

11.2 DESIGN FACTORS AND DETAILS TO BE ADDRESSED IN THE STUDY PLAN

No trial should be undertaken without:

- A concise statement of its objective(s)
- A specification of the outcome measure(s) to be used for evaluating the study treatments
- Agreement on the treatments to be tested
- A sample size calculation that indicates the required number of patients, or a calculation of the power provided with a prestated sample size
- Specification of the required length of patient follow-up
- A specified set of patient entry and exclusion criteria
- A method for randomization
- A specified baseline and follow-up examination schedule
- A set of data intake procedures, including specification of the methods for data entry, editing, and quality control
- An established organizational and decision-making structure

Agreement on the design and operating features of a trial cannot be ensured unless they have been written down and have been reviewed and accepted by investigators responsible for the trial.

11.3 OBJECTIVE AND SPECIFIC AIMS

The statement of the primary objective is by far the most important specification in the trial. It must be formulated and agreed upon before a data collection scheme can be developed. The statement should indicate the:

- Type of patients to be studied
- Class of treatments to be evaluated
- Primary outcome measure

Sample statements of objectives follow:

University Group Diabetes Program (UGDP)

Evaluation of the efficacy of hypoglycemic treatments in the prevention of vascular complications in a long-term, prospective, and cooperative clinical trial (University Group Diabetes Program Research Group, 1970d).

Coronary Drug Project (CDP)

Evaluate the efficacy of several lipid-influencing drugs in the long-term therapy of CHD in men ages 30 through 64 with evidence of previous myocardial infarction (Coronary Drug Project Research Group, 1973a).

National Cooperative Gallstone Study (NCGS)

To determine the efficacy of oral administration of a high and low dose of CDC acid in dissolving or reducing the size of cholesterol gallstones, as compared with placebo treatment (National Cooperative Gallstone Study Group, 1981a).

The statement from the CDP comes closest to satisfying the three requirements stated above. It indicates the type of patients to be treated and the class of treatments to be used. However, it is ambiguous with regard to outcome, other than to suggest that it is related to coronary heart disease (CHD). The UGDP statement indicates nothing about the study population and is ambiguous with regard to chosen outcome measure. The NCGS statement names the treatment and outcome measure, but says nothing about the study population.

It is not uncommon for a large-scale trial to have secondary objectives as well. They are illustrated for the three trials cited above.

UGDP

- To study the natural history of vascular disease in maturity onset, noninsulin dependent diabetics.

- To develop methods applicable to multicenter clinical trials.

CDP

- To obtain information on the natural history and clinical course of CHD.
- To develop more advanced technology for the design and conduct of large, long-term, collaborative clinical trials.

NCGS

- To determine whether either a high or low dose of chenodeoxycholic acid could be safely used to dissolve cholesterol gallstones.
- To determine the rate of recurrence of gallstones in those patients in which chenodeoxycholic acid feeding has successfully dissolved gallstones.

Whenever multiple objectives are stated, it is wise to rank them in order of importance. The ranking will have important design implications, especially if data requirements for the objectives differ. The investigators should state the specific aims to be pursued in conjunction with each objective. The methods and data collection requirements of the trial should then be constructed to satisfy the stated aims.

11.4   THE TREATMENT PLAN

General considerations involved in choosing the test and control treatments were discussed in Chapter 8. Once they have been selected, it is necessary for investigators to address a series of practical issues concerning treatment administration. One issue in drug trials concerns whether the treatments are to be administered using a fixed- or variable-dosage schedule. Ideally, the administration schedule should be as near that used in actual practice as feasible. A variable dosage schedule, tailored to the needs of individual patients, should be used if the test drug is ordinarily used in this way. A fixed-dosage schedule may be used if the drug is normally used in this way or if the variation in dosages used is small.

The choice may be constrained by masking requirements. The desire to individualize treatment in order to achieve some desired effect (for example, to normalize blood glucose levels in the case of a hypoglycemic drug) may have to be

abandoned if there is to be double-masked administration of the treatments. The manipulations required for dosage titrations can be hazardous to patients if they are done in a masked fashion and may in any case render the masking ineffective.

Another issue in drug trials has to do with the formulation of the test treatment. Whenever feasible, it should be used in the same form as in normal practice. However, here again some compromises may be necessary. For example, investigators may choose to use capsules for dispensing study medications even though the test drug is normally dispensed in tablet form in order to mask the taste and appearance of the study drugs. Modification in the form or route of administration is acceptable only if it does not affect the bioavailability or pharmacological action of the study drugs.

A key design decision in trials involving two or more treatments that may be used alone or in combination concerns whether a factorial treatment structure should be used (see Glossary for definition). Table 11-1 illustrates use of this design for a two-drug study. Separate placebos for each drug tested are necessary when the test drugs are to be dispensed on different time schedules or in different forms (e.g., capsules for one test drug and tablets for the other test drug). Patients in the cell designated AB would receive both drug A and B, those in cell A$\bar{\text{B}}$ would receive drug A and the placebo for drug B, and so on. A trial involving three different drugs, each administered at a single, fixed-dose level and suitable for use alone or in combination, would involve eight (i.e., 2^3) treatment combinations: ABC, AB$\bar{\text{C}}$, A$\bar{\text{B}}$C, $\bar{\text{A}}$BC, A$\bar{\text{B}}\bar{\text{C}}$, $\bar{\text{A}}\bar{\text{B}}\bar{\text{C}}$, $\bar{\text{A}}\bar{\text{B}}$C, and $\bar{\text{A}}\bar{\text{B}}\bar{\text{C}}$.

The main advantage of a factorial treatment structure lies in the opportunity it provides for estimating both individual and combined treatment effects via the same experiment. A full factorial treatment structure (see Glossary for definition) should be considered whenever there is a reason to suspect additive or synergistic treatment effects. It should not be used with treatments that are incompatible, or where there is no interest in some of the treatment combinations. A partial factorial treatment structure (see Glossary) may be considered in the latter case, as in the Persantine Aspirin Reinfarction Study (PARIS). Persantine was not used alone, because of the high dose level required in the absence of aspirin and because of previous animal work suggesting that the combination of aspirin and.persantine had a more profound effect on blood platelets than either drug alone (Persantine Aspirin Reinfarction Study Group, 1980b). The primary aim of the study was to provide a comparison of the combination of persantine and aspirin against aspirin alone. A secondary aim was to measure the usefulness of this combination against a placebo treatment. This difference in interest is reflected by the fact that the number of patients assigned to the placebo treatment was only half the number assigned to either of the other two treatment groups (Table 11-2).

The methods for administering the treatments and ground rules under which treatments may be altered or stopped should be set down in the treatment protocol. Table 11-3 provides a list of the items that should be included in this document.

The details of the protocol should be subjected to careful review before implementation. Lack of agreement can lead to unacceptable variation in the data collection or treatment process. Establishing standards for data collection and treatment administration is important whenever multiple investigators are involved in a trial, whether they are located in a single clinic or in multiple clinics.

Medical conditions that may require a study physician to depart from the assigned treatment should be detailed. It is also wise to outline side effects that are a normal part of a drug's pharmacological effect. For example, the treatment protocol for the NCGS warned physicians

Table 11-1 Example of a factorial treatment design for a two-drug study

Drug	B	$\bar{\text{B}}$
A	AB	A$\bar{\text{B}}$
$\bar{\text{A}}$	$\bar{\text{A}}$B	$\bar{\text{A}}\bar{\text{B}}$

Table 11-2 Numbers of patients by treatment group in PARIS

Drug	Persantine	Persantine placebo
Aspirin	810	810
Aspirin placebo	0	406

Table 11-3   Major items to be included in the treatment protocol

- Specification of the test and control treatments to be tested and rationale for the choices
- Review of previous research on the safety and efficacy of the proposed treatments
- Description of the methods for administering the test and control treatments
- List of contraindications for the proposed treatments
- Specification of the clinical conditions that may necessitate termination of the assigned treatment
- Specification of side effects that may require termination of the assigned treatment, as well as those that should not
- Methods, in the case of masked drug trials, for packaging and dispensing drugs, including a general outline of the conditions under which the masking may have to be revealed to clinic personnel or to a study patient
- General scheme to be used for assigning patients to the study treatments

against stopping a patient's treatment because of mild diarrhea, since such problems were a recognized side effect of chenodeoxycholic acid therapy and were not considered to be serious (National Cooperative Gallstone Study Group, 1981b).

The conditions under which a treatment assignment is revealed to clinic personnel in a double-masked trial should be specified. As a rule, there are few valid reasons for unmasking assignments during the course of the trial, since the assigned treatments can be terminated without revealing their identity to patients or clinic personnel. For example, provisions for unmasking in the CDP were limited to emergencies involving life-threatening uses of a medication by a patient or a member of his family or when a patient required emergency surgery and the surgical team needed to know his treatment assignment. Patients undergoing elective surgery simply stopped taking their study medicine before the surgery and during the recovery period.

11.5 COMPOSITION OF THE STUDY POPULATION

The formulation of patient selection criteria for the study represents a balance of two opposing forces: one designed to produce a highly homogeneous study population and the other designed to minimize the restrictions on the study population and hence maximize the opportuni-

ties for patient recruitment. On the one hand, the more homogeneous the population, the more precise the study, and hence the smaller the number of patients needed to detect a given difference. On the other hand, the greater the heterogeneity, the broader the basis for generalizing findings at the end of the study. The advantages and disadvantages of different selection strategies are summarized in Table 11-4.

Investigators must agree on selection and exclusion criteria before patient recruitment starts. Often they fail to appreciate the impact the criteria will have on recruitment. Estimates of patient availability made during the design stage of the trial are likely to be unrealistically high unless they are based on actual patient surveys using the proposed criteria. Factors that are not likely to influence outcome should not be used for exclusion, since they do nothing to improve the precision of the trial while they make patient recruitment more difficult. Table 11-5 lists the main selection criteria used in the trials sketched in Appendix B.

Socioeconomic status is usually not a valid basis for patient selection. Neither the scientific nor the lay community is likely to look kindly on such forms of selection. Selection on the basis of ethnic origin, religion, or race should also be

Table 11-4   Advantages and disadvantages of opposing selection strategies

Highly restrictive selection criteria

- **Advantages**
  - Provides more precise comparison of the test and control treatments
  - Results of the trial less likely to be effected by population variability
- **Disadvantages**
  - Increases the cost and time required for patient recruitment
  - Limits the generalizability of the study findings

Minimally restrictive selection criteria

- **Advantages**
  - Makes patient recruitment easier
  - Provides base for wider generalization of findings
- **Disadvantages**
  - May obscure treatment effects because of variability in composition of study population
  - Results of the trial may be confusing, especially if an observed effect appears to be associated with a subgroup of patients in the study and the subgroup is too small to yield a reliable treatment comparison

Table 11-5 Primary selection criteria of trials sketched in Appendix B

Trial	Sex	Age limits on entry	Disease state
AMIS	Both	30–69	Prior MI
CASS	Both	None	Prior MI
CDP	Males	30–64	Prior MI
HDFP	Both	30–69	Diastolic blood pressure ≥95 mm Hg
HPT	Both	25–49	Diastolic blood pressure ≥78 but <90 mm Hg
IRSC	Both	<10	Grade III or IV vesicoureteral reflux
MPS	Both	≥50 for SMD, ≥18 for HISTO, None for INVM	Evidence of neovascularization for all three conditions
MRFIT	Males	35–57	High risk for CHD
NCGS	Both	None	Radiolucent gallstones
PARIS	Both	30–74	Prior MI
PHS	Males	40–75	Absence of MI history
POSCH	Both	30–64	Hypercholesterolemia
UGDP	Both	None	Newly diagnosed diabetes
VACSP 43	Males	None	Evidence of gangrene of either foot

avoided. A possible exception relates to diseases or conditions concentrated primarily, if not exclusively, in individuals of a particular religious, ethnic, or racial background. However, even if one avoids use of such factors, the study population of a clinic may be quite homogeneous with regard to them. The socioeconomic, ethnic, or racial spectrum covered by a study population will be a function of where and how it is recruited. The racial mix of clinics in the UGDP varied from being nearly all white to being nearly all black (University Group Diabetes Program Research Group, 1970e). This variation stands in marked contrast to that observed in the Coronary Artery Surgery Study. The population in that study was virtually all white—a reflection, undoubtedly, of the nature of the patients served by the participating clinics and of the popularity of bypass surgery in white middle-class America (Coronary Artery Surgery Study Research Group, 1981).

Of the 14 trials listed in Table 11-5, 4 used sex as an exclusion. The sex restriction in the CDP was required because estrogen—one of the drugs tested in that trial—was contraindicated for females. The Veterans Administration Cooperative Study Program No. 43 (VACSP 43) and the Physicians' Health Study (PHS) excluded females from enrollment simply because of the small number of females contained in the populations approached for study. The rationale for the restriction in the Multiple Risk Factor Intervention Trial (MRFIT) is less clear. There is no question that even if the trial had been open to females that the majority of enrollees would have been male. However, that fact alone does not provide a sufficient rationale for the exclusion. Valid treatment comparisons can be made so long as the proportionate mix of males and females is the same across study treatments.

Ten of the 14 trials used age as a selection criterion. Generally, practical considerations figured in the limits used. For example, this was the case in the choice of the lower age limit for the Hypertension Prevention Trial (HPT). The original design called for a lower limit of 18. Ultimately, however, the limit was raised to 25 before the study started because problems were anticipated in recruiting and following people aged 18 to 25.

The use of upper age limits, especially in studies involving adult populations, is less easy to justify. CDP investigators arbitrarily imposed an upper limit of 65 primarily as a means of excluding individuals who had experienced their first MI relatively late in life. The limit made recruitment more difficult and in all probability did little to improve the precision of the trial, since there is no reason to believe the study treatments are any more or less effective in individuals over 65 than for those under 65.

11.6   THE PLAN FOR PATIENT ENROLLMENT AND FOLLOW-UP

The study plan should include a description of methods to be used for patient recruitment and an outline of the data collection schedule (see Chapters 12 and 14). Ideally, there should be at least two separate patient contacts before randomization with adequate time between the contacts to:

- Allow clinic staff time to consider the suitability of the patient for study
- Facilitate the identification of "faint of heart" patients
- Allow a staged approach to the informed consent process (see Section 14.6)

The study design should provide for a landmark that when passed marks entry of a patient into the trial (e.g., the point at which the treatment assignment is divulged to clinic personnel). A patient should be counted as part of the study population, regardless of his subsequent course of treatment, once the landmark has been passed.

After enrollment, patients will be required to return for one or more scheduled follow-up visits. The timing of these visits will depend on the data collection requirements of the study. The frequency is usually highest right after the initiation of treatment. The CDP required a clinic visit of each patient at one month and again at two months after enrollment for dosage increases. The next required visit was at four months after enrollment and then every four months thereafter (Coronary Drug Project Research Group, 1973a).

Except in special cases, the frequency of required data collection visits should be the same for all patients. A difference in the visit rates can bias the study results if it influences the rate at which clinical events are diagnosed and reported. This kind of bias was of concern in the Hypertension Detection and Follow-Up Program (HDFP) because of more frequent contacts with patients assigned to stepped-care than with those assigned to usual care (Hypertension Detection and Follow-Up Program Cooperative Group, 1979a).

The possibility of bias is not eliminated by use of identical schedules for required visits if the rate of interim unscheduled visits between scheduled visits is different for the study groups. A differential rate of unscheduled observations can still bias the way in which events are diagnosed and reported in the trial. Most long-term trials keep track of such contacts, if for no other reason than to provide a means of comparing the study groups for differences in contact rates.

The study plan should include provision for some minimal form of follow-up for dropouts (see Glossary for definitions). The follow-up may be for mortality only or for other kinds of outcomes, depending on the trial. See Chapter 15 for more details.

11.7   THE PLAN FOR CLOSE-OUT OF PATIENT FOLLOW-UP

An important design issue concerns disengagement of a patient from the trial when it is finished. Two general models are used for this purpose. One model is characterized by a common closing date for all patients, regardless of the date of enrollment. Another involves close-out after a specified length of follow-up. The latter approach requires as much time for close-out as for enrollment, whereas close-out takes place at the same time for all patients, regardless of when they were enrolled, when the former approach is used (see Section 15.4 for added discussion).

The CDP is an example of a trial using a common close-out date. All patients were separated from the study during June through August of 1974 (Coronary Drug Project Research Group, 1975). The NCGS provides an example of close-out after a specified period of follow-up—two years (National Cooperative Gallstone Study Group, 1981a).

12. Data collection considerations

Investigators seem to have settled for what is measurable instead of measuring what they would really like to know.

Edmund D. Pellegrino

12.1 INTRODUCTION

Decisions regarding the data collection schedule and related forms are among the most important in the trial. They will determine both the amount and quality of data generated in the trial.

There must be adequate time, once the study is funded and before data collection starts, for investigators to agree on the details of the data collection process. They must be concerned first with setting the schedule at which patients are seen, both before and after entry into the trial, and then with outlining the specific items of information to be collected each time the patient is seen. The investigators should allow adequate time after these steps are completed for developing and testing required data forms and for receiving and reacting to suggestions from clinic personnel who must use them.

The form development process should be undertaken by personnel who are experienced in form construction and who are familiar with methods for data collection and data processing in prospective studies. The development of data

119

forms can be facilitated by review of sample forms used in other trials, especially those from trials with design and operating features similar to the one in question. Some of the desired samples can be obtained through the published literature (e.g., see appendixes in Coronary Drug Project Research Group, 1973a, and Coronary Artery Surgery Study Research Group, 1981) or via a central respository (e.g., see National Cooperative Gallstone Study Group, 1981a, for reference to forms placed on file at the National Technical Information Service). Others will have to be obtained by direct request to investigators involved in the trials of interest.

The reference list in Appendix I includes a number of citations pertinent to data collection and the construction of forms. Several of the references are from interview and survey literature but are relevant to clinical trials as well. A classic book by Payne (1951), although focused on opinion polling, is useful reading for anyone involved in data collection. The *Teacher's Word Book of 30,000 Words* (Thorndike and Lorge, 1944) indicates the expected level of comprehension of words as a function of education level. It is a useful resource, especially when forms are being designed for use in patient interviews.

Also included are several textbooks with chapters on forms design (Backstrom and Hursh-César, 1981; Kidder, 1981; Marks, 1982; Sudman and Bradburn, 1983), as well as a number of journal articles. The three articles by Wright and Haybittle (1979a,b,c) and a chapter from a monograph from the Coronary Drug Project (Knatterud et al., 1983) have direct relevance to the field of clinical trials. Papers by Collen and co-workers (1969), Helsing and Comstock (1976), Hochstim and Renne (1971), Holland and co-workers (1966), and Milne and Williamson (1971) deal with data collection via questionnaires. Other papers of interest include those by Barker (1980), Barnard et al. (1979), Bishop et al. (1982), Duncan (1979), Edvardsson (1980), Finney (1981), Layne and Thompson (1981), McFarland (1981), Romm and Hulka (1979), Roth et al. (1980), Schriesheim (1981), Smith (1981), and Zelnio (1980).

12.2   FACTORS INFLUENCING THE CLINIC VISIT SCHEDULE

12.2.1   Introduction

Every clinical trial must provide for data collection at a minimum of two time points: at or just before randomization and the initiation of treatment to provide baseline data, and at least once after randomization for collection of follow-up data. It is possible to collect all the required data for a patient during a single clinic visit if it is possible to collect the necessary baseline data, issue the treatment assignment, administer the treatment, and make the required follow-up observations all on the same day. However, the usual situation is one in which a patient is required to make one, two, or even more visits to the clinic on different days before he or she can be enrolled and assigned to treatment. Thereafter, the patient may need to make a series of return visits, extending over a period of weeks, months, or even years, to receive the assigned treatment and for follow-up data collection.

The discussion throughout this book deals with trials in which data collection is performed on an outpatient basis. If any hospitalization is required, it is assumed to be a small portion of the total time the patient is expected to be under study.

Patient visits that take place before the randomization visit are herein referred to as prerandomization visits. Enrollment into the trial occurs at the randomization visit and is marked by some explicit act (e.g., the opening of the treatment allocation envelope). Thereafter, the patient is a member of the treatment group to which he or she was assigned.

It is conventional to consider data collected at the prerandomization and randomization visits as baseline data and to refer to both types of visits as baseline visits (see Glossary). This convention will be followed in this book. It is reasonable if all data collected at the randomization visit are collected before initiation of treatment. Post-randomization visits include all visits that take place after the randomization visit. All such visits will be referred to as follow-up visits in this book, whether they are done on a scheduled or ad hoc basis.

12.2.2   Baseline clinic visit schedule

Baseline visits (prerandomization and randomization visits) are needed to:

● Determine a patient's eligibility for enrollment
● Provide baseline data for assessing changes occurring after the initiation of treatment
● Explain the purpose of the study to the patient and to obtain consent for participation in the trial
● Issue the treatment assignment

Whenever possible, it is useful to have the patient make at least two visits to the clinic before enrollment. The visits may be only a few days apart, especially when there is an urgent need to initiate treatment, or they may extend over a period of weeks, or even months. The repeat visits make it possible to replicate certain key baseline measurements. A time separation between visits may be needed as well to:

- Perform the necessary screening and diagnostic procedures for determining patient eligibility
- Allow sufficient time for a patient to recover from a procedure performed at one visit and to go through the preparatory steps required for the next clinic visit
- Provide adequate time for the informed consent process
- Allow adequate time for clinic staff to evaluate the data collected on the patient before enrollment

The Coronary Drug Project (CDP) required two prerandomization visits. The first visit was used to make an initial determination of a patient's eligibility for enrollment into the study, to obtain serum for lipid and other determinations, to perform a general physical examination, and to provide the patient with a preliminary explanation of the study. The second visit, scheduled approximately 1 month after the first visit, was used to assess a prospective patient's adherence to the prerandomization treatment schedule,[1] to obtain additional serum for a repeat set of laboratory determinations, and to obtain the patient's signed consent to participate in the trial. The randomization visit, scheduled approximately 1 month after the second prerandomization visit, was used for a final asessment of the patient's suitability for enrollment into the trial, including a further assessment of his adherence to the assigned medication schedule, and verification that the patient was indeed willing to be randomized. If so, the treatment allocation envelope was opened and the assigned treatment was initiated (Coronary Drug Project Research Group, 1973a).

Required diagnostic and data collection procedures should be designed to minimize patient inconvenience and exposure to unnecessary procedures, particularly those entailing risks to the patient. Hence, whenever feasible, the simplest procedures with the least risk should be performed first so that patients who then prove to be ineligible can be spared the inconvenience (and risks, if any) of the more complex and time-consuming procedures.

12.2.3 Follow-up clinic visit schedule

A follow-up visit is any visit, either required or nonrequired, to the study clinic by a patient who has been enrolled into the trial (i.e., assigned to treatment) that takes place after the randomization visit. Required visits should be specified in the study protocol and should be scheduled to take place at specified time points after the randomization visit. They are herein variously referred to as scheduled follow-up visits, required follow-up visits, or, in contexts where the meaning is clear, simply as follow-up visits. Visits of this class are needed to:

- Carry out procedures specified in the study protocol, including those for treatment administration and treatment adjustment
- Evaluate the patient's response to treatment
- Assess patient and physician adherence to the assigned treatment
- Collect information on the treatment process and outcome and related data needed for evaluation of the treatments

The timetable for required follow-up visits will be dictated by various factors, including:

- Requirements for treatment administration and for assessing adherence to treatment
- Rate of occurrence of the outcome(s) of interest
- Patient health care needs
- Cost of a patient visit
- Patient convenience considerations

The schedule for required follow-up visits may be designed to allow for more frequent visits immediately after enrollment of a patient into the trial to permit clinic personnel to initiate and administer the assigned treatment. The interval between visits may be increased to some maximum and held constant thereafter once the initial treatment process is completed.

Follow-up visits that are made on an ad hoc basis because of special problems experienced by the study patients after enrollment into the trial will be variously referred to as unscheduled follow-up visits, nonrequired follow-up visits, or interim follow-up visits.

---

1. Patients considered eligible for enrollment into the CDP at the end of the first prerandomization visit were given a single-masked placebo medication (three capsules per day) which they were to take until the randomization visit.

Investigators should construct the data collection schedule so as to be able to distinguish between required and nonrequired follow-up visits. The data system should be designed to yield a count of both types of visits. Differences among the treatment groups in the number of interim follow-up visits can lead to biases in the diagnoses and reports of clinical events used to evaluate the study treatments (see Section 11.6 and Question 68 of Chapter 19 for further discussion).

12.2.4   Visit time limits

Ideally, the entire set of scheduled baseline and follow-up visits for a patient should be done at precise time points relative to the time of randomization. However, such precision is generally not possible in a free-living population, nor is it necessary for most of the observations required in the typical clinical trial. The usual approach is to consider a visit and related data collection as valid if the visit took place within a defined interval on either side of the desired time point. The permissible length of this time window (see Glossary) will depend on the number of required data collection visits and on the amount of variation that can be tolerated in the timing of observations.

The CDP allowed a maximum of 4 months for completion of the three baseline examinations. After enrollment, the patient was required to return to the clinic 1 month after randomization and again at 2 months after randomization for scheduled dosage increases in his assigned medication. Regular follow-up visits were scheduled to take place at 4-month intervals thereafter. Each of these visits had to be within 2 months of the preferred date, as dictated by the date of randomization. Visits not carried out within the time window were counted as missed. The coordinating center for the study provided clinics with computer-generated appointment schedules that indicated the preferred date and the permissible time window for each required follow-up visit (Table 12–1).

12.3   DATA REQUIREMENTS BY TYPE OF VISIT

12.3.1   General considerations

The development of data forms cannot be started until:

- A baseline and follow-up visit schedule has been established by the study investigators

- The purpose(s) of each visit has been outlined
- There is general agreement among the investigators on the specific procedures to be carried out at each visit

A key step in form construction is identification of the specific items of information to be collected during each clinic visit. The process required for the step should be designed to guard against errors of omission as well as errors of commission (see Table 12–2 for a list of precautions). Probably the single most common cause of errors of omission is haste in the development of the data forms. The process of identifying required data items and then constructing and testing them takes time and patience. Efforts to shorten this process in order to get started with patient recruitment and data collection are usually unwise.

The desire to create forms that, in addition to meeting the research aims of the study, provide data needed for routine patient care is probably the single most important contributor to errors of commission. The fact that certain measurements need to be made in providing routine care for patients is not sufficient reason to justify inclusion of them in the study data system.

Before starting form construction, the types of data needed and the procedures for generating them should be outlined. Once developed, the outline should be reviewed by personnel not directly involved in constructing the data forms as a check against the two kinds of errors mentioned above. Further, there should be general agreement on the ordering of the procedures to be performed at any given data collection visit before the forms are constructed. The ordering will influence the sequencing of items on the forms.

One of the last steps in the construction process is to carry out an item-by-item review of each form against a list of data needs and goals, as set down by the leadership of the study. Data items that cannot be justified in this review should be deleted from the final data forms. All follow-up forms should also be checked against each other and against the baseline set of forms for consistency and as a safeguard against errors of omission.

12.3.2   Data needed at baseline visits

The first step in the design of any set of forms is to enumerate the types of data needed (see Section 12.2.2). Baseline data are needed:

Table 12-1 Sample appointment schedule and permissible time windows, as adapted from the Coronary Drug Project

Patient Name: John D. Doe   Patient ID No.: 59–0021
Date of entry: Oct. 31, 1966
Bottle number assigned: 2

The indicated visits should be done within the time windows specified and as close to the desired date as possible. Visits not completed within the sepcified time window should be skipped and will be counted as missed.

Visit	Desired date	First possible date	Last possible date	Interval length in days
Dosage adj. Visit 1	Dec. 1,66	Nov. 16,66	Dec. 16,66	31
Dosage adj. Visit 2	Dec. 31,66	Dec. 17,66	Jan. 15,67	30
Follow-up visit 1	Mar. 2,67	Jan. 16,67	May 1,67	106
Follow-up visit 2	July 1,67	May 2,67	Aug. 31,67	122
Follow-up visit 3	Oct. 31,67	Sep. 1,67	Dec. 31,67	122
Follow-up visit 4	Mar. 2,68	Jan. 1,68	May 1,68	122
Follow-up visit 5	July 1,68	May 2,68	Aug. 31,68	122
Follow-up visit 6	Oct. 31,68	Sep. 1,68	Dec. 31,68	122
Follow-up visit 7	Mar. 2,69	Jan. 1,69	May 1,69	121
Follow-up visit 8	July 1,69	May 2,69	Aug. 31,69	122
Follow-up visit 9	Oct. 31,69	Sep. 1,69	Dec. 31,69	122
Follow-up visit 10	Mar. 2,70	Jan. 1,70	May 1,70	121
Follow-up visit 11	July 1,70	May 2,70	Aug. 31,70	122
Follow-up visit 12	Oct. 31,70	Sep. 1,70	Dec. 31,70	122
Follow-up visit 13	Mar. 2,71	Jan. 1,71	May 1,71	121
Follow-up visit 14	July 1,71	May 2,71	Aug. 31,71	122
Follow-up visit 15	Oct. 31,71	Sep. 1,71	Dec. 31,71	122

Source: Reference citation 104. Adapted with permission of the American Heart Association, Inc., Dallas, Texas.

- To establish patient eligibility through items that indicate the presence of required eligibility conditions and the absence of exclusion conditions
- To characterize the demographic and general health characteristics of patients eligible for enrollment into the trial
- To establish a baseline for assessment of changes in variables to be measured over the course of follow-up
- For any stratification required in the randomization process
- For post-stratification
- To aid in contacting and tracing patients
- To assess clinic performance in carrying out the informed consent process
- To assess adherence to the study protocol
- To link baseline and follow-up records
- To address other topics unique to the study in question

The second step is to list the specific data items and forms needed for each visit. Some items will appear only once in the list; others will appear under several categories.

The need for record linkage can usually be satisfied by use of a unique number that identifies the patient and type of visit performed. The data needed for stratification will be satisfied by collection of information necessary for making the classifications called for in the stratification. Variables that are to be tracked over time must be observed during the prerandomization or randomization visit to provide the necessary baseline information. The same is true for variables that are to be used in risk-factor or subgroup analyses to be carried out later on in the trial. Investigators must have a thorough knowledge of the epidemiology of the disease being treated and of the conditions likely to influence the selected outcome measures to make an intelligent choice of baseline variables for use in such analyses.

Table 12-2 Methods for avoiding errors of omission and commission in the data form construction process

A. Safeguards against errors of omission

- Allow adequate time for developing and testing data forms before starting data collection
- Solicit content advice and input from persons not directly involved in the development process
- Review data forms used in similar trials
- Ask persons not directly involved in the developmental process to review proposed data forms for deficiencies
- Test data forms under actual study conditions before use in the study

B. Safeguards against errors of commission

- Distinguish between data needed for patient care and those needed to address the objectives of the trial
- Make certain every data item scheduled for collection is of direct relevance to achieving a stated aim or objective of the trial
- Establish an appropriate set of review and approval procedures in order for new items to be added to existing data forms

12.3.3 Data needed at follow-up visits

Data collected during follow-up are needed to:

- Assess changes in variables that are or may be affected by treatment
- Characterize the nature of treatment over the course of follow-up
- Characterize departures from the treatment protocol and the reasons for them
- Characterize patient adherence to the assigned treatment(s)
- Characterize the nature of treatment effects observed, including side effects and patient complaints related to treatment or believed to be related to treatment
- Characterize the state of a patient's health and quality of life
- Maintain up-to-date patient locator information
- Assess adherence of clinic staff to required procedures, as set down in the study protocol
- Link baseline and follow-up records obtained on the same patient
- Address other topics unique to the study in question

The same process as outlined for baseline forms should be used to construct the follow-up forms. It should begin with an enumeration of items related to the above categories. It is wise to identify all the variables on the baseline set of forms that are to be updated at one or more follow-up visits before starting construction of the follow-up forms. Once this is done, it is necessary to indicate the visit or visits at which specified variables are to be observed.

A series of items will be required to provide data on treatment administration. Trials involving technically complicated treatment procedures, such as in some surgical trials, may require an entire set of forms for characterizing the treatment process.

The follow-up data system must also provide information on treatment compliance and on the amount of exposure a patient has had to competing treatments. The latter information is needed to characterize the extent of cross-treatment contamination present in the various treatment groups when the results of the trial are analyzed. The follow-up forms must also include items for recording real or imagined treatment side effects reported by the study patients. A thorough knowledge of the treatments being tested and of pertinent medical literature is needed to formulate suitable items.

A category of major interest in some trials (e.g., cancer chemotherapy trials) concerns the effect of treatment on a patient's quality of life. The outcome measure, whether it be death or some nonfatal clinical event, may be only part of what is needed for treatment assessment. A test treatment, even if known to prolong life, may be rejected by patients because of its noxious side effects. Information on changes in a patient's employment status, recreational activities, exercise habits, ability to care for himself, etc., will be needed if quality of life measures are to be used in evaluating the study treatments.

12.4 CONSIDERATIONS AFFECTING ITEM CONSTRUCTION

12.4.1 Implicit versus explicit item form

A key consideration in item construction has to do with wording of the items and whether they are stated in explicit or implicit terms. Examples of the two forms are given below.

Explicit item form

What is your present age? ___ ___

Age in
Years

What is your birthdate? ___ ___ – ___ ___ – ___ ___
Mo   Day   Yr

Implicit item form

Age . . . . ___ ___

Birthdate ___ ___ – ___ ___ – ___ ___
Mo   Day   Yr

The wording chosen will depend upon the nature of the information being collected and on the level of sophistication of the person responsible for completing the items. An explicit form is needed when the wording of an item can effect the information to be obtained. Survey researchers have long recognized the importance of standardized wording for questions when the information is collected via an interview.

An implicit form may be satisfactory for items completed by clinic personnel. However, even in this case, care must be taken to make certain the item is constructed so as to avoid misinterpretation among staff responsible for completing the item.

12.4.2 Interviewer-completed versus patient-completed items

The data forms may be designed to be completed by clinic staff or by the patients themselves. Most of the forms will be completed by clinic personnel in a clinical trial. Hence, the remainder of this chapter and Appendix F is written from this point of view. However, many of the same points outlined in Sections 12.5 and 12.6 apply to forms completed by patients as well.

Items used as a reminder to clinic personnel to obtain certain information should be distinguished from those that are to be read or presented to the patient exactly as they appear on the form. The Hypertension Prevention Trial (HPT) preceded all items of the latter type by letter codes of AAW—Ask-as-Written—or SAW—Show-as-Written (see examples below). Items that had a long list of possible answers or were considered too complicated to comprehend via a verbal presentation were presented in the SAW fashion using specially prepared flashcards. The participant selected his response from among those listed on the card, either by point-ing to the proper line on the card or by reading his reply from the card.

Example of Ask-as-Written item

(*AAW*) *Are you presently taking vitamins or minerals regularly?*

( ) ( )
Yes No

Example of Show-as-Written item

(SAW) Have you taken any of the following drugs in the last month? (Use HPT Flashcard 04 and check as many as apply)

( )   Anacin
( )   Appedrine
( )   Bromoquinine
( )   Coryban D
( )   Dexatrim
( )   Dristan
( )   Excedrin
( )   Midol
( )   Nodoz
( )   Permathene-12
( )   Prolamine
( )   Triaminicin
( )   Vanquish

The SAW approach can be useful in the collection of sensitive information involving personal income, sexual behavior, or the like. A patient may be more willing to indicate his reply by pointing to the appropriate reply or by referring to a letter or number code on a flashcard than to answer the question verbally. Other techniques have been developed for collection of sensitive information. A particularly interesting one involves a "random response" technique. The technique is not discussed herein, but descriptions and illustrations of it can be found in papers by Bégin et al. (1979), Bégin and Boivin (1980), Frenette and Bégin (1979), Himmelfarb and Edgell (1980), Martin and Newman (1982), and Zdep et al. (1979).

12.4.3 Questioning strategy

The designers of the data forms must decide where general, nondirective, questions are to be used to elicit subjective information and where more specific, directive ones are to be used. Clearly, the type and amount of information obtained can be influenced by the questioning strategy used. For example, the number of patients reporting gastrointestinal distress in an aspirin study can be expected to be higher if the count is based on responses to a specific question concerning such problems (e.g., Have you had any gastrointestinal distress since you started treatment?), as opposed to a general question (e.g., Have you had any problems since you started treatment?). The two strategies may be used in tandem in situations in which it is appropriate to begin an area of inquiry with a general question followed by one or more that are specific and direct.

12.4.4   Single versus multiple-use forms

The organization and content of the forms will be influenced by whether they are designed to be completed over a series of clinic visits or at a single visit. Multivisit forms are more efficient to use in that there are fewer forms to complete and process than is the case with single-visit forms. Further, since there is some administrative overhead associated with the completion and processing of any form, the fewer the forms, the lower the total overhead.

A disadvantage with multivisit forms is the time and inconvenience involved in filing and retrieving partially completed forms. Further, their use can slow the flow of information in the study since a form cannot be sent to the data center until it is complete. The delay can be lengthy if the visits to be covered are widely separated in time. Hence, if they are used at all, their use should be limited to sets of visits that are completed over short time intervals.

Data generated at different sites, whether within or outside the clinic, even if part of the same visit, should be recorded on separate forms. This is particularly true for forms used to record results of procedures or measurements that are done by personnel who are not under the direct control of the study clinic and that cannot be provided on the day of the patient's visit to the clinic (e.g., as is usually the case with most laboratory determinations and with expert readings of biopsy materials, coronary angiograms, ECGs, eye fundus photographs, and the like). The only exceptions are those in which the data in question flow back to the study clinic within a day or two of the patient's clinic visit.

12.4.5   Format and layout

Decisions need to be made regarding the general format and layout of the data forms. Issues to be

addressed include (see Section 12.6 for discussion):

- Full-page versus multicolumn layout
- Paper size, quality, and color
- Use of boxes, parentheses, or lines for recording responses to designated items
- Location of check spaces for responses
- Printed versus photocopied forms

12.5   ITEM CONSTRUCTION

This section and the next contain a series of detailed comments and suggestions concerning item and form construction. Many of the points are supported with illustrations contained in Appendix F.

12.5.1   General

1. Every item and item subpart should have a unique identifying number (Appendix F.1).
2. Items should always be constructed to require a response, regardless of whether a condition is present or absent. The practice of allowing a blank or unanswered item to indicate the absence of a condition can cause confusion. Once the form is completed there is no way to distinguish between items purposely left blank because the condition in question was not present from those accidentally left blank (Appendix F.2).
3. The conditions under which an item is to be skipped should be part of the item or should be included in the instructions for the item (Appendix F.2.4).
4. Items or sections on a form that may be skipped in certain instances should be preceded by items that document the legitimacy of the skip. For example, a form should include an item for recording the patient's age if parts of the form are to be skipped for patients in a specific age range.

12.5.2   Language and terminology

5. Use simple, uncomplicated language.
6. Avoid the use of esoteric terms and abbreviations. This is especially important in situations where there is likely to be a turnover in the personnel responsible for completion of the study forms, or in multicenter trials where the level of staff familiarity with the study forms may vary.

7. Avoid the use of terms that may have different meanings to the different people involved in completing the forms.

8. Provide necessary definitions on the forms or indicate where they may be found.

9. Use simple sentences in the construction of items and instructional materials. Phraseology should be consistent with the educational level of the individuals responsible for completion of the forms.

10. Avoid unnecessary words (Appendix F.3).

11. Avoid the use of double negatives (Appendix F.4).

12. Avoid the use of compound questions by dividing them into a series of specific questions (Appendix F.5).

13. Items requiring a comparative judgment should indicate the basis for the comparison (Appendix F.6).

14. Language research suggests that positive terms, such as better, bigger, or more, are less subject to interpretation error than negative terms, such as worse, small, or less (Wright and Haybittle, 1979a) (Appendix F.6.3).

15. Items requiring an affirmative or negative response are confusing when an affirmative reply indicates the absence of a condition (Appendix F.7).

16. For the same reason as indicated in 15, questions concerning disease state or history are easier to understand if stated in a way which requires a yes or positive reply when the condition is present, rather than when it is absent (Appendix F.8).

17. The time point or interval to be used in answering an item should be explicitly stated in the item. A time point may be defined by a specified date, by some event or condition, or simply as the "present." A time interval may be defined by two calendar dates or from some date to the present (Appendix F.9).

18. Variation in the direction of response from question to question (e.g., stating some questions that require a comparative assessment in positive terms and others in negative terms) should be avoided (Appendix F.10).

19. Avoid leading questions (Appendix F.11).

12.5.3 Use of items from other studies

The item construction process can be facilitated by a review of existing forms from related studies. The review may help identify data items that should be included on the data forms as well as aid in their construction and format.

20. Assemble sets of forms from other related studies and order by topic (e.g., smoking history, exercise habits, disease history, and so on).

21. Do not use an item *simply* because it has been used before in other studies.

22. Do not construct an item de novo if a suitable version of the item already exists, has been used in other studies, and has seemingly produced reliable information.

23. Do not modify the wording of an item taken from another study if the item has been shown to produce useful information and if information generated from it is to be compared with findings from studies in which the item was used.

24. Do not use an entire form or section of a form that has been copyrighted without the written approval of the copyright holder.

25. Do not reproduce an entire form or section of a form used in another study without permission from the study, even if the form is not copyrighted.

12.5.4 Closed- versus open-form items

A closed-form item is one that is completed using a defined list of permissible responses. An open-form item is characterized by the absence of a defined list of permissible response options.

Closed-form examples

Indicate the highest grade completed in school:

( ) 6th grade or less
( ) 7th, 8th, or 9th grade
( ) 10th or 11th grade
( ) 12th grade
( ) 2 or 3 years of college
( ) 4 years of college
( ) 5 or more years of college

Have you had any of the following diseases or conditions diagnosed in the last year? (check all that apply)

( ) Heart attack
( ) Stroke
( ) Congestive heart failure
( ) Emphysema
( ) Cancer
( ) None of the above

Open-form examples

What is the highest grade you have completed in school?

_____

Use the space below to list serious illnesses that you have had. (Enter "none" if you have never had a serious illness.)

_____

_____

26. An open-form item should be used when it is difficult to anticipate the different responses that may be given, or when there is a desire to avoid leading the respondent by indicating permissible replies.

27. An open-form item should be used to record continuous data, unless a closed form, with designated categories, is considered to provide adequate detail (see Section 12.4.2). An open form should be used even if data are to be subsequently tabulated into designated categories (e.g., age <25, 25–49, and ≥50). The opportunity to categorize in different ways is lost whenever continuous data are collected and recorded in categorical form.

28. Closed-form items, with a predefined list of response options, should be used when there is a need to structure the responses obtained (e.g., when it is desired to present the respondent with all possible options when answering a question or when it is desirable to remind him of the permissible response options).

29. The time required to code and process information from open-form items is usually greater than for closed-form items.

30. A closed-form item will do little to facilitate coding and processing if most of the responses fall into a general catchall category, such as the "other (specify)" category, included at the end of the response list.

12.5.5   Response checklist

A response checklist defines the permissible or acceptable responses to an item. The simplest checklist is one for items requiring a binary response, such as yes or no, present or absent, or the like. This list should cover all possible responses and may be constructed to allow only one response or multiple responses, depending on the item.

31. A response checklist is preferable to an unformatted written reply, except as indicated in Section 12.5.4. An item involving a long list of possible response options (see Section 12.4.2 for flashcard alternative) will require more space for layout than an item designed to elicit an unformatted written reply, but the information generated will be easier to process and interpret than is the case with an unformatted written reply.

32. Vertical checklists are easier to use and are subject to less confusion with regard to the location of appropriate check spaces than are horizontal checklists (Appendix F.12).

33. A response checklist that is not exhaustive should include an "other" category that can be used to record responses not covered in the list.

34. There should be adequate space on the form for respondents to write out responses that fall into the catchall category. The space provided will influence the amount and legibility of the information recorded.

35. Frequent use of a catchall category for an item increases the time required for completion of the item and for coding and processing the information generated by it (assuming the written responses are to be coded and processed).

36. It may be wise or necessary to expand the list of permissible response options for an item during the trial. Any expansion should be based on a review of the responses provided in the catchall category and should be done as soon after the start of data collection as is feasible. Expansion may not be practical in short-term trials or in situations in which it can be expected to cause major coding or analysis problems.

37. A condition is more likely to be recorded as present if it appears in a checklist than if it does not. Hence, list expansions during the trial may appear to "increase" the prevalence of certain conditions. However, the expansion will not influence treatment comparisons unless the changes were implemented at different times for the various treatment groups under study.

38. It is sometimes convenient to include a summary check position at the head or end of a list that may be used in lieu of checking each individual entry for the list (see Appendix F.12.2.4 for example).

12.5.6 *Unknown, don't know,* and *uncertain* as response options

39. The three options are interrelated and are to a large extent used as if they were interchangeable. The particular option listed will depend on the context of the question.
40. The operational implications are about the same. All three options imply the lack of information needed to answer a question.
41. *Don't know* or *uncertain* should not be listed as a response option if the aim of the item is to require the respondent to record his best guess even if he does not know or is uncertain regarding the accuracy of his reply. The form should have written instructions when guesses are required.

12.5.7 Measurement and Calculation items

A measurement item is one that requires the respondent to record some measurement. A calculation item is one that requires the respondent to carry out an arithmetic calculation using other information on the form. The examples that follow are taken from the HPT.

Height and weight measurement and calculation example

Height (shoes off): ___ ___
inches

Weight (outdoor garments and shoes off): ___ ___ ___
lbs

Q.I. = Wt/Ht²   0. ___ ___ ___ ___   *lbs/in²*

Blood pressure measurement and calculation example

	BP in mm Hg	
	SBP	*DBP*
1st RZ BP		
a. Reading	___ ___ ___	___ ___ ___
b. Zero value	___ ___	___ ___
c. a−b	___ ___ ___	___ ___ ___
2nd RZ BP		
d. Reading	___ ___ ___	___ ___ ___
e. Zero value	___ ___	___ ___
f. d−e	___ ___ ___	___ ___ ___
Average RZ BP		
g. Sum (c + f)	___ ___ ___	___ ___ ___
h. Avg (g ÷ 2)	___ ___ ___	___ ___ ___

42. The unit of measurement should be specified on the form (Appendix F.13).
43. Measurements should be made and recorded in units familiar to the personnel responsible for making them. Use of an unconventional unit may lead to data collection and recording errors (Appendix F.13.4)
44. Whenever feasible, all recordings of a specified variable should be made using the same unit. Use of different units may occur when different laboratories are used (e.g., as in a multicenter trial in which each clinic relies on its own laboratory for making required laboratory determinations).
45. Space should be provided on the form for the respondent to indicate the unit of measurement when it is not practical to specify the unit in advance (Appendix F.13.2.2, F.13.2.3).
46. Continuous variables, such as age, blood pressure, laboratory values, and the like, should not be recorded in categorical form (see statement 27).
47. The precision required for a measurement should be specified on the data form (Appendix F.14).
48. The amount of precision required for a measurement should not exceed the error involved in making the measurement (see comment regarding item F.14.1 in Appendix F).
49. The raw data used to make any summary calculations should be recorded on the form.
50. Data forms should be constructed to minimize the number of arithmetic calculations required during a patient visit. All calculations except those needed to perform a patient examination or to carry out some other treatment or data collection function during the examination should be performed at the data center as part of the data entry and analysis processes.
51. Calculations needed on data forms made by clinic staff, even relatively simple ones, should be made using a pocket calculator or a computer.
52. Items requiring a series of arithmetic operations during completion of a data form should be arranged in a format that facilitates those operations. For example, numbers that must be added or subtracted should be arranged vertically and with adequate space for recording intermediate calculations (Appendix F.15).

53. Arrange the calculations for a given item in a single unbroken column, if possible. Avoid arrangements in which calculations are started on one column of a form and continued on the next column or page.

12.5.8 Instruction items

An instruction item is one that is included on a form to instruct the individual completing the form as to how to deal with a given question. The two types of instruction items discussed are STOP and SKIP items (Appendix F.16).

54. A STOP item is used to indicate conditions that, when encountered during the course of a patient visit, require clinic personnel to temporarily or permanently halt some procedure or process. The stop will be permanent unless the conditions that require the stop can be removed.
55. STOP items on any given form should be arranged to allow the respondent to terminate all work on the form as soon as a stop is checked. This requires an arrangement in which essential information, required on all patients, is obtained before any stops are allowed.
56. A common use of STOP items during the prerandomization series of clinic visits is to indicate conditions that exclude a patient from enrollment into the trial. Stops of this sort will halt further work-up of the patient.
57. It is wise to arrange prerandomization stops for procedures in ascending order with regard to the risk or general discomfort they entail for patients. The goal should be to carry out the lowest risk, least expensive, most productive procedures first.
58. A SKIP item may be used whenever there is an item or series of items on a form that can be skipped depending on the answer to the item.
59. A SKIP item should indicate the conditions under which the skip can occur and the item or items to be skipped.

12.5.9 Time and date items

A time item is one that requires the respondent to record the actual clock time at which some step, procedure, or measurement was carried out.

A date item is one that indicates the date some step, procedure, or measurement was carried out (see items in Section F.13.1 of Appendix F for examples).

60. Items requiring a clock time should indicate whether the time recordings are for A.M. or P.M. if a 12-hour recording system is used. The use of A.M. and P.M. will cause confusion for recording 12 noon and 12 midnight, unless instructions given on the form indicate how these times are to be recorded.
61. Times should not be recorded on a 24-hour basis unless personnel responsible for the recordings are thoroughly familiar with 24-hour timing schemes or the readings are made directly from 24-hour clocks.
62. The order to be used in recording the date should be specified on the form (e.g., see items in Section F.13.1 in Appendix F). The two most common conventions are:

> Month, Day, Year
> Day, Month, Year

63. Failure to specify the convention to be used dates if they are recorded in digital form. For example 1-9-82, could be read as January 9, 1982, or 1 September 1982, depending on the convention used.

12.5.10 Birthdate and age items

64. The baseline data forms should include both an age and birthdate item if age is to be used either as an eligibility condition for enrollment into the trial or in subsequent data analyses.
65. Date of birth is a key piece of information in many trials. It may be needed for making accurate age calculations or for record search and linkage operations in the follow-up of dropouts for mortality via the National Death Index and other similar files. Birthdate may also be useful in linking different records for the same individual if name is not collected.
66. A patient's reported age should be checked against his reported birthdate on entry into the trial, as illustrated in Appendix F.17. This is particularly important if age is used as an eligibility condition. Discrepancies should be resolved.
67. The age that is reported may differ depending on the source it is taken from. For

example, insurance companies consider a person to have attained the next year of age one-half year beyond his last birthday anniversary, whereas a person reporting his age will give it as of his last birthday anniversary.

12.5.11 Identifying items

Every data form should contain space for recording the patient's ID number and name (or name code). Once these two items have been entered into the data system, a cross-check should be made on all new data to be entered. Information from a form should not be added to the data system if the ID number and name (or name code) do not agree. See Section 12.6.9 for further comments.

68. It is wise to construct a name code, made up of some combination of letters from the patient's first, middle, and last name, for use as a patient identifier. This identifier is in addition to ID number and should not be changed once it has been issued, even if the patient has a subsequent name change. The name code may be used in addition to name or in place of it depending on whether the study forms are designed to preclude collection of name.

69. Each follow-up data form should include an item for recording visit number. The number is typically checked against the patient's appointment schedule (see Table 12-1 for example) to determine if the visit occurred within the permissible time window.

70. Patient identifiers useful for mortality follow-up include:

- Social Security number
- Date of birth
- Place of birth
- Father's name
- Mother's maiden name
- Patient's maiden name for females
- Date and place of death (if applicable)

71. A unique identifier should be assigned to each member of the clinic staff involved in data collection. This number may be used in place of name or initials (or in combination with name) to identify the individual responsible for completing or reviewing a form, or a series of items on a form.

12.5.12 Tracer items

A tracer item is one that is used to obtain information needed to locate a patient. In some cases the information provided by such items is used to locate and recontact a patient who has dropped out of the study to try to persuade him to return to the clinic for examination and subsequent follow-up. In other instances the items are used to facilitate the collection of mortality or morbidity data.

72. Tracer data should be collected on all patients upon entry into the trial and should be updated at periodic intervals over the course of the trial.

73. Useful patient tracer data include:

- Current address and telephone number (home and work if patient has both)
- Employer's name, address, and telephone number
- Name, address, and telephone number of a close relative
- Name, address, and telephone number of a friend or neighbor
- Name and address of patient's private physician

74. Other tracer items, especially for mortality follow-up, are listed in Section 12.5.11, Statement 70.

12.5.13 Reminder and documentation items

A reminder item is one that is intended to remind clinic personnel to perform an indicated procedure or task (Appendix F.18.1). A documentation item is one that is used to indicate that a step or condition required in the data collection, enrollment, treatment, or follow-up process has been performed (Appendix F.18.2).

75. Reminder items are useful in trials with complicated data collection schemes, or in which there is a good chance that some of the personnel involved in data collection will be unfamiliar with details of the data collection protocol.

76. Reminder items should be used in conjunction with steps or procedures that are essential to the data collection, enrollment, treatment, and follow-up processes.

77. Key data items that are to be completed by a designated individual should be followed by documentation items for recording the

date the items were completed and the name or certification number of the individual who was responsible for their completion.

78. There should be space at the end of each form to record the date the form was completed.

79. Documentation items should be included at the end of each form for recording the name or certification number of the person responsible for review of information on the form and for recording the date of the review (Appendix F.18.2).

12.6 LAYOUT AND FORMAT CONSIDERATIONS

12.6.1 Page layout

80. Choose a layout that permits use of a single page size for all forms (e.g., $8\frac{1}{2}'' \times 11''$).

81. Use a layout in which all pages within a form are oriented in the same way. That is, with pages laid out either portrait style (i.e., with lines of print running across the short axis of the page) or landscape style (i.e., with lines running across the long axis of the page).

82. If possible, use the same page orientation for all forms of a given type (e.g., all those used at the clinic for follow-up data collection).

83. Use a layout that is uncluttered and that facilitates use of the forms by both clinic and data processing personnel.

84. Choose between a full page or two-column layout (Appendix F.19).

85. Generally, two-column layouts are more space efficient than full page layouts.

86. The layout chosen should be compatible with the data entry needs of the study; clinic needs should take precedence over those for data entry if meeting both needs leads to conflicting layout requirements.

87. Avoid a layout such as that displayed in Appendix F.19.1.1, where check spaces are scattered over the page. The layout increases the time required to complete and key a form and may contribute to errors in those processes as well.

88. Use layouts such as those illustrated in Appendix F.19.1.2 and F.19.2. Standardizing the location of check positions within and across forms facilitates completion of the forms and reduces the time and errors involved in keying data from them.

89. Whenever feasible, choose a layout that facilitates entry of data directly from the form, such as illustrated in Appendix F.19.2.

90. Items should be arranged so as to minimize the number that are split across columns or pages of a form.

91. The pages of a form should be printed or typed on only one side. The reverse side of the pages may be used to print instructional material or should be left blank.

92. Page layout should be designed to help respondents identify items or sections of a form that are to be skipped under specified conditions. This may be done by setting key words or phrases in boldface type or by use of special instructions or other aids to direct the respondent to applicable items or sections (Appendix F.20).

93. The space between subparts of an item should be less than the space between items.

94. The space separating items should be uniform unless variation in spacing has operational significance.

95. Similarly, the space separating one part or section of a form from another should be the same and should be greater than the space separating individual items.

96. Right-hand justification of typed or printed text should be avoided if it results in noticeable variation in the spacing between words.

12.6.2 Paper size and weight

97. Use a good quality paper with enough gloss to avoid bleeding through from ink or felt pens.

98. Use the same size paper for all forms (see statements 80, 81, and 82).

99. A paper size of $8\frac{1}{2}'' \times 11''$ is preferable to other sizes, especially when forms are to be photocopied and filed using standard office equipment.

12.6.3 Type style and form reproduction

100. The print or type font used should be large and crisp enough to allow for image degradation when forms are photocopied.

101. Use a print or type font at least the size of newsprint.

102. Avoid capitalization of long phrases or sentences. Text written in capital letters is more difficult to read than a mixture of upper- and lower-case letters (Wright and Haybittle, 1979b).
103. Use a different print or type font for emphasizing specific words, phrases, and headings and for distinguishing instructional material from data collection items (e.g., see items F.21.1 in Appendix F).
104. Printed forms are generally easier to read and are esthetically more pleasing than typewritten forms.
105. Consideration should be given to printing forms that are to be used in large numbers or that are difficult to photocopy because of their size or the way in which they are assembled. Forms should not be printed until they have been thoroughly tested and are no longer subject to revision. It may be less costly to photocopy forms that are used in small numbers. The same may be true for forms used in relatively large numbers if they are likely to undergo changes. Forms may be photo-reproduced from either typed or professionally printed masters.

12.6.4 Location of instructional material

106. Instructional material on the first page of the form should indicate when the form is to be used and who is responsible for completing it (Appendix F.21.2.1).
107. Instructional material relating to specific items or sections of a form should be located next to those items or sections (Appendix F.21.2.2).
108. All instructions needed for completion of a form should be included on the form. This is especially important in long-term trials in which personnel may change over the course of the trial, and in multicenter trials.
109. All instructional material should be as concise and simple as possible.
110. Instructional material should be identified by use of a special type font or in some other way (Appendix F.21).
111. Instructional material that is too extensive for inclusion next to the item or section to which it pertains should be contained in a separate booklet or should appear on the back side of the page adjacent to the one in question.

112. Key definitions needed for completion of an item should appear on the form.
113. The instructions should identify items that are to be read verbatim to the patient, as discussed in Section 12.4.2.
114. Items with a list of permissible responses that are not mutually exclusive should contain an instruction to indicate whether or not the respondent may check more than one response.
115. Items which include *unknown, don't know,* or *uncertain* as response options should include instructional notes to indicate if any special procedures are required before these categories are checked (e.g., an instruction to remind clinic staff to check specific medical records before checking the uncertain category for a designated item).
116. The instructions should indicate the steps to be followed in performing a particular measurement or procedure. Reference to the appropriate section of the study handbook or the manual of operations should appear on the form if the measurement or procedure is too complicated to be outlined on the form.
117. There should be an instruction at the end of each form that indicates where the form is to be sent after completion and the steps to be followed in preparing the form for transmission.

12.6.5 Form color coding

Color coding is useful if there is a need to distinguish among different types of forms (e.g., pre-randomization forms versus follow-up forms, or forms completed in the laboratory versus those completed in the clinic) or among different copies of the same form (e.g., white for the original, green for the first copy, and pink for the second copy).

118. The color-coding scheme should be simple, logical, and easy to remember.
119. The colors chosen should be limited to a few distinct shades.
120. A particular color should have the same meaning throughout the study (e.g., pink always identifies the second copy of an original).
121. As a rule, forms printed on pastel-colored paper are easier to read and will produce better quality photocopies than those

printed on dark-colored paper. The legibility of photocopies produced from pages using the colors proposed should be checked before making the final color selection.

122. Color coding should never be used as the sole means of identifying a form or its use. Written information should appear on the form to designate its use and should be sufficient to identify a particular form if individuals are unable to distinguish among the colors.

123. It may not be practical to use multicolor forms if a clinic is responsible for maintaining its own supply of forms from photocopy masters.

12.6.6   Form assembly

124. Multipage forms may be supplied to clinics collated and bound (e.g., stapled), collated and unbound, or uncollated. The latter method of supply is preferable when the number of pages making up a form varies depending on the patient or examination. Forms that are collated should be supplied unbound if it is likely that they will have to be disassembled for completion or to make photocopies of them after completion.

125. The individual pages of a form should be sequentially numbered and should indicate the total number of pages in the form (e.g., by using the following kind of numbering scheme: page 1 of 10, page 2 of 10, etc.).

126. Paper clips or similar kinds of fasteners are not acceptable for securing the pages of completed forms. They are likely to come off as the forms are handled in copying, coding, or filing.

127. Forms may be developed with specially designed answer pages that may be detached from the main body of the form. The Lipid Research Clinics used this approach to reduce the volume of paper flowing to the coordinating center. Detachable answer pages may be used only if all information required for data entry can be recorded on the answer sheets and adequate documentation is provided on the answer sheet to identify the patient and type of examination performed.

12.6.7   Arrangement of items on forms

Thought should be given to the ordering of items within and across forms. The arrangement

should be compatible with the needs of patients and clinic staff. Arrangements that are not may result in missed or poor quality data.

128. Place items calling for a particular frame of reference next to one another.

129. The nature, quality, and quantity of information obtained on a form may be influenced by the order of the items on it.

130. The number of positive responses to a list of questions will be higher for lists that are read or shown to the patient than when the list is simply used by clinic staff to record information volunteered by the patient (see Section 12.4.3).

131. The order of procedures should remain fixed over the duration of the trial, especially if there is any chance that one procedure (e.g., ingestion of iopanic acid in order to perform cholecystograms) affects the results of another procedure (e.g., serum cholesterol determinations; see National Cooperative Gallstone Study Group, 1981a, for additional details). A fixed order does not necessarily eliminate this problem, but it does control the effect over time and across treatment groups. Further, not all variations in sequencing can be avoided if the number of procedures performed differs from examination to examination.

132. The arrangement of items within a form should be compatible with the preparation required for a particular examination (e.g., the items to be completed with the patient in a fasting state should appear before those that are to be completed after the patient has been allowed to eat or has been given a glucose load).

133. Group items into sections with headings indicating the general content of the sections. Use a different type font to facilitate identification of section headings.

134. The numbering and identification schemes used on a form should be designed to facilitate the identification of items and their subparts.

135. Use different spacing to indicate transition from one item to another and from one section to another.

136. Devise a numbering system for identification of individual items on a form. Items should be numbered sequentially over the entire form or within sections of the form. The former system is preferable. The latter one has the advantage of allowing for addition or deletion of items in a section with-

out disrupting the numbering system for other sections. However, the disadvantage is that both a section and item number are needed to locate a specific item on a form.

137. Items should be arranged among forms so that any given form can be completed in a single session, as discussed in Section 12.4.4.

138. The time lag between collection of a block of information and transmission of that information to the data center should be minimized. This generally requires use of different forms for recording data that are generated at different clinic visits. Different forms may be needed as well for data generated at the same visit, but by people at different locations in the clinics.

139. Data items that are considered confidential or that deal with sensitive information should appear on separate pages of a form or on a different form so that it is possible for the page or form to be stored apart from the remainder of the patient's file.

12.6.8   Format

12.6.8.1   Items designed for unformatted written replies

Items in this class should provide space for handwritten replies without any restriction on the number of characters of information that may be provided (Appendix F.22).

140. The amount of space provided on the form will influence the quantity and quality of information supplied.

141. The space provided should be consistent with the amount of detail desired and should be large enough to prevent the respondent from having to resort to use of cryptic abbreviations or unnaturally small handwriting.

142. Designate the area where the reply is to be recorded. If lines are used, the space between them should be at least ¼″ (e.g., see item F.22.2 in Appendix F).

143. An unlined space, such as shown in item F.22.3, may be preferable to use of lines, especially if responses are typed.

12.6.8.2   Items requiring formatted written replies

Items in this class require the respondent to fit the response into a designated number of char-

acter spaces. The restriction is ordinarily imposed to facilitate processing of the information.

144. The number of allowable characters per item will be dictated by the code format established when the item was developed.

145. Formatted items should indicate the number of data characters allowed or required. This may be done in the instructions accompanying such items (e.g., by asking the respondent to make certain his reply does not exceed more than a specified number of characters) or by using character boxes or lines, as illustrated in Appendix F.13.1 and F.23.

146. Character lines are preferable to character boxes, especially if the lines that form the boxes serve to camouflage characters contained in the boxes. The weight of the lines or color of the ink used to form the boxes should be distinctly different from the line weight or color of the characters appearing in the boxes when boxes are used.

147. Forms to be completed by hand should have character line segments that are $\geq$¼″ long. The line segments may be shorter if the forms are to be completed using a typewriter.

148. The precision requirements for numeric data should be indicated in the item, as illustrated in Appendix F.14.1 or F.14.2.

12.6.8.3   Items answered by check marks

149. The order of responses (e.g., yes followed by no, or vice versa) should be uniform throughout a form and across forms (Appendix F.24).

150. Inadequate space for checking the proper response (Appendix F.24.4) may lead to errors when items are completed or keyed. The separation of check spaces when arranged vertically may have to be fairly sizable if multiple copies of a form are to be made using carbon or NCR (no carbon required) paper. Variation in the registry of the copies relative to the master can render entries recorded on the copies ambiguous.

151. The space used for checking a response should be as near the items as possible. A dashed or dotted line should be used to associate the check space with the response category when the latter is widely separated from the former (see Appendix F.24.8 and F.24.9).

152. A long list of response options should be broken by a blank line after every third or

fourth entry in the list to aid the eye in locating the appropriate check space (Appendix F.24.9 and F.24.10).

153. Forms requiring a check mark to indicate the appropriate reply to a question are preferable to those in which the respondent reads a list of items associated with the question and then records the code number(s) of the item(s) selected. The latter approach should be considered only when the same list of responses applies to several different questions on the form, or when the list of possible responses is inordinately long.

154. Use of lists that are not part of a form, or that are located elsewhere on it, may increase the time needed to complete the form.

12.6.9   Location of form and patient identifiers

155. Each form should bear the name of the study, the name of the form, a form number, version number, and version date.

156. The form number, version number, and version date should appear on each page of the form. The version date is useful if individual pages are revised during the study.

157. There should be space on each page for recording the patient ID number and visit number (see Section 12.5.11).

158. The space for recording patient ID number should appear in the same relative position on all forms (e.g., upper right-hand corner). A standard location helps to minimize the risk of the item being left blank when forms are completed and facilitates use of the information for filing and retrieval.

12.6.10   Format considerations for data entry

159. If possible, data forms should be designed to allow for data entry directly from the form, without intervening transcription of the data. This generally requires designation of codes and fields on the form (Appendix F.25), except where data entry is done via CRT screens that display the required fields.

160. It may be useful to reserve space on each form for office use. The space may be used

to record transactions involved in the completion of the form and entry of information into the data system.

161. Coding and data entry operations should be designed to minimize the number of times a form is handled. Ideally, all information should be keyed at the same time, including any handwritten unformatted information.

162. A special code should be entered into the data system to identify items that contain data that are not keyed (e.g., uncoded handwritten replies). The code is useful if it is ever necessary to retrieve forms containing unkeyed information.

163. The location of check spaces should be standardized to facilitate the data entry process.

164. Coding conventions should be uniform across forms (e.g., use the same letter or number code to denote a yes reply).

165. The layout of a form should take account of coding and data entry requirements, but should not be dominated by them, especially if the layout complicates use of the form in the clinic.

166. The coding layout should permit data entry personnel to proceed through a form in an orderly fashion with few, if any, references to items already keyed or to items still to be keyed.

167. The form number, version number, or version date appearing on a completed form should be keyed. The information may be needed to interpret changes in the data that occur as a result of forms or coding changes.

12.7   FLOW AND STORAGE OF COMPLETED DATA FORMS

Data forms should flow to data entry for keying and storage as they are completed. (See Chapters 16, 17, and 24 for additional discussion concerning data flow, editing, and storage procedures.) Continuous unrestricted flows are preferable to those that are constrained by batching requirements (e.g., such as those imposed by requiring a clinic to forward forms for processing only at specified time intervals).

Intermediate stops as a form moves from the clinic to the data center for processing should be avoided, if at all possible. Many of the Veterans Administration multicenter trials have procedures in which forms are sent from clinics to the study chairman's office for a preliminary review and edit, and then to the data center for keying, editing, and storage. The intermediate stop delays receipt of the forms at the data center, thereby reducing the usefulness of the edits and analyses carried out by the center. Further, intermediate stops complicate communications with clinics concerning missed visits or deficient forms, since the inventorying and editing responsibilities are shared by the chairman's office and the data center.

The requirements for form storage should be addressed early in the course of the trial, ideally before any forms have been completed. The storage plan should be designed to protect the records from any unauthorized use and against loss or destruction. Protection of the latter type may require maintenance of duplicate files—one at the clinic and the other at the data entry site. Large or important files may be microfilmed to reduce the space required for storage or as a further safeguard against loss.

Part III. Execution

Chapters in This Part

The four chapters of this Part are concerned with execution of the trial. Chapter 13 outlines the steps required in executing the trial, with emphasis on the steps to be carried out in getting started. Chapters 14 and 15 concentrate on the recruitment, treatment, and follow-up processes. The last chapter details general procedures needed to ensure the quality of the data generated in a trial.

13. Preparatory steps in executing the study plan

The lame man who keeps the right road outstrips the runner who takes a wrong one. Nay, it is obvious that when a man runs the wrong way, the more active and swift he is the further he will go astray.

Sir Francis Bacon

13.1 ESSENTIAL APPROVALS AND CLEARANCES

All trials require completion of a series of steps before they can be started. The steps outlined in this chapter are in addition to those discussed in Chapters 11, 12, and 21 with regard to preparation of the study plan, data forms, and funding request.

13.1.1 IRB and other approvals[1]

One set of approvals has to do with those provided by the institutional review boards (IRBs)

1. See Section 14.6 for additional comments.

of individual centers in a trial (clinics, as well as the data center and any other resource center concerned with data collection or patient care). The main function of the board is to provide assurance that the proposed research meets accepted standards of ethics and medical practice. Technically, the assurance is needed only for federally funded studies. However, most institutions require reviews for all research involving humans, regardless of the source of funding. The impetus for the boards grew out of concerns in the 1960s regarding the nature and extent of research involving humans. A memo dated February 8, 1966, from the Surgeon General of the United States Public Health Service mandated creation of the local boards as a prerequisite for continued funding. The structure for IRBs, their composition, and their domain of responsibility has subsequently been spelled out in federal regulations on protection of human subjects (Office for Protection from Research Risks, 1983).

Each board, in order to comply with current regulations, must:

- Have at least five members
- Not be made up exclusively of members of one sex or of one profession
- Include at least one member whose primary concerns are in a nonscientific area (e.g., law, ethics, theology)
- Include at least one member who is not otherwise affiliated with the institution and who is not part of the immediate family of a person who is affiliated with the institution
- Exclude any member from review of a specific proposal who has a conflict of interest (e.g., is an investigator in a study under review)

Individual IRBs have their own rules regarding time schedules for submissions, formats for proposals, and the nature and amount of materials to be supplied. Table 13-1 lists the information requirements as envisioned for a "typical"

Table 13-1   Information required for IRB approval

- Statement of study objectives and rationale
- Description of the study treatments and methods of administration
- Recap of prior evidence concerning safety and efficacy of the study treatments
- Type and source of study patients
- Primary outcome measure for assessing the study treatments
- Length of patient follow-up
- Number of patients to be enrolled and rationale for proposed sample size
- Risk-benefit analysis of trial
- Method of treatment assignment (e.g., random, physician choice, etc.)
- Summary of methods for protecting patients from needless or prolonged exposure to a harmful study treatment
- Summary of safeguards to protect patient privacy and confidentiality
- Consent statement and related material

IRB in relation to clinical trials. Specifics will vary from board to board.

The material submitted to the IRB should indicate the nature and extent of safety monitoring to be performed (see Chapter 20). The individual or group responsible for this function should be identified in the submission along with sufficient details to enable members of the IRB to make an informed judgment regarding the statistical credentials and expertise of the individual or group named. The submission should include a general description of the methods to be used for safety monitoring, the frequency of interim analyses for monitoring purposes, and the procedure to be followed in communicating with local investigators and the IRB regarding proposed treatment changes emanating from the monitoring. Details regarding the communication process are especially important in trials in which monitoring responsibilities are vested in an individual or group that is not under the control of the local clinical investigator, as in most multicenter trials and some single-center trials.

The National Institutes of Health (NIH) will not review a research proposal involving humans without assurance from the proposing investigator's IRB. The assurance is supplied via completion of form HHS 596 (Protection of Human Subjects Assurance/Certification/Declaration)

that is signed by a responsible official of the IRB.

Proposals for clinical trials may require at least two IRB reviews before initiation of patient intake. The first will be required in conjunction with the submission of the funding proposal to the sponsor. The second will be required after the proposal is funded and before the initiation of patient intake, after the details of the study protocol and consent process have been set.

The proposing investigator is responsible for communications with his IRB. He must be prepared to address their concerns in a forthright manner and to revise consent statements in accordance with their requests. Concerns regarding the rights of patients to privacy and confidentiality, as well as safety issues, must be addressed. The entire review and clearance process may take months and may be complicated by the need to clear changes through the leadership of the study, in the case of multicenter trials (see Section 14.6.2 for added details).

Additional reviews and approvals will be needed if the trial involves use of hazardous materials, such as radioactive isotopes, or laboratory animals.

13.1.2   IND and IDE submissions

Most drug trials will require submission of an Investigational New Drug Application (INDA, also referred to as an IND) to the Food and Drug Administration (FDA) before they can be started (Food and Drug Administration, 1981). Table 13-2, Part A, lists general items of information required for an INDA.

An INDA is required for any drug that is not approved by the FDA for the indication proposed. The requirement extends to established drugs that are to be used in ways that depart from prescribed practice, as indicated in the label insert. For example, the University Group Diabetes Program (UGDP) needed an INDA for both tolbutamide and phenformin even though they had been approved by the FDA as hypoglycemic agents. Even a nonprescription drug requires an INDA if it is used like a prescription drug. For example, one was required for aspirin in both the Coronary Drug Project Aspirin Study (CDPA) and Aspirin Myocardial Infarction Study (AMIS).

The FDA approval process can delay the start of the trial and lead to alterations in its design. Investigators in the National Cooperative Gallstone Study (NCGS) were required to carry out

Table 13–2 Items of information required for IND and IDE submissions to the FDA

A. Investigational New Drug Application (Summarized from FDA Form 1571, 10/82, Notice of Claimed Investigational Exemption for a New Drug)

- Details concerning the drug, including drug name, composition, source, method of preparation, quality control procedures in production and packaging

- Summary of previous investigations involving the drug

- Copies of informational material (including information on label and labeling) about the drug to be supplied to investigators involved in administering the drug

- Name and qualifications of each investigator to be involved in proposed studies

- Name and qualifications of personnel responsible for monitoring progress of proposed studies and for safety monitoring

- Description of the study plan, including details, in the case of proposed clinical trials, regarding sample size, duration of the study data collection, methods of treatment, as well as details concerning the IRB responsible for reviewing the proposed work, and details regarding informed consent

- Assurances from the IND sponsor that:
  - The FDA will be notified if the investigation is discontinued and of the reasons for the action
  - Each investigator associated with the IND will be notified if an NDA for the drug is approved, or if the investigation is discontinued
  - If the drug is to be sold, an explanation will be supplied to the FDA as to why sale is required and why sale should not be regarded as commercialization of the drug
  - Clinical studies in humans will not be initiated prior to 30 days after receipt of the Notice of Claimed Investigational Exemption for a New Drug by the FDA, unless otherwise indicated by the FDA
  - An environmental impact statement will be provided to the FDA, if so requested

  - All nonclinical laboratory studies have been or will be conducted in accordance with the Good Laboratory Practice regulations of the federal government, or that reasons why they have not or cannot be followed will be supplied to the FDA

B. Investigational Device Exemption (Summarized from reference 189, Appendix I)

- Name and address of sponsor of IDE along with names and addresses of all other investigators to be involved in the IDE

- Summary of prior investigations of the device

- Description of the methods, facilities, and controls used for the manufacture, processing, packaging, storage, and, where appropriate, installation of the device

- Certification that all investigators have signed an agreement to be involved in the IDE and that no new investigators will be added without signed agreements

- Name and address of the chairperson of each IRB associated with the IDE request

- Details regarding price of the device if it is to be sold and an explanation of why sale does not constitute commercialization of the product

- An environmental impact statement when requested

- Details concerning labeling of the device

- Copies of all forms and informational materials to be provided to patients in relation to the consent process

- Description of the study plan including:
  - Statement of purpose
  - Study protocol
  - Risk analysis
  - Description of the device
  - Methods for monitoring the investigation (progress as well as safety), including names and addresses of monitors

---

biopsy studies of patients treated with chenodeoxycholic acid before they were allowed to proceed with a full-scale trial of the drug (National Cooperative Gallstone Study Group 1981a, 1981b, 1984).

Amendments to the Federal Food, Drug, and Cosmetic Act of 1938, passed in 1976, extended the regulatory authority of the FDA to medical devices. A medical device is defined as (Food and Drug Administration, 1983):

Any instrument, apparatus, implement, machine, contrivance, implant, in vitro reagent, or other similar or related article,

including component, part, or accessory, which:

- *Is recognized in the official National Formulary, or the United States Pharmacopeia, or any supplement to them;*

- *Is intended for use in the diagnosis of disease or other conditions, or in the cure, mitigation, treatment, or prevention of disease, in man or other animals; or*

- *Is intended to affect the structure or any function of the body of man or other animals; and*

- *Does not achieve any of its principal intended purposes through chemical action within or on the body of man or other animals and which is not dependent upon being metabolized for the achievement of any of its principal intended purposes.*

The definition covers approximately 1,700 devices that range from blood collection tubes and tongue depressors to heart valve replacement materials and pacemakers.

The FDA has established three classes of devices, based on the degree of control deemed necessary for assuring the safety and efficacy of the device (Food and Drug Administration, 1983). All three classes are subject to the Good Manufacturing Practices Regulations. In fact, the only controls required for Class I devices (e.g., capillary blood collection tubes, tongue depressors, crutches, and arm slings) are via these regulations. Added assurances for Class II devices (e.g., hearing aids, blood pumps, catheters, and hard contact lenses) and Class III devices (e.g., life-support or life-sustaining devices, such as pacemakers, intraocular lenses, and heart valve replacements, as well as devices considered of importance in preventing impairment of health) are provided via performance standards plus clinical trials for Class III devices. Permission to carry out trials of Class III devices is obtained via an Investigational Device Exemption (IDE), granted by the FDA. Part B of Table 13–2 lists items of information required in conjunction with an IDE application (Food and Drug Administration, 1980).

13.1.3   OMB clearance

The Office of Management and Budget (OMB), one of the offices in the executive branch of the United States government, has the authority to review and approve data forms used by all branches of the federal government, including the NIH. Technically, any data form to be administered or distributed to ten or more people that is produced by a governmental agency, or by a group under contract to it, requires OMB clearance—even draft versions of data forms developed simply for testing purposes. Forms developed under NIH grants are not subject to the order.

The review can delay the start of data collection, especially if staff at OMB regard certain forms or items as unnecessary or to constitute an invasion of a person's privacy. Usually, however, the review and approval process is not a major stumbling block. In fact, many areas of clinical investigations are exempt from review and those that are required may be achieved in short order if the project officer of the sponsoring agency maintains an effective working relationship with OMB staff and allows sufficient lead time for clearance.

13.2   APPROVAL MAINTENANCE

13.2.1   IRB

The approval granted by the IRB prior to the start of the trial and for each renewal will be for a one year period, unless otherwise indicated. The submission accompanying a renewal request should indicate the nature and extent of progress made since the initial request or last renewal request, the reasons for continuing the study, and proposed changes in the study protocol or consent procedures. Changes must be cleared before they can be implemented. Those that cannot wait for the annual review will require special reviews.

The IRB may require a synopsis of interim results for renewals of trials requiring safety monitoring (see Table 22–1 in Chapter 22). Complying with this request will pose problems in trials in which clinical investigators are denied access to interim results for reasons discussed in Chapter 22. The results portion of the renewal submission will have to be prepared and submitted by nonclinical personnel in such cases. The boards may be willing to forego looks at interim results if they are satisfied with the safety monitoring done in the study, as discussed in Section 13.1.1. They may have no choice in multicenter trials if clinics are not given access to interim results. Theoretically, they could still insist on synopses of results for the clinic in question, but they would be of little value because of the numbers of patients involved.

Investigators are obligated to report unexpected adverse events as they occur. Those reports are reviewed as they are received and may lead to immediate suspension or withdrawal of the approval until or unless changes mandated by the IRB are made.

13.2.2   FDA

The individual (or agency) to whom the INDA or IDE is granted is required to report unexpected adverse events to the FDA as they occur. There is also a requirement to provide summaries of study results as the trial progresses. The latter reporting requirement may be satisfied by simply supplying the FDA with copies of reports prepared for the treatment effects monitoring committee (see Chapter 23). Both the CDP and NCGS satisfied the majority of their FDA reporting requirements in this way.

13.2.3 Other approvals

Other approvals granted at the start of the trial, such as for use of radioactive compounds or controlled substances, will have to be updated as the trial proceeds. Changes to the data forms may have to be cleared through OMB if the study is funded via a government contract. Sponsoring agencies, such as the NIH, will require interim progress reports to continue funding for the trial.

13.3 DEVELOPING STUDY HANDBOOKS AND MANUALS OF OPERATIONS

Any trial requires two basic sets of documents: one that describes clinic operations and another that describes the data intake and processing procedures in the trial. These two sets of documents may constitute separate sections in the same handbook or manual or may be contained in separate documents (see Appendix G).

A large multicenter trial may require several other documents in addition to the two mentioned above. Studies with a central laboratory will need a document that describes its methods and procedures. Other resource centers, such as those needed for performing special reading or coding functions, will also need documents detailing their practices.

The groundwork needed for production of the required handbooks and manuals is laid when the trial is planned. The work involved in writing and maintaining these documents will start shortly after the trial is funded and continue until it is finished. Table 13–3 contains a list of suggestions concerning their development and maintenance.

A handbook, as used in this context, is a document that contains a series of tables, charts, figures, and specification pages that detail the design and operating features of the trial. A manual, as discussed herein, is a document that

details the methods and procedures of the entire trial or some aspect of it largely through written narrative and accompanying tables, charts, and figures. The two kinds of documents serve somewhat different functions and, hence, are not necessarily interchangeable. The primary virtue of a handbook lies in its organization and in the tabular nature of the material presented. It is designed for use as a ready reference for study personnel. Manuals are designed to document procedures used in the trial. They are most useful to persons who want a detailed description of the actual procedures used.

The two kinds of documents may be developed simultaneously or in sequence, starting with the handbook. The latter approach was used in the Hypertension Prevention Trial (HPT). Work on the manual of operations was delayed until the handbook was developed. The development of the handbook simplified the task of preparing the study manual of operations. Further, the fact that the trial had been under way about 9 months when the work started allowed its developers to reference existing study documents and task specific manuals, thereby avoiding the need for inclusion of those details in the main document.

13.4 TESTING THE DATA COLLECTION PROCEDURES

Three general assurances should be satisfied before data collection is initiated:

- Essential data collection and patient examination procedures have been reviewed and approved by the study leadership
- Data forms needed for patient enrollment and for the initial phase of treatment and follow-up have been tested and are ready for use
- Projected time requirements for developing, testing, reviewing, and approving data collection procedures and related data forms for use in the later stages of treatment and follow-up are consistent with the data collection schedule of the trial

Satisfying the last condition may require a delay in the start of patient recruitment, even though the initial data intake procedures have been tested and approved. Once the first patient is enrolled, the rest of the data collection schedule is lockstep. It is better to delay the start of patient recruitment than to be forced into postponing follow-up visits because of the lack of

Table 13-3 Suggestions for development of study handbooks and manuals of operations

A. General

- Identify major topics or functions for which handbooks or manuals are required (e.g., clinic operations, data intake and processing, laboratory procedures, etc.)
- Develop a draft table of contents for each required handbook or manual and submit for review and comment by the leadership group of the trial before development
- Develop methods and procedures for data collection with input from key study personnel, including clinicians, statisticians, clinic coordinators, laboratory technicians, and the like
- Ensure that written material contained in handbooks or manuals is concise and devoid of complex sentences and esoteric language
- Test the adequacy of each handbook or manual by having it reviewed by individuals who will be using it
- Release a handbook or manual for use only after it has been reviewed and approved by the leadership of the study

B. Organization

- Each handbook or manual should have an official name and should be easily distinguished from all other handbooks or manuals in the study (e.g., through use of different colored binders)
- The name of the handbook or manual, date of release, version or edition number, and the name of the individual or group responsible for its distribution should be indicated on the title page
- Include a detailed table of contents, along with a listing of all tables and figures in the document
- Include a subject index and glossary
- Chapters in manuals should be divided into numbered subsections; the accompanying numbers and titles should appear in the table of contents of the document
- Left-hand page margins should be wide enough to keep text from being obscured or lost when pages are photocopied or bound (e.g., at least 1¼" for standard 8½ x 11" pages assembled in loose-leaf notebooks or pressure binders)

- Right-hand page margins should be wide enough to allow room for user notes (e.g., at least ¾" for standard 8½ x 11" pages). The same is true of top and bottom margins
- Pages should be typed using high resolution type fonts to allow for image degradation in photo-reproduction without a serious loss of legibility
- Boldface type, underlining, or other methods should be used to identify key phrases, definitions, and important procedural statements
- Ideally, pages should be numbered sequentially from the beginning to the end of a document, without regard to chapter or subsection. Numbering systems that recycle by chapter or section allow for page updates without disrupting the entire numbering system. However, such systems are not as convenient for users as are continuous numbering systems
- Placement of page and other identifying information should appear in a standard location on all pages (preferably upper right-hand corner) and should not be too near the edge of the page

C. Suggested maintenance aids

- Responsibility for periodic review and revision of a manual should be assigned to a specific individual or group
- A specific individual should be given responsibility for keeping track of revisions made to a handbook or manual and for making certain that all users of the handbook or manual are supplied with updates as they are produced
- Each new version of a handbook or manual should be identified with a revision date and should indicate the date and version number of the document it replaces
- Large documents that are subject to frequent updates should be kept in loose-leaf binders (facilitates page replacements and simplifies photo-reproduction of the document)
- Individual pages that are updated and inserted in an existing version of a document as replacements for outdated pages should include the revision date in the top or bottom right-hand corner of the pages.

---

data forms or to use forms that have not been adequately tested.

The construction of the data collection instruments is one of the most important tasks in the entire study. General rules for item construction and forms development have already been discussed in Chapter 12. The paragraphs that follow deal with methods for testing the data forms.

It is probably fair to say that any item on a data form that can be misinterpreted will be. Some of the interpretation problems can be

avoided by a careful review of all forms before any field testing is done. The next review should involve use of the forms on a few "practice" patients. Ideally, the forms should be completed for persons as similar to study patients as possible, but friends, colleagues, or spouses, instructed to behave and respond like "typical" patients, may suffice for some of the testing.

The entire set of data forms and accompanying procedures should be submitted to "walk-throughs," involving the staff who will be responsible for completing them, before they are tested on real patients. The "walk-throughs" invariably identify items or sections that need to be relocated or rewritten to eliminate confusion or to streamline the way forms are to be completed.

Once these steps have been completed the forms are ready for field tests involving real patients. The test conditions should be as similar to those for the actual trial as feasible. The best approach is one in which the entire set of study procedures are carried out. However, this may not be possible for procedures that entail risks or that are justified only in special circumstances. The forms used should be in near final form, with one or two exceptions. They should make generous use of open-ended response categories, such as discussed in Section 12.5.4, in order to collect information useful in constructing response checklists for the final versions of the forms. They may also include alternative versions of the same item in order to determine the preferred wording of the item.

The number of patients used for the test should be large enough and heterogeneous enough to provide a reliable basis for preparation of final versions of the forms. The number will depend on available resources and on the complexity of the data collection scheme proposed. The penalties for undetected deficiencies are greatest in trials involving large numbers of patients.

The deposition of data collected in the test run should be settled before the run is undertaken if study-eligible patients are to be used in the test. The temptation in such cases is to reserve the option of adding the test data to the main data file if the number of changes mandated by the test is "small." The best approach is to preclude this option from the outset for several reasons. First, the desire to preserve the option may reduce the value of the test itself if investigators limit the changes they are willing to make simply as a means of maintaining the option. Second, the effort involved in merging test data into the main file may not be worth the return, especially if the merger requires a lot of recoding and reprogramming. Third, the absence of a stated policy can open the trial to criticism later on if the decision on use of test data appears to have been motivated by a desire on the part of the investigators to accentuate or ameliorate the observed treatment effect.

The intelligibility of any material that is read or given to patients in the trial should receive special scrutiny during the testing process. Particular attention should be paid to the patient consent statement and related materials. They should be tested on sample patients and then modified where necessary to ensure a clear and accurate presentation of the trial.

13.5 DEVELOPING AND TESTING THE DATA MANAGEMENT SYSTEM

Ideally, the development of computer programs needed to inventory completed data forms, and to edit, store, and retrieve data contained on those forms, should be started as soon as the forms have been developed for testing. However, this ideal is rarely achieved in reality. For one reason, even experienced investigators can underestimate the time required to develop a functioning data management system. Inexperienced investigators may not even recognize the need for one until well into the trial. Other reasons have to do with time and resource limitations. Of necessity, most of the work in the initial phase of a trial is devoted to development of the study protocol, data forms, and the data system. The pressures to complete these tasks and to get started with patient recruitment makes it difficult to find the time needed to develop a working data management system. The problem is compounded by the fact that it is not feasible to develop a working system until data collection procedures for the trial have been set—something that may not be done until patient recruitment is ready to start.

It is the responsibility of the data center to make sure that essential data management routines are available when needed. Basic routines, such as those needed for randomization, must be available by the time the first patient is randomized. Others, such as for inventorying data forms, should be available as soon as forms begin arriving at the center. The same is true for the editing routine to be applied to completed forms. Work on programs needed for performance and safety monitoring should begin soon thereafter (see Chapters 16 and 17).

The decision to start data intake before the data management system is in place can jeopardize its subsequent development. A good data center will keep this from happening by insisting on adequate lead time for its development before the start of data collection.

13.6 TRAINING AND CERTIFICATION

As a minimum, data collection personnel should be required to work through a sample set of data collection forms and to familiarize themselves with study procedures before being allowed to start data collection. Obviously, training cannot be started until data forms are in final form and needed documents, such as the study handbook or manual of operations, are available. This familiarization effort may be followed by workshops for demonstrating specific procedures and for observing personnel performing assigned data collection tasks. The training may be part of a formal certification process in which personnel are required to pass proficiency tests before they are allowed to start data collection, for example, as used in the DRS (Diabetic Retinopathy Study Research Group, 1981). This process should be started well before the projected start of data collection in order to avoid delays due to certification failures.

The training and certification processes are an essential part of quality control. They should be maintained over the course of data intake. Existing personnel should be required to undergo refresher training and recertification at intervals over the course of the trial. New personnel, recruited during the course of the trial, should be required to go through essential training and certification procedures before starting data collection in the trial.

The need for training and certification is most apparent in multicenter trials. Special efforts are required in such cases to make sure that all clinics are operating under the same ground rules and that they are adhering to established data collection procedures. However, the need is not unique to such trials. It extends to single-center trials as well. The opportunity for variation and misunderstanding with regard to data practices can be as great, sometimes greater, than in multicenter trials.

13.7 PHASED APPROACH TO DATA COLLECTION

Once the necessary testing and certification have been completed, patient enrollment may begin. There is a temptation, once this point is reached, to proceed as rapidly as possible. However, some initial restraint is wise, since live study conditions can be expected to reveal heretofore undetected defects. The larger the number of patients already enrolled when the defects are discovered, the greater the costs involved in correcting them.

A phased approach to data collection is especially important in multicenter trials involving a large number of clinics. Allowing all clinics to start data collection at the same time can swamp the data center before staff have had a chance to develop a functional data system. This problem can be minimized in one of two ways. One way is to fund only a skeleton set of clinics to begin with. The full complement of clinics can be recruited and funded once data collection is under way in the initial set of clinics. This approach was used in the CDP. The study started with just 5 clinical centers in 1965. A second set of 29 clinics was added in 1966. A third set of 21 clinics was added in 1967 to bring the total to 55 (Zukel, 1983).

The other way, when a full complement of clinics is identified from the outset, is to authorize only one or two clinics to start data collection. Other clinics are not phased in until essential support systems have been developed and tested. This approach was used in the Multiple Risk Factor Intervention Trial, MRFIT (Sherwin et al., 1981). The sponsoring agency must have the flexibility needed to determine when funding for data collection is to start in the individual clinics to make this approach viable.

14. Patient recruitment and enrollment

Seek, and ye shall find.

Matthew 7, verse 7

14.1 RECRUITMENT GOALS

The recruitment goal in fixed sample size designs should be set before the trial is started. As noted in Chapter 9, it may be based on a formal calculation or on practical considerations. It serves as a landmark for gauging progress during patient recruitment when accompanied by a timetable to indicate when it is to be achieved.

It is not uncommon for trials to fall short of their stated goal, even when the recruitment period is extended well beyond the date originally set for achieving the goal. The Coronary Artery Surgery Study (CASS) extended the recruitment time and even then enrolled fewer patients than originally planned. The same was true for the Program on the Surgical Control of Hyperlipidemia (POSCH). Their recruitment experiences are similar to those outlined for trials carried out as part of the Veterans Cooperative Studies Program (Collins et al., 1980). Unfortunately, it is not easy to assess the recruitment performance of many of the completed trials because of the absence of details in published reports concerning the original recruitment goal and timetable for achieving it.

Investigators may set a number of secondary recruitment goals or quotas in addition to the main one. Some may relate to the mix of patients within a clinic (e.g., the number of males versus females). Others, in the case of the multicenter trials, will relate to the numbers of patients to be enrolled per clinic. All secondary goals should be viewed as general guidelines rather than as absolute for practical reasons. For example, it is more efficient to allow all clinics in a multicenter trial to recruit to a common cutoff date than to a set number per clinic. The same is true with regard to goals or quotas regarding the mix of patients within a clinic. Certain kinds of patients will be harder to find than others. Insistence on a specified mix will increase the time needed for patient recruitment.

14.2 METHODS OF PATIENT RECRUITMENT

Table 14-1 lists methods of patient recruitment. The methods have been divided into those that rely on direct patient contact and those that do not. Each method has specific strengths and weaknesses that must be considered when a choice is made among them (Table 14-2). Any method of recruitment requires the support of colleagues to succeed. An investigator should not undertake a trial without this support.

Studies relying on patient referrals can expect to experience difficulties meeting their recruitment goal if referring physicians are not in sympathy with the study or if they are reluctant to make referrals for fear of "losing" their patients to the study. The National Eye Institute distributed letters to ophthalmologists announcing the start of the Diabetic Retinopathy Study (DRS),

Table 14-1   Methods of patient recruitment

Recruitment method	Trials using method*
A. Direct patient contact	
• Clinic contacts	AMIS, CDP, UGDP
• Screenings	HDFP, MRFIT
• Direct mailings	HPT, LRC
B. Indirect patient contact	
• Referring physicians	AMIS, CASS, CDP, DRS, MPS, UGDP
• Retrospective record reviews	POSCH, UGDP
• Spot radio and TV ads	AMIS, MRFIT

*See Glossary for name corresponding to acronym.

Table 14-2   Comments concerning the choice of recruitment methods

Recruitment method	Comments
A. Direct patient contact	
Via primary care clinic	• Clinic must be large enough to yield the required number of patients if it is to serve as sole source of patients
	• The study investigator should be responsible for the primary care clinic or play a major role in its operation
	• Fellow colleagues in the clinic must subscribe to the tenets of the study and be willing to follow the prescribed treatment
	• Generally, only viable for relatively common diseases or conditions. Not viable if most patients seen at the clinic are ineligible for the study
Via screening	• Method of choice for identification of patients with a disease or condition that can be diagnosed with a simple and inexpensive test and that is not routinely diagnosed via regular patient care channels
	• May be used to supplement other recruitment methods when the disease or condition of interest is rare (e.g., a certain type of hyperlipemia)
	• Study clinic should have facilities to treat identified patients or must be prepared to refer patients not suitable for study to appropriate sources for care
Via mailings or telephone calls	• Best limited to recruitment for primary prevention trials or trials focusing on treatment of a disease or condition not presently being treated by the medical community
	• Not recommended for recruitment of patients with a disease or condition routinely diagnosed and treated. Direct appeals in this case may be viewed as efforts to "steal" patients
	• Method usually used in combination with screening procedures carried out at the clinic to determine the eligibility of those who respond to the direct mail or phone appeal. Screening is essential if a respondent is not likely to know whether he has the disease or condition of interest

Table 14-2 Comments concerning the choice of recruitment methods (*continued*)

Recruitment method	Comments
B. Indirect patient contact	
Via referring physician	• Required mode of recruitment if study clinic located in tertiary care facility. May be used as the primary method of recruitment or as an adjunct to other methods
	• Study clinic should be located in an established referral center for the disease or condition of interest
	• Patient's primary care must be compatible with study tenets
	• Not a reliable method of recruitment if the disease or condition is routinely treated by a primary care physician
	• Method works best for a disease or condition for which there is no recognized form of therapy and when the referring physician has no concern about "losing" referred patients
	• It may be necessary to augment the referral process by:
	– Mailing letters to referring physicians to inform them of the study and of the type of patients needed
	– Journal articles outlining the design and purpose of the trial
	– News articles in the medical or lay press concerning the trial
	– Presentations at medical meetings to acquaint referral physician with the trial
Via retrospective record reviews	• May be preferred method for rare disease or condition, if routinely diagnosed and noted in clinic records
	• Not useful if newly diagnosed patients are required, or where most patients identified by the reviews are likely to be ineligible for enrollment (e.g., because they have received a form of treatment that disqualifies them from consideration)
	• May have to be used:
	– When it is impractical or too costly to mount a screening effort to identify patients
	– When there is no risk-free low-cost screening procedure available
	– If eligible patients are unlikely to be referred to the study clinic
	– If the disease or condition is so rare as to make it impractical to consider any of the recruitment methods outlined above
Via radio or TV spot ads and the news media	• Usually used as an adjunct to other methods of recruitment
	• Often used to acquaint members of the lay and medical community with the trial

which outlined the type of patients desired for the trial. Care was taken in the letter to note that patients who were referred for study would remain under the care of the referring ophthalmologist for their regular eye care.

Some trials have used the news media to facilitate patient recruitment. Recruitment publicity may take the form of news stories appearing in area newspapers, may be aired on radio or television, or may consist of paid advertisements aimed at certain types of patients. Some of the clinics in the Multiple Risk Factor Intervention Trial (MRFIT) used spot television ads to inform potential study candidates of the trial. Such direct appeals are only practical in settings where patients can be expected to know they have the disease or condition of interest and are not under treatment for it (see Chapter 24 for further discussion of study information policy issues). The need to have newly diagnosed, untreated patients can be a major stumbling block to recruitment if most of the patients arriving at a clinic are already under treatment. This was one of the difficulties in recruiting patients in the University Group Diabetes Program (UGDP).

Studies may be forced to establish their own screening and referral procedures if existing sources of patients are inadequate. Various trials, such as the Hypertension Detection and Follow-Up Program (HDFP), Coronary Primary Prevention Trial (CPPT) of the Lipid Research Clinics (LRC), and MRFIT, had to develop special screening procedures to find suitable patients. The LRC had to make over 436,000 patient contacts in order to find the 3,810 ultimately enrolled into the CPPT (Lipid Research Clinics Program, 1982). The MRFIT screened over 361,000 to find the 12,866 enrolled in that study (Multiple Risk Factor Intervention Trial Research Group, 1982). The HDFP screened over 158,900 to identify the 10,940 patients enrolled in that trial (Hypertension Detection and Follow-Up Program Cooperative Group, 1979a).

The systematic review of hospital records can offer a useful means of patient identification if the records can be expected to contain the needed information. However, it is not useful if most of the patients are ineligible because of their disease history or treatments received. The review is fairly easy to carry out if it is restricted to the investigator's own institution, but not if it involves other institutions as well, as in POSCH. That study relied on record searches at several hundred different hospitals. Special personnel were required to negotiate the agreements needed to make the searches (Matts et al., 1980).

14.3   TROUBLESHOOTING

The period of patient intake is crucial in the life of a trial. Special efforts are needed over the entire period to spot and correct problems that impede patient intake. Recruitment performance should be monitored closely by comparing the rate of enrollment with that required to achieve the stated recruitment goal in the time period specified. An extremely low recruitment rate may call for a relaxation of some of the selection criteria or cancellation of the entire study or of support for one or more of the clinics in it. The monitoring process may be facilitated by screening logs. The logs may help to pinpoint reasons for exclusions and, hence, may suggest ways of modifying selection criteria to increase patient yield. They may also help to characterize the ways in which the population enrolled differs from the population screened, as in CASS—information that may be useful when generalizing results of the trial (Coronary Artery Surgery Study Research Group, 1984; see also Question 9 in Chapter 19).

Study leaders should conduct formal visits to clinics for on-site inspections. The first round of visits should be as soon after the start of patient recruitment as possible. Subsequent visits may be carried out at intervals over the life of the trial (see Section 16.8.3). The visits can be helpful in identifying and correcting problems and in bolstering the morale of clinic staff (see Cassel and Ferris, 1984, for discussion of site visiting procedures in the Early Treatment Diabetes Retinopathy Study, ETDRS).

14.4   THE PATIENT SHAKE-DOWN PROCESS

The process of evaluating a patient for entry into a trial may require several examinations. The longer the evaluation period, the easier it will be to identify uncooperative or otherwise unsuitable patients. Patients who fail to keep appointments or who do not comply with data collection requirements for baseline visits are not likely to become more compliant after enrollment.

Some drug trials (e.g., the CDP, Coronary Drug Project Research Group, 1973a) require use of a single-masked placebo during the pre-randomization evaluation period to help identify noncompliant patients (see Question 37, Chapter 19). No medication, not even a placebo, should be given without explanation. Of necessity, the explanation must be less than forthright if clinic staff are to conceal its nature in the case of single-masked placebos. The evasive nature of the explanation required can strain the patient-physician relationship at a crucial point in the enrollment process.

14.5 THE ETHICS OF RECRUITMENT

The methods used for recruitment should be devoid of any procedures that may be construed as coercive. Cash payments as inducements for enrollment or for patients to continue in a trial should be used with caution, especially if the trial involves risks. They may be necessary in trials involving healthy volunteers who will not realize any direct benefit from the trials, but not in trials involving treatment of some health condition. In those cases, the benefits derived from the care provided should serve as a sufficient inducement for enrollment.

The recruitment process should not involve any restrictions on the demographic, social, or ethnic characteristics of the patient population, except those needed for scientific reasons (e.g., restriction of age to allow concentration on a high-risk group of patients, or restriction to the sex group with the preponderance of the disease) or for practical or ethical reasons (e.g., exclusion of non-English-speaking patients because of concern regarding adequacy of the informed consent process). However, this is not to say that the study may not end up with a preponderance of one sex or ethnic group, or with patients largely from the same social class. The composition will depend on patient sources available to clinics.

The recruitment procedures used in a trial may come under scrutiny long after enrollment has been completed. The Tuskegee Syphilis Study is a case in point (Schuman et al., 1955; Tuskegee Syphilis Study Ad Hoc Advisory Panel, 1973; Vonderlehr et al., 1936). Critics of the study have suggested that the concentration on poor, uneducated blacks led to a climate of complacency in the way it was run (Brandt, 1978; Jones, 1981; Rothman, 1982).

14.6 PATIENT CONSENT[1]

14.6.1 General guidelines

It is unethical to carry out any experiment that entails risks to humans without their voluntary consent. The Nuremberg Code[2] and all codes since then have been explicit on the need for voluntary consent (Levine and Lebacqz, 1979; Levine, 1981). However, relatively little attention

---

1. See Section 13.1.1 for additional comments.
2. The code was an outgrowth of the war crimes trials in Nuremberg following World War II. The code is reproduced in Levine, 1981.

was devoted to the actual consent process in medical research until the Surgeon General of the United States Public Health Service (USPHS) addressed the issue in a memo (dated February 8, 1966) to heads of institutions conducting research under Public Health Service grants. The memo ultimately led to detailed regulations, including the creation of institutional review boards (IRBs), as a means of ensuring adherence to ethical practices in the design and conduct of research on humans. Table 14-3 provides a summary of the pertinent points concerning the consent process, as contained in the most recent set of regulations. The regulations read in part:

Except as provided elsewhere in this or other subparts, no investigator may involve a human being as a subject in research covered by these regulations unless the investigator has obtained the legally effective informed consent of the subject or the subject's legally authorized representative. An investigator shall seek such consent only under circumstances that provide the prospective subject or the representative sufficient opportunity to consider whether or not to participate and that minimize the possibility of coercion or undue influence. The information that is given to the subject or the representative shall be in language understandable to the subject or the representative. No informed consent, whether oral or written, may include any exculpatory language through which the subject or the representative is made to waive or appear to waive any of the subject's legal rights, or releases or appears to release the investigator, the sponsor, the institution or its agents from liability for negligence (Office for Protection from Research Risks, p. 9, 1983).

The requirement for consent, when first introduced, led to fear that it would make recruitment of patients for studies impossible. This fear has not been justified, although the burden imposed by the regulations is unfair in one regard. An investigator is required to make certain that a patient about to enter a trial understands the nature of the risks and benefits that may accrue from the treatments to be offered. Yet that same patient, when seen by his regular physician, may be offered similar treatments without any discussion of their risks or benefits (Chalmers, 1982a).

Table 14–3 General elements of an informed consent

- A statement that the study involves research, an explanation of the research and the expected duration of the subject's participation, a description of the procedures to be followed, and identification of any procedures that are experimental

- A description of any reasonably foreseeable risks or discomforts to the subject

- A description of any benefits to the subject or to others that may reasonably be expected from the research

- A disclosure of appropriate alternative procedures or courses of treatment, if any, that might be advantageous to the subject

- A statement concerning the extent, if any, to which confidentiality of records identifying the subject will be maintained

- For research involving more than minimal risk, an explanation as to whether any compensation or medical treatments are available if injury occurs and, if so, what they consist of, or where further information may be obtained

- An explanation of whom to contact for answers to pertinent questions about the research and research subjects' rights, and whom to contact in the event of research-related injury to the subject

- A statement that participation is voluntary, refusal to participate will involve no penalty or loss of benefits to which the subject is otherwise entitled, and the subject may discontinue participation at any time without penalty or loss of benefits to which the subject is otherwise entitled

- When appropriate, one or more of the following elements of information shall also be provided to each subject:

  - A statement that the particular treatment or procedure may involve risks to the subject (or to the embryo or fetus, if the subject is or may become pregnant) that are currently unforeseeable

  - Anticipated circumstances under which the subject's participation may be terminated by the investigator without regard to the subject's consent

  - Any additional costs to the subject that may result from participation in the research

  - The consequences of a subject's decision to withdraw from the research and procedures for orderly termination of participation by the subject

  - A statement that significant new findings developed during the course of the research that may relate to the subject's willingness to continue participation will be provided to the subject

  - The approximate number of subjects involved in the study

Source: Reference citation 365.

14.6.2 The consent process

Table 14–4 provides a list (prepared by the author) of items that should be covered in the consent process. It differs from the list in Table 14–3 in that it is specific to the area of clinical trials. Appendix E contains sample consent statements from three of the trials sketched in Appendix B.

The consent process, to be valid, must be based on factual information presented in an intelligible fashion and in a setting in which the patient, or his guardian, is able to make a free choice, without fear of reprisal or prejudicial treatment. Meeting these conditons may be impossible in cases where the patient is highly vulnerable, either because of his medical condition or physical surroundings. Extra precautions are needed whenever minors, mental patients, or prisoners are approached. The class action suit for damages brought against investigators at the University of Maryland on behalf of Maryland state prisoners had to deal with questions concerning the nature of free consents obtained in prison settings (United States District Court for the District of Maryland, 1979). No damages were awarded, but the suit took years to complete.

Reservations concerning the adequacy of the consent process in institutionalized populations have all but eliminated these populations as patient sources for research studies. They have also tended to discourage trials in children. The latter trend is unfortunate. Some trials must be done in children to obtain information pertinent to their illnesses or treatments.

The consent process must be completed before the treatment assignment is issued (except with the method proposed by Zelen; see Section 14.8). No patient should be randomized who expresses a reluctance or unwillingness to accept whatever treatment is assigned. The process should include an explicit statement regarding a patient's right to withdraw from the trial at any time after randomization. The statement may be balanced with a discussion of the effect withdrawals have on the trial and the responsibility a patient has, within limits, to continue in the trial if he decides to enroll (Levine and Lebacqz, 1979).

It is best to avoid exact time specifications regarding the anticipated length of follow-up in long-term trials. The time, even if seemingly fixed at the outset, may have to be extended later for reasons unanticipated at the outset. Similarly, promises as to when the study treatment will be offered to patients assigned to the control treatment should be avoided if there is any chance of having to renege on them later, as was the case in the NCGS (National Cooperative Gallstone Study Group, 1981a).

Table 14-4 Suggested items of information to be imparted in consents for clinical trials

General descriptive and design information	Patient responsibilities and safeguards
• Description of the disease or condition being studied and how the patient qualifies for the study • Type of patients being studied and the number to be enrolled • Anticipated length of follow-up • Description of data collection schedule and procedures	• Outline of responsibilities of patients enrolled in the trial, including discussion of the importance of continued follow-up • Outline of what is expected of the patient in following the examination schedule and in carrying out special procedures between visits • Outline of safeguards to prevent continued exposure of a patient to a harmful study treatment or denial of a beneficial one
Treatment information	• Outline of safeguards for protecting a patient's right to privacy and confidentiality of information
• List of the treatments to be studied and rationale for their choice • Treatment alternatives available outside the study • Nature of the control treatment • Method of treatment administration • Method of assigning patients to treatment • Level of treatment masking • Nature of information regarding treatment results that will be made available to patients during and at the conclusion of the trial	• Indication of a patient's right to withdraw from the trial at any time after enrollment without penalty or loss of benefits to which he is otherwise entitled • Statement of the policy of the investigator's institution on compensation for, or treatment of, study-related injuries • Statement of the patient's right to have questions answered regarding the trial and indication of items of information that will not be disclosed (e.g., the treatment assignment in a double-masked trial)
Risk-benefit information	• Statement of the length of time personal identifiers will be retained after the close of the trial, where such information will be retained, and the reasons for keeping it (e.g., for use in contacting or recalling the patient after close of the trial). Statement should also indicate ways in which the information may be used (e.g., to access the National Death Index or other information sources for determining mortality status after the close of the trial)
• Description of the risks and benefits that may accrue to a patient from participation in the trial • Enumeration of the potential risks and benefits associated with the study treatments, as well as an enumeration of common side effects • Description of any special procedures that will be performed, including an enumeration of the risks and benefits associated with those procedures, and the time points at which they are to be performed	

Most clinical trials involve the collection and storage of personal information, such as name and address, on study patients (see Section 15.3 for uses of the information in tracing patients). Some investigators engaged in epidemiological studies have indicated the exact date at which such information will be purged from patient files. The commitment is unwise in long-term clinical trials for two reasons. First, it may be impossible to meet because of unexpected delays in the conduct of the trial. Second, and more important, there may be a need to contact patients after the trial is completed, especially if any of the study treatments appear to be producing late and unexpected adverse effects.

The mechanics of obtaining the informed consent must be individualized to the population to be studied. Information may be presented in various ways so long as there is adequate opportunity for a patient (or his guardian) to have all questions regarding the study answered before

he is asked to make a decision on enrollment. Hard sells are to be avoided. First, because they represent subtle forms of coercion. Second, because they can lead to enrollment of uncooperative patients.

Whenever feasible, it is wise to carry out the consent process in two stages with a time separation of a day or more between the first and second stages. Many trials lend themselves to this approach, especially those that require multiple visits to establish a patient's eligibility for enrollment. Exceptions are cases in which treatment must be started on the spot.

The first stage should be designed to acquaint the patient with the study and its requirements. It should involve a conversation with the patient in a setting that is conducive to a two-way exchange. The information imparted should be supplemented with written material, including a copy of the consent statement for the patient to take home to review at his leisure. The second stage should be used to answer questions raised by the patient and to review what would be required of him if he agrees to enroll. The consent statement should be signed at the end of this stage.

Both stages should allow ample opportunity for the patient to question clinic personnel regarding the study and his role in it. A patient should not be asked to sign the consent statement if he has any doubts about enrolling or if the clinic staff believes he does not understand what his participation would involve. The patient should be asked to reaffirm his willingness to accept whatever treatment is assigned before he signs the statement.

The time point at which the consent process is initiated is important. If it is initiated too early in the recruitment process, a good deal of time may be wasted explaining the trial to individuals who are subsequently found to be ineligible for enrollment on medical grounds. However, delaying the start of the process until the eligibility assessment is complete may not allow enough time for an orderly two-stage consent, especially if there is any urgency to start treatment once eligibility has been established.

The treatment assignment should be issued on the same day the consent is signed. The treatment should be initiated as soon thereafter as feasible, preferably on the day of assignment. A large time gap between consent and initiation of treatment will tend to increase the patient's anxiety regarding treatment and may increase the chance of his withdrawing before treatment is started.

The consent statement used in multicenter trials should be standardized to the extent possible. Some variation in language may be unavoidable because of local IRB wording requirements. However, the amount can be minimized by providing clinics with a prototype statement that covers the items listed in Table 14-4. Individual clinics may not reduce or abridge information contained in the statement, but may add to it if required to do so by local IRBs.

14.6.3   Documentation of the consent

Federal regulations require that:

Informed consent shall be documented by use of a written consent form approved by the IRB and signed by the subject or the subject's legally authorized representative. A copy shall be given to the person signing

the form (Office for the Protection from Research Risks, p. 10, 1983).

The IRB must approve the consent statement and will want to review all information (written as well as verbal) presented to patients in conjunction with the consent process. The statement presented for signature may contain a written description of all pertinent information needed in the consent process, or may refer to materials presented orally or in an accompanying document, such as in a patient information booklet. The patient's signature should be witnessed by a third party, regardless of how the presentation is made. The patient should be given a copy of the consent form after it has been signed. The original should be kept in the patient's file.

The responsibility for obtaining informed consent goes beyond the simple mechanics of presenting and signing documents. It is the responsibility of all those connected with the study to ensure that the process is carried out in a responsible manner. This responsibility extends beyond the clinics in multicenter trials. The approved statements should be collected by the coordinating center for review and storage. The review should be done by the study leadership and should be aimed at making certain that the statements meet study standards. In addition, the center should set up procedures to withhold treatment assignments until signed consents have been obtained.

Clinic site visits (see Section 16.8.3) should include checks on the consent process. This can be done via a walk-through for a hypothetical patient or by witnessing the process being carried out with an actual patient. The visiting team may also talk to patients who have gone through the process to learn what they know about the trial. The Beta Blocker Heart Attack Trial (BHAT) assessed the quality of the consent process by interviewing a sample of patients (Howard et al., 1981).

14.6.4   What constitutes an informed consent?

The question of what constitutes an informed consent is complex. It depends on the information to be conveyed and on how it is perceived by the patient. The formal nature of the doctor-patient relationship, coupled with the patient's anxieties regarding his condition, can be major blocks to meaningful communication. Studies of the consent process suggest that patients may fail to comprehend much of what they are told (Howard et al., 1981).

Consent materials should be simply written. It is important for design concepts, such as randomization, placebos, and masking, to be explained in lay terms. Some investigators have chosen to exclude patients who do not comprehend fundamental aspects of the study design. The Hypertension Prevention Trial (HPT) required patients to correctly answer a series of questions on the trial before they could be enrolled. A vaccine study research group at the University of Maryland requires volunteers to pass a test on the trial prior to enrollment (Levine, 1976; Woodward, 1979).

The failure to cover important items of information in the consent statement can cause a dilemma later on. A case in point is the failure to specify the nature of follow-up that will be carried out on indivduals who drop out after enrollment. It is common in a long-term trial to employ special procedures to obtain up-to-date mortality data on all study patients, including dropouts, at the time of final data analysis (see Chapter 15). Normally, these procedures are carried out unobtrusively. Nevertheless, the preferred approach is to make the patient aware of the ways in which his personal identifying information may be used for tracing and mortality follow-up before he is enrolled. A patient who is uncomfortable with what is proposed should not be enrolled.

14.6.5 Maintenance of consents

Consents given at the time of enrollment may have to be updated to remain valid. Patients should be informed of any decision or action that is likely to affect their willingness to continue in the trial, such as a decision to stop a study treatment in another group of patients because of an adverse effect or to add a data collection procedure that is inconvenient, uncomfortable, or risky. The CDP informed all study patients of the decision to terminate use of the high-dose estrogen treatment, even though less than one-quarter of them were on that treatment.

Changes in the federal regulations regarding the informed consent process during a trial may require addendums to the consents. For example, investigators in the UGDP were required to obtain signed consent statements from patients after recruitment had been completed. Undocumented oral consents, obtained at the start of the trial, were not considered sufficient after the February 8, 1966, memo from the Surgeon General of the USPHS. More recently, addendums have been required to inform patients of local policy on compensation for and care of study related injuries.

14.7 RANDOMIZATION AND INITIATION OF TREATMENT

Patients judged eligible and who are willing to participate in the trial are ready for enrollment. The point at which the treatment assignment is disclosed to the treating physician should be used to mark formal entry of a patient into the trial. Once enrolled, a patient should be counted as part of the study population (see Chapter 18).

The randomization procedure should be set up to make certain that assignments remain masked until they are needed for initiation of treatment (see Chapters 8 and 10). As already noted in Section 14.6.2, treatment should be started as soon after enrollment as practical, ideally on the day of randomization.

14.8 ZELEN CONSENT PROCEDURE

The usual approach is to obtain a patient's consent before he is randomized. The sequence is reversed in a modification proposed by Zelen (1979). In that method, eligible patients are randomized before consent is obtained. Those assigned to the control (standard) treatment are given that treatment without discussion of the alternative treatment(s) under evaluation. Only patients assigned to the test treatment(s) are given an opportunity to refuse the treatment assignment. Patients who refuse are given the control treatment.

The appeal of the approach lies in the fact that only patients assigned to test treatments are presented with information on treatment alternatives. The others are spared the anxiety that may be aroused by such discussions. However, in actual fact, most IRBs are reluctant to accept the approach, except under very special circumstances (such as in a trial involving a high-risk treatment on patients with a poor prognosis for life), and then only where cogent arguments can be made in its favor.

The approach has a number of limitations. Of necessity, it is limited to unmasked trials since the treating physician must know the assignment to identify patients with whom choices are to be discussed. In addition, refusals after randomization, if sizable, will make it difficult to reach any conclusion from the trial. Further, the procedure can lead to subtle forms of coercion. Patients assigned to the test treatment may be coaxed by study personnel to accept the assignment simply as a means of avoiding the data analysis and interpretation problems that can arise if there are a lot of treatment refusals. Finally, the method is unfair in that only patients assigned to test treatments are allowed a choice.

15. Patient follow-up, close-out, and post-trial follow-up

> There are only two classes of mankind in the world—doctors and patients. . . . you [doctors] have been, and always will be exposed to the contempt of the gifted amateur— the gentleman who knows by intuition everything that it has taken you years to learn.
> Rudyard Kipling

15.1 INTRODUCTION

Before approaching the subject matter of this chapter it is necessary to provide working definitions of three different processes. They are:

Patient follow-up
   A process involving periodic contact with the patient after enrollment into the trial for the purpose of administering the assigned treatment, observing the effects of treatment, modifying the course of treatment, and collecting data to evaluate the treatment.

Patient close-out
   A process carried out to separate a patient from the trial, involving cessation of treatment and termination of regular follow-up.

Patient post-trial follow-up
   A process that involves patient follow-up after completion of the close-out stage of the trial and that is designed to yield information on the primary or a secondary outcome measure.

This chapter deals with the steps involved in carrying out these three processes (see also Appendix D).

15.2 MAINTENANCE OF INVESTIGATOR AND PATIENT INTEREST DURING FOLLOW-UP

The follow-up process requires a dedicated and committed staff to schedule and carry out the required examinations and a willing patient population. Both are needed if the trial is to succeed.

15.2.1 Investigator interest

Investigator commitment to the trial and interest in its activities must be high throughout if it is to succeed. Interest will be easy to maintain in a short-term trial, where the initial enthusiasm that usually accompanies the start of any new activity is enough to carry it through to completion. However, even in such cases spirits can sag before the data analyses are done and the final paper has been written. They can sag long before that point in long-term trials. Table 15–1 lists some of the aids that can be used to maintain investigator interest. The list is written with long-term multicenter trials in mind. However, morale problems are not unique to multicenter trials. They can be just as great in single-center trials.

   Periodic meetings of study personnel are essential in maintaining a cohesive investigative group. They are needed before the start of the trial to outline the treatment and data collection procedures for the trial, and they are an essential

Table 15–1 Aids for maintaining investigator interest

- Periodic meetings of all study personnel
- Distribution of periodic progress reports on patient recruitment and follow-up, data collection, and other performance characteristics of the trial for review by all members of the investigative group
- Periodic newsletters distributed to study personnel designed to inform them of study progress, protocol changes, and so forth
- Investigator participation in the analysis of results and in writing or presenting papers concerning the trial
- Preparation of reports and papers during the course of the trial summarizing the design, organizational, and operating features of the trial
- Execution of ancillary studies
- Certificates of appreciation from the sponsor, and signed by key study leaders, to staff reaching important milestones (e.g., their five-year anniversary with the study)

part of the quality assurance process once it is under way. Meetings should include clinic coordinators, technicians, and other support staff important to the trial, as well as senior personnel.

The long-term multicenter trial will require a variety of other ways to maintain investigator interest. The chance for investigators to engage in ancillary studies (see Glossary for definition and Section 22.7.3 for discussion of management issues related to such studies) can help maintain their interest and general commitment to the trial. The opportunity to carry out analyses on data collected during the trial can also help morale. In reality, the opportunities for such analyses may be limited in settings in which there is a desire to mask clinic staff to treatment results, as discussed in Chapter 22. However, this policy does not preclude access to data unrelated to treatment outcome. The Coronary Drug Project (CDP) allowed access to baseline data for all the treatment groups as well as follow-up data for the placebo-treated group of patients. The follow-up data were used to generate several papers on the natural history of coronary heart disease (see Table B–3 of Appendix B for list).

Access to adherence or process measures by treatment group is also acceptable. Staff in the Multiple Risk Factor Intervention Trial (MRFIT) were provided with data indicating the level of risk reduction achieved as the study progressed. These summaries included data on clinic performance in terms of achieving stated treatment goals and were used by study leaders to assess the intervention procedures.

15.2.2 Patient interest

A patient's interest in the trial and willingness to continue in it can be expected to diminish with time. The longer the period of follow-up the greater the need for measures to counteract waning interest and participation levels. Table 15–2 lists factors and approaches that can help sustain patient interest in the trial. However, by all odds, the most important factor is the attitude of clinic staff. Uninterested or discourteous staff will lead to an uninterested patient population.

15.3 LOSSES TO FOLLOW-UP

A loss to follow-up occurs whenever an item of information required as part of a scheduled follow-up examination is not obtained in the permissible time window (see Glossary for definition). The loss may be due to:

- Failure of the clinic staff to complete an item on an otherwise properly completed data form
- Failure of the patient to agree to certain procedures during an examination
- Failure of the patient to return to the clinic for an examination within the time window specified for it

Losses due to missed examinations or to examinations that are not done within the specified time window, and hence are counted as missed, are more worrisome than the losses resulting from failure to complete specific items or procedures during an examination. Further, an occasional missed examination for a patient has different implications than does a sequence of missed examinations. The longer the sequence, the greater the uncertainty regarding the outcome status of the patient.

Patients who are no longer able or willing to return to the clinic for scheduled follow-up examinations are dropouts. The declaration may be made by the patient (e.g., by announcing an intent to leave the study because of a lack of interest or because of a forthcoming move to another city) or by clinic staff. The latter will be the case with a patient who disappears or who does not, for whatever reason, keep his scheduled appointments. However, a clinic declaration should not be made until (1) clinic staff have made a concerted effort to locate the patient if

Table 15-2 Factors and approaches that enhance patient interest and participation

- Clinic staff who treat patients with courtesy and dignity and who take an interest in meeting their needs
- Clinic located in pleasant physical surroundings and in a secure environment
- Convenient access to parking for patients who drive, and to other modes of transportation for those who do not
- Payment of parking and travel fees incurred by study patients
- Payment of clinic registration fees and costs for procedures required in the trial
- Special clinics in which patients are able to avoid the confusion and turmoil of a regular out-patient clinic
- Scheduled appointments designed to minimize waiting time
- Clinic hours designed for patient convenience
- Written or telephone contacts between clinic visits
- Remembering patients on special occasions, such as Christmas, birthday anniversaries, etc.
- Establishment of identity with the study through proper indoctrination and explanation of study procedures during the enrollment process; through procedures such as use of special ID cards to identify the patient as a participant in the study, and by awarding certificates to recognize their contribution to the trial

he has disappeared, and to try to convince him to return to the clinic for a follow-up examination; and (2) the patient has missed a specified number of follow-up clinic visits. The date of the patient's last completed follow-up examination should be used as the date of dropout. The patient should remain classified as a dropout until or unless he returns to the clinic for a follow-up examination.

Patients who are classified as dropouts may or may not be lost to follow-up for the outcome of interest. They are when the diagnosis or measurement of the primary outcome can only be done at follow-up examinations performed in study clinics. They are not when it can be done outside study clinics (e.g., as in trials with death as the primary outcome). Similarly, conversion of a patient from active to dropout status may or may not affect his treatment compliance (see Glossary for definition). It will not if the conversion occurs after treatment has been completed and if the treatment cannot be reversed or nullified. It will be tantamount to creating a state of noncompliance if the conversion requires termination of an ongoing treatment process (e.g., as in most chronic drug treatment trials).

The willingness of a patient to remain under active follow-up will depend on a variety of factors, including:

- The amount of time and inconvenience involved in making follow-up visits to the clinic
- The perceived importance of the procedures performed at follow-up visits from a health maintenance point of view
- The potential health benefits associated with treatment versus potential risks
- The amount of trauma and discomfort produced by the study treatment or procedures performed
- The number and type of side effects associated with treatment

The dropout rate may well change over the course of follow-up, as illustrated in Figure 15-1 for the three treatments continued to the end of the CDP. The rate declined with time, but only slightly. The niacin treatment group had the highest 5-year rate. It was also the group that had the largest number of patients with treatment-related complaints (Coronary Drug Project Research Group, 1975).

The procedures carried out in conjunction with follow-up examinations may influence dropout patterns. For example, a spurt in dropouts may occur just before an examination involving a noxious procedure. Similarly, there may be a peak after patients pass a specified time point in the trial, especially if they perceive that their time commitments to the trial are satisfied.

A certain number of dropouts in long-term trials will occur simply because of patient relocations. Such losses can be reduced in multicenter trials by transfer of follow-up responsibilities to sister clinics. The CDP was able to maintain the clinic visit schedule for several patients in this way (Coronary Drug Project Research Group, 1973a).

Dropouts should be contacted at periodic intervals. The contacts may be made via home visits, telephone, or mail and should be made even if they cannot be used to collect outcome data since they may be useful in persuading patients to return to active follow-up.

Patients who cannot be contacted should be traced so that contact may be re-established. The tracing process should be initiated as soon as possible. Table 15-3 provides a list of some of the methods that can be used for tracing (see Section 12.5.12 for a discussion of the types of identifying and locator information that should

Figure 15-1   Lifetable cumulative dropout rates for the clofibrate, niacin, and placebo treatments in the CDP.

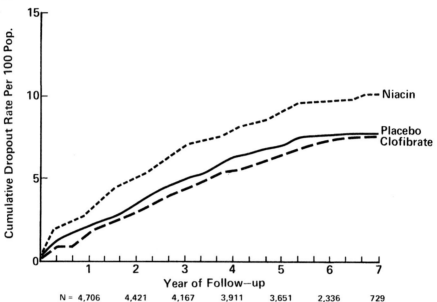

Note: N denotes total number of patients in clofibrate, niacin, and placebo groups combined. Approximate numbers for individual treatment groups are 2/9, 2/9, and 5/9 times N for clofibrate, niacin, and placebo, respectively.

Source: Reference citation 107. Adapted with permission of the American Medical Association, Chicago, Ill. (copyright © 1975).

be collected). Simple steps (Part A, Table 15–3), such as those involved in checking phone and address directories, may enable clinic staff to locate most of the "lost" patients, and they should be carried out before any of the approaches listed in Part B of Table 15–3 are considered.

Searches carried out by agencies retained for that purpose should be done discreetly, without patient contact. This proscription should extend to the coordinating center or other resource centers in the trial as well, unless the patient has had prior contact with the center in question or consented to such contact when he was enrolled.

The cost of searches carried out by firms, such as Equifax,[1] will vary from a few dollars to several hundred, depending on the extent of the search. Relatively inexpensive searches may locate the majority of lost patients, whereas a fairly large investment may be needed to locate those that are especially hard to find. Some help in the location process may be provided by governmental agencies. As a rule, they will not re-

lease address information but they may reveal whether their record indicates that the patient has died or may agree to send letters to study patients that are alive, suggesting that they recontact the study clinic.

Table 15-3   Methods for relocating dropouts

A. Ordinary

- Via check for address change through the post office, city directories, telephone books, etc.
- Via contact with known friends or relatives of the patient
- Via other sources, such as the patient's most recent employer, church group, etc.

B. Special

- Via a private agency specializing in locating people
- Via firms maintaining large address files and that market a tracing or follow-up service
- Via departments of motor vehicles*
- Via a government agency, such as the Social Security or Veterans Administration*
- Via a private or public institution, such as a hospital*
- Via the patient's private doctor*

1. Equifax is an Atlanta-based firm that was established to provide credit and related information for clients of the banking and insurance industry. A branch of the firm was established in the 1970s for marketing a locator service for follow-up studies.

*May not yield direct contact with patient if the agency or individual is unwilling to supply the desired address information or is legally constrained from doing so.

Contact with the patient or his family is essential for most forms of follow-up. One notable exception is for mortality follow-up using the National Death Index—NDI (National Center for Health Statistics, 1981). Table 15–4 lists the items of information needed for such searches. The Index contains deaths recorded in the U.S. since 1979. It contains basic identifying information for each deceased person, including the death certificate number and state in which the certificate is located.

It should be possible, with the search methods described above, to provide mortality data on virtually every patient enrolled in a trial. Both the CDP and UGDP were able to achieve this goal (without the NDI since it was not operational when these studies were done). The CDP had vital status on all but a few of the 5,011 patients covered in the final report on clofibrate and niacin (Coronary Drug Project Research Group, 1975). The 1970 publication from the UGDP on tolbutamide provided mortality data on all but 5 of the 823 patients included in that report (University Group Diabetes Program Research Group, 1970e).

15.4 CLOSE-OUT OF PATIENT FOLLOW-UP

The process of disengaging patients from a trial may require as much skill and care as the enrollment process. Recent papers have addressed aspects of the close-out process (e.g., Hawkins and Canner, 1978; Klimt and Canner, 1979; Klimt, 1981). Table 15–5 provides a summary list of considerations that should be addressed in planning for close-out. (See Chapter 3 and Appendix D for additional information.)

Table 15–4 Data items that may be used in searches of the National Death Index

- Last name*
- First name*
- Middle initial

- Social security number*
- Month,* day, and year* of birth
- Father's surname* (for females)

- Age at death (actual or estimated)
- Sex
- Race

- Marital status
- State of residence
- State of birth

*Considered to be key in checking for a possible record match

Table 15–5 Study close-out considerations

- Time schedule (i.e., whether to close-out follow-up for all patients at the same calendar time or after a fixed period of follow-up, see Section 11.7)
- Information to be collected (see Section 15.4)
- Phased treatment disengagement (usually applicable only to drug trials, see Section 15.4)
- Nature of recommendations given to patients regarding subsequent treatment
- Method for ensuring proper transfer of patient care responsibilities to alternate clinic or physician when appropriate
- Ensuring patients have ample opportunity to make alternative arrangements for care and to have any questions answered regarding the trial and its outcome before separation
- Method of summarizing baseline and follow-up data for subsequent use by patient's private physician
- Nature of patient contact required to document separation from trial
- Update of patient locator information and consent (applicable only if there is any possibility of having to contact patients later on to check their status or to recall them for examination)
- Masked trials: Time at which treatment is to be unmasked for study staff; for patients
- Masked trials: Amount of information to be collected on the efficacy of the mask (see Section 15.4 and Section 8.5)

The separation can be an emotional experience for both patients and clinic staff. It should be based on a detailed plan that has been constructed and reviewed before the start of close-out. The details of the separation should be discussed with patients well before separation occurs. Clinic staff must spend whatever time is necessary to answer questions and to help find suitable alternative sources of care. The latter step is imperative in any trial that has been providing patients with routine medical care, as in the UGDP. Investigators in that study discussed care requirements with each patient before departure and made certain of continued care after the close of the trial. The study clinic provided the new clinic or physician with a summary (prepared by the coordinating center) of key baseline and follow-up data assembled on the patient when transfers of care were involved.

The record generated in conjunction with separation should contain:

- The name of the treatment the patient was on
- The date the patient was informed of the treatment assignment (for masked trials)

- The date treatment was discontinued (when appropriate)
- The date of the final close-out visit
- The name of the clinic or physician responsible for future care of the patient
- The treatment recommendation and prescription (when appropriate)
- A list of materials and information given to the patient on departure

Close-out provides an opportunity to assess the adequacy of the mask in masked trials. Theoretically, such checks could be made at various time points throughout the trial. However, usually they are not carried out because of a desire to discourage speculation concerning the treatment assignments since the assessment involves asking the masked individual(s) to state a guess regarding treatment assignment (see also Section 8.5 and Krol, 1983).

A key consideration at close-out has to do with whether to carry out added data collection on patients as they are separated from the trial (the same consideration may arise in conjunction with protocol changes involving termination of a particular treatment during the trial). The wisdom of making such provisions depends on the importance of the data generated in relation to the aims of the trial. Results obtained for tests or procedures for which there are no corresponding baseline values will be of limited use in making treatment comparisons if the treatment groups differ because of losses due to dropouts or deaths. Investigators in the CDP opted against introduction of special data collection schemes during close-out, except for the addition of a few items to facilitate relocation of patients (Krol, 1983).

The method of terminating therapy in masked drug trials must be given special consideration. A dosage step-down scheme may be necessary if an abrupt cessation of one or more of the drugs is considered unsafe. In addition, a patient will want to know the treatment he was on. Hence, study physicians must be supplied with treatment codes well in advance of close-out visits, especially in trials where time is needed to consider alternative courses of therapy before making a treatment recommendation.

Ideally, any treatment recommendation given to patients at close-out should be based on findings from the trial. However, often this is not possible, since the final analysis of the results may not be completed by the time of close-out. Recommendations may have to be qualified or simply withheld, especially in designs involving close-out after a fixed period of follow-up (see Section 11.7). In such cases, the close-out process will extend over a period of time as long as that required for patient enrollment. It may not be advisable to unmask treatment assignments in such designs until all patients have been separated from the trial, unless it is possible to lift the mask on a per-patient basis (see Section 10.5).

Patients should be told at close-out if the clinic plans to keep in touch with them and, if so, the reason for doing so and the way in which contact will be maintained (e.g., via mail, telephone, or home visits). They should be asked to sign a consent authorizing the contacts and to provide updated locator information if contacts are planned. In fact, it is a good idea to alert patients to the possibility of future contacts and to obtain consents for them even if subsequent contacts are not planned, if there is any chance they will be needed later on.

15.5   TERMINATION STAGE

Close-out of patient follow-up is only the first stage in shutting down the trial. It is normally followed by a series of activities (see Table 15–6 and Section VI of Appendix D) beginning with completion of the close-out visits and ending with termination of all funding for the trial. The time needed for termination is variable and depends on the trial. A period of a year or longer is common for trials of the type sketched in Appendix B.

As a rule, clinics will require financial support for a period of time beyond the patient close-out stage to complete data transmissions to the data center and to respond to edit queries from that center. Support for the data center will have to extend beyond that for clinics to allow adequate time for the center to complete analyses of the results and to prepare them for publication. The UGDP Coordinating Center continued to receive funding through April 1982, nearly 7 years after completion of the last close-out examinations. The coordinating center in the CDP continued to operate through 1983, over 9 years after termination of the closeout stage of that trial.

One of the last steps in the termination stage has to do with record storage and disposition. All study forms and related documents to be retained (especially those with personal identifiers on them) should be stored in a secure location. Forms and related documents should be

Table 15-6 Activities in the termination stage

A. General

- Revise organizational structure (at the start of the termination stage) to meet special needs of the termination stage. Discharge committees no longer needed

- Update mortality follow-up for all patients, including dropouts

- Carry out final data edit checks

- Establish cutoff date beyond which changes to the data system are no longer allowed (needed so data files can be "frozen" for final analysis)

- Develop and implement plan for the final disposition of the study data forms and related documents, such as x-rays, fundus photographs, ECGs, etc.

- Develop plan for dealing with requests for special analyses or for access to the study data after termination of study funding (see Chapter 24)

- Disseminate study findings and conclusions to study investigators and to referral physicians (may be done by distributing preprint or reprint of main study manuscript)

- Discharge all remaining committees at the end of the termination stage

B. Additional activities in drug trials

- Collect sample of study drugs for future laboratory analysis in case of questions regarding drug purity

- Dispose of remaining unused study drugs

- Submit final report to the FDA if trial involved an INDA or IDEA; cancel INDA or IDEA after acceptance of the report by the FDA

destroyed (in compliance with local statutes for disposition of medical records) if secure storage cannot be assured and the required period of storage has passed (see Section 17.6). General factors to consider in arranging for record storage and policy questions concerning access to study data are discussed in Chapter 24.

15.6 POST-TRIAL PATIENT FOLLOW-UP

Post-trial follow-up, by definition, takes place after the termination stage of the trial (see Chapter 3, Appendix D, and Glossary for further details). Ideally, the patient personal identifiers needed for the follow-up should be deposited at a central location before the trial terminates, especially in multicenter trials. If this is not done, the task of assemblying the information after the trial has terminated may make subsequent follow-up difficult, if not impossible. The repository should be established at a center that can assure secure storage, and that is likely to remain functional into the foreseeable future. Federal agencies, such as the National Institutes of Health (NIH), generally are not suitable as a repository because of their susceptibility to requests under the Freedom of Information Act (see Chapter 24).

There should be a sound rationale for any post-trial follow-up involving direct patient contact. The prime motivation for most post-trial follow-ups stems from a desire to extend the period of observation for death or some other serious but nonfatal event. Another reason may be to observe patients for a disease or condition that may be caused or aggravated by treatments administered during the trial. The usefulness of the information obtained will depend on the completeness of the follow-up and the nature of intervening treatments administered after closeout. Interpretation of the results will be easiest if patients have not been exposed to any additional treatment after separation from the trial. It will be problematic if they have been.

The CDP provides an example of post-trial mortality follow-up. The follow-up was performed by the coordinating center, with help from clinics still in operation when the follow-up started in 1981. Addresses and other identifying information on patients were used for tracing them and for accessing the National Death Index and other files.

Some trials have provided a form of post-trial follow-up during the trial. For example, this was the case for the two discontinued treatments in the UGDP. Patients assigned to both the tolbutamide and phenformin treatments were followed for mortality (as well as for other nonfatal events) until separation of all patients in August of 1975. There has been no further post-trial follow-up of any of the UGDP treatment groups since then (University Group Diabetes Program Research Group, 1982).

16. Quality assurance

If it ain't broke, don't fix it.

Old American Adage

16.1 INTRODUCTION

Quality assurance, as applied to clinical trials, is any method or procedure for collecting, processing, or analyzing study data that is aimed at maintaining or enhancing their reliability or validity. Examples include (see Table 16–1):

- Edit procedures to check on the accuracy of items on completed data forms
- Repeat of a laboratory determination to check on reproducibility
- Rekeying data as a check for errors in the entry process
- Carrying out analyses by clinic in a multicenter trial to detect performance variations
- Reprogramming an analysis procedure as a means of checking on its accuracy

Deficiencies anywhere in the chain of events from data generation to publication of the results can reduce the quality of the finished product and the conclusions reached from the trial. Everyone involved in data collection, analysis, and manuscript writing must perform effectively to produce a quality end result.

This chapter deals with the mechanics of quality assurance. Other chapters of this book touch upon issues related to quality assurance. They include:

- Treatment masking (Chapter 8)
- Randomization (Chapters 8 and 10)
- Data form construction (Chapter 12 and Appendix F)
- Production and maintenance of study handbooks and manuals (Chapter 13)
- Testing the data intake and processing system (Chapter 13)
- Database maintenance (Chapter 17)
- Review procedures for study publications (Chapter 24)
- Activities staging (Appendix D)

16.2 ONGOING DATA INTAKE: AN ESSENTIAL PREREQUISITE FOR QUALITY ASSURANCE

Most of the quality assurance procedures outlined in Table 16–1 require a continuous and timely flow of data from the clinic to the data center to be useful. The data edits and analyses carried out during the trial to assess data quality and clinic performance will lose much of their value if there is a large time gap between data generation and conversion into computer-readable formats.

The ideal data intake system is one in which data are edited and entered on the day of genera-

Table 16-1 Quality assurance procedures

- Visual check by a member of the clinic staff after a data form is completed for illegible responses and for unanswered or incorrectly answered items
- Ongoing data processing
- Replication of the coding and data entry process as a means of error detection
- Computer edit of keyed data for inadmissible codes or missing values
- Data edit queries (directed from the data center to the clinic) concerning completed data forms
- Generation of periodic status reports concerning the data collection process
- Repeat laboratory determinations
- Multiple independent readings of ECGs, fundus photographs, X rays, tissue slides, etc.
- Independent review of patient death records for classifying cause of death
- Submission of masked duplicate specimens or records to check on the reproducibility of a measurement or reading procedure
- Generation of periodic reports assessing the compliance of clinics to the treatment protocol
- Comparison of the performance of clinics in a multicenter trial to detect differences in the quality or completeness of the data generated, as reflected by such characteristics as number of missed follow-up examinations, number of dropouts, number of deficient data forms, etc.
- Reprogramming of a data editing or analysis procedure as a check on program accuracy or on the quality of program documentation
- Interim analyses of study data for treatment effects that can be used to reveal inadequacies or inconsistencies in the data collected

tion, or very shortly thereafter. Theoretically, the entry process could take place as patients are examined using video displays to remind physicians and technicians of items to be entered. However, on-line data entry of this sort is usually not practical. The need to do so during an examination may distract both the patient and physician and may complicate the examination. Further, it is unlikely that all data could be entered on the spot since much of it may not be available until some time after the examination is completed (e.g., as with results of certain laboratory tests or readings from biopsy material, ECGs, X rays, etc.). However, even if these problems could be overcome, documentation of the data collection process argues against on-line entry. The data forms and related paper records are needed to document the data collection and

entry processes, to say nothing of their use in patient care. Hence, discussion throughout this book is predicated on the assumption that data collection always involves completion of paper forms and records, regardless of where and how data entry is done.

One viable approach to on-site data entry involves completion of a paper form during the patient examination and then entry of the information contained on that form as soon after the examination as possible—ideally, on the same day or within a few days after the examination. The entry should be done by clinic personnel who are familiar with the data collection requirements of the trial, and should be subjected to edits during the entry process. The keyed data may remain at the clinic for subsequent analyses or may be transferred to a central data facility for additional edits, analysis, and storage. The transfer may take place on-line as the data are keyed, or may be done off-line either on a fixed schedule or on demand, as dictated by the data center. On-line transfer may be via hard-wired or telephone connections to the central facility. Off-line transfers may be done by telephone or by mailing the magnetic records to the central storage facility.

Systems involving on-site data entry and multiple data generation sites, as in multicenter trials, are herein referred to as distributed data entry systems. Those in which data forms are sent to a data center for entry are referred to as centralized data entry systems. All but two of the 14 trials sketched in Appendix B had systems of the latter type. Only the Coronary Artery Surgery Study (CASS) and Hypertension Prevention Trial (HPT) had distributed data entry systems.

A trial in which each data generation site is responsible for maintaining its own database with programs provided from the data center is herein referred to as having a distributed database (e.g., the HPT). A trial in which the only electronic database that exists is the one maintained at the central data facility is herein referred to as having a centralized database.

The main advantages of distributed data entry have to do with the potential for eliminating the time lag between the data generation and data entry processes, and with the ability to involve data collection personnel in the data entry process. However, in order to work well, the approach requires skilled personnel at the data center who have the patience and know-how to select the equipment needed for the system, to supervise acquisition and installation of it at the clinic, to train clinic personnel in its operation, and to develop and maintain the software packages needed for on-site data entry and editing.

The lag time between the generation of a form and data entry should never be more than a week or two, regardless of the type of entry system. The goal should be to establish and maintain the discipline needed to ensure a timely flow of forms from the point of origin through data entry. Designs that allow forms to accumulate over a specified time interval or in batches of a certain size before they are forwarded for data entry should be avoided. The best design is one in which individual forms proceed to data entry on a per-form basis without regard to other forms or conditions. Batching increases the time from completion of a form to data entry. If some batching is required for reasons of efficiency, it should be minimal and should never allow forms to accumulate for more than a week or two. The same is true for accumulation of forms at the data entry site.

16.3 DATA EDITING

The term *data editing* refers to the process of detecting, querying, and, when appropriate, correcting values in a data set that are invalid. The normal editing process involves a series of edit checks and edit queries. An edit check is an operation carried out on an item or series of items on a completed data form for the purpose of identifying possible errors (see Table 16–2). An edit query is a question generated from review of a completed data form that concerns the accuracy or adequacy of some item of information on the form and that requires someone at the generation site to review the information in order to respond to the query. The query may be generated by a clerk checking a completed form for deficiencies, or by a CRT or printer driven by edit programs.

Edit queries that are written will be referred to as edit messages. Any edit message that requires review and possible corrective action should be printed on hard copy. This does not preclude use of a CRT for a preliminary display of messages, but this procedure is not adequate if messages must be sent to various places in the clinic for review and action. Special care must be taken to make certain that the messages are intelligible. Table 16–3 gives suggested edit message rules.

A sample of such messages, as taken from the Macular Photocoagulation Study (MPS), is reproduced in Figures 16–1 and 16–2 for a fictitious clinic and patient. The two pages relate to

Table 16–2   Types of edit checks

Type	*Edit check*
• Patient identification and record linkage	• Check of ID number and name code for transposition errors
	• Check of name for spelling errors
	• Check to make certain all pages of a given form carry the same ID number
• Legibility	• Check for illegible handwritten replies, spelling errors, etc.
	• Check for response checkmarks placed outside designated spaces
• Form admissibility	• Check to determine if the form was completed within the specified time window
	• Check to make certain the form completed is the correct one for the indicated examination
• Missing information	• Check for unanswered items or sections of an otherwise completed form
	• Check to make certain all required forms have been completed
• Consistency	• Check of information supplied in one section against another section on the same form for inconsistencies
	• Check of information supplied on the same patient on one data form with that from another form completed at the same or at a different examination as a check for possible data inconsistencies
• Range and inadmissible codes	• Check to identify items with values that exceed specified ranges
	• Check for undefined alphabetic or numerical codes

Table 16-3 Edit message rules

- Use a format that facilitates use by clinic personnel, even if the format is not ideal for data entry
- Test the intelligibility of the messages on personnel who must deal with the messages
- Avoid the use of esoteric codes, abbreviations, and other symbols that are not readily understood by personnel who must respond to the statements
- Identify the patient, examination, form, and item number on the edit statement
- Allow space on the statement for the respondent to indicate the action taken
- Group messages for a given patient examination in such a way so as to simplify the task of dealing with them (e.g., list all laboratory-related edit messages for a given examination on one page and all messages concerning clinical evaluation of the patient on another page, if different personnel are required to deal with the two types of edit messages)
- Generate duplicate copies of the edit messages to allow clinics to retain a copy of answered queries

patient 03–072–S, with name code MARV, seen on July 6, 1983, in connection with his fifth follow-up clinic visit (second annual examination). The message dated August 3, 1983, relates to inconsistencies noted in visual acuity measurements done on the patient. The message dated October 4, 1983, relates to discrepancies in readings of fundus photographs done at the clinic with those done at the MPS Fundus Photography Reading Center. Clinic personnel are required to indicate corrected values on the edit message sheets and to return them to the MPS Coordinating Center for processing.

The first set of edit checks should be done by hand at the clinic shortly after a form is completed. A second set of checks, involving a combination of hand and computer checks, may be performed when the data are keyed. The main advantages of computer checks lie in the ease and accuracy with which they can be made and in the ability to use the computer to write and

Figure 16-1 MPS Coordinating Center edit message of August 3, 1983.

```
Clinic : 03  Eye Research Clinic              Study: SMD

Patient : 03-072-S    Code : MARV             Visit: fv05   07/06/83
                                              (Follow-up Visit 05)


   ** COMPONENT   0702   Visual Acuity Measures (Follow-up)


        ITEM                OLD VALUE              CORRECTED VALUE
        ====                =========              ===============



        4AR                 10                     --

        4BR                 99                     --

        4CR                 00                     --


There is a problem with one or more of the above answers.  Question 4AR
must be answered with either a '10' or a '05', and the answers to Questions 4BR
and 4CR must indicate the smallest line read at THAT distance and the number
of additional letters read at THAT distance.
Please supply the correct answers for all three questions.
```

PERSON COMPLETING THIS FORM: _____ DATE: _____

Figure 16-2   MPS Coordinating Center edit message of October 4, 1983.

```
*** MPS READING CENTER ***

Clinic : 03  Eye Research Clinic                    Study: SMD

Patient : 03-072-S    Code : MARV                   Visit: fv05   07/06/83
                                                    (Follow-up Visit 05)

      ** COMPONENT   5511   Annual Follow-up Grading Form (PT, FV01, FV03 ...)

            ITEM                  OLD VALUE              CORRECTED VALUE
            ====                  =========              ===============


            1a                    n                      —

            5b                    5                      —

            6b                    n                      —

If there is no blood, there is no blood !
In other words, if question 1a is 'n' then questions 5b and 6b must also be 'n'.




            10a                   9                      —

            10b                   n                      —

If photos or FA are present then questions 10a and 10b MUST be answered.
If there is no RPE atrophy (Question 10a = 'n') then question 10b must also be 'n'.




         PERSON COMPLETING THIS FORM: ---------------------- DATE: --------
```

keep track of the queries. Clinics need periodic reminders of outstanding queries to ensure they are addressed (see Chapter 17 for a discussion of file updates based on edit changes). The computer, however, should never be a substitute for the checks performed by staff at the clinic before forms are forwarded for data entry. An experienced clinic coordinator, with an eye for errors and an encyclopedic knowledge of the study protocol, can do more to enhance the quality of the data generated than any set of computer checks.

There should be an audit trail for any change made to a completed data form, regardless of when and how the change was initiated. The nature of the deficiency, when it was detected, the change, and when the change was made should be noted. Once recorded on a form, data should not be erased or obliterated. Entries that are incorrect should be lined out and the new entries added to the form. Any change, regardless of when it was made, should be dated and

should carry the initials of the person making the change.

Data entry personnel should be given explicit instructions regarding the types of data changes they may make. Sound practice dictates that data should be entered as recorded, even if an item is "clearly" in error and the change required seems obvious. The temptation is to make an "obvious" change on the spot, without any checking. However, there are at least two reasons to resist the temptation. First, there is always the chance that the item has been correctly recorded even though it appears to be in error. Second, on-the-spot changes will lead to discrepancies between the computer data file and the original study records. Such discrepancies, if sizable, may lead to serious questions concerning the integrity of the data collection and processing activity. Both audits of the University Group Diabetes Program (UGDP) focused on the accuracy of the data collection and entry processes, as evidenced by comparisons of values recorded on the original study forms with entries appearing in the computer data file of the study (Committee for the Assessment of Biometric Aspects of Controlled Trials of Hypoglycemic Agents, 1975; Food and Drug Administration, 1978). Fortunately, procedures in the UGDP Coordinating Center required all changes to the computer file to originate with the original data forms. It would not have been possible to maintain a one-to-one correspondence between the original records and computer file without such a rule.

A series of identification and linkage checks should be performed before any form is added to the computer file. The ID number recorded should be checked for transposition errors (e.g., via a check digit; see Glossary). No form should be added to the file unless the ID number and other identifiers agree (e.g., such as name or name code).

Admission of a record to the data file may also depend on time window (see Glossary) checks needed to ensure that the information in question was obtained within a specified time interval. Examinations performed outside the specified window may either be rejected or assigned to the appropriate time slot, depending on the philosophy of the study.

Computer checks made during data entry should be designed to detect use of inadmissible codes (e.g., entry of an alphabetic character when only numeric codes are permissible or use of an undefined or inadmissible numeric code). These errors should be corrected before the generation of edit messages.

Most editing systems are designed to deal with one item at a time. There may be some cross checking of items, but it is usually limited to items on the same form. Cross checking of items across forms is generally not done because of the logistical difficulties involved in making such checks and because of the limited return in added undetected errors and deficiencies.

The foundations for data editing should be laid when the study is designed. The edit requirements should be specified in the handbooks and manuals needed for operation of the trial. The data forms used in the trial, as suggested in Chapter 12, should include reminder and documentation items (see Section 12.5.13) that require clinic personnel to carry out essential checks while the forms are being completed and that remind them of the steps that must be per-

formed in conjunction with specified data collection procedures.

16.4 REPLICATION AS A QUALITY CONTROL MEASURE

Replication of an observation or reading is frequently used as a check on the quality of the data obtained. Examples of replication used in this way are:

- Comparison of two independent measurements, such as a laboratory test, to determine if the difference observed is outside a specified range
- Use of two independent readings of an ECG to identify items of disagreement for adjudication by a third reader
- Comparison of cause of death codes assigned by two different individuals to identify areas of disagreement for adjudication by a third reader
- Averaging two or more consecutive blood pressure readings made on a patient during a given clinic visit in order to have a more reliable estimate of the patient's "true" blood pressure
- Rekeying data as a check for errors in the entry process
- Use of a computer program, written specifically to duplicate the tasks performed by another program, to check the accuracy of results provided with the original program

Replicate values obtained from repeat readings or from aliquots of the same laboratory specimen are usually combined by averaging to yield a single composite value. However, this approach is not suitable for combining independent readings made from the same record involving binary measures (e.g., presence or absence of S-T depression on ECGs). Some form of adjudication is necessary when the readings disagree. It may be done by having an "expert" make the judgment or by asking the individual readers to reach agreement. It is important to select readers who work well together and who interact on a peer basis if the latter approach is used.

A common problem in trials involving laboratory determinations has to do with the detection and disposition of outlier values (see Glossary). Explicit rules are required to indicate the conditions under which a determination is to be repeated and the value or values to be reported in such cases. The procedures of the laboratory performing the determinations should be reviewed when the rules are constructed. Laboratories differ with regard to the practices they follow in making repeat determinations because of suspected errors. Some of those practices can bias the results reported, for example, as is the case with a laboratory that does three determinations per sample, but reports only the two most concordant values. The same is true for a laboratory that opts to make repeat determinations when the observed inter-aliquot difference for the first set of determinations exceeds a prespecified limit and then reports only the results of the second set.

The easiest, and often the best, rule to follow is one that requires the laboratory to report all determinations made, without any censoring. Outlier values which, if retained in the data file, would have undue influence on means and variances may be eliminated or trimmed when the analysis tape is written (see Section 17.7).

16.5   MONITORING FOR SECULAR TRENDS

A secular trend in the readings made from records, such as ECGs, X rays, fundus photographs, and the like, or from laboratory determinations, can be troublesome, especially if differential by treatment. The possibility of this happening is minimized when the ordering of the readings or determinations is independent of treatment assignment (e.g., in schemes in which readings or determinations are done on an ongoing basis and in the order of generation). However, even so, it is wise to monitor for trends. The information is useful in characterizing the magnitude of the trend and in indicating whether it is differential by treatment. Assurance in the latter regard is especially important for readings or determinations that are not masked with regard to treatment assignment or that are ordered by treatment assignment. In addition, characterization of the trend, even if not needed for making treatment comparisons, is useful when evaluating follow-up results for a particular treatment group in natural history studies.

The number of repeat determinations or readings that are made should be dictated by the importance attached to detecting time trends and the total resources available for quality control. The cost of maintaining systems designed to detect secular trends can be sizable. Only a small part of the cost may be associated with making the actual readings or determinations. The larger costs will be associated with managing the monitoring system.

Monitoring a laboratory or reading center for secular trends requires use of known standards that are subjected to repeat analyses or readings over the course of the trial. To be useful, the repeat specimens should be indistinguishable from other specimens received at the laboratory or reading center.

Developing a reliable set of standards, at least for laboratory determinations, is not a trivial task. The problem would be easily solved if a single set of standards could be used throughout the trial. However, most biological substances degrade with time and, hence, more dynamic approaches are needed. The Coronary Drug Project (CDP) created a pool of donor serum. The pool was aliquoted and then frozen (Canner et al., 1983c; Hainline et al., 1983). Specimens from the pool were submitted to the central laboratory on a time schedule designed to coincide with actual patients in the trial, using ID numbers of deceased patients.[1] When a given pool was near depletion, or the time limit set for its use was about to expire, a new one was created. Use of specimens from the new pool overlapped use of specimens from the old pool, so as to provide a basis for estimating concentration differences between the two pools.

Similar monitoring is needed for readings of ECGs, fundus photographs, X rays, biopsy materials, etc. However, the mechanics of setting up and maintaining systems for this purpose are even more complicated than those required for laboratory determinations. The CDP used a system for making repeat ECG readings to monitor for time-related shifts in reading standards (Coronary Drug Project Research Group, 1973a). However, the system was difficult to manage, and it was not easy to keep readers from identifying repeat tracings, especially those with distinctive patterns. In any case, the system was only effective in detecting short-term trends since the tracings chosen for rereading were selected from batches of tracings that had been read in the recent past. Inclusion of records read in the distant past was not practical because of date information contained on the tracings. There was concern that lack of homogeneity of

---

1. Use of fictitious ID numbers would have caused the central laboratory to reject the specimens because of edit checks performed by it prior to admitting specimens for analysis.

dates within a reading batch would enable readers to identify repeat tracings.

Another method sometimes used to control a reading process involves use of reference measurements or records to help readers gauge the degree of abnormality seen in actual records. This approach was used in the MPS for grading the severity of certain kinds of eye abnormalities, as seen in fundus photographs. The severity of an observed abnormality was graded by selecting the photograph from an ordered set of standard photographs that was most similar to the one in question.

Concerns regarding secular trends are obviated if records are read over a short period of time at the end of the study and in a random order with regard to the time of generation and treatment assignment. However, this approach suffers from two major disadvantages. First, postponing readings until the end of data collection means that results from the records in question will not be available for interim analyses during the trial (see Chapter 20). Second, waiting for the readings may delay preparation of the final report. Both disadvantages are avoided with an ongoing reading program that runs over the course of the trial.

16.6 DATA INTEGRITY AND ASSURANCE PROCEDURES

An editorial by Meinert (1980b) discusses factors that may contribute to dishonest practices in the field of clinical trials. They do occur, but there is no reason to believe their incidence is higher in this field than in other areas of research. In fact, it may be lower because of the general emphasis on error detection and quality control. However, even so, there are good reasons for constant vigilance against shady practices. The luxury of replication, used so effectively in the laboratory sciences to confirm or refute findings, is not always feasible in clinical trials for practical as well as ethical reasons. For example, it would be difficult to justify additional placebo-controlled trials of hypertensives in the light of the conclusions from those done by the VA (Veterans Administration Cooperative Study Group on Antihypertensive Agents, 1967, 1970) or to replicate the Multiple Risk Factor Intervention Trial in view of its cost and the time required to complete it (Multiple Risk Factor Intervention Trial Research Group, 1982).

Table 16–4 Data integrity checks

- Comparison of information on a patient's medical chart with that recorded on a study data form
- Comparison of information on data forms with that in the computer
- Interviews with support personnel for identification of questionable or undesirable data practices
- Review of methods for issuing treatment allocations to check for discrepancies in the administration of the allocation schedule
- Review of analysis procedures used by the data center for evidence of a bias for or against a particular treatment
- Comparison of the distribution of inter-aliquot differences to detect clinic differences in reading or reporting procedures
- Independent audit of published reports to determine if the conclusions are supported by the raw data.

Table 16–4 provides a list of checks that can be performed to help identify questionable data practices, whether due to honest errors, careless oversights, or purposeful acts. The checks, like others in the trial, should be ongoing since the problems they are aimed at detecting can occur at any time over its course.

The best preventive measure is a staff that appreciates the importance of honesty and integrity in all aspects of the trial. The responsibility for instilling the proper philosophy rests with the leaders of the trial. They must, by the statements they make and the actions they take, set a tone and standard that permeates the entire investigative group.

16.7 PERFORMANCE MONITORING REPORTS

It is good practice to prepare reports summarizing performance characteristics of the trial as it proceeds. The reports should be prepared by the data center and should be designed to provide up-to-date information on all relevant activities of the trial. Some of the performance characteristics that should be monitored are listed in Table 16–5. See also Appendix G for sample reports.

The information in the report should be reviewed by the leadership of the trial (e.g., the steering committee) and should be used as a basis for initiating corrective action, where appropriate. To be useful as a monitoring tool, reports should indicate the relative standings of

Table 16-5 Performance characteristics subject to ongoing monitoring

A. Clinic characteristics

1. Patient recruitment

- Number of patients screened for enrollment; proportion rejected and tabulation of reasons for rejection*
- Current rate of recruitment compared with that required to achieve a prestated recruitment goal

2. Patient follow-up

- Distribution of enrollment times and median length of follow-up
- Number of completed follow-up examinations*
- Number of missed examinations and number past due*
- Rate of missed examinations*
- Number of dropouts*
- Total number of dropouts and estimated dropout rate
- Number of patients who cannot be located for follow-up

3. Data quantity and quality

- Number of forms completed since last report and number that generated edit messages
- Current edit message rate per form contrasted with rates from previous time periods
- Number of forms received with missing parts or missing supporting records
- Number of unanswered edit queries*
- Number of patients enrolled with incomplete baseline information*

4. Protocol adherence

- Number of ineligible patients enrolled*
- Number of patients who did not accept the assigned treatment*
- Number of patients who received a treatment other than the one assigned*
- Summary of data on pill counts and other adherence tests by treatment group*
- Number of departures from the treatment protocol*
- Summary of other treatment or data collection protocol violations

B. Data center characteristics

- Number of allocations issued*
- Number of allocations returned unused
- Number of forms received*
- Total number of forms awaiting data entry*
- List of coding and protocol changes implemented since last report
- List of data processing and programming errors and likely impact on study results
- Summary of major events, such as computing malfunctions, necessitating use of backup tapes to restore the data system
- Timetable for unfinished tasks

C. Central laboratory characteristics

- Number of samples received*
- Number of samples received improperly or inadequately identified*
- Number of samples lost or destroyed*
- Number of samples requiring reanalysis and tabulation of reasons for reanalysis*
- Backlog of samples remaining to be analyzed*
- Summary of major events affecting laboratory operations, such as power outages, particularly those resulting in possible degradation of frozen samples
- Mean and variance of inter-aliquot differences over time for specified tests
- Secular trend analyses based on repeat determinations of known standards

D. Reading center characteristics

- Number of records received and read*
- Number of records received that were improperly labelled or had other deficiencies (tabulate deficiencies)*
- Analyses of repeat readings as a check on reproducibility of readings and as a means of monitoring for time shifts in the reading process

E. Other performance characteristics

- Status of papers being written
- Progress in locating patients lost to follow-up
- Labelling errors made in drugs dispensed from the central pharmacy

*Report should contain results for the entire study period, for the time period covered since production of the last report, and for the last one or two preceding time periods.

clinics in multicenter trials with regard to important functions such as patient recruitment, completeness of follow-up, number of error-free forms, etc. The tabulations may be for the entire study period or for defined time intervals (e.g., the last 3 months, 4 to 6 months ago, etc.). The rankings can be helpful in identifying problem clinics. However, they should be viewed with caution when used as a basis for taking corrective or punitive action involving individual clinics. The range of the difference between the best and worst clinics with regard to a performance statistic is more important than clinic rankings.

Members of the entire investigative group should have access to the performance monitoring reports to enable them to gauge their standing in the study. Peer pressure, exerted via dissemination of the information, can be helpful in encouraging clinics with poor performance records to improve.

16.8 OTHER QUALITY CONTROL PROCEDURES

16.8.1 Site visits

A site visit, used in this context, is:

A visit to a center in a trial made by personnel from outside that center for the purpose of assessing its performance or potential for performance.

Those making the visit may be from other centers in the trial or from outside the trial. The size of the visiting team will be dictated by the nature of the visit. It may be done by just one person or it may involve a half dozen or more people depending on needs and circumstances. (See Cassel and Ferris, 1984, for details regarding clinic visiting procedures in an ophthalmic study.) The "typical" clinic visit in a multicenter trial may involve the chairman of the study (or his representative), a director of another clinic in the trial, the director of the data coordinating center (or his representative), and the project officer, as well as other selected resource people (e.g., a clinic coordinator if there are problems in the way forms are completed, or a person knowledgeable in laboratory methods if there are problems in this area).

The head of the visiting team should prepare a written report of the visit, based on input from the entire team. It should indicate when the visit took place, who made it, who was seen, the areas of activities reviewed, and the strengths and weaknesses of the center. When appropriate, it should contain a list of specific recommendations. It should be sent to the director of the center visited and to the appropriate leadership body of the study for review (usually the steering committee).

Clinic visits may be made on an as-needed basis or on a set time schedule. The CDP used a combination of the two approaches. The steering committee requested visits of clinics considered to have performance problems. Clinics that were not visited on this basis were visited routinely over the course of the trial.

The visits should include contacts with senior staff as well as essential support staff in the clinic and may involve any or all of the following activities:

- Private meeting of the site visitors with the clinic director
- Meeting of the site visitors with members of the clinic staff
- Inspection of examining and record storage facilities
- Comparison of data contained on selected data forms with those contained in the computer data file
- Review of file of data forms and related records to assess completeness and security against loss or misuse
- Observation of clinic personnel carrying out specified procedures
- Check of handbooks, manuals, forms, and other documents on file at the clinic to assess whether they are up-to-date
- Physical or verbal walk-through of certain procedures (e.g., the series of examinations needed to determine patient eligibility, or the steps followed in the informed consent process
- Conversations with actual study patients during or after enrollment as a check on the informed consent process
- Private conversations with key support personnel to assess their practices and philosophy with regard to data collection
- Private meeting with the clinic director's chief concerning special issues

The visiting process should not be limited to clinics. It should include the data center as well as other key resource centers in a trial. A "typical" data center visit may include many of the activities mentioned above as well as:

- Review of methods for inventorying forms received from clinics
- Review of methods for data entry and verification
- Assessment of the adequacy of methods for filing and storing paper records received from clinics, including the security of the storage area and methods for protecting records against loss or unauthorized use
- Review of available computing resources
- Review of method of randomization and of safeguards to protect against breakdowns

in the randomization process (see Chapter 10)

- Review of data editing procedures
- Review of computer data file structure and methods for maintaining the analysis database
- Review of programming methods both for data management and analysis, including an assessment of program documentation
- Comparison of information contained on original study forms with that in the computer data file
- Review of methods for generating analysis data files and related data reports
- Review of analysis philosophy, especially in relation to the principles discussed in Chapter 18
- Review of methods for backing up the main data file
- Review of methods for restoring the main data file or original study records if lost or destroyed
- Review of master file of key study documents, such as handbooks, manuals, data forms, minutes of study committees, etc., for completeness

Some studies, such as the National Cooperative Gallstone Study (NCGS), have gone a step beyond the process outlined above in monitoring data center operations. It established a special monitoring committee, made up of people from outside the study, with first-hand experience in data coordinating center operations to review operations in the center (National Cooperative Gallstone Study Group, 1981a). The committee was responsible for carrying out periodic reviews of the center and for reporting results of those visits to the NCGS Steering Committee and Advisory-Review Committee.

16.8.2   Quality control committees and centers

Certain of the quality control functions in some of the larger-scale multicenter trials may be performed by specifically constituted committees, as already stated above for the NCGS. For example, the CDP had a laboratory committee to review laboratory standards and methods (Coronary Drug Project Research Group, 1973a). The Aspirin Myocardial Infarction Study (AMIS) created a committee that was responsible for monitoring the performance of all centers in the trial, primarily via performance monitoring reports prepared by the AMIS Coordinating Center (Aspirin Myocardial Infarction Study Research Group, 1980b). Various other committees in the structure of a trial will have quality control functions.

A few studies, such as the Persantine Aspirin Reinfarction Study (PARIS), have funded a quality control center (Persantine Aspirin Reinfarction Trial Research Group, 1980a). The function of the PARIS center was to carry out data audits by comparing data from original study forms with those in computer files at the PARIS Coordinating Center. A second function was to check on the accuracy of analyses performed by the Coordinating Center. A third was to serve as a second analysis center for the study, using tapes provided by the PARIS Coordinating Center.

16.8.3   Data audits

A data audit, as used herein, involves an item-by-item comparison of information recorded on an original study form with that contained in the computer file for that form. Such audits, as mentioned in Section 16.3, were carried out by groups reviewing the UGDP, after the study was finished. To be useful as a quality control measure they must be carried out during the trial. Ongoing audits of this sort are especially important in studies with distributed data systems where forms are keyed at the clinic and, hence, may never be sent to the data center, as in the HPT. Clinics in that study are required to forward a random sample of completed data forms to the data coordinating center. Staff at the center compare entries on the forms with those in the data file. Discrepancies are noted for review. A less systematic approach might involve on-the-spot audits carried out during clinic site visits and done by arbitrarily selecting a few forms for comparison with data listings prepared by the data center in conjunction with the visit.

Part IV. Data analysis and interpretation

Chapters in This Part

The four chapters in this Part deal with issues involved in the analysis and interpretation of results from trials. The first chapter details issues concerned with database management. Chapter 18 details general principles to be followed when results are analyzed. It also contains brief descriptions of commonly used methods of analysis for trials involving a binary event as the outcome measure. Chapter 19 contains a list of questions and short answers concerning the design, analysis, and interpretation of clinical trials. Chapter 20 addresses issues involved in treatment monitoring and provides a brief description of some of the analysis approaches used for that purpose.

17. The analysis database

Round numbers are always false.

Samuel Johnson

17.1 INTRODUCTION

This chapter contains a discussion of issues involved in the development and maintenance of the analysis database. The analyses may be for the purposes of quality control (Chapter 16), safety monitoring, (Chapter 20), or for preparation of publications at the end of the trial (Chapters 18 and 25).

The study database, as defined herein, consists of all data contained on official data forms of the study. It includes data from all baseline and follow-up forms, as well as data from laboratory tests and other procedures (e.g., ECGs, fundus photographs, liver biopsies, etc.) that are a required part of the study protocol. It does not include data that are part of a patient's general medical record, except to the extent that such information overlaps that which is needed for the study.

The analysis database is constructed from the study database, and consists of all codified information contained in the latter database. Ideally, there should be a one-to-one correspondence between the paper forms generated from a study and the analysis database. There will be when all entries on study forms are made in codified form. However, this is not always practical, especially if some of the information collected is recorded in narrative form and is not coded.

17.2 CHOICE OF COMPUTING FACILITY

Most trials will require use of electronic files to facilitate analysis of the study results. The choice of the electronic medium (e.g., tape or disk) and facility is not as crucial in a short-term trial as in a long-term one. The choice of the facility will be between a dedicated one, operated by study personnel for the exclusive use of the study, or a general-use facility, operated by someone else and shared with other users, or a combination of the two kinds of facilities. Table 17-1 outlines the pros and cons of the two classes of facilities.

Once the type of facility has been chosen, the next decision has to do with hardware selection within the class (Table 17-2). The options available may be limited if the decision is to rely on a general-use facility, especially if the selection is limited to facilities within the investigator's own institution. However, even in such cases there is usually room for a choice if the institution has multiple general-use facilities. A comparative evaluation, including the use of benchmarking techniques to assess the computing power and cost of candidate facilities, is needed to make an informed choice. Consideration should be given to the experience of staff in the computing facilities in database management and data analysis and to the kinds of software packages available for those activities.

The existence of good database management packages, along with standard analysis packages, such as provided in BMDP, SPSS, and SAS (Devan and Brown, 1979; Dixon, 1981; Norusis, 1983; Ray, 1982), can markedly reduce

Table 17-1   General-use versus dedicated computing facilities

---

I. General-use facility

  A. Pros and cons

  - Likely to provide more computing power for the study than is feasible with a dedicated facility, but access to the facility may be limited

  - Investigators are freed of responsibilities for operation of the facility; however, the operators of a general-use facility may be insensitive to specific needs of the trial

  - Number of programming options on a general-use facility is likely to be greater than on a dedicated facility

  - Generally provides a wider array of hardware than available on a dedicated facility

  - Protection of data files on the system may be more difficult than with a dedicated facility

  B. Factors favoring choice of general-use facility

  - Existence of good general-use facility operated by staff responsive to user needs and equipped with hardware needed for the study

  - Total duration of the trial, including the period of final analysis, relatively short (e.g., ≤ 3 years)

  - Programming and data processing staff needed for the trial is small (e.g., ≤ 1 FTE)

  - No one in the data center staff has the interest or talents needed for operation of a dedicated facility

II. Dedicated facility

  A. Pros and cons

  - Access to computer can be limited to study personnel, thereby avoiding competition with other users

  - Limited access may make it easier to protect data files against unauthorized entry

  - Amount of computing power and number of hardware and software options likely to be more limited than on large general-use facilities

  - Responsibility for operation of the facility rests with study personnel. May be a disadvantage depending on the skills and interests of the personnel involved

  B. Factors favoring choice of dedicated facility

  - No general-use facility in the institution housing the data center, or the facilities that exist are overloaded

  - Data processing needs are sizable and will continue over a long period of time (e.g., > 3 years)

  - Programming and data processing staff needed for the trial is fairly large (e.g., ≥ 4 full-time equivalents)

  - The existence of staff with the interest and talents needed for operation of a dedicated facility

---

Table 17-2   Considerations in choosing among computing facilities

---

A. Considerations in choosing among different general-use facilities

  - Type and amount of staffing available for advice and consultation

  - Hours of operation and modes of access (e.g., only on-site batch entry versus entry via remote job entry station or via CRT work station)

  - Record of mainframe hardware supplier (e.g., firm with an established record for sales and service versus one that is a recent entry into the hardware field)

  - Primary use of the facility (e.g., research versus administration)

  - Compatibility of hardware and software features with other facilities (especially important if there is a need to switch facilities during the trial)

  - Array of available hardware and software packages, particularly for data management and data analysis

  - Past history of operation, including record of past hardware upgrades

  - Level of satisfaction expressed by other research users of the facility

  - Charging policy for computer time, on-line data storage, printing, etc.

B. Choosing among different dedicated facilities

  - Available hardware and software features, especially those related to computing power, response time, database maintenance, and construction of files for data analysis

  - Compatibility of programming languages with other operating systems

  - Past history of vendor in producing and servicing small-scale dedicated computers

  - Nature of details contained in manuals for operating the facility

  - Vendor method of providing updates to the system and their costs

  - Expertise of vendor sales and service personnel

  - Level of access to vendor systems personnel for answering questions having to do with operation of the system

  - Cost and maintenance charges

---

the amount of programming time required for both kinds of activities.

The options available if a dedicated facility is chosen are greater and more varied. Making an informed judgment may require months of work to collect the necessary cost and operating information. Highly specialized items of equipment, requiring use of esoteric programming languages, should be avoided. The cost and inconvenience involved in converting programs to operate on some other system may make it impractical to consider conversions later on.

A crucial cost issue is whether to purchase or lease the required hardware. Generally, purchase is cheaper than lease for items used at least three years. The disadvantage is that purchase may make it impractical to take advantage of subsequent upgrades, especially if the upgrades involve new product lines.

17.3 ORGANIZATION OF PROGRAMMING RESOURCES

The requirements for the data system should be developed by data processing personnel, in collaboration with the clinical investigators. Development of programs should not be started until there is general agreement on the requirements for data flow and editing. It may be efficient to vest responsibility for the development and maintenance of programs needed for operation of the database and those needed for data analysis with different groups (e.g., see Meinert et al., 1983). The majority of programming work early in the trial will be related to development of the data management system. The demand for this will diminish once the basic database management systems are in place. Programming efforts thereafter will be limited to those needed for maintenance of the system and for implementing changes dictated by hardware or software changes or by modifications to the study protocol. The demand for analysis programming will begin once recruitment is under way. The first efforts in this regard will relate to analyses needed for performance and safety monitoring and later on for manuscript preparation. The overall demand for programming is likely to increase over the course of the trial.

The time spent in improving the efficiency of operating programs should depend on the number of times they are likely to be used over the course of the study, the amount of time required to run them, and the way computer charges are billed. Most general-use computing centers have charges for on-line data storage, number of lines printed, tape or disk I/Os, etc. Minor changes in the charging algorithm can have major cost implications for the trial. Reprogramming may be necessary to lessen their impact.

A major issue in the development of any system has to do with the amount of testing that is done before programs are released for use in the trial. Many flaws can be detected via the reviews that are part of any good programming effort. On-line testing should not be started until there has been a successful "walk-through" of the program. A number of test runs should be made thereafter. The data sets used for this purpose should be typical of data likely to be collected as part of the trial. A number of different data sets should be used to reflect a variety of conditions.

Operating programs should be sufficiently well documented to allow someone unfamiliar with the programs to operate them. The need for good documentation, although greatest in long-term trials because of the changes in programming personnel that can occur, is important for all trials. Use of a structured programming language, such as PL/I, can help in this process; however, there is no substitute for the critical review of others in testing the adequacy of the documentation.

17.4 OPERATIONAL REQUIREMENTS FOR DATABASE MAINTENANCE

Data will be added to the analysis database in blocks. Keyed data are usually stored in a temporary file until a defined data entry session has been completed or until after the close of a defined time period. Thereafter, the resulting data block is transmitted to the analysis database for storage and subsequent manipulation. The update schedule will depend on the rate of data flow and on how and where data are keyed. The data center in the Coronary Artery Surgery Study (CASS) gathered information keyed and temporarily stored at the clinics, by polling clinic workstations (usually at night) on a weekly basis. The Coronary Drug Project (CDP) updated its main database about every two weeks (Meinert et al., 1983).

The prime function of the updating process is to link new data with that already in the analysis file. This may be accomplished by physically locating new data for a patient next to that already on file for the patient or by use of directories in which new data are added to the end of the file without regard to location of other data pertinent to a particular patient. The approach used will be determined by the type of computing hardware and software features available and the cost of data retrieval under one structure versus another.

The computer data file should be designed to minimize the amount of sorting and hand processing preparatory to an update, as well as the amount of computer time needed for the update. Generally, files that are constructed for easy updating are not easy to use for data analysis. Hence, it is usually necessary to reorganize them preparatory to any analyses.

A crucial issue in the updating process has to do with the disposition of data items that are still in a state of flux because of outstanding edit queries (see Chapter 16). Should such items be added to the analysis database or should they be excluded until the edit queries have been resolved? The CDP analysis database excluded all such data items. They were added to the file, on an item-by-item basis, as they cleared the edit process. They were included in the Aspirin Myocardial Infarction Study (AMIS) analysis database. However, items with outstanding edit queries were flagged. The flags remained in place until the edit queries were resolved and were used to eliminate questionable data for certain of the analyses performed.

17.5   DATA SECURITY PRECAUTIONS

The database of the study must be safeguarded against loss or unauthorized use (see the next section and Sections 15.5 and 24.4 for comments concerning storage of the original study records). Table 17-3 provides a list of the general precautions and safeguards that should be taken in any data operation (Part A), a list of safeguards applicable to files containing patient identifying information (Part B), general methods for protecting data files against misuse (Part C), and methods for protecting files against loss or destruction (Part D).

It is the responsibility of the study leadership to outline data security guidelines for the trial and to make certain that they are followed. Staff should be instructed as to their duties and responsibilities regarding data safeguards before they are allowed access to any study data. They should be cautioned against the release of data

to anyone except authorized individuals, and then only through approved channels. All employees concerned with data processing should be given instructions regarding data security and should be informed (perhaps via statements they sign) of the types of disciplinary actions, including immediate dismissal, that can be expected if those safeguards are ignored or willfully violated.

Several of the large-scale multicenter trials (e.g., Aspirin Myocardial Infarction Study, Macular Photocoagulation Study, and Persantine Aspirin Reinfarction Study) have data systems that preclude collection of any personal identifiers, such as patient name and address, at the data center. The proscription provides a means of eliminating any chance for breaches of patient confidentiality in the data center (see Part B of Table 17-3 for safeguards used when patient identifying information is collected).

The data center has a responsibility to protect data in its custody against loss or destruction, whether caused by mistakes, accidents, or purposeful acts. A good data center will have the capability of regenerating the analysis database via backup files. Ideally, the tapes or disks containing these files should be stored in a building remote from the one housing the main database. At least two sets of backup tapes (or disks) should be maintained so that one set can be held in reserve while the other is used to restore the system. The schedule for generation of updated tapes or disks for backup purposes will be a function of the rate at which new information is added to the analysis database. (See Meinert et al., 1983 for a description of the CDP backup system.)

17.6   FILING AND STORING THE ORIGINAL STUDY RECORDS

The clinic should retain a copy of all data forms and related records generated in the trial until all essential work, including final analysis of the results, has been completed. This file may be the only hard copy of study records that exists. This will be the case in single-center trials without data centers and in multicenter trials with distributed data entry (see Section 16.2). Generally, a second paper file is needed if data entry is done outside the clinic, especially in multicenter trials. The file used for data entry should be considered the official file of the study and should contain the original copy of all paper forms and related records.

Table 17-3 Precautions and safeguards for database operations

A. General precautions and safeguards

- Study leadership that is sensitive to needs for data security
- Staff experienced in the operation of a database and in protecting it against loss or misuse
- Signed assurance from each employee authorized to work on the database, stating he understands the safeguards and precautions to be followed and the consequences of a willful disregard of them
- Periodic staff meetings to remind database personnel of required operating procedures and safeguards
- Periodic review of required operating procedures and established safeguards by study leaders
- Monitoring for adherence to precautions and safeguards via periodic on-site checks

B. Patient confidentiality safeguards

- Data flow procedures from the clinic to the data center that exclude transmission of patient identifying information
- Electronic storage of patient identifying information in enciphered form or in a separate file
- Separation of the file containing patient identifying information from other files
- Physical separation of pages containing personal identifying information from other pages of the data forms (especially if forms contain highly sensitive information)
- Proscription against distribution of data listings that contain patient name, name code, or any other identifiers easily associated with a specific patient
- Proscription against use of patient name, name code, hospital chart or record number, or other unique identifiers, such as Social Security number, in any published data listing. Study ID number should not be published if it is possible for people outside the study to use that number to identify a patient. Published UGDP patient listings (University Group Diabetes Program Research Group, 1970e, 1975, 1977, 1982) were devoid of both clinic and patient ID number for this reason.
- Secure procedures for disposing of computer output

from aborted runs that contain patient identifying information

- Denial of access to any patient record stored in the data center to persons outside the center without the express written consent of the patient

C. Safeguards against misuse

- Limit the number of persons in the data center who have access to the original study forms or any related data file, especially those containing patient identifying information
- Restrict access to the analysis computer files containing study results through use of passwords or other means
- Proscribe release of any data listing, tape, etc., without approval of the study leadership committee
- File completed study forms, data tapes, and disks, in an attended, locked area

D. Loss safeguards

- Maintain a duplicate file of the original study records (e.g., by requiring clinics to maintain a copy of forms and records sent to the data center)
- Microfilm original data forms, computer listings, study manuals, meeting minutes, etc., for storage in a secure location
- Establish and maintain a series of backup tapes (or disks) for the analysis database that will allow restoration of it in the event of a system malfunction
- Store copies of backup tapes (or disks) of the main analysis database in an off-site location or in an on-site fireproof vault
- Establish strict rules to safeguard access to backup tapes (or disks) to avoid unauthorized use in restoration efforts
- Provide backup tapes (or disks) of all essential programs, such as those needed for editing, inventorying, storage, retrieval, and analysis of the study data, as well as programs used for the operating systems
- Carry out occasional "fire drills" to test the ability of the staff in the data center to restore the main analysis database from backup tapes (or disks)

Decisions must be made as to where to house records that cannot be easily or reliably reproduced, such as X rays. Records that are needed for patient care should remain in the clinic or be returned to it as soon as they are read and the information from them has been codified and keyed. Some records, such as ECG tracings, can be "duplicated" by making a second tracing when the patient is examined. However, this option does not exist if the "duplication" entails added risks for the patient (e.g., as with X rays).

Both the official and backup paper files should be stored in locked cabinets in a secure area. The files should be checked periodically to make certain needed updates are made and that they do not become cluttered with superfluous materials.

The organization of the file will depend on where the file resides and how it is to be used. Those housed in the clinic will almost certainly be organized along patient lines. Those housed at the data center may be organized in other ways. For example, the CDP Coordinating Center found it convenient to arrange paper records by form type and by edit period (i.e., time period in which the forms were received). This ordering was more efficient than an arrangement by patient ID number and visit because of the data entry and editing process used by the center.

Data forms and related records stored at the clinic and data center may be retained in their original state or on microfilm. If microfilm is used, the original records should be retained until microfilm images have been checked for legibility and proper identification. Destruction of study forms and related records should be in accordance with local statutes for medical records. Data forms, medical records, computer listings, or microfilm images that contain patient identifying information should be burned or shredded. They should not be moved to the disposal site unless they can be destroyed upon receipt.

General National Institutes of Health guidelines require investigators to retain raw study documents (or microfilm copies of them) for a minimum of two to three years after expiration of funding (Department of Health, Education and Welfare, 1976; Department of Health and Human Services, 1981, 1982b). Requirements may extend beyond these limits in any case where there are legal challenges to the study, or where the results are under review by some official government agency. Prudent investigators will retain study records well beyond the required legal limit for scientific reasons alone.

17.7 PREPARATION OF ANALYSIS TAPES

Most data analyses will be done from a tape or disk created from the analysis database. There are several reasons for doing so, especially for interim analyses done for performance or safety monitoring (see Section 16.7 and Chapter 20). The principal ones are:

- To allow database maintenance personnel to continue making updates to the database without altering the analysis database

- To reduce the number of times the database is accessed for data analyses (in order to minimize the chances of programmer errors)
- To enable analysis personnel to rearrange data, including application of data reduction and special coding routines, in order to create a file that is more compact and suitably arranged for use with data analysis programs

Theoretically, the updating process could be terminated while data analyses are being done. However, termination of the updating process is not always practical, particularly when data analyses take weeks to carry out, as may be the case when preparing complex reports for patient safety monitoring (see Chapter 20). In any case, the interruption of data flow into the database complicates management of the updating process and reduces the usefulness of edits carried out in conjunction with the updating process.

It is wise to decide on a target date for generation of the analysis tape. The date chosen should correspond to the last major update or change to the analysis database or to some other event in the trial, such as close-out of follow-up or termination of a treatment. The format of the analysis tape or disk requires careful thought. Organization of data may be quite different from that of the analysis database. A decision must be made as to whether to array data by patient or by variable. Thought is also needed regarding the degree to which data are to be reduced as they are written onto the analysis tape or disk. Verbatim listings from the analysis database will provide the analyst with the greatest amount of flexibility, but they are also more complicated to use. Generally, some reduction, in which codes are combined to reduce the number of categories and by averaging aliquot determinations or repeat readings, will be necessary.

A decision is also needed regarding the amount of editing to be done on data written onto the analysis tape (or disk). Outlier values or values known to be in error should be identified when the tape is written to keep the analyst from having to perform these checks each time a variable is used.

18. Data analysis requirements and procedures

Another difficulty about statistics is the technical difficulty of calculation. Before you can even make a mistake in drawing your conclusion from the correlations established by your statistics you must ascertain the correlations.

George Bernard Shaw

18.1 BASIC ANALYSIS REQUIREMENTS

The essence of a trial emanates from comparisons of the treatment groups for differences in outcome. Those comparisons should be made following ground rules listed below.

Ground rule number 1 Patients used in treatment comparisons should be counted in the treatment group to which they were assigned.

Ground rule number 2 The denominator for a treatment should be all patients assigned to that treatment.

Ground rule number 3 All events should be counted in the comparison of primary interest.

Clearly, there are situations in which the first rule is followed, but the second is violated (e.g., certain patients are excluded from analyses because their treatment was not in "accordance" with the study protocol). The third rule is an admonition against analyses in which investigators elect to present results only for events believed to be related to the disease process under

185

Table 18-1 Examples of analysis ground rule violations

Violation	Example
Counting only a portion of the events observed	Carrying out the primary analysis for cause specific mortality, ignoring all cause mortality
Counting only those events that occur after a specified period of treatment	Restricting the database for the primary analysis to 30-day postsurgical deaths in a surgery trial, or by ignoring deaths that occur within a specified time period after the initiation of treatment in a drug trial
Using only those patients who received their assigned treatment or who had perfect (or suitably high) adherence to the assigned treatment	Exclusion of patients from the database who did not receive the "full" course of treatment in a drug trial
Allowing the treatment actually administered to determine the group in which a patient is counted	Counting a patient allocated to control treatment as a member of test-treated group because he received the test treatment
Using only "evaluable" patients	A cancer trial that ignores results for patients who failed to develop tumors of a certain size
Exclusion of ineligible patients enrolled in the trial	Elimination of patients who were judged ineligible after enrollment by personnel who were aware of treatment assignment and course of treatment

treatment (e.g., cardiovascular deaths in a heart study). See Table 18-1.

An unsophisticated investigator can be expected to rebel at the notion of using data from patients who refused the assigned treatment or who were not treated in accordance with the study protocol for making treatment comparisons. One temptation is to ignore such patients and to proceed with analyses as if they were never enrolled—a violation of the second ground rule. The only clue offered to readers to indicate that this was done may be a single telltale sentence, such as "The analyses in this paper have been restricted to evaluable patients." Of equal concern are cases where data from all patients are used, but where the primary analysis is done by the treatment administered rather than by the one assigned— a violation of the first ground rule. The main reason for randomizing in the first place, as noted in Chapter 8, has to do with the desirability of establishing treatment groups that are free of patient and physician selection bias. There is no assurance in this regard if patients are arbitrarily excluded from consideration after randomization.

Even if investigators accept the need for analyses based on the first two ground rules, they may willfully violate the third one. Counting rules that call for exclusion of certain events are, at best, difficult to defend because of their arbitrary nature. Further, their use can open the

study to serious criticism. The Anturane Reinfarction Trial (ART) is a case in point. The published report from the trial drew criticism because of the failure of study investigators to count deaths occurring within 7 days of the initiation of treatment (Anturane Reinfarction Trial Research Group, 1978; Temple and Pledger, 1980). These exclusions made it difficult to interpret the mortality results. The concern of critics stemmed from uncertainty regarding the validity of the assumption underlying the exclusions (i.e., that deaths occurring in this time period were not treatment-related) and the apparent post hoc nature of the 7-day rule. Clearly, rules for exclusions devised after the start of data collection must be viewed with skepticism. The same is true for any exclusion rule, regardless of when it was written, which is administered by personnel who have access to patient treatment assignments, especially if subjective judgments are required in administering the rule.

Adherence to the above ground rules can lead to an underestimate of the true treatment effect, especially if treatment compliance is low, there are a lot of treatment crossovers (see Glossary for definition), or the denominators for the treatment groups include a lot of patients who could not be followed for the outcome of interest. The latter should not be a problem in trials using mortality as the outcome (see Chapter 15), but can be in trials with a nonfatal event or a laboratory or physiological measure as the outcome. A prudent investigator will carry out supplemental analyses aimed at quantifying the degree of conservatism implied. Certainly, there is no proscription against such analyses so long as they are accompanied by the primary ones suggested above. They may include analyses by level of treatment adherence and for a number of secondary outcomes as well.

18.2 BASIC ANALYTIC METHODS

This section provides a review of analytic methods used for making treatment comparisons in trials with a clinical event as the primary outcome. Readers may consult textbooks such as those by Armitage (1971), Brown and Hollander (1977), Bulpitt (1983), Buyse et al. (1984), Elandt-Johnson and Johnson (1980), Fleiss (1981), Ingelfinger et al. (1983), Kalbfleisch and Prentice (1980), Lee (1980), Pocock (1983), Shapiro and Louis (1983), and Tygstrup et al. (1982); and papers by Cutler and Ederer (1958), Kaplan and Meier (1958), Mantel and Haenszel (1959), Mantel (1966), and Peto et al. (1976, 1977), among others, for additional details.

18.2.1 Simple comparisons of proportions

The simplest and often most useful analysis involves a comparison of the proportion of patients in the two treatment groups who have experienced the event of interest. This method of analysis is valid so long as:

- Patients in the treatment groups were enrolled over the same time period and are subject to the same intensity of follow-up
- The loss to follow-up is low and is the same across treatment groups
- The treatment groups have comparable baseline characteristics

Outcome analyses based on comparisons of proportions appear throughout publications of the trials sketched in Appendix B. Figure 18–1 is based on UGDP mortality data reported in a 1970 publication on tolbutamide (University Group Diabetes Program Research Group, 1970e).

This method of analysis, while best suited to binary data, need not be limited to such data if investigators are willing to convert a polychotomous or continuous outcome measure to binary form, as in the National Cooperative Gallstone Study (NCGS). Investigators in that study chose to categorize gallstone dissolution data as an all-or-none phenomenon for the primary analysis, even though the underlying measure was continuous (National Cooperative Gallstone Study Group, 1981a). Investigators in the Macular Photocoagulation Study (MPS) used a binary outcome (based on a comparison of base-

Figure 18-1   Number of deaths in the UGDP through October 7, 1969, by treatment group.

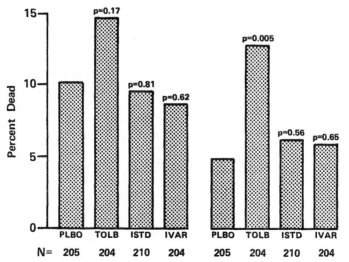

Note: p values recorded above the bars are based on $\chi^2_{(1\ df)}$ for the indicated drug-placebo comparison. The numbers of patients in the treatment groups are indicated below the bars.

Source: Reference citation 468. Adapted with permission of the American Diabetes Association, Inc., New York.

Table 18–2   Percentages of UGDP patients with indicated baseline characteristics (denominators given in parentheses)

Baseline characteristic	PLBO	TOLB	p-value*
Age at entry ≥55	41.5(205)	48.0(204)	0.18
Male	30.7(205)	30.9(204)	0.97
Nonwhite	49.8(205)	47.1(204)	0.59
Fasting blood glucose ≥110 mg/100 ml	63.5(203)	72.1(204)	0.07
Relative body weight ≥1.25	52.7(205)	58.8(204)	0.21
Visual acuity (either eye ≤20/200)	4.3(188)	5.2(192)	0.66

Source: Reference citation 468. Adapted with permission of the American Diabetes Association, Inc., New York.

*Probability of chi-square value as large as or larger than the one observed under the null hypothesis

line and follow-up visual acuity readings) instead of mean change in visual acuity as the principal outcome measure (Macular Photocoagulation Study Group, 1982, 1983a, 1983b).

Furthermore, use of this mode of summary is not limited to outcome measures. It is useful in characterizing differences in the baseline composition of treatment groups and for comparisons of various kinds of follow-up data as well. Table 18–2 is an example of a comparison of the distribution of selected baseline variables that have been converted to binary form (University Group Diabetes Program Research Group, 1970e). Table 18–3 illustrates use of proportions in summarizing follow-up data on observed side effects (Persantine Aspirin Reinfarction Study Research Group, 1980b).

Statistical evaluation of the difference observed via a comparison of proportions can be performed using Fisher's exact test (Fisher, 1946; see also Chapter 9). The *p*-value for the test corresponds to the probability of obtaining a test-control difference as large or larger than the one observed under the null hypothesis of no difference. The *p*-value may be obtained using packaged computer programs for the test or from

Table 18–3   Percentages of PARIS patients with indicated complaint during follow-up

Complaint	Treatment group		
	PR/A	PLBO	Z-value
Stomach pain	15.8	7.7	3.74
Heartburn	9.6	5.2	2.58
Vomiting	2.5	1.0	1.59
Denominator	810	406	

Source: Reference citation 376. Adapted with permission of the American Heart Association, Inc., Dallas, Texas.

tables, such as those constructed by Lieberman and Owen (1961).

The continuity corrected chi-square approximation to the test can be used if the numerators for the two percentages being compared are both ≥ 5 and the denominators are ≥ 30. The *p*-values obtained in such cases are indistinguishable from those obtained with Fisher's exact test. In fact, the approximation is reasonably good even if denominators are as small as 20 (Cochran, 1954).

18.2.2   Lifetable analyses

The typical trial involves patient recruitment over an extended period of time and follow-up through a common calendar time point. Hence, any analysis done during or at the end of the trial will involve patients with varying lengths of follow-up, depending on when they were enrolled. Simple counts of events, such as shown in Figure 18–1, are not designed to take account of follow-up time and hence are insenitive to the way events accumulate over time. The cumulative proportion of patients experiencing events can be the same even though there are marked differences between the treatment groups as to when events occur over the course of follow-up, as illustrated in Table 18–4 for a hypothetical trial. Note that comparisons of the percent dead based on tabulations done at the end of calendar year 6 or before favor treatment B. Those done at the end of calendar year 7 and thereafter favor treatment A.

One way of tracking changes over time via proportions is illustrated in Figure 18–2. This method of analysis, while useful for safety monitoring (see Chapter 20), does not give a means of characterizing the treatment groups with regard to the rate of occurrence of events. Rate calculations are ordinarily made using lifetable meth-

Table 18-4 Hypothetical trial involving comparison of percentage of patients dead at indicated time points*

Calendar time from start of trial	Cumulative number of patients enrolled		Cumulative percent dead	
	Treatment A	Treatment B	Treatment A	Treatment B
1 year	100	100	10.0	2.0
2 years	200	200	13.6	3.5
3 years	300	300	16.2	6.5
4 years	300	300	21.0	12.3
5 years	300	300	24.2	19.4
6 years	300	300	26.7	25.8
7 years	300	300	28.9	31.7
8 years	300	300	31.1	37.2
9 years	300	300	33.1	42.2

*Percentages calculated assuming annual mortality rates (per 100 population) of 10, 8, 5, 4, 3, 3, 3, 3, and 3 for years 1 through 9 of follow-up, respectively, for treatment group A and 2, 3, 8, 8, 8, 8, 8, 8, and 8 for treatment B. Enrollment is assumed to have taken place on the first day of years 1, 2, and 3.

ods (such as described by Elandt-Johnson and Johnson, 1980; Kalbfleisch and Prentice, 1980; Lee, 1980), as illustrated in Figures 18–3 for the UGDP and 18–4 for the CDP. Other examples may be found in publications from the Aspirin Myocardial Infarction Study (AMIS), Hypertension Detection and Follow-Up Program (HDFP), Multiple Risk Factor Intervention Trial (MRFIT), and PARIS (see Appendix B for references).

The main advantage of the lifetable approach is that it provides a means of dealing with varying lengths of follow-up, as illustrated in Table 18–5. The cut-off date for the analysis was October 7, 1969. All patients by that time had been under follow-up for a minimum of 3 years, 8 months and a maximum of 8 years, 8 months. Hence, the only attrition during the first 3 years of follow-up was that due to death. Thereafter, it was due to both deaths and withdrawals because of when patients were enrolled. For example, there were five patients in the tolbutamide-treated group who were enrolled after October 7, 1965, and who were still alive on October 7, 1969. They were counted as withdrawals during the fourth year of follow-up since they had not

Figure 18-2 Plot of observed ESG1-placebo difference in percent of CDP patients dead from lung cancer.

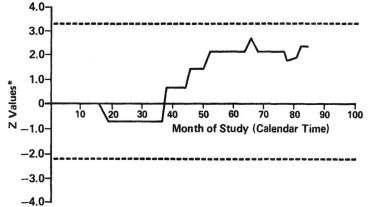

*Z values plotted are for observed ESG1-placebo differences in proportions of deaths from lung cancer. Dotted lines denote Z values corresponding to 0.05 level of significance taking into consideration there were repeated evaluations of the data for treatment differences over the course of the trial.

Source: Reference citation 105. Adapted with permission of the American Medical Association, Chicago, Ill. (copyright © 1973).

Figure 18-3   UGDP cumulative lifetable mortality rates by year of follow-up and by treatment assignment.

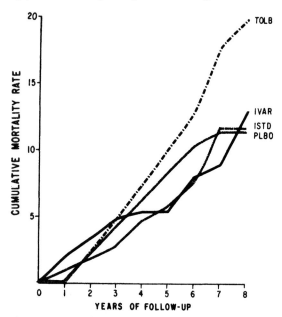

Source: Reference citation 468. Reproduced with permission of the American Diabetes Association, Inc., New York.

been in the study long enough to have completed the fourth year of follow-up.

Statistical comparisons of lifetable rates may be done using confidence estimation or log rank tests. The plot of lifetable rates reproduced in Figure 18–5 uses two standard error limits (i.e., approximate 95% confidence intervals) about the line of no difference to assess the statistical importance of the DT4-placebo mortality difference. The log rank test summarized in Table 18–6 is for data given in Table 18–5. (See Mantel and Haenszel, 1959, Mantel, 1966, and Peto et al., 1977 for general details regarding the test.) Ideally, the calculations should be based on exact time to death, rather than on grouped data, as given in Table 18–5. However, the difference between the two methods of calculation will be small provided the deaths are uniformly distributed within the intervals and that they are not concentrated in just one or two of the intervals. The difference in this example is trivial. Use of exact time to death yielded a log rank test value of 1.82 as contrasted with a value 1.78 for grouped data.

Figure 18-4   Lifetable cumulative dropout rates for the clofibrate, niacin, and placebo treatments in the CDP.

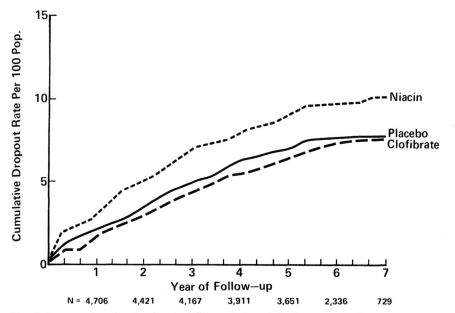

Note: N denotes total number of patients in clofibrate, niacin, and placebo groups combined. Approximate numbers for individual treatment groups are 2/9, 2/9, and 5/9 times N for clofibrate, niacin, and placebo, respectively.

Source: Reference citation 107. Adapted with permission of the American Medical Association, Chicago, Ill. (copyright © 1975).

Table 18-5 Lifetable cumulative mortality rates for the placebo and tolbutamide treatments in the UGDP, as of October 7, 1969

Year of follow-up	Number of deaths in		Number of survivors in			Estimated probability of death in interval	Observed rate per 100 population at risk		Mortality rate standard error
	Patients due for withdrawal in interval	Patients not due for withdrawal in interval	Patients due for withdrawal in interval	Patients not due for withdrawal in interval	Total number starting interval		Mortality rate	Survival rate	
Placebo treatment group									
First	0	0	0	205	205	0.0	0.0	100.0	0.6
Second	0	5	0	200	205	0.024	2.4	97.6	1.1
Third	0	4	0	196	200	0.020	4.4	95.6	1.4
Fourth	0	4	4	188	196	0.021	6.4	93.6	1.7
Fifth	0	4	23	161	188	0.023	8.5	91.5	1.8
Sixth	0	3	43	115	161	0.022	10.4	89.6	2.1
Seventh	0	1	50	64	115	0.011	11.4	88.6	2.5
Eighth	0	0	36	28	64	0.0	11.4	88.6	2.8
Tolbutamide treatment group									
First	0	0	0	204	204	0.0	0.0	100.0	0.6
Second	0	5	0	199	204	0.025	2.4	97.6	1.1
Third	0	5	0	194	199	0.025	4.9	95.1	1.4
Fourth	0	5	5	184	194	0.026	7.4	92.6	1.7
Fifth	0	5	24	155	184	0.029	10.1	89.9	1.8
Sixth	1	3	41	110	155	0.030	12.8	87.2	2.1
Seventh	0	5	47	58	110	0.058	17.8	82.2	2.5
Eighth	0	1	33	24	58	0.024	19.8	80.2	2.9

Source: Reference citation 468. Adapted with permission of the American Diabetes Association, Inc., New York.

Figure 18-5 CDP lifetable plot of the DT4-placebo mortality differences and 2.0 standard error limits for the differences.

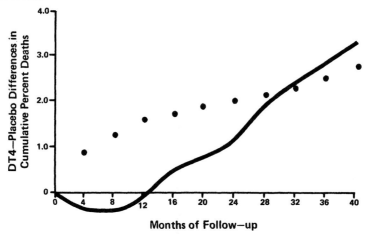

Source: Reference citation 103. Adapted with permission of the American Medical Association, Chicago, Ill. (copyright © 1972).

18.2.3 Other descriptive methods

Any comparison of outcome by treatment group should be accompanied by other analyses to help in interpretation of the results of the trial. Tables 18-2 and 18-7 and Figure 18-6 provide examples of supporting analyses, as taken from the UGDP (University Group Diabetes Program Research Group, 1970e). The results in Table 18-2 are useful for assessing the baseline comparability of the treatment groups. Table 18-7 was used to characterize differences among treatment groups with regard to treatment adherence. Figure 18-6 provides a plot of changes in fasting blood glucose levels for the cohort of patients followed through 4.75 years (i.e., through 19 follow-up examinations). Only patients who remained under active follow-up over this time period were included in the analysis. A plot of means, based on the number of patients observed at each follow-up examination, might have been used instead. However, the two forms of analyses are not necessarily interchangeable. They will yield different results if the composi-

Table 18-6 Log rank test for comparing lifetables in Table 18-5

Year of Follow-up	Number starting interval			Observed deaths			Expected deaths		
	PLBO	TOLB	Total	PLBO	TOLB	Total	PLBO	TOLB	Total
0–1	205.0	204.0	409.0	0	0	0	0.00	0.00	0.00
1–2	205.0	204.0	409.0	5	5	10	5.01	4.99	10.00
2–3	200.0	199.0	399.0	4	5	9	4.51	4.49	9.00
3–4	194.0	191.5	385.5	4	5	9	4.53	4.47	9.00
4–5	176.5	172.0	348.5	4	5	9	4.56	4.44	9.00
5–6	139.5	134.5	274.0	3	4	7	3.56	3.44	7.00
6–7	90.0	86.5	176.5	1	5	6	3.06	2.94	6.00
7–8	46.0	41.5	87.5	0	1	1	0.53	0.47	1.00
Total				21	30	51	25.76	25.24	51.00

Source: Reference citation 441.

Log rank $\chi_1^2 = (21 - 25.76)^2/25.76 + (30 - 25.24)^2/25.24 = 1.78$, *p*-value = 0.18

Figure 18-6 Percent change in fasting blood glucose levels for cohorts of patients followed through the nineteenth follow-up visit.

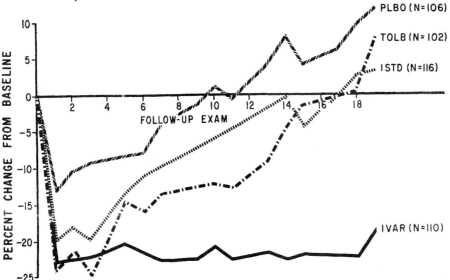

Source: Reference citation 468. Reproduced with permission of the American Diabetes Association, Inc., New York.

tion of the study population enrolled, with regard to the variable of interest, changed over the course of patient recruitment.

18.3 ADJUSTMENT PROCEDURES

To be valid, the evaluation of treatment effects must be performed on treatment groups that are comparable with regard to baseline characteristics. Usually, the comparability provided by randomization is adequate. However, randomization does not guarantee comparability. As noted in Chapter 10, stratification can be used to assure comparability for a few variables, but the distribution with regard to others must be left to chance. As a result, there can be minor, and sometimes even major, differences in the baseline composition of the study groups. The impact of such differences on treatment comparisons should be removed using procedures such as those outlined below.

18.3.1 Subgrouping

The simplest approach involves making the required treatment comparisons in subgroups of patients that are homogeneous for selected entry characteristics. This method of adjustment is illustrated in Table 18–8. All of the subgroups were formed using measures observed before the start of treatment. The table indicates the size of each subgroup and the percentage of patients in the subgroup who had died as of the analysis cut-off date, October 7, 1969.

This approach, while simple, has obvious limitations. Thirty-two (i.e., 2^5) different subgroups would be required to simultaneously categorize patients for the presence or absence of the five measures represented in Table 18–8. The number

Table 18–7 Percentage distribution of UGDP patients by level of treatment adherence

	Treatment group			
Level of adherence *	*PLBO*	*TOLB*	*ISTD*	*IVAR*
Low	10.2	10.3	12.8	14.8
Intermediate	20.0	15.7	29.6	39.9
High	69.8	74.0	57.6	45.3
Number of patients	205	204	210	204

Source: Reference citation 468. Reproduced with permission of the American Diabetes Association, Inc., New York.

*Defined as follows:

Low Patient took all of prescribed study medication <25% of all follow-up periods

Intermediate Patient took all of prescribed study medication 25–74% of all follow-up periods

High Patient took all of prescribed study medication ≥75% of all follow-up periods

Table 18-8   Percentages of patients dead within specified subgroups created using selected baseline characteristics

	Number		Percent dead	
Entry risk factor	*PLBO*	*TOLB*	*PLBO*	*TOLB*
Definite hypertension				
Absent	127	139	11.0	12.9
Present	74	60	9.5	16.7
History of digitalis use				
No	193	183	8.3	13.1
Yes	9	15	55.6	33.3
History of angina pectoris				
No	192	187	9.4	13.9
Yes	10	14	30.0	21.4
Significant ECG abnormality				
Absent	193	193	9.3	13.0
Present	6	8	33.3	50.0
Cholesterol				
<300 mg/100ml	181	169	10.5	14.8
≥300 mg/100ml	17	30	11.8	13.3
Any of above cardiovascular risk factors				
None	98	100	9.2	11.0
One or more	88	92	12.5	17.4

Source: Reference citation 468. Adapted with permission of the American Diabetes Association, Inc., New York.

of patients in many of the subgroups would be too small for meaningful comparison.

In addition, the method requires use of arbitrary cut-points for subgroupings involving continuous variables. The arbitrary nature of the cut-points selected can raise questions concerning the validity of the analyses presented, especially if there is any suspicion that they were chosen to minimize or maximize observed treatment differences.

18.3.2   Multiple regression

An alternative approach that avoids some of these problems and provides a means of controlling for several sources of variation simultaneously involves use of regression models represented by Equations 18.1 and 18.2. (See Cox, 1958, Draper and Smith, 1966, and Kleinbaum et al., 1982, for details on methods of estimation using the models.) The models are used to estimate the probability that a patient experiences the outcome of interest, given a particular set of entry characteristics. One drawback to the linear regression model has to do with the possibility of obtaining probability estimates that lie outside the range of 0 to 1. This possibility is avoided with the logistic model.

Linear[1] multiple regression model

$$y_i = A + \epsilon_i \tag{18.1}$$

Logistic multiple regression model

$$y_i = \frac{1}{1 + e^{-A}} + \epsilon_i \tag{18.2}$$

where

$A = \beta_0 + \beta_1 x_{1i} + \cdots + \beta_j x_{ji} + \cdots + \beta_k x_{ki}$

y_i = outcome observed for the ith patient (either 0 or 1 for binary outcome measures)

x_{ji} = value observed for the ith patient and jth entry characteristic ($j = 1, \cdots, k$)

ϵ_i = error associated with y_i

and

$\beta_0, \beta_1, \ldots, \beta_k$ = regression coefficients (parameters) to be estimated from observed data

The UGDP used a logistic regression model to adjust observed mortality results for differences in the distribution of 14 different entry charac-

1. Referred to as linear because the model does not involve any parameter raised to a power other than unity. The term is not a comment on the shape of the curve arising from the analysis. The model may yield a curved line or surface depending on the form taken by the independent variable(s) in the model.

teristics (University Group Diabetes Program Research Group, 1970e). Results are summarized in Table 18–9. The CDP used both multiple linear and multiple logistic regression models to adjust observed mortality for as many as 54 different baseline characteristics (Coronary Drug Project Research Group, 1974, 1975).

The use of regression procedures for adjustment has been extended to event rates calculated from lifetables (Cox, 1972). The method has been used in studies such as AMIS (Aspirin Myocardial Reinfarction Study Research Group, 1980b) and PARIS (Persantine Aspirin Reinfarction Study Research Group, 1980b).

18.4 COMMENT ON SIGNIFICANCE ESTIMATION

The *p*-values resulting from conventional tests of significance are often used by investigators to decide whether to characterize a particular result as being statistically significant. Clearly, *p*-values can help in the statistical quantification of a result, but they should not become a substitute for rational thought. The acceptance or rejection of a treatment rarely hinges on whether a difference reaches some arbitrary level of significance. In fact, the amount of evidence required to conclude that a test treatment is no better than the control treatment may be less than that required to conclude that it is better. Generally, there is need in the latter case to make certain the beneficial effects observed persist—a judgment that

Table 18-9   Observed and adjusted tolbutamide-placebo difference in percent of patients dead

	TOLB	PLBO	TOLB-PLBO difference
Observed percent dead	14.7	10.2	4.5
Adjusted* percent dead	14.5	10.2	4.3

Source: Reference citation 468. Adapted with permission of the American Diabetes Association, Inc., New York.

*Based on logistic regression model using 14 different baseline characteristics.

can be reached only by continuing follow-up for some time after the emergence of an important difference.

The question of what constitutes statistical significance is complex. Methodological problems involved in the interpretation of conventional tests of significance for safety monitoring are outlined in the next chapter. However, even if those problems are ignored, it is still necessary to use a good deal of caution in the interpretation of *p*-values. Most trials, even if designed to focus on a single outcome, will provide data on a variety of other outcome measures as well. For example, the CDP provided data on the rate of occurrence of myocardial infarctions, strokes, and several other nonfatal cardiovascular events, in addition to death. The *p*-values obtained for one outcome measure will not be independent of those obtained using another outcome measure.

19. Questions concerning the design, analysis, and interpretation of clinical trials

There are three kinds of lies: lies, damned lies and statistics.

Benjamin Disraeli

19.1 INTRODUCTION

This chapter focuses on questions concerning the design, analysis, and interpretation of study data. Material is presented in the form of questions and answers and is organized in categories related to the various aspects of a clinical trial.

19.2 QUESTIONS CONCERNING THE STUDY DESIGN

1a. *Question:* Can a new study treatment be added during the course of the trial?

Answer: Yes, but not without impact on the study design. The University Group Diabetes Program (UGDP) elected to add a fifth treatment, phenformin, 18 months after the start of patient enrollment (University Group Diabetes Program Research Group, 1970d). The allocation ratio of phenformin to tolbutamide to insulin standard to insulin variable to placebo was fixed at $3:1:1:1:1$ and was satisfied after enrollment of every 14, 28, 42, etc., patient in each of the 6 clinics administering phenformin. Patients in

the other 6 UGDP clinics and the first 32 patients in one of the clinics included in the phenformin portion of the study were allocated using a ratio of $0:1:1:1:1$ in blocks of 16.

The two different allocation schemes created problems when treatment comparisons were made involving phenformin-treated patients (University Group Diabetes Program Research Group, 1975). The decision in the Coronary Drug Project (CDP) to study aspirin late in the trial avoided these design problems by setting up a separate trial using patients from discontinued treatments (Coronary Drug Project Research Group, 1976).

1b. *Question:* Can a treatment be deleted from the study design once the trial has started?

Answer: Yes. Use of the test treatment will have to be stopped if it is shown to be inferior to the control treatment. The control treatment will have to be stopped if it is inferior to the test treatment. The UGDP provides examples of the former kind of change (University Group Diabetes Program Research Group, 1970e, 1975). The Diabetic Retinopathy Study (DRS) provides an example of the latter type of change (Diabetic Retinopathy Study Research Group, 1976, 1978).

A treatment may also be deleted for reasons unrelated to treatment results. The original design of the DRS included a test treatment involving photocoagulation with both xenon arc and argon laser. The treatment was abandoned early in the course of the trial for practical reasons.

2a. *Question:* Do all clinics participating in a multicenter trial have to be in the trial from the outset?

Answer: No. Results from clinics can be combined regardless of when they were added to the trial, provided all clinics followed the same treatment protocol and all treatment assignments were made using a common allocation ratio. See question 1a.

2b. *Question:* What if a clinic in a multicenter trial resigns after it has started patient enrollment? Will the resignation affect treatment comparisons?

Answer: Clinic resignations are not uncommon. There were two in both the CDP and the National Cooperative Gallstone Study (NCGS) (Coronary Drug Project Research Group, 1973a; National Cooperative Gallstone Study Group, 1981a). They may be initiated by the clinic because of the death, illness, or departure of a key person or by the study leadership because of performance problems.

The loss of a clinic will reduce the overall precision of the trial unless other clinics are recruited to make up for the loss. The loss will be minimal if few patients are involved and if responsibility for the continued care and surveillance of patients already enrolled can be assumed by another clinic in the trial. It will be sizable if the clinic had a large number of patients that cannot be transferred to other clinics in the trial. Such patients will have to be counted as dropouts and treated as such for data analyses in the trial. A large number of dropouts caused by clinic resignations will make it difficult to detect treatment effects, but they should not invalidate treatment comparisons provided the allocation ratio in clinics that have resigned was the same as in the remaining active clinics. Incidentally, the possibility of clinic resignation in a multicenter trial is one reason why it is wise to construct the allocation schedule with clinic as a stratification variable.

3. *Question:* Is it proper to make modifications to the treatment protocol during the trial?

Answer: Many times it is not so much a question of propriety as of necessity. Changes must be made if patient safety is in question. Other changes may be necessary simply to clear up ambiguities in the protocol. All changes should be noted and reported in publications from the trial.

4a. *Question:* If the required sample size cannot be achieved, should it be reduced to bring it in line with reality?

Answer: It is always possible to find some combination of α, β, and Δ which yields the "desired" result (see Chapter 9). Reduction

of the sample size via such manipulations, simply to bring it in line with expectation, is game playing.

4b. *Question:* How about revising the sample size calculation during the trial?

Answer: Revised sample size calculations, based on observed outcome and dropout rates, can help the investigators and sponsor decide if more clinics are needed or if the period of follow-up should be extended to achieve the desired statistical precision. The calculations should be made using the α, β, and Δ specified when the trial was planned (see Chapter 9).

4c. *Question:* Is it all right to change the outcome measure after the start of the trial as a means of reducing the sample size requirement?

Answer: Such maneuvers are open to the same criticism as mentioned in the answer to question 4a. One kind of maneuver involves a switch from a single event as the prime outcome measure to a composite event (see Glossary). The expected rate of occurrence of such an event will be higher than that for any of its component parts. The higher the expected rate, the easier it will be to detect a specified relative difference with a given sample size. However, the "gain" in precision is achieved at the expense of clinical relevancy. It is more difficult to interpret the meaning of a finding based on combinations of events than one that is based on a single set of events.

5. *Question:* Is it permissible to extend the period of patient follow-up to compensate for a lower than expected event rate in the control-treated group or for a shortfall in patient recruitment?

Answer: Yes.

6. *Question:* Is it necessary to specify stopping rules for the trial before it is started?

Answer: No. In fact, many trials are done without any formal stopping rules for reasons discussed in Chapter 20.

Other related questions: 7, 42, 43, and 47.

19.3 QUESTIONS CONCERNING THE SOURCE OF STUDY PATIENTS

7. *Question:* Is it all right to change patient eligibility criteria once the trial has started?

Answer: Ideally no, but some changes may be necessary. The likelihood of change is greatest in trials involving long periods of recruitment and in those in which investigators are having trouble meeting their sample size goals within the stated time periods. The changes will not affect the validity of treatment comparisons if they are independent of the observed treatment results and if the proportion of patients allocated to the different treatment groups remains unchanged over the course of patient enrollment.

8. *Question:* Will changes in the composition of the study population enrolled have an impact on treatment comparisons?

Answer: No, assuming the proportion of patients assigned to a particular treatment, relative to the total number of allocations made, remains constant over the course of the trial. This is usually assured with randomization procedures designed to balance the number of assignments made to the treatment groups at various points over the course of patient recruitment.

9. *Question:* Is it useful to collect data on patients screened for enrollment?

Answer: It is if there is a reliable way to define the base population at risk of enrollment, as in the Coronary Artery Surgery Study (CASS). The only patients considered for enrollment were those who had had a heart catheterization at a study clinic (Coronary Artery Surgery Study Research Group, 1981). It is not useful when the base population is ill defined, as in the UGDP. Investigators in that trial tried to maintain screening logs, but abandoned the effort because of lack of agreement among them as to who should be listed in the logs.

Other related questions: 73.

19.4 QUESTIONS CONCERNING RANDOMIZATION

10. *Question:* Is randomization needed for a valid trial?

Answer: Not necessarily, provided the method of assignment is free of treatment-related selection biases. In fact, some people have even argued that randomization is unnecessary (Harville, 1975; Lindley, 1982). Indeed, it

would be if all extraneous sources of variation could be identified before the start of the trial and then controlled in the assignment process. However, this is rarely, if ever, possible. The main virtue of randomization is the protection it provides against patient or physician selection biases in the treatment assignment process.

11a. *Question:* Is it acceptable to use an informal, nonauditable method of random assignment, such as a coin flip?

Answer: Not if it can be avoided. Such methods, even if properly administered, are difficult to defend if questions are raised concerning the assignment process. There is no satisfactory way to dispel doubts concerning the possibility of selection bias with any nonauditable allocation scheme.

11b. *Question:* How about methods of randomization that base treatment assignment on a specified digit of the patient's Social Security or medical record number? Are they acceptable?

Answer: Again, not if they can be avoided. Most of these methods fail to satisfy the conditions needed for a sound allocation scheme, as discussed in Chapters 8 and 10.

12. *Question:* Are schemes such as those based on day of the week, time of day, or order in which patients are seen all right to use?

Answer: No. All such methods are susceptable to selection biases and, as a result, may not provide a valid basis for comparisons in the trial. It is too easy for patients or clinic staff to discover the assignment rules and then to alter the time or order in which patients are seen simply to achieve the "desired" assignments.

13. *Question:* Should the treatment assignment be blocked?

Answer: Yes. There can be subtle changes in the composition of the study population as the trial proceeds. Blocking helps to eliminate the impact secular changes may have on treatment comparisons (see Chapter 10).

14a. *Question:* Are the number adaptive schemes, such as the biased-coin method of randomization in which assignment probabilities change as a function of previous assignments, a substitute for blocking?

Answer: Yes. They can serve the same function, as suggested in Section 10.2.

14b. *Question:* Are such schemes better than those that rely on blocking to achieve the desired allocation ratio?

Answer: Yes and no. On the one hand, such methods avoid the problem of predictability as discussed in Chapter 10—a serious problem with small blocks of uniform size, especially in unmasked trials. On the other hand, they can yield longer unbroken runs of patients who are all assigned to the same treatment. Further, the schemes are more complicated to administer than schemes involving blocking.

15. *Question:* Should one use blocks of variable size if blocking is used?

Answer: Generally, yes, particularly in unmasked trials. The variation reduces the likelihood that clinic personnel will be able to predict a treatment assignment.

16. *Question:* Is it necessary to stratify on all important baseline variables in the randomization process?

Answer: No. Valid treatment comparisons can be made without any stratification.

17. *Question:* Is there a limit to the number of variables that can be controlled via stratification during the randomization process?

Answer: Definitely. Generally, it is not practical to stratify on more than two or three variables.

18. *Question:* Should one use clinic as a stratification variable in multicenter trials?

Answer: Generally yes, except in a situation in which there are so few patients per clinic (as in some multicenter trials involving an extremely rare disease) that it is impractical to do so. The characteristics of patients enrolled can vary widely from clinic to clinic. These differences, if uncontrolled, can confound treatment comparisons.

19. *Question:* Is there a way to determine whether randomization has "worked"?

Answer: No. A random process is defined by the methods underlying the process. The demographic and baseline characteristics of patients enrolled in the various treatment groups can be compared. However, the existence of a large difference involving an arbitrarily small *p*-value does not necessarily mean that the assignments were "nonrandom," nor that there was a breakdown in the way in which they were issued. The difference may be due to chance.

20. *Question:* Does the lack of baseline comparability among the treatment groups indicate a breakdown in the randomization process?

Answer: Not necessarily. It may be due to chance, as noted in question 19.

21a. *Question:* Is it all right for the data center to take back a treatment assignment once it has been revealed to the clinic?

Answer: No. The assignment and the patient for whom it was intended should be counted in the study once it has been disclosed. Care should be taken to make certain that the patient is eligible and willing to participate in the trial before the assignment is revealed (see Section 10.7).

21b. *Question:* Should returned assignments (assuming the envelopes in which they are contained have not been opened) be reissued?

Answer: They can be, but often are not because of the difficulties involved in reissuing them.

21c. *Question:* Can the returned assignments result in measurable departures from the desired allocation ratio?

Answer: Not if the number returned is small. They could if the number is large, but even in this case the chance of a sizable departure is small, unless the number is differential by treatment group—not likely except in cases where decisions to return assignments are made by personnel who know the treatment assignments when the decisions are made.

21d. *Question:* What if a mistake is made in preparing the assignment and the wrong one is disclosed to clinic personnel? Should it be taken back?

Answer: No. The assignment should stand as issued once it is disclosed.

21e. *Question:* Can such mistakes lead to a departure from the desired allocation ratio?

Answer: They should not, provided they are independent of treatment assignment. However, they can raise doubts regarding the integrity of the study if they occur frequently.

22a. *Question:* What if the clinic wants to return an assignment because it was used by mistake?

Answer: The assignment should stand as issued once it has been disclosed to clinic personnel.

22b. *Question:* What if a clinic wishes to switch a treatment assignment?

Answer: The assignment should stand as issued once it has been revealed to clinic personnel.

23a. *Question:* What if a clinic administers the wrong treatment to a patient. Should the assignment be changed to correspond to the treatment used?

Answer: No. The assignment should stand as issued. The mistake should be noted when the results of the trial are published.

23b. *Question:* Will mistakes of the type referred to in Question 23a affect the validity of the trial?

Answer: They may, depending on their frequency and whether they are treatment related.

24. *Question:* What if the observed allocation ratio departs from the one specified in the study design?

Answer: Small departures are to be expected, even with small block sizes, few allocation strata, and no returned assignments. Bigger departures can occur with large blocks and multiple strata. Generally, other than detracting from the esthetic quality of the allocation design, the departures will not affect the validity of the trial. An obvious exception is where the departures are treatment related.

25. *Question:* Is it a good idea to have a large number of allocation strata?

Answer: Yes and no. On the one hand, the greater the number of strata the greater the control of extraneous sources of variation. On the other hand, numerous strata will complicate management of the allocation process (see Section 10.3.2).

Other related questions: 7, 8, 49, 50, 51, and 56.

19.5 QUESTIONS CONCERNING MASKING

26. *Question:* Is an unmasked trial valid?

Answer: Masking per se is not an indicator of validity. Valid treatment comparisons can be made without masking. The issue is whether the data collection process, especially as it relates to outcome assessment, is subject to treatment-related biases.

27. *Question:* What if it is impossible to mask?

Answer: This is often the case. The trial should be designed recognizing the opportunities for treatment-related bias. Bias control procedures, such as those discussed in Chapter 8, should be considered.

28. *Question:* Are there circumstances in masked drug trials in which the treatment assignment for a specific patient must be revealed during the course of the trial?

Answer: Yes, a few. However, as noted in Section 8.5, they should be limited to emergency situations. The preferred approach is to terminate use of the assigned treatment without revealing its identity.

29. *Question:* Are there cases in which an entire set of assignments must be unmasked during the trial?

Answer: Yes, when a treatment is discontinued during the study. Clinic personnel will need to identify patients affected by the change in order to implement it.

30. *Question:* Should a patient be informed of the treatment assignment if he is separated from the trial before it is over?

Answer: The answer depends on when the separation occurs, on the arrangements agreed upon when the patient was enrolled, and on the health care needs of the patient. Unmasking individual patients as they depart from the study can create problems in maintaining the mask for other patients, as discussed in Section 15.4.

31. *Question:* Should patients in a masked trial be told of the treatments they were on when the trial is terminated?

Answer: Yes.

32. *Question:* Should the effectiveness of the treatment masking be assessed when the trial is over?

Answer: Yes, as discussed in Section 15.4. Guesses made by clinic staff and patients regarding treatment assignments can be used to make the assessments.

Other related questions: 40, 62, 63, and 64.

19.6 QUESTIONS CONCERNING THE COMPARABILITY OF THE TREATMENT GROUPS

33. *Question:* Are tests of significance helpful in identifying differences in the baseline characteristics of the treatment groups?

Answer: Yes, but the results of such tests must be viewed with caution because of the problems associated with making multiple comparisons, as mentioned in Section 9.3.12.

34. *Question:* When assessing treatment effects, is there a need to be concerned with differences in the baseline comparability of the treatment groups if the differences are small?

Answer: Probably not, but as noted in Section 18.3, it is a good idea to adjust for baseline differences even if small.

35a. *Question:* Is it reasonable to expect the treatment groups to have identical baseline distributions?

Answer: No. The groups will be identical only for those variables controlled in the randomization process. Differences of varying sizes will exist for the other variables.

35b. *Question:* What if at the end of the study one discovers that an important baseline characteristic was overlooked in the data collection process? Is it reasonable to expect that variable to explain the observed treatment difference?

Answer: No. The expected difference among treatment groups for an unobserved baseline characteristic is the same as that for an observed characteristic, assuming the groups are the product of a properly administered randomization scheme.

Other related questions: 7, 8, 57, 71, and 73.

19.7 QUESTIONS CONCERNING TREATMENT ADMINISTRATION

36. *Question:* What should be done about treatment protocol violations detected during the trial?

Answer: Corrective action should be taken to avoid future violations. The departures noted and actions taken should be reported in publications from the trial.

37. *Question:* Is there a reliable way to measure treatment adherence in drug trials?

Answer: Not really, except in inpatient settings. Various methods have been used to assess drug adherence in studies involving outpatient populations. However, all of them have shortcomings. One method involves use of a tracer substance that is added to the study drugs and that can be assayed in the blood or urine of study patients. One of the shortcomings of this method has to do with formulary problems that arise from the addition of any tracer substance to existing drugs. The choice of substances must be limited to those approved by the Food and Drug Administration and that do not affect the bioavailability or pharmacology of the drugs. Another problem has to do with the mechanics of obtaining blood or urine samples for the adherence test. They are normally collected as part of scheduled follow-up visits. As a result they can provide a biased view of adherence if patients change their medicine-taking behavior in preparation for a forthcoming clinic visit.

Blood or urine tests, designed to detect the presence of the drug itself, can be used when it is not feasible to use a tracer substance. However, results from such tests can be quite variable and may not be specific for the drug. In addition, they suffer from the same problem mentioned above if tests are performed as part of a regular clinic visit.

The advent of miniaturized electronic devices has led to development of electronic pill dispensers that automatically record the times at which medicines are withdrawn from them. Comparison of the observed time record with the one prescribed provides an indirect measure of compliance. Pill counts, based on medications returned to the clinic by the patient, are sometimes used as crude measures of adherence. However, these measures have limited use, especially when patients realize that they are used to check on adherence.

38a. *Question:* Should a patient who either refuses to take his assigned treatment upon entry into the trial or who refuses to continue the treatment after entry be retained in the trial?

Answer: Yes. All patients enrolled in the trial should be retained for follow-up regardless of treatment course.

38b. *Question:* Should patients who are started on their assigned treatment and subsequently found to be ineligible for enrollment be retained for followup?

Answer: Yes, particularly if the assigned treatment is continued. However, even if a treatment change is required the patient should continue to be followed.

39. *Question:* Should patients found to be ineligible for the trial after randomization be continued on treatment?

Answer: The answer depends on the nature of the treatments involved. Obviously, treatment should not be continued if there are contraindications for doing so.

Some study designs require the initiation of treatment before a final assessment of eligibility is made (e.g., a trial involving MI patients who are started on treatment in the emergency room). Treatment may have to be stopped if subsequent tests indicate that the individual did not have the condition under study.

Termination of treatment may not be sensible if the final eligibility assessment occurs some time after the start of treatment and if there is no reason to stop the treatment, as was the case in the UGDP (University Group Diabetes Program Research Group, 1970d).

40. *Question:* Should clinic personnel be provided with a supply of placebo tablets for use in single-masked fashion if it is necessary to stop a patient's assigned treatment temporarily because of a suspected drug reaction in a double-masked trial?

Answer: Single-masked administration of a placebo may be of value when the complaints leading to the termination are vague and there is a desire to determine whether they are due to a real or an imagined cause. The procedure is of less value when the reaction can be documented with laboratory tests or by some other objective means.

The CDP allowed study physicians to use a single-masked placebo on patients who appeared to be having drug reactions (Coronary Drug Project Research Group, 1973a). However, their use created a dilemma for physicians when they were called upon to answer questions from patients concerning their use. Often they were placed in the position of having to tell "white lies" to preserve the mask. The wisdom of this deception is questionable because of the impact it may have on patient-physician relations.

Other related questions: 26, 27, 28, and 29.

19.8   QUESTIONS CONCERNING PATIENT FOLLOW-UP

41. *Question:* Should follow-up of a patient be terminated once he experiences the event of interest?

Answer: No, except when the event itself precludes further follow-up. Added follow-up through the close of the trial for new events can provide additional data for comparison of the treatment groups.

42. *Question:* Is there any way to compensate for losses to follow-up due to dropouts or lack of treatment compliance?

Answer: Yes and no. As noted in Chapter 9, there are ways to increase the sample size to compensate for anticipated losses. However, the increases do not protect against bias if the losses are differential by treatment group.

43. *Question:* Some studies are designed to add a new patient for each one who refuses the assigned treatment, or whenever one drops out. Is this a useful maneuver?

Answer: It can serve the same purpose as the sample size adjustment alluded to in the answer to question 42. However, the practice can lead to a false sense of security if it is perceived as a solution to treatment compliance or dropout problems.

The practice is only useful in preserving the statistical precision of the trial if patient recruitment continues over the entire course of follow-up. It is not a practical means of maintaining the desired type I and II error protection if most of the losses are from patients who drop out after recruitment has been completed.

44. *Question:* Does it pay to try to get patients back under follow-up once they have dropped out?

Answer: Yes, especially in a long-term trial. Periodic contact with patients who have dropped out can be useful in convincing some to resume treatment and to return to active follow-up (see Section 15.3 for further discussion).

45. *Question:* Is it reasonable to assume that patients who remain under active follow-up have the same risk of developing the event of interest as those who do not?

Answer: Often no. Patients who drop out may have different risk factors than those who continue in the study. These differences may place them at a higher (or lower) risk of developing the event of interest.

Other related questions: 5, 38, and 65.

19.9 QUESTIONS CONCERNING THE OUTCOME MEASURE

46. *Question:* Is it all right to use a composite outcome measure as the primary outcome measure for a trial?

Answer: Yes, but it is much better to use a single outcome measure for the primary measure. It is difficult to determine the clinical relevancy of most combinations of outcomes, particularly those due to a mixture of disease processes.

47. *Question:* Should an outcome measure not used in the original sample size calculation, or mentioned in the design documents for the trial, be ignored when results of the trial are analyzed?

Answer: No. All available data should be used in the evaluation of the study treatments. While it is desirable to be as explicit as possible in the design stage regarding the primary outcome measure, failure to designate a variable as an outcome measure does not preclude its use in data analysis. (See Section 20.5 for general precautions.)

48. *Question:* What if the outcome measure is subject to a treatment-related ascertainment bias?

Answer: An effort should be made to assess the nature and magnitude of the bias, and a summary of the problem should be included in the study publication.

Other related questions: 4, 45, 58, 72, 75, and 76.

19.10 QUESTIONS CONCERNING DATA INTEGRITY

49. *Question:* What should be done if someone has tampered with the randomization process?

Answer: The entire set of results from the trial may have to be discarded if the tampering was widespread. The extent of the problem, the way the tampering was done, the way in which it was detected, and the action taken should be reported in the study publication. It should also indicate if the problem led to a data purge and, if so, the amount of data purged. If no purge was made, the paper should indicate why the investigators believe none was required. It is good practice to perform two sets of treatment comparisons when purges involving sizable numbers of patients are made: one set for purged patients and the other set for all remaining patients. The results of the two analyses should be included in a publication from the trial.

50. *Question:* Can exclusion of patients judged to be ineligible after randomization affect the credence placed in the results?

Answer: It can. Elimination of patients who are randomized and subsequently found to be ineligible can bias the results if the judgments on eligibility are made by persons who know the treatment assignments. Exclusions, if allowed at all (see answer to question 39), should be based on data collected before randomization and should be made by individuals masked to treatment assignment.

51. *Question:* What should be done with the data from a clinic in a multicenter trial that withdraws during the course of the trial?

Answer: The answer depends on the reason for the withdrawal. The data should be purged from the database if it was due to questionable data practices. Otherwise they should be retained. Whenever possible, an effort should be made to continue follow-up of patients affected by the withdrawal. Sometimes this can be accomplished by transferring care responsibilities to another clinic, as suggested in the answer to question 2b.

The elimination of data from a clinic will not necessarily have any impact on treatment comparisons, provided the proportionate mix of patients by treatment group in the clinic eliminated is the same as for the remaining clinics.

52. *Question:* Is it possible to change data collection or coding practices during the course of the trial and still have a valid trial?

Answer: Yes, so long as the changes are independent of observed treatment effects. However, it is desirable to minimize these changes for practical as well as scientific reasons.

53. *Question:* What should be done with contrived data?

Answer: The answer depends upon the extent of the problem and on whether the contrivance was treatment related. The results of the entire trial may have to be discarded if the problem is extensive and treatment related, whereas no purge may be required if it is restricted to a few isolated cases.

The Multiple Risk Factor Intervention Trial (MRFIT) elected to retain data from one clinic in which personnel were alleged to have falsified blood pressure data for patients being screened for enrollment (Presberg and Timnick, 1976). On the other hand, the data center in the Eastern Cooperative Oncology Study (ECOG) elected to purge all data contributed by one of its clinics because of the serious nature and extent of the falsification (*Boston Globe,* 1980a, 1980b, 1980c, and 1980d; *Boston Sunday Globe,* 1980).

Manuscripts generated from trials in which data falsification has occurred should indicate the nature of the problem and the action taken, if any, to eliminate the questionable data.

Other related questions: 4.

19.11   QUESTIONS CONCERNING DATA ANALYSIS

54. *Question:* What is the basis for pooling treatment results across clinics in a multicenter trial?

Answer: It stems from the use of common treatment and data collection procedures, and from the ongoing quality assurance procedures designed to detect and minimize procedural differences among study clinics.

55. *Question:* Is randomization required for a valid analysis?

Answer: No. The main purpose of randomization is to provide a method of assignment that is free of selection bias. Randomization theory has been used to form the basis for some tests of significance, but the theory, per se, is not crucial for most of the data analyses carried out in the typical clinical trial.

56. *Question:* Is one obligated to make treatment comparisons in subgroups defined when the trial was designed?

Answer: No. In fact, the first analysis should be without regard to any subgrouping. Secondary analyses may be done within various subgroups, including randomization strata.

57. *Question:* Can differences in the baseline composition of the study groups invalidate treatment comparisons?

Answer: It depends on how large they are and how they occurred. They can if the differences are an expression of a treatment-related bias resulting from a breakdown in the assignment process, but not if they are relatively small and unrelated to treatment.

Much of the discussion concerning the UGDP results published in 1970 (University Group Diabetes Program Research Group, 1970e) centered on the comparability of the treatment groups at the time of randomization. Critics argued that the constellation of baseline entry characteristics present in the tolbutamide-treated patients automatically predisposed them to a higher risk of mortality than was the case for control-treated patients (Feinstein, 1971; Schor, 1971; Seltzer, 1972). Arguments concerning comparability persisted in spite of the fact that the observed differences were within the range of chance, that adjustment for the differences did not materially affect the size of the tolbutamide-placebo difference in mortality, and that analyses by others outside the UGDP reached similar conclusions regarding tolbutamide therapy (Committee for the Assessment of Biometric Aspects of Controlled Trials of Hypoglycemic Agents, 1975; Cornfield, 1971).

58. *Question:* Is it appropriate to consider more than one outcome measure in the analysis of the data?

Answer: Yes. As a matter of fact it is often an essential part of the analysis process. See question 47.

59. *Question:* Are there dangers in analyses that focus simply on patients who received the assigned treatment?

Answer: Yes, they can lead to overestimation of the treatment effect (see Section 18.1).

60. *Question:* Where should data on patients who did not receive the assigned treatment be counted?

Answer: The primary analysis should be based on the original treatment assignment (see Section 18.1). Other analyses, including those based on classification of patients by treatment received, may be carried out.

61. *Question:* How does one take account of changes in a patient's adherence to treatment over the course of the trial?

Answer: The problem with varying levels of adherence is common in drug trials in which patients are expected to remain on their assigned treatment for long periods of time. The primary analysis should be by the initial treatment assignment, without regard to adherence. This analysis can be followed by others that are designed to take account of observed adherence levels (e.g., see University Group Diabetes Program Research Group, 1970e).

62. *Question:* What should be done with data from a patient whose treatment is unmasked for medical reasons?

Answer: They should be analyzed in the treatment group indicated by the randomization. Other analyses may be performed and reported in which data for such patients are excluded to determine if doing so affects the magnitude of the observed treatment effect.

63. *Question:* What if the treatment masking was ineffective? Are the data still worth analyzing?

Answer: Masking is never 100% effective. Treatment-related side effects may reveal the treatment assignment to both patients and physicians. The validity of treatment comparisons will depend on whether or not the deficiencies in masking allowed introduction of treatment-related biases.

64. *Question:* What should be done with data for patients whose treatment assignment was needlessly unmasked?

Answer: The analysis approach should be similar to that outlined for question 61. However, the frequency of frivolous unmaskings should be noted in the published report. A large number may be indicative of a lack of regard for the study protocol by investigators in the trial and may raise general questions regarding the validity of the study.

65. *Question:* How does one deal with missing data caused by losses to follow-up?

Answer: While there is no substitute for complete follow-up, the usual approach is to carry out a series of analyses, each requiring a different set of assumptions regarding the rate of outcome events after patients are lost to follow-up. One of the analyses should be done assuming a zero event rate over the periods patients are lost to follow-up. Other analyses may be done in which all patients lost to follow-up are assumed to have had the event after loss to follow-up, or alternatively, in which they are assumed to have experienced the event at the same rate as a defined portion of the study population (e.g., the control-treatment group of patients who remained under active follow-up). Losses are not a serious source of concern if the various analyses all support the same basic conclusion and if they are not differential by treatment group.

66. *Question:* How should aberrant laboratory results be handled?

Answer: Outlier values, whether they are a legitimate indicator of some underlying biological problem or are due to a laboratory or recording error, may have to be trimmed or eliminated in analyses involving means or variances. The rules for trimming or elimination should be constructed and administered without regard to treatment assignment or effect and should be specified in published reports from the trial.

67. *Question:* What if there is a secular trend in the laboratory data generated in a trial? Will this affect comparisons between treatment groups?

Answer: It should not, assuming that patients in all treatment groups were enrolled over the same time frame and that the time sequence in which laboratory determinations were performed was independent of treatment assignment.

68. *Question:* How should data obtained from interim unscheduled examinations be handled?

Answer: The first analysis should be done ignoring the results. A second one may be done with the results included. A differential rate of interim unscheduled examinations by treatment group can influence the rate at which nonfatal events are diagnosed and reported. CDP investigators were sufficiently concerned about this possibility as to virtually ignore results from unscheduled examinations when analyzing the dextrothyroxine results (Coronary Drug Project Research Group, 1972; 1981).

69. *Question:* Is it permissible to perform analyses during the course of the trial to detect treatment effects?

Answer: Yes. They are not only permissible but required in any trial in which the treatments are hazardous, or in which early detection of a treatment effect may prove beneficial to patients already in the trial or to those yet to be enrolled (see Chapter 20).

70. *Question:* What if there is a major time lag in the flow of data from the clinic to the data center? Can this have an impact on the detection of treatment differences during the trial?

Answer: Yes, especially if the time lag is differential by treatment group. Procedures should be established to ensure data flows that are timely and uniform with regard to treatment assignment (see Chlebowski and co-workers, 1981).

71a. *Question:* Is it reasonable to argue that imbalance in the distribution of an important but unobserved baseline risk factor could account for an observed treatment difference or lack of one in a randomized trial?

Answer: Not really. As noted in the answers to questions 35a and 35b, the expected distribution of an unobserved characteristic is the same as for an observed characteristic.

71b. *Question:* Is a trial invalid if there are differences among the treatment groups with regard to key baseline variables?

Answer: Generally no, unless the differences are due to selection biases arising from a breakdown in the way treatment allocations were made.

72. *Question:* Is it appropriate to use a subset of deaths as the prime outcome measure?

Answer: The trial may be designed for detection of a specified difference for a subset of deaths, as was the case in MRFIT (Multiple Risk Factor Intervention Trial Research Group, 1982). However, the initial analysis should be for mortality from all causes (see question 75b).

Other related questions: 4, 8, 34, 35, 45, 47, 48, 51, 53, 75, and 76.

19.12 QUESTIONS CONCERNING CONCLUSIONS

73. *Question:* Is it really possible to draw any conclusions from a clinical trial because of the select nature of the study population involved?

Answer: Yes. Comparisons between treatment groups are valid so long as all groups have been exposed to the same selection factors.

74. *Question:* Is it possible to generalize findings beyond the population studied and the treatments used?

Answer: Any generalization that goes beyond the study population must be made with caution and is judgmental rather than statistical in nature. Treatment effects observed in a specified population with a particular dosage of a drug may not be generalizable to a broader population. Similarly, an effect produced with one formulation of a compound may not be produced by a sister product. For example, it is tempting to generalize the UGDP findings on tolbutamide to other sulfonylurea compounds. However, the study included only one member of the family (University Group Diabetes Program Research Group, 1970d). The question of scientific validity versus generalizability is touched upon by the National Diet-Heart Study Research Group (1968).

75a. *Question:* Is it appropriate to base conclusions from a trial on a nonfatal event if there is differential mortality by treatment group?

Answer: No. Conclusions based on differences in a nonfatal outcome are only valid if there is no difference among the study groups with respect to mortality. A differential mortality by treatment group may influence the rate of occurrence of nonfatal events. The treatment group with the highest mortality rate may have the lowest nonfatal event rate if death occurs before patients have a chance to develop the nonfatal event of interest.

75b. *Question:* Is it appropriate to base conclusions on deaths due to a specific cause (e.g., cardiovascular deaths)?

Answer: Only if the conclusion is consistent with the one reached when all deaths are considered.

76. *Question:* Is it appropriate to base conclusions on an outcome measure that was not

expected to yield a difference when the trial was designed?

Answer: Yes, especially when the measure has more clinical relevance than the one used in the design of the trial. The focus on mortality in assessment of the tolbutamide and phenformin results in the UGDP, even though the study was designed to look for differences in nonfatal outcomes, is a case in point (University Group Diabetes Program Research Group, 1970d, 1970e, 1975).

Other related questions: 10, 26, 52, 54, 55, 57, 71, and 72.

20. Interim data analyses for treatment monitoring

Pigs is pigs, data is data.

Jerome Cornfield (1975)

20.1 INTRODUCTION

An interim analysis is any assessment of data done during the patient enrollment or follow-up stages of a trial for the purpose of assessing center performance, the quality of the data collected, or treatment effects. The kinds of tabulations and interim analyses needed for performance monitoring and data quality control are discussed in Chapter 16. Those discussed in this chapter relate to the treatment monitoring (also referred to as safety monitoring; see Glossary) carried out during the trial.

Major ethical questions arise if investigators elect to continue a medical experiment beyond the point at which more prudent people would have stopped. A case in point is the Tuskegee Syphilis Study, initiated in 1932 and continued into the early 1970s. The study involved enrollment and follow-up of 400 untreated latent syphilitic black males (and 200 uninfected controls) in order to trace the course of the disease. Criticism of the study stemmed from the fact that the syphilitics remained untreated after penicillin, an accepted form of treatment for the disease, became available (see Chapter 14 for references).

The need for treatment monitoring extends to most trials, whether they are done to assess a therapeutic, prophylactic, or diagnostic procedure, and whether they involve a fixed sample or sequential design, crossed or uncrossed treatment structure, short-term or long-term follow-up, or single or multiple clinics. Further, it extends over the life of the trial, beginning with enrollment of the first patient and continuing to the end of follow-up, regardless of how and when treatments are administered and even if patients are no longer being exposed to the study treatments.

Investigators have a responsibility to notify patients as well as the medical community of the preferred course of treatment once the choice is clear. Patients assigned to the inferior treatment should be removed from it (and offered the superior treatment if appropriate) as soon as the choice is clear.

The general need for treatment monitoring has been noted by the National Institutes of Health (National Institutes of Health Clinical Trials Committee, 1979). Published guidelines specify that:

- Every clinical trial should have provisions for treatment monitoring
- The mechanism proposed should be approved by responsible Institutional Review Boards
- Multicenter trials should have an independent treatment monitoring committee that:
  - Includes clinicians with expertise in the disease under study, biostatisticians, and scientists from other relevant disciplines
  - Excludes physicians caring for patients in the trial

A good rule of thumb is to design the trial with treatment monitoring unless there are overriding reasons to the contrary. (See Table 22–1 for classes of trials requiring safety monitoring.) Arguments concerning the logistical difficulties involved in carrying out the monitoring, or that are based on the assumption that the treatments are safe are not acceptable. The same is true for arguments based on the assumption that the treatment differences will be small.

All of the trials sketched in Appendix B include provisions for treatment monitoring. The picture appears to be different when viewed through the published literature. Very few of the papers reviewed in Chapter 2 contained any evidence of such monitoring, even those involving fairly long periods of follow-up. Either none was done or the investigators simply failed to mention it in their reports.

Interim analyses for treatment effects can be useful even if not needed for treatment monitoring. They help to ensure the orderly development of methods and procedures needed for analyses when the study is finished. In addition, they may reveal data deficiencies that can be corrected by modification of the data forms or study procedures.

20.2 PROCEDURAL ISSUES

Several questions must be addressed before any treatment monitoring can be done. One has to do with designation of the individual or group responsible for carrying out the analyses needed for monitoring and for generating the treatment monitoring reports. Normally, the responsibility is vested in the data center for the trial.

A second issue has to do with selection of the individual or group having responsibility for reviewing the monitoring reports and for deciding whether or not the trial should be allowed to continue. This review may be carried out by the same individual or group that was responsible for generation of the reports in the first place, or by someone else. The latter is the case for all the trials sketched in Appendix B and is the preferred mode of operation (see Chapter 23 for a discussion of treatment monitoring committees).

A third issue has to do with the schedule for interim analyses. They may be done on a fixed time schedule (e.g., after every six months) or on one determined by occurrences in the trial (e.g., after a certain number of deaths). All of the trials sketched in Appendix B had schedules (see item 29.g, Table B–4, Appendix B) that called for generation of two or three monitoring reports per year in conjunction with scheduled meetings of the safety monitoring committee. The staffs in the data coordinating centers were responsible for alerting members of the safety monitoring committees to unexpected changes occurring between meetings. In fact, the data coordinating centers in several of the studies (e.g., Coronary Drug Project and Veterans Administration Cooperative Study No. 43) distributed interim reports between meetings to allow members of the committees to call special meetings when appropriate. The frequency of meetings can be expected to increase as a study nears a decision point. For example, the Macular Photocoagulation Study (MPS) required two extra meetings of its safety monitoring committee before it decided in favor of photocoagulation for patients with senile macular degeneration (Macular Photocoagulation Study Group, 1982).

The usefulness of the monitoring process depends on a timely flow of primary outcome data from the generation site to the analysis center. It will be reduced by delays in the flow (e.g., see Chlebowski et al., 1981). It can also be diminished by delays in receiving or processing secondary outcome data based on reading of records, such as ECGs, X rays, or fundus photographs.

The general steps oulined in Section 17.7 concerning preparation of the analysis tape pertain to interim as well as final analyses. Each monitoring report should be based on a defined data set that is used to generate all tables in the report. The analysis tape(s) or disk(s) should be retained for a time following review of the report. Some tapes (disks), especially those used for generation of reports leading to a treatment change, should be kept indefinitely.

20.3 TREATMENT MONITORING REPORTS

The discussion that follows assumes that the reports are generated for review by committees, as described in Chapter 23. Table 20–1 provides a stylized outline of a "typical" report. The outline assumes that other tabulations needed for performance monitoring are contained in a separate report (see Section 16.7 and Table 16–5). Appendix G contains sample tables from the MPS treatment monitoring report and the list of tables appearing in a Persantine Aspirin Reinfarction Study (PARIS) treatment monitoring report.

The report should contain a table of contents

Table 20-1 Content of treatment monitoring reports

A. Table of contents
- List of tables and figures in report and associated page numbers

B. Narrative section
- Summary of main findings
- Discussion of special problems influencing interpretation of results
- Procedures used for preparation of report, including cutoff date for analysis, editing rules, etc.

C. Design summary section
- Purpose of the trial
- List of participating clinics
- Location of data center and other resource centers
- Recruitment goal and sample size specifications
- Study treatments
- Level of treatment masking
- Randomization or treatment unit
- Summary of patient admission criteria
- Prerandomization and follow-up examination schedule
- Projected timetable for the trial, including time for patient recruitment, follow-up, and final analysis

D. Data quality and quantity
- Number of patients randomized by treatment group and clinic
- Summary of missing information as reflected by:
  - Number of missed prerandomization and follow-up visits by treatment group and clinic
  - Number of patients classified as dropouts by treatment group and clinic
  - Number of patients lost to follow-up by treatment group and clinic
  - Number of missing items of information on completed data forms by treatment group and clinic
- Distribution of patients by time of entry (used to indicate the amount of follow-up information being generated and for predicting the amount of data that will be available at some point in the future, e.g., the number of patients who will have at least two years of follow-up by the next time the report is generated)
- Number of delinquent data forms by clinic (and by treatment group if there is concern regarding a differential delinquency rate, e.g., as in unmasked trials)
- Number and percent of deficient data items by clinic (and by treatment group in unmasked trials)
- Inter-aliquot differences in laboratory tests by clinic (and by treatment group in unmasked trials)
- Coding and data entry error rates by clinic with distributed data entry systems (and by treatment group in unmasked trials)
- Enumeration of special data problems that may influence interpretation of the treatment results

E. Population description summary section
- Frequency distribution of selected baseline demographic characteristics, such as age at entry, sex, race, etc., by treatment group

(Section A, Table 20-1). Pages in the report should be numbered and stapled or bound in some other fashion. The tables and graphs in the report should have titles that are self-explanatory. Axes of graphs should be labelled. All information in the report should be checked for accuracy prior to inclusion.

Section B, the narrative section, should indicate who prepared the summary, the amount of data included in the report (by indicating the cut-off date for data), and should include a summary of the key findings contained in the report. This section should also be used to remind committee members of any deficiencies in the quality of data and of coding or editing procedures that might affect the way in which results are interpreted.

Section C should contain a digest of the key design features of the trial. The section may not be necessary if committee members have an intimate knowledge of the study and meet regularly. It is useful for complicated trials and for committees that meet only a few times a year.

Section D should provide data on the nature of the database. Tabulations indicating the number of missed follow-up visits, the number of dropouts, and number of patients lost to follow-up are important indicators of the completeness and adequacy of the database and should be included in each report.

Section E serves two functions. It should indicate the baseline comparability of the treatment groups and provide a description of the study population. Knowledge of the study population

Table 20-1 Content of treatment monitoring reports (*continued*)

- Descriptive tabulations for selected baseline laboratory and physiological measures (e.g., cholesterol, body weight, diastolic blood pressure, etc.) by treatment group
- Other summary tabulations of entry characteristics needed to provide a baseline for evaluation of subsequent changes by treatment group, with particular emphasis on known or suspected risk factors for the disease or outcome of interest

F. Treatment administration summary section

- Number of patients assigned to each treatment group
- Number of ineligible patients enrolled by treatment group
- Number of patients who refused the assigned treatment by treatment group
- Number of patients who received a treatment other than the one assigned by treatment group
- Summary tables describing the level of adherence over the course of follow-up by treatment group
- Number of instances in which treatment assignments were unmasked (in the case of masked trials) by treatment group

G. Treatment effects summary section

- Number and percent of patients dead by treatment group
- Percent of patients who experienced the primary outcome at, or before, a specified cut-off date by treatment group

- Lifetable analysis of the primary outcome to provide event rates by treatment group over the course of follow-up
- Percent of patients experiencing an indicated secondary outcome by treatment group
- Lifetable analysis of each secondary outcome of interest by treatment group
- Subgroup analyses by treatment group, using selected entry characteristics as a means of adjustment for baseline differences in the composition of the study group and for identification of treatment effects within subgroups
- Multiple linear or logistic regression and Cox regression analysis (see Chapter 18) as a means of adjusting outcome data for differences in the baseline composition of the treatment groups
- Treatment comparisons involving the outcome of primary interest by treatment group and level of treatment compliance
- Summary table of percentages and rates for the primary and secondary outcomes as contained in current report as well as corresponding values from previous reports
- Summary tabulation of patients experiencing indicated side effects by treatment group

H. Special analysis section

- Listing of special problems not covered in other sections of the report, especially any that may temper interpretation of the treatment results
- Special tabulations designed to provide information on the natural course of the disease under study

characteristics is important for generalization of treatment findings.

Information on the treatment process is summarized in Section F. It should provide data on patient and physician compliance to the treatment protocol. The treatment results are summarized in Section G. It is the most important and largest part of the report.

A typical report may contain a number of other tabulations distributed throughout the sections already mentioned, or contained in a special section at the end of the report. Some of them may be standard and appear in each report, whereas others may be prepared in response to a specific request and may appear only once.

Reports, after they have been reviewed,

should be stored at a central repository (usually the data coordinating center). The written record (minutes of the meeting) generated during review of the report (also stored in the repository) should indicate when the report was reviewed and the specific actions recommended, if any, as a result of review.

20.4 SPECIAL STATISTICAL PROBLEMS

The need to make periodic treatment comparisons of the outcome data over the course of patient enrollment and follow-up gives rise to what is termed herein as the multiple looks problem. Two other problems, termed herein the multiple outcomes problem and the multiple comparisons problem, are likely to be encountered as well. The first problem is unique to interim analyses. The other two can arise in conjunction with any data analysis, whether done during, or at the end of the trial.

20.4.1 The multiple looks problem

This problem has been addressed by various authors (e.g., Abt, 1981; Anscombe, 1953, 1954; Armitage et al., 1969; Bailey, 1967; Brown, 1983; Canner, 1977a, 1977b, 1983a, 1983b; Cornfield, 1966a, 1966b, 1969, 1976; Coronary Drug Project Research Group, 1972, 1973b, 1981; Dupont, 1983a, 1983b; National Cooperative Gallstone Study Group, 1981a; Seigel and Milton, 1983; O'Brien and Fleming, 1979; Royall, 1983; University Group Diabetes Program Research Group, 1970e, 1971b, 1975). Some investigators have ignored the problem by behaving as if each look is the only one to be performed and have followed conventional rules for interpreting p-values (i.e., have behaved as if a test result is statistically significant at the 5% level if its p-value is ≤ 0.05). This approach has obvious shortcomings, forcefully illustrated by Anscombe (1954). He has shown that the probability of obtaining a "significant" result approaches unity when a test of significance is performed at various points over the course of a study.

Cornfield (1976) has commented on the same problem in more picturesque terms:

> *Just as the Sphinx winks if you look at it too long, so, if you perform enough significance tests you are sure to find significance, even when none exists.*

He relied on the likelihood principle to address the problem (Cornfield, 1969). Crudely stated, the principle specifies that the information contained in a data set is independent of the way in which the set is ordered (Dupont, 1983a, 1983b). Cornfield's method of analysis yields two probability calculations—one under the null hypothesis of no treatment effect and the other under a specified alternative to the null hypothesis. The ratio of the two probabilities has been referred to as the relative betting odds (RBOs) by Cornfield, since the resulting value provides a measure of the support for the null hypothesis, relative to a specified alternative. (See the University Group Diabetes Program Research Group, 1970e, 1971b, 1975 for illustrations of the method.)

Another approach involves use of simulation techniques to produce monitoring bounds, such as those used in the UGDP and CDP (University Group Diabetes Program Research Group, 1970e, 1975; Coronary Drug Project Research Group, 1973b). Figure 20–1 is a reproduction of the bounds used for the tolbutamide-placebo mortality comparisons in the UGDP. Figure 18–2 is an illustration of the same concept, as used in the CDP. The bounds pictured represent, in effect, the 95% statistical limits of variability that one would expect in the observed test-control treatment differences for the method of comparison used if it were possible to repeat a trial many times under the null hypothesis and assuming a set number of data looks over the course of the trial. Viewed as a decision-making tool, a trial continues so long as the observed test-control difference for the specified outcome remains within the bounds. The test or control treatment is terminated if the observed difference crosses one of the boundaries.

20.4.2 The multiple outcomes problem

This problem arises whenever two or more outcome measures are used to assess the study treatments. The need to look at multiple outcomes exists in most trials, even those designed to focus on a primary outcome measure. Analyses are rarely restricted to that measure alone.

Among the three problems listed, this one is the most difficult to address. It is complicated by the fact that the primary and secondary outcomes of interest are likely to be interdependent (Cupples et al., 1984). The usual approach is to ignore the interdependence and to make comparisons involving the different outcome measures as if they were independent of one another. The practice can lead to erroneous conclusions unless results are interpreted with caution. For example, one might be impressed with a statistically significant difference in nonfatal MI rates favoring the test treatment in a heart study with mortality as the primary outcome. However, the result is only of interest if there was no test-control difference in mortality or if the difference favored the test treatment.

A common practice in trials involving death as the outcome measure is to focus on cause-specific mortality, for example, cardiovascular deaths in MRFIT (Multiple Risk Factor Intervention Trial Research Group, 1982). The tests of significance obtained in such cases must be interpreted in conjunction with those obtained for overall mortality. For example, the lack of a statistically significant tolbutamide-placebo dif-

(a) All cause mortality

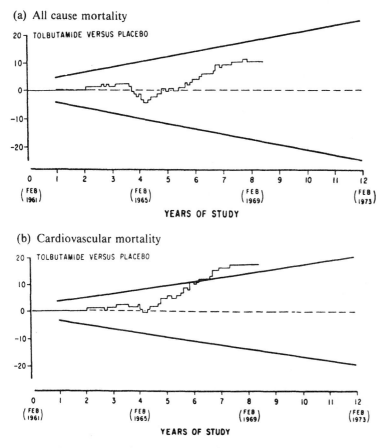

(b) Cardiovascular mortality

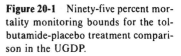

Figure 20-1 Ninety-five percent mortality monitoring bounds for the tolbutamide-placebo treatment comparison in the UGDP.

Source: Reference citation 468. Adapted with permission of the American Diabetes Association, Inc., New York.

ference for overall mortality in the UGDP (*p*-value = 0.17) made the study investigators reluctant to draw any conclusion about the excess cardiovascular mortality observed, despite its size (University Group Diabetes Program Research Group, 1970e).

Certainly, a practice to be frowned upon is one in which results for only a subgroup of outcomes are reported, as noted in Chapter 18 in connection with discussion of analysis ground rule 3. Readers should be provided with results for the entire set of outcomes (e.g., all deaths) from which the subset (e.g., cardiovascular deaths) was derived or, failing that, for complementary subsets (e.g., cardiovascular versus noncardiovascular deaths).

20.4.3 The multiple comparisons problem

The multiple comparisons problem arises when an investigator chooses to make several different treatment comparisons all involving the same outcome measure (and all done at the same time

point). It has been addressed by various authors, including Bégun and Gabriel, 1981; Dawkins, 1983; Duncan, 1955, 1975; Duncan and Godbold, 1979; Duncan and Brandt, 1983a; Duncan and Dixon, 1983b; Dunnett, 1955, 1964; Miller, 1966, 1977; O'Brien, 1983; Scheffé, 1953; and Tukey, 1951, 1977.

The need arises in two general settings. In the first, the investigator is interested in determining subgroups of patients within the test-treated group that appear to be benefited (or harmed) by the treatment. It can give rise to an indeterminant number of comparisons if the subgroups are identified as a result of data dredging (see Section 20.5). In the second setting, the investigator is interested in comparing each of several different test treatments with the control treatment or with one another. It will give rise to a minimum of *t* test-control comparisons—one for each test treatment. Other comparisons will be required if the investigator wishes to establish the superiority (or inferiority) of one test treatment relative to other test treatments.

Various frameworks have been developed to deal with the statistical problems involved in making multiple comparisons. A particularly simple one is based on Bonferroni's inequality. The inequality states that the probability of one or more k independent events occurring simultaneously is $< kp$, where p, the probability of a given event, is the same for all k events (Abt, 1981; Feller, 1968). The statement can be used to provide an upper bound on the combined type I error for making k simultaneous comparisons. The probability of rejecting the null hypothesis when it is true with tests of significance for the k comparisons is $k\alpha'$ if each of the k comparisons is made at an α' type I error level. The combined type I error level for all k tests will be less than α if α' is set equal to α/k. The NCGS used the inequality to adjust p-values for individual test-control comparisons presented in that study (National Cooperative Gallstone Study Group, 1981a).

20.5   DATA DREDGING AS AN ANALYSIS TECHNIQUE

Data dredging is a term used to characterize analyses that are done on an ad hoc basis, usually without benefit of a prestated hypothesis, as a means of identifying differences of note within specified subgroups of patients. The subgroups are typically formed by subdividing patients into mutually exclusive subgroups using observed baseline characteristics, as illustrated in Table 18–8.

The practice of data dredging is common and is not unique to clinical trials. In fact, it is the hallmark of most epidemiological research concerned with identifying etiological factors of diseases. Data dredging arises in clinical trials from the desire to identify subgroups of patients who are benefited or harmed by the study treatment. It can occur during the trial or when it is finished. CDP investigators spent a great deal of time doing such analyses in an effort to understand the dextrothyroxine (DT4) treatment results (Coronary Drug Project Research Group, 1970b, 1972). The same was true of MRFIT investigators trying to decide if antihypertensive drug therapy for hypertensive men with an abnormal resting ECG is dangerous (Multiple Risk Factor Intervention Trial Research Group, 1982).

The main concern with data dredging has to do with the statistical interpretation of differences found in this way. Table 20–2 lists general

Table 20–2   Ground rules for data dredging via subgroup analyses

- Limit choice of subgrouping variables to baseline characteristics
- Present results for all subgroups defined with a subgrouping variable
- Distinguish between a priori and a posteriori selected subgrouping variables
- Choose cutting points that are independent of observed treatment differences
- Avoid conventional interpretation of significance tests
- When possible, validate findings before reporting on subgroups identified via data dredging
- Report methods and procedures
- Be cautious regarding conclusions.

rules that should be followed. They are in addition to those outlined in Section 18.1.

As noted in Table 20–2, the choice of subgrouping variables (see Glossary for definition) should be limited to data collected before randomization (i.e., baseline data). Variables observed after randomization may be influenced by the study treatments and, hence, the subgroups created using them may be subject to selection biases, especially those formed using measures of treatment compliance.

All subgroups formed with a subgrouping variable (two if a single cut-point is used as in Table 18–8, more if multiple cut-points are used) should be looked at and reported. Failure to do so can lead to erroneous impressions if a difference observed in one subgroup is offset by a difference in the other direction in the other subgroup(s).

The fourth point—independence of the choice of the cut-point and observed treatment differences—listed in Table 20–2 is basic. It may be taken for granted when cut-points are set before the start of data collection or when they are dictated by the data collection process. It cannot be if the cut-points are chosen after the start of data collection.

Investigators should be wary of any "significant" differences that are found via data dredging. Conventional rules for interpreting a p-value do not apply to dredged results. Precautions are needed to avoid false proclamations of significance. The precautions may take one of two forms. The first involves use of some method for "adjusting" the p-values for the fact that multiple comparisons were done, as discussed in Section 20.4.3. The second involves a form of internal cross-validation in which only a portion of the data (say half) are used to identify subgroup treatment differences (e.g., see Coronary Drug Project Research Group, 1981). The remaining portion is used to replicate the analysis to determine if both portions of the data identify the same subgroups.

The emphasis here has been on data dredging involving different subgroupings of the patient. A variation involves using different outcome measures. The ultimate form of dredging is to use the two forms in combination.

20.6 THE PROS AND CONS OF STOPPING RULES IN MONITORING TRIALS

A stopping rule is one, usually established before or shortly after the start of patient recruitment, that specifies a limit for the test-control outcome difference which, if exceeded, automatically leads to termination of one or the other treatments depending on the direction of the observed differences (see articles by Dupont, 1983a, 1983b, and related discussion by Brown, 1983; Canner, 1983a, 1983b; Greenhouse, 1983; and Royall, 1983). An example of a stopping rule, using mortality as the outcome and based on a standardized comparison of two proportions, is outlined below. The steps are carried out at each of a series of designated time points over the trial until a stopping point is reached or until the trial is completed.

Sample stopping rule

Step 1. Calculate the proportion of patients dead in the test and control treatment groups, p_t and p_c, respectively, at the first time point at which an interim analysis is required, as specified when the rule was constructed.

Step 2. Evaluate the test statistic:

$$t = \frac{p_t - p_c}{\sqrt{\text{Var}\,(p_t - p_c)}}$$

Step 3. Stop the test treatment and conclude it is inferior to the control treatment if $t > Z$. Stop the control treatment and conclude the test treatment is superior to it if $t < -Z'$. Continue the trial if $-Z' < t < Z$. (The values for Z and Z' will be set by the study investigators. Their size will be a func-

tion of the degree of statistical certainty desired before stopping and the amount of "adjustment" to be made for multiple looks. The two values will be equal if symmetry in the decision-making process is desired. Z will be $< Z'$ if more evidence is required to accept the test treatment as beneficial than for stopping it because of possible harmful effects.)

Step 4. Repeat steps 1 through 3 for each subsequent time point until the trial is stopped or until it is finished.

Stopping rules have some appealing features. They are easy to use and they force investigators to think about the analysis process and to specify the outcome measure to be used in evaluating the treatments before the trial starts (see Section 8.3 and Section 9.3.2). However, they also have serious limitations. A major one is that it is virtually impossible to construct rules that deal with all of the contingencies that can arise during the course of the trial. Sometimes it may be necessary to terminate use of a treatment even though the test-control difference is well within the range specified by the rule. For example, just three cases of chronic active hepatitis in the NCGS were enough to raise serious questions as to whether to continue the trial, even though the test treatment showed promise with regard to the primary outcome measure. Further, even if one were clairvoyant enough to anticipate the various conditions that would require stopping the trial, it is not wise to use statistical tests of significance as the sole decision-making tool in the treatment monitoring process. Other factors that will enter in involve judgments concerning:

- The merits of the treatment
- The availability and usefulness of alternative treatments
- The seriousness of the conditions being treated
- The acceptability of the treatment to patients, as evidenced by their willingness to use it, and by the number of side effects it produces
- The clinical importance of the observed difference
- The consistency of the results with other findings in the trial and with other studies

The amount of evidence required for investigators to give up on an elective treatment for which there are alternatives may be less than that required for a treatment considered to be life sustaining for which there are no alternatives. UGDP investigators terminated use of both tolbutamide and phenformin simply because the treatments were no better than the placebo (University Group Diabetes Program Research Group, 1970e, 1971b, 1975). They did not consider it appropriate to continue an elective treatment that failed to show any promise of benefit.

The judgment as to how long the trial should be continued in the face of a positive result will be influenced by the size of the difference, the length of time it took to emerge, and the degree of certainty investigators have as to the stability of the results. Investigators in both the Diabetic Retinopathy Study (DRS) and MPS continued treatments in those trials for some time after emergence of a positive result (Diabetic Retinopathy Study Research Group, 1976; Macular Photocoagulation Study Research Group, 1982, 1983a). They were concerned that the benefits observed might be offset by subsequent adverse effects. Long-term follow-up data were needed before they felt comfortable offering photocoagulation for untreated control eyes.

20.7 STEPS IN TERMINATING A TREATMENT

Once the decision has been made to stop the test or control treatment a series of steps will be required to implement it (see Section 15.4 for details on patient close-out and Sections 23.6 and 23.7 for comments on procedures for recommending treatment changes). The first step will be to present the results to the clinic staff responsible for implementing the decision. The presentation should be done as soon after the decision to stop as possible and should be designed to acquaint clinic staff with the findings and the reasons for stopping. It may be done from slides or handouts prepared from the treatment monitoring report leading to the decision and should include a discussion of the implications of the results and of the advice to be given patients affected by the change.

Clinic staff should be provided with guidance as to how rapidly they are to proceed in implementing the change. Treatments regarded as dangerous will require deliberate and immediate action. However, even if this is not the case, it is a good idea to proceed with implementation as soon as possible. It is not a good idea to wait until the results are ready for publication, especially if the delay entails continued exposure of patients to a harmful or inferior treatment.

Records should be kept to indicate when each patient was contacted regarding the change and what he was told. Documentation of this sort is important regardless of whether the patient is being taken off an ineffective treatment or is being offered a beneficial one.

Obviously, patients affected by the change should be told of the reasons for the change. However, it is also a good idea to inform other patients in the trial of the change, even though they are not affected by it. They may need reassurance and may be asked to give a new consent for continuation in the trial (see Section 14.6.5).

Patients removed from a treatment but who remain associated with the trial may or may not be given alternative forms of therapy, depending on the treatment options available. Patients in the UGDP and assigned to tolbutamide or phenformin therapy were not offered any other oral hypoglycemic agent when these treatments were terminated. Untreated eyes still eligible for treatment in the DRS were considered for photocoagulation treatment when study investigators were told of results in that trial (Diabetic Retinopathy Study Research Group, 1976).

Patients should be told if they are expected to continue under follow-up after a treatment protocol change. The data may be of some value in characterizing long-term treatment effects. However, their usefulness in this regard will depend on the extent to which patients are exposed to other treatments after the change. Investigators in both the UGDP and CDP elected to have patients continue on the same clinic visit schedule they had before the change. They did so, in part, for the reason mentioned above and also to avoid the morale problems and disruption that might have resulted if some patients had been separated while others were required to continue.

Part V. Management and administration

Chapters in This Part

The first chapter in this Part details the nature of funding vehicles for clinical trials, with emphasis on NIH grants and contracts. It also contains specific budgeting suggestions for the various centers in a multicenter trial. Chapter 22 contains an outline of the general principles and practices to be followed in managing a trial. The last chapter contains a review of organizational structures used in mulitcenter trials. The chapter discusses a number of practical issues concerned with the formation and operation of committee structures.

21. Funding the trial

The hypothesis is unencumbered by any supporting evidence. The budget is the only part of the application which seems to have any substance whatsoever.

Anonymous NIH study section member

21.1 INTRODUCTION

An essential step in the execution of a trial is the acquistion of funding to carry it out. The approach taken is influencd by whether the investigator or sponsor is responsible for initiating the trial. In practice, some trials, at least the larger-scale trials, are initiated through the joint efforts of the sponsor and investigator(s). The Coronary Drug Project (CDP) is a case in point. A special committee was convened by the National Heart Institute (now the National Heart, Lung, and Blood Institute, NHLBI) in early 1961 to explore the desirability, feasibility, and methods needed to initiate a large-scale trial to evaluate the role of lipid-influencing drugs in the treatment of post-myocardial-infarction patients. A group of investigators worked in concert with staff at the Institute to design the study as envisioned by the committee. Funding for the trial started in 1965, about four years after the initial meeting of the special committee (Coronary Drug Project Research Group, 1973a; Zukel, 1983).

The trials sketched in Appendix B represent a mix of investigator (7 out of 14), sponsor (5 out of 14), and sponsor-investigator initiated (2 out of 14) trials. See item 6, Table B-4, Appendix B, for specifics.

No inference can be made as to how a trial was initiated from the type of vehicle used to fund it. The Diabetic Retinopathy Study (DRS) was investigator-initiated but was contract-supported over most of its course. The Diabetic Control and Complications Trial (DCCT), initiated by the National Institute of Arthritis, Metabolism, and Digestive Diseases—NIAMDD (now the National Institute of Arthritis, Diabetes, and Digestive and Kidney Diseases, NIADDK) has both grant and contract funding. Clinics are funded via grants and the data coordinating center is funded via a cost-reimbursement contract (National Institute of Arthritis, Metabolism, and Digestive Diseases, 1981a, 1981b).

Table 21-1 provides information on the use of grants and contracts for the National Institutes of Health (NIH) extramural trials listed in the 1979 Inventory of Clinical Trials (National Institutes of Health, 1980). See Section 2.1, for details on how the Inventory is compiled.

21.2 NIH GRANT PROPOSALS

21.2.1 Deadlines and review process

Deadlines for unsolicited new applications are February 1, June 1, and October 1 of each year. Deadlines for unsolicited continuation and supplemental applications are March 1, July 1, and November 1. Deadlines for applications solicited by the NIH via requests for application (RFAs) are announced in the solicitations.

All applications are received by the Division of Research Grants (DRG), where they are assigned to specific institutes for administration

and payment if they are funded. The assignments may be made in consultation with personnel from the institutes in question, but the final decisions are made by DRG staff. The DRG is also responsible for assigning the applications for initial review. The reviews are carried out by the 80 or so chartered study sections,[1] or by special ad hoc study sections. This review structure is in addition to reviews managed by the various bureaus, institutes, and divisions (BIDs) of the NIH.

The primary responsibility of the study sections is to assess the scientific merit of research proposals received by NIH. Meritorious proposals receive a priority score based on scores assigned by individual members of the study section (1.0 for highest scientific merit through 5.0 for lowest scientific merit). This score, along with a written critique of the application (summary statement), prepared by the executive secretary of the study section (from written comments provided by members of the review group), is forwarded to the institute(s) designated by DRG to administer the grant.

The recommendations of the study section are reviewed by the advisory council (board) of the

---

1. A publication, *NIH Public Advisory Groups*, produced by the Committee Management Staff of the NIH, lists the chartered study sections and their membership.

Table 21-1 Number and percent of NIH extramural sponsored trials, by type of support

Type	Grant		Contract		Mixed*		All	
	Number	%	Number	%	Number	%	Number	%
A. Cancer Institute								
Single center	75	46.9	82	51.2	3	1.9	160	100.0
Multicenter†	340	88.3	38	9.9	7	1.8	385	100.0
All cancer	415	76.1	120	22.0	10	1.8	545	100.0
B. All other institutes								
Single center	153	76.5	47	23.5	0	0.0	200	100.0
Multicenter†	24	33.8	46	64.8	1	1.4	71	100.0
All other	177	65.3	93	34.3	1	0.4	271	100.0
C. Total (A + B)								
Single center	228	63.3	129	35.8	3	0.8	360	100.0
Multicenter†	364	79.8	84	18.4	8	1.8	456	100.0
All	592	72.5	213	26.1	11	1.3	816	100.0

*Includes trials with both grant and contract support and trials with both an intramural and extramural component
†The NIH definition of a multicenter trial is not as specific as the one used in this book and hence includes some studies that would be classified as single center

designated institute. The council is composed of health researchers plus others from outside the health field. Members are appointed by the Secretary of Health and Human Services (HHS) for a specified term, usually four years. The meeting of the council is held about three to four months after the initial review of an application and about six to eight months after the deadline for receipt of the application.

As a rule, only applications recommended for approval by a study section and approved by an advisory council will be funded. Most institutes have the authority to fund a small percentage of approved applications in the absence of council approval. However, such actions are rare. The number of proposals that are actually funded by any given institute will be a function of the priority scores assigned during the initial reviews, the size of the institute's budget, and existing funding commitments.

An applicant will receive a written summary of the results of the initial review, complete with priority score, as soon after the review as is practical. He will receive written notification of the action taken on his proposal after the council has met. This notification will be accompanied by a letter indicating the likelihood of funding in the case of an approved application. An applicant with a proposal recommended for funding that does not have a priority score above the payline (see Glossary) will receive notice to this effect and information concerning prospects for funding in the future. All such applications are kept under active consideration for three consecutive council meetings. They are removed from consideration if they have not been funded within that time.

21.2.2 Application outline

The outline below is based on details provided in the NIH grant application package (PHS 398, revision 5/82).

Section 1: General

- Face page containing project title and other identifying information
- List of key professional personnel to be engaged in proposed project
- Abstract of proposed project (must not exceed designated space)
- Table of contents
- Detailed budget for first 12 months of project
- Budget for total period of support requested

- Budgets pertaining to consortium or contractual arrangements
- Biographical sketch of principal investigator/ program director (not to exceed two pages)
- Biographical sketches for other key professional staff (not to exceed two pages per sketch)
- Sources of salary support (including support covered in pending applications) for the principal investigator/program director, as well as for all other key professional staff listed in the proposal
- Description of available resources, facilities, and general research environment

Section 2: Research plan

A. Specific aims (not to exceed one page)
B. Significance of the proposed research (not to exceed three pages)
C. Progress report/preliminary studies (not to exceed eight pages)
D. Experimental design and methods
E. Human subjects
F. Vertebrate animals
G. Consultants
H. Consortium arrangements
I. Literature cited

Section 3: Appendix

This section will contain supplementary materials pertinent to the application. Documents may include published papers, manuscripts still in preparation, proposed forms for data collection, procedure manuals, etc.

21.2.3 Content suggestions

The grant application kit, aside from the general outline provided above, does not specify content requirements. The suggestions contained in Table 21–2 are those of the author. The applicant will have to decide how the material outlined in Table 21–2 will be organized vis-à-vis the general outline given in Section 21.2.2. Most of the items listed in Table 21–2 relate in some way or other to the research plan.

A well-written application will contain an outline of the study design, its rationale, and the procedures that will be used to carry it out. While it may not be practical to provide a detailed protocol and a polished set of data collection forms, sufficient details should be provided to give reviewers an accurate assessment of the data collection approaches to be used.

Table 21-2   Grant application content suggestions for clinical trials

1. **Aims and objectives**
   - Clear statement of the objective of the trial and the outcome measure to be used to judge the success of the treatment
   - Secondary aims to be pursued in the trial

2. **General design specifications**
   - Method of randomization
   - Level of treatment masking
   - Outcome measure of primary interest
   - Proposed length of patient follow-up
   - General procedures to be used for bias control in the data collection process
   - Baseline and follow-up examination schedule and rationale for the schedule
   - Outline of data collection quality control procedures

3. **Significance of the study**
   - Importance of the treatment evaluation proposed
   - Potential impact of the trial on future patient care procedures

4. **Timetable**
   - Anticipated length of the trial, including start-up period and final analysis
   - Time required for protocol development, patient recruitment, patient follow-up, and final data analysis

5. **Treatment specifications**
   - Description of the test and control treatments
   - Rationale for choice of treatments, supported with appropriate literature references
   - Summary of previous evidence on the safety and efficacy of the proposed treatments
   - Method of treatment administration and level of masking

6. **Study population**
   - Patient eligibility and exclusion criteria
   - Proposed source of study patients
   - Methods of patient recruitment
   - Realistic appraisal of ability to meet specified recruitment goal using the stated eligibility and exclusion criteria, preferably done with counts of eligible patients seen in the clinic(s) over a specified time period

7. **Sample size specifications**
   - Patient recruitment goal and anticipated time required to achieve it

   - Rationale for stated goal
   - Statistical properties of the proposed recruitment goal (e.g., type I and II error protection provided)

8. **Data intake**
   - Specification of types of data to be collected, complete with sample copies of data forms, when possible
   - Staff responsible for data collection
   - Quality assurance procedures for the data intake process
   - Method of data entry and for verification of the accuracy of the data entry process

9. **Data processing and analysis**
   - General methods for receiving, coding, storing, and processing study data
   - Quality assurance procedures used to detect deficient data and approach to be used in correcting deficiencies
   - Approach to monitoring for treatment effects
   - Methods for detecting departures from the study protocol and for monitoring the performance of participating clinical centers
   - Outline of general data analysis plans

10. **Study organization**
    - List of centers to be included in the trial and description of responsibilities to be performed by specialty resource centers, such as the data coordinating center, central laboratory, etc.
    - Composition of the key leadership group and description of its method of operation
    - Method of creating key committees, including an outline of membership qualifications

11. **Other procedures**
    - Outline of patient informed consent process
    - Methods of protecting patient confidentiality
    - Provisions for secure data storage

12. **Facilities description**
    - Description of clinic facilities, data coordinating center, and other resource centers
    - List of special items of equipment required for data collection and analysis
    - Description of any other facilities key to execution of the trial

13. **Budget and justification**
    - See Sections 21.4 and 21.5.10

Defects to be avoided include:

- Vague and unsubstantiated claims regarding patient recruitment
- Unrealistic timetable
- Absence of a rationale for the stated sample size
- Clumsily written and fragmented proposal that lacks cohesion and that conveys the impression that it was written in haste by several people who had different perceptions of the work required
- Lack of organizational details concerning methods for carrying out the trial

Investigators should be realistic regarding the time required for patient recruitment. Experienced reviewers are likely to be skeptical of claims regarding patient availability and rate of recruitment unless they are supported with appropriate data.

Care should be taken to make certain that essential data intake and analysis functions are covered in the proposal. A general discussion, unrelated to the specifics of the proposal, is likely to be perceived as a weakness. This is particularly true if study section members perceive a lack of statistical input in the writing effort.

An area often overlooked is the organizational structure of the trial. Organization is important for any activity involving large numbers of people, whether located at a single center or multiple centers. The written proposal should outline the leadership structure proposed and the methods to be used for coordinating trial activities.

21.3 NIH REQUESTS FOR CONTRACT PROPOSALS

21.3.1 Deadlines and review process

As a rule, NIH contract-supported projects will be initiated by the sponsoring institute, via release of a request for proposals (RFP). Unsolicited proposals for contract funding are usually not accepted by the NIH.

Institutes within the NIH are required to advertise their intention to release an RFP in the *Commerce Business Daily* at least ten business days in advance of the projected date of release. It is also announced in the *NIH Guide for Grants and Contracts*. In addition, solicitations may be advertised in selected scientific journals and periodicals.

The RFP will indicate the deadline for response. Responses received after the deadline will not be considered, unless it is in the government's best interest to do so. Requests for extension of the deadline are unlikely to be granted unless the extension applies to all applicants.

The RFP will indicate where responses are to be sent—generally, in the case of NIH-released RFPs, the contracting or review office of the institute that released the RFP. The technical merit review of the responses received by the NIH are either managed by BID review personnel or, for the smaller institutes, by DRG. The review process is similar to that described for grant applications.

21.3.2 Factors to consider when deciding whether or not to respond

A prospective respondent must decide whether or not to prepare a response to an RFP. This decision must be made within a short time period because of the constraints imposed by the deadline for response. Questions to consider when assessing the merits of responding to an RFP are listed in Table 21–3. The questions are written from the perspective of an investigator considering applying for a center in a multicenter trial. The questions in Part A are general and are not related to any particular RFP. Those in Part B are specific to the RFP in question.

A single, or even a few, negative answers to the questions listed need not preclude responding to an RFP, but negative answers to key questions should. The same is true for any RFP that yields a large number of negative or equivocal answers, even if they are not related to key questions.

A major frustration in preparing a response to an RFP can be the amount of time available for response. Most NIH solicitations require a response within 60 to 90 days. The time between the date of release and the deadline for response was as short as 40 days for some of the proposals reviewed by the Coordinating Centers Models Project—CCMP (Coordinating Center Models Project Research Group, 1979b). An investigator should bear in mind that the actual time for response is always less (sometimes a great deal less) than the difference between the date of release and the deadline for response because of time needed to clear adminstrative channels in his institution after the response has been written.

Table 21-3 Questions to be considered when deciding on the merits of a response to a Request for Proposal (RFP)

Part A. General questions

Career goals

- Is the role proposed compatible with your career goals and interests?
- Do you have sufficient time to carry out the study?
- Do you enjoy collaboration with others?
- Are your opportunities for promotion likely to be adversely affected by participation in the project, especially if there are few if any opportunities for recognition as a key author on publications generated from the study?
- Can you function in a committee setting, and are you willing to accept the dictates of such a committee or the sponsor for execution of the trial?

Environment

- Are the stipulations in the business portion of the RFP compatible with the policies of your institution?
- Is the institution in which you work likely to continue in operation for the period of the trial?
- Are the personnel recruitment practices, pay scales, and promotion criteria of your institution compatible with those needed for execution of the trial?
- Is the business office of your institution capable of administering the contract?
- Is the trial compatible with the goals of your institution?
- Would colleagues view your activities in the trial in a favorable light?
- Will you be able to obtain the necessary signatures from administrative personnel in your institution if a proposal is submitted?

- Will you have the active support of your chief if you are selected to carry out the proposed work?
- Will there be adequate space, office equipment, and facilities to do the work if you are funded?
- Does your institution have staff with the required expertise for execution of the study and will you have access to them if you are funded?

Part B. Specific questions concerning the RFP

- Is there sufficient time to prepare an adequate response?
- Is the problem posed worthy of investigation?
- Is the project likely to achieve its stated aim?
- Does the project have a realistic timetable and is it subject to modification if necessary?
- Does the sponsoring institute desire strong investigator input in the operation of the trial (i.e., does it desire more than a service role from applicants)?
- Will there be adequate lead time for development of the study protocol and data forms before the trial is started?
- Are the suggested staffing guidelines realistic?
- Are the suggested funding levels realistic?
- Will it be possible to amend the design and proposed operating tenets of the trial, if necessary?
- Are the duties of the project officer in the sponsoring agency compatible with your perceived role in the trial?
- Are there adequate provisions for data processing and analysis outlined in the RFP?
- Is the reporting schedule for progress summaries during the trial reasonable?

21.3.3 The response

The RFP will contain an outline of required workscope along with a list of general methods and procedures to be used in carrying out the work. It may indicate the level of staffing needed for the study and whether the level stated is to be considered as an absolute or suggested upper limit. The limit may be exceeded if the latter is the case.

The respondent should indicate how the work outlined in the RFP is to be accomplished. Deletions or additions to the workscope as outlined in the RFP and reasons for the changes should be noted in the response. Minor changes may be acceptable if they do not alter the main purpose or aim of the study. Major modifications are likely to cause the sponsor to reject the response.

Instructional material accompanying the RFP should be read before starting work on the response and should be reviewed during its preparation. The material provided will indicate the way in which the response is to be assembled, the number of copies required, the deadline for response, and where it is to be sent.

21.4 THE STUDY BUDGET

21.4.1 Grants

The budget categories for NIH grant applications are listed below. Indirect costs (see Glossary) associated with execution of an NIH grant-supported project are not included in the budget request, except for indirect costs that are to be paid to other institutions (e.g., contractual arrangements with other institutions that are outlined in the application).

NIH grant application cost categories

1. Personnel
2. Consultants
3. Equipment
4. Supplies
5. Travel
6. Patient care costs
7. Alterations and renovations
8. Consortium/contractual costs
9. Other expenses
10. Total direct costs

The budget proposed should be a realistic appraisal of what is needed to carry out the study. It should not conform to a preconceived limit, unless a limit has been set by the sponsor. Requests that extend over multiple years should anticipate normal salary increases. The same is true for anticipated increases in the cost of fringe benefits for personnel. Some institutes of the NIH have escalation ceilings that relate to salary increases in the second and subsequent years of a budget request (e.g., 6% for NHLBI-supported projects).

NIH grant applications require a detailed breakdown of costs for the first year of requested support and a summary of costs for each subsequent year. The detailed breakdown should include the planned time commitment (listed as hours per week or as a percentage based on a full-time effort) and projected salary support for each person or position listed. Detailed information is not required for subsequent years; however, it may be included if the applicant wishes to do so. The added detail can be particularly important if there are large cost increases in the second or subsequent years due to staff additions.

Appendix H contains a sample set of budget tables, as contained in the budget request for the Data Coordinating Center in the Hypertension Prevention Trial (HPT). Only Table H–2 was required. Tables H–3 through H–7 were constructed to facilitate the budgeting process and to provide the reviewers with detailed budgetary data.

Construction of the budget requires specification of an anticipated starting date for the proposed work. This will be stated by the sponsor in the case of a sponsor-initiated study and by the investigator in an investigator-initiated study.

The starting date selected should be at least nine months after the submission deadline in the case of investigator-initiated NIH grant applications. This much time will be required for the review and approval process, as outlined in Section 21.2.1.

The proposed expenditures should be justified (see Section 21.5.10). While it is true that the initial review, in the case of NIH funding requests, is designed to focus on scientific merit, budget details and their justification cannot help but influence the review.

21.4.2 Contracts

Most NIH RFPs contain suggested budget categories. The categories below are from Optional Form 60—a form produced by the General Services Administration of the federal government and which is a standard part of most NIH-released RFPs.

NIH contract cost category

1. Direct material
2. Material overhead
3. Direct labor
4. Labor overhead
5. Special testing
6. Special equipment
7. Travel
8. Consultants
9. Other direct costs
10. Total direct costs and overhead
11. General and administrative expense
12. Royalties
13. Total estimated cost
14. Fee or profit
15. Total estimated cost and fee or profit

Most institutes of the NIH require respondents to separate the business and research portions of the response. The separation ensures that the initial review focuses on the technical merit of the proposal without regard to budgetary considerations.

21.5 BUDGET BREAKDOWN

Table 21–4 provides a list of items included under each of the categories listed in Section 21.4.1 for grant applications. The list is intended primarily as a reminder of the type of items to be considered in the budgeting process.

Table 21-4 Direct cost items, by budget category

1. **Personnel** (Individuals with a direct involvement in the trial and with a stated time commitment. Funds requested should be for salaries plus fringe benefits.)
   - Center director and co-director
   - Study physicians
   - Clinic coordinator
   - Laboratory technicians
   - Biostatisticians
   - Programmers
   - Data coordinator
   - Data entry personnel
   - Research assistants
   - Administrative assistant
   - Secretaries
   - Clerks
   - Other personnel

2. **Consultants** (Individuals paid on a fee-for-service basis and who are not part of any center in the trial.)
   Consultants may be needed to:
   - Provide expert advice in the diagnosis, classification, or treatment of patients in the trial
   - Perform a specialty function, such as reading ECGs, biopsy material, etc.
   - Provide expert advice to a resource center in the trial, such as to the data coordinating center for data analysis
   - Serve as an expert advisor to the study leadership or sponsor of the trial

3. **Equipment** (Purchased or leased)
   - General office equipment
     Typewriters
     Word processors
     Transcribing and dictating machines
     Filing cabinets
     Desks, chairs, and tables

   Photocopying machines
   Telephone equipment
   Miscellaneous office equipment, such as heavy-duty staplers, paper cutter, 3-hole punches, electric staplers, etc.
   - Clinic equipment
     Furniture for examining and waiting rooms
     Required items of equipment needed for data collection such as a random-zero sphygmomanometer or laboratory equipment for special readings or analyses
     Items of equipment needed for data collection such as ECG recorder, fundus camera, etc. (Requests for standard equipment, regarded as essential to any nonstudy clinic setting, may not be allowed when the budget is reviewed unless the requests are adequately justified. The justification should indicate why existing equipment will not meet the needs of the study).
   - Data center equipment
     Data entry equipment such as key-to-tape or key-to-disk units, intelligent terminals, etc.
     Computing and related hardware such as tape and disk drives, printers, remote job entry stations, CRTs, portable terminals, etc.
     Computing software for database management and analyses
     Mailing equipment, such as postage meter, postage scale, envelope opener, envelope stuffer and sealer, etc.
     Machines for assembling and binding reports
     Paper shredder (for disposing of confidential records)

4. **Supplies**
   - General office supplies
     Paper, pencils, notebooks, typewriter supplies, dictation tapes, etc.
     Postage
     Photocopy supplies (e.g., toner, developer, etc.)

No single trial will necessarily include all the items listed.

21.5.1 Personnel

A major portion (from 50 to 80%) of the requested support will be for personnel. Actual salaries expected to apply at the start of funding should be used for personnel named in the budget. Salary estimates, using prevailing figures at the applicant's institution, should be used for positions to be filled during the study. The time commitments for personnel should be realistic. That for the center director should be large enough to represent a meaningful role in the operation of the center. Padding the budget by including unnecessary personnel or needlessly large time commitments is unwise and may lead reviewers to question the competence or integrity of the applicant. In addition, it may cause them to make drastic cuts in the budget.

Table 21-4 Direct cost items, by budget category (*continued*)

Supplies for special items of equipment, such as word processors

- Clinic

    Drugs, syringes, etc.

    Laboratory reagents and supplies

    Data forms

    Patient informational material

    Mailers for laboratory specimens

    Supplies for special items of equipment, such as film for fundus camera, etc.

- Data center

    Computer supplies, such as paper, printer ribbons, magnetic tapes, disks, etc.

    Data entry supplies, such as punch cards, floppy disks, tape cassettes, etc.

    Supplies for special items of equipment, such as graphics terminal, plotter, microfilm camera, etc.

5. Travel

- Study staff

    Local (for mileage charges incurred as part of patient recruitment and home visits)

    National (for travel and living expenses incurred in conjunction with study-related activities, including clinic site visits and study committee meetings, as well as for travel to selected professional meetings, especially for presenting study-related papers)

    International (for travel and living expenses for foreign travel required for study and related activities, and for selected professional meetings* related to the needs and goals of the study)

- Consultants (for travel to study center or to study-related meetings)

- Committee members (for travel of members of the advisory-review committee and the treatment effects monitoring committee to study-related meetings)

6. Patient care costs* (Funds in this category are used to pay for procedures carried out on patients that are done primarily for their research value and that are not considered necessary for routine medical care. Hence, they cannot be charged to the patient or his insurance carrier.)

7. Alterations and renovations*

- Renovation of a clinic area

- Air conditioning for computing equipment

- Renovations to accommodate special items of equipment needed in the trial

8. Consortium/contractual costs (Funds in this category are used to cover payments to individuals or groups outside the investigator's institution who have formal agreements to perform specified functions in the study.)

9. Other expenses

- Patient travel to and from clinic

- Equipment maintenance charges

- Telephone installation and monthly usage charges

- Copying and reproduction charges

- Computing time charges

- Data entry charges

- Study insurance

- Books and journals

- Journal page and reprint charges

- Charges for printing and distributing study forms, manuals, etc.

- Fee-for-service charges, such as for laboratory determinations, reading ECGs, etc., if not covered under a consultant or contractual agreement

- Space rental

- Moving charges

- Indirect costs for associated contractual services included in item 8

10. Total direct costs (Sum of cost in above nine categories)

*Categories or items that may not be allowed, or that require special justification.

Ideally, applications should carry named investigators in key support positions. This is especially true for the position of deputy director. An alternative, when a deputy is not named, is to indicate the approach to be followed in replacing the center director, should that become necessary. A list of qualifications the individual to be recruited should have and the mechanism for screening and selecting a replacement should be outlined.

Another key support position, vital to data collection, is that of clinic coordinator. The person who fills this position provides a link between patients and physicians in the clinic and between the clinic and the data center.

Large centers may also require a part-time or full-time administrator. Generally, the administrative services available through the investigator's business office will not be adequate to meet the day-to-day administrative needs of the study. The justification should indicate why the position is needed, and why the duties cannot be performed by personnel in the investigator's business office.

21.5.2 Consultants

Normally, consultants are required to provide services or fulfill functions that cannot be met by salaried personnel in the study. They should not be used to perform essential day-to-day tasks because of their peripheral role in the study. By definition, they should be located outside the applicant's institution. When they are not, they should be listed in the personnel section of the budget.

21.5.3 Equipment

Items of equipment requested may be purchased or leased. The approach proposed will depend on the expected duration of the trial and the anticipated useful life of the items in question. Purchase is usually cheaper than lease if the item is required for three years or longer. Leasing should be considered for equipment needed for less time or when there is a chance it may have to be replaced before the trial is finished. Costs for equipment maintenance and repairs should be included in the "other expenses" category.

The request may include funds for office equipment, such as typewriters, transcribers, and office furniture, except where such costs are proscribed by the sponsor. The request, especially for large-scale trials, may also include equipment needed for data processing as well (see Section 5.2.4 and Table 5–4 for more details).

21.5.4 Supplies

See Part 4 of Table 21–4 for list.

21.5.5 Travel

The need for money for staff-related travel may be nil in a trial carried out in a single institution, but may be sizable in a multicenter trial. Review groups may question the need for the proposed travel by study staff. Hence, the applicant must take pains to explain why it is necessary. Foreign travel, unless directly related to the study, is not likely to be approved. The budget of one center, usually the coordinating center in a multicenter trial, may carry funds for travel costs not covered in the budgets of the other centers, such as for study consultants and for members of the treatment effects monitoring committee.

The budget may include funds to cover transportation for patients who cannot provide their own. Trials requiring long-term patient follow-up may even include funds to cover transportation and related living expenses of patients who must travel long distances to continue in the study. Costs for patient travel are listed in the "other expenses" category in NIH grant applications, since they are not considered a part of the cost for patient care.

21.5.6 Patient care costs

The budget for the study should include funds for experimental procedures that are of no direct benefit to the patient and that are done simply for research purposes. Ordinary patient billing and collection practices should be used to recover costs for procedures that are considered to be an essential part of a patient's care (i.e., those that would be required whether or not the patient was enrolled in the study). It is prudent, when in doubt as to whether costs for a procedure should be billed to a patient or his insurance company, to include costs for the procedure in the study budget.

21.5.7 Alterations and renovations

Budget requests for alterations or renovations can be expected to receive close scrutiny by the sponsor. Normally, funds are not awarded for such purposes, at least via the NIH, unless they are absolutely essential to the study and are well justified. The guidelines stated for grant requests, or as listed in the particular RFP in question, should be consulted before requesting funds for this purpose.

21.5.8 Consortium/contractual costs

The typical application may not require any funds in this category. Funds should be requested only in instances in which the applicant proposes to have certain functions fulfilled outside his own institution (e.g., certain laboratory tests). The group(s) proposed to perform these functions and the reasons for selection should be indicated in the budget request. A contractual or subcontractual[2] arrangement should not be considered if the functions to be performed can be done better or at a lower cost in the applicant's own institution.

2. The term used depends on whether the parent application is a grant or a contract.

All costs in this category should include direct as well as indirect contractor or subcontractor costs. This is true for grant applications as well as contract proposals. A detailed budget, using the categories listed in Section 21.4.1 or 21.4.2, should be provided if the contract or subcontract represents a significant fraction of the total funds requested.

21.5.9 Other expenses

This category, as seen in Table 21–4, includes a variety of items. Several of them, such as computing and laboratory determinations, may be billed either on a fee-for-service basis or under a fixed sum agreement. The cost under fee-for-service agreements is determined by the amount of service rendered, whereas it is fixed in advance under a fixed sum agreement. Agreements of the latter type are easier to administer than fee-for-service agreements. However, the options available in any given case may be limited. For example, most general-use computing facilities will be reluctant to provide computing for a predetermined fixed sum.

Most offices will have photocopying equipment that can be used to meet the copying needs of the project. If so, the budget may simply include an item for copying charges incurred for using that equipment. If not, funds should be included for renting or purchasing needed photocopying equipment.

Some of the budgets for large-scale multicenter trials, such as the CDP and the Hypertension Detection and Follow-up Program (HDFP), included funds for study insurance. The protection provided was over and above that available via an investigator's own institution and extended to all centers in the trial, including the data center, as well as all study committees, including the advisory-review and treatment effects monitoring committees.

21.5.10 Budget justification

All categories and major items within those categories should be justified. The need for some items, such as general office supplies and some of the items in the "other expenses" category, will be self-evident. However, other items, such as proposed renovations or alterations, purchase of costly pieces of equipment, and most travel, will need careful justification. The personnel budget, because of its importance, requires detailed justification. It should be supported with a

brief description of the duties and responsibilities of each staff member or position listed and the rationale for the stated time commitment.

It may be useful to provide summary tabulations, such as illustrated in Tables H–6 and H–7, Appendix H, to indicate the way in which funds have been apportioned. The percentage distribution of funds by category of expenditure can help reviewers judge the appropriateness of the allocations proposed. Budgets that are top-heavy with funds for personnel, relative to funds for other categories, should be re-examined before submission. Similar tabulations that break down personnel costs by function to be performed (e.g., data generation versus data analysis) may help to determine whether the proposed distribution of personnel is adequate.

21.6 PREPARATION AND SUBMISSION OF THE FUNDING PROPOSAL

The preparation of the funding proposal involves a great deal more than simply writing the application and assembling it. Some of the preparatory steps include:

- Contacting colleagues to determine if they are willing to participate in the study and to reach agreements with them on time commitments for the work outlined
- Preparation of updated biographical sketches for each professional listed in the proposal
- Collection of salary and fringe benefit information for use in preparing the personnel budget
- Collection of cost information for items of equipment, supplies, travel, computing, and the like
- Collection of letters of agreement from consultants and contractors or subcontractors mentioned in the proposal

Once the application is completed, it should be reviewed to make certain it is properly paginated, that the table of contents is accurate and complete, and that all essential materials, such as biographical sketches and support letters, are included. The budget should receive special attention. Figures should be checked and rechecked for accuracy before the application is submitted.

The application will not be reviewed by the NIH without the proper signatures and assurances. Grant applications must be signed by the applicant as well as by the senior administrative officer of the applicant's institution. Written assurance (provided by forwarding a properly executed Form HHS 596 to the NIH) from the applicant's Institutional Review Board (IRB) regarding the adequacy of the proposed patient consent procedures and methods for treatment and follow-up must be received within 60 days following the deadline for receipt in order for review to proceed (see Chapter 13).

21.7 NEGOTIATIONS AND AWARD

The size of the award will be determined by the sponsor, using input received during the review process. In rare cases it can exceed the amount requested if the sponsor elects to add funds for expenses overlooked by the applicant. It is more likely that the sponsor will impose cuts, often without consulting the applicant. Agencies, such as the NIH, have formal appeal processes that can be followed if the applicant feels the cuts are unjust or that they jeopardize the success of the project. The appeal may not result in a full restoration of funds, but some redress may be possible if the applicant makes a convincing case.

A greater opportunity for negotiation exists under the contract mode of funding. The peer review process described in Section 21.3.1 is designed to assess scientific merit. Once the reviews are completed, the proposals are ranked on the basis of priority scores. Those with the best scores will be singled out for a second-stage review. These offerors will be given an opportunity to make their best and final offer and may be asked to respond (usually in writing) to a series of questions raised during the initial review. Final contract negotiations will be undertaken with the offeror(s) selected.

Expenditures cannot be made against a pending grant or contract until all necessary documents have been received and signed by the applicant's institution. These include the Notice of Grant Award for NIH grants and a signed agreement bearing all required signatures for contracts. Job commitments should not be made until all the required documents are in hand.

21.8 GRANT AND CONTRACT ADMINISTRATION

The applicant's business office is responsible for receiving money from the sponsor and for making all payments under the award. Administrative questions concerning use of study funds

must be cleared through this office. Questions that cannot be answered should be forwarded to the sponsor for resolution. The day-to-day administrative needs of the project, such as preparation of purchase orders, payroll entries, and the like, will be met by general staff in the applicant's department or by staff hired specifically for this purpose using study funds, depending on the size of the project.

21.9 SPECIAL FUNDING ISSUES

21.9.1 Direct versus indirect funding for multicenter trials

A key issue that must be resolved in any multicenter trial deals with the dispersal of funds to the individual centers in the trial. In one case, each participating center submits an application containing design documents common to the entire study, plus operational and budgetary information specific for the center. The award is made to each successful applicant, directly from the sponsor. An alternative approach involves a consortium award (see Glossary) in which one investigator submits a proposal designed to cover the budgetary needs of all the participating centers. If the proposal is funded, that same individual, in conjunction with his business office, assumes responsibility for dispersing funds to individual centers in the trial. Both approaches are used by the NIH for grant- as well as contract-funded trials. The applicants have prime responsibility for choosing the method of fund dispersal in investigator-initiated multicenter trials. The sponsor will have the primary say in sponsor-initiated multicenter trials.

The advantages and disadvantages of the two approaches are summarized in Table 21-5. The factors influencing the choice of one approach over the other are outlined in Table 21-6.

The main advantage of consortium funding is the opportunity it provides for reallocation of funds among centers during the trial. A second advantage has to do with the mechanics of preparing the budget request during the application process. It is usually much easier for one or two key investigators to develop a composite budget for the trial than it is to coordinate development of a series of budgets needed when each center is to be funded directly from the sponsoring agency.

The consortium approach may be necessary in an investigator-initiated proposal if it is not practical to identify all centers to be included in the

Table 21-5 Direct versus indirect (consortium) funding for centers in multicenter trials

A. Direct funding (Individual awards to each center direct from sponsor)

Advantages

- Vests all fiscal responsibilities with the sponsor and thereby helps to maintain a clear separation of the fiscal and scientific affairs of the trial

- All centers have identical relationship to the sponsor (i.e., avoids the unbalanced relationship of indirect funding where the lead center has direct funding and all others receive funding via that center)

- Grant or contract administration done through sponsor, usually by experienced personnel

- May be perceived by recipients as a more desirable mode of support than support provided via another center

Disadvantages

- Requires a detailed funding proposal from each participating center

- May preclude the sponsor from redistributing funds among centers once the awards have been made (especially true for NIH grant-supported trials)

- Difficult to coordinate the preparation of individual budget requests, especially if there are only limited opportunities for contacts among applicants when the budgets are being prepared, as in some investigator-initiated trials

B. Indirect funding (Awards to individual centers via a lead center)

Advantages

- Simplifies logistics of preparing the funding request

- Provides flexibility in amount of funds that may be dispersed to any given center

Disadvantages

- Places a heavy administrative burden on the lead center

- Fiscal control exercised by the lead center may have adverse effect on its working relationships with other centers in the study

- Quality of administration provided by lead center highly dependent on experience and competence of the center's business office

- May be viewed by recipients as a less desirable mode of support than support provided direct from the sponsor

---

trial at the time the proposal is submitted. However, review groups can be expected to have trouble recommending funding for any study with unnamed centers, unless they are satisfied with the process proposed by the applicant for center selection.

A disadvantage with the consortium approach has to do with the difficulties any investigator has in directing both the scientific and fiscal affairs of a trial. The investigator responsible for administration of the consortium award must make fiscal decisions affecting individual centers in the trial, while at the same time playing a key role in the scientific conduct of the trial.

The overall administrative cost of either approach is probably about the same. In the one case the sponsor assumes the major portion of the administrative burden, whereas in the other it is assumed by the director of the lead center.

21.9.2 Work unit payment schedules

Payments for clinics may be a function of the number of patients seen or enrolled. Work unit payment schedules, while not common in NIH-sponsored trials, are used in industry-sponsored trials. PARIS, one of the trials sketched in Appendix B, had clinic payment schedules that were based, in part, on the number of patients seen (Persantine Aspirin Reinfarction Study Research Group, 1980a).

The danger with any payment schedule based on patient load is the temptation it provides for the enrollment of questionable patients, or even for falsifying patient reports to maintain a certain income level. Such payment schedules should not be considered without a monitoring plan designed to guard against such possibilities.

Table 21-6 Factors influencing the choice between direct versus indirect (consortium) funding

Direct funding

Considered when:

- All centers are to be selected before funding is initiated

- The amount of support required for each center is above some minimum

- A leadership structure exists to ensure proper coordination of the individual funding requests

Indirect funding

Considered when:

- Individual centers require only minimal levels of funding

- It is not possible or practical to select all centers before funding is initiated

- It is not practical to coordinate the preparation of a series of individual funding requests

22. Essential management functions and responsibilities

You cannot manage soldiers into battle: you must lead them.

Source unknown

22.1 MANAGEMENT REQUIREMENTS

Any research activity that involves multiple investigators requires a defined structure for performing necessary activities. The need is most apparent in multicenter trials, but it exists in single-center trials as well, especially if they involve various people performing different functions. A sound structure will provide:

- Delineation and separation of responsibilities
- A communications structure for disseminating essential information needed by personnel to discharge their responsibilities
- Checks and balances in the decision-making process
- Specified goals for measuring progress and performance during the trial
- Ongoing quality assurance and performance monitoring to detect and correct deficiencies in the data generation and processing procedures in the trial
- Appropriate administrative support to implement and carry out functions needed for execution of the trial

22.2 MANAGEMENT DEFICIENCIES

22.2.1 Failure to delegate authority with responsibility

A common deficiency is one in which a member of the research team is expected to perform a specific function but is not given the authority needed to carry it out. This deficiency can result in bottlenecks in decision making. Position-by-position reviews, with the goal of matching authority to responsibility, are necessary at periodic intervals over the course of the trial if the problem is to be avoided.

22.2.2 Inadequate provisions for personnel backup

Key positions in the study must be backed up to assure continuity of operations. Failure to do so can jeopardize the entire study if a key position is vacated at an inopportune time. The backup should be accomplished by designating deputies who are empowered to act in the absence of the persons they represent. The concept applies to committee positions as well as to positions within individual centers. The designations may be via informal understandings for secondary positions, but not for key leadership personnel. Formal appointments are required in such cases to avoid confusion as to the succession of authority. It is interesting to note in this context that only 8 of the 14 trials sketched in Appendix B had a designated vice-study chairman (line 28.b, Table B–4).

22.2.3 Ill-defined decision-making structure

Ambiguity in the decision-making structure of a group is almost always due to the failure of the group leaders to empower specific members of the group with the authority needed to perform designated tasks. Structures with multiple committees or centers that have overlapping domains of responsibility are at greatest risk of having obscure lines of authority. The reluctance of members of the steering committee of a multicenter trial to vest a designated center or defined set of individuals with the authority needed to perform specified tasks in the trial can lead to chaos. The need to obtain approval from the committee before each new step is taken increases the time required to perform a task and is demoralizing to those who must perform it.

22.2.4 Inadequate funding

Attempting to carry out a trial without adequate financial support is a serious mistake, especially if doing so leads to poor quality data or requires patients to assume risks that could be avoided with adequate support. Responsible investigators will not start a trial without adequate financial support. Failing that, they will scale down their efforts to bring them in line with available funding.

22.2.5 Lack of performance standards

There is no way to monitor performance in a trial in the absence of standards for making such assessments. A well-designed and well-managed trial will have a timetable indicating when key activities, such as patient recruitment, are expected to begin and finish. It will have a patient recruitment goal and standards of performance relating to various aspects of the data collection and analysis processes as well.

22.2.6 Failure to separate essential activities

Sound leadership requires separation of essential roles in the trial. Some of these separations are discussed in Section 22.6. Failure to provide needed separations can result in duplication of effort, internal squabbles, and biases in the data collection or analysis of results.

22.2.7 Ill-defined communication structure

The information flow in the trial should proceed through designated channels. Structures involving two or more communication routes, such as in trials with both a data and treatment coordinating center (see Chapter 5 for general discussion and Sketch 13, Appendix B, for specific example), must take special pains to make certain that the structure does not produce conflicting communiques or allow lapses in the communication process.

22.3 PATIENT SAFETY MONITORING: AN ESSENTIAL FUNCTION

Patient safety monitoring, or simply safety monitoring, is any process carried out during a trial that involves the review of accumulated outcome data for groups of patients to determine if any of the treatment procedures practiced should be altered or stopped. This type of monitoring is in addition to that which is done on a per-patient basis by each patient's own study physician.

Safety monitoring may be done by a single person, usually a statistician, in a small trial or by a committee in a large one (see Chapters 20 and 23). It is essential in any trial of treatments that carries risks (see Table 22–1 for classes of trials requiring safety monitoring). Continuation

Table 22–1 Classes of trials requiring safety monitoring

- Trials with a clinical event as the primary outcome measure
- Trials involving treatments that carry potential short-term or long-term risks
- Trials involving treatments with the potential for producing serious side effects
- Any trial that has the potential of generating definitive results before the scheduled conclusion of the trial
- Any trial involving data collection procedures or schedules that either entail risks or inconvenience to the patients or that are costly to carry out

of such trials is justified only so long as there is no reliable way to choose between the test and control treatments. Once data have accumulated to indicate the superiority of one treatment over another, the inferior treatment should be stopped. Ethically, the need for safety monitoring is greatest so long as patients continue to be enrolled and treated in the trial. However, the need exists even after recruitment and treatment is finished (e.g., as in a surgical trial where patients are followed after surgery). Patients who received the inferior treatment by virtue of randomization should have an opportunity to receive the superior treatment (assuming they are still treatable). In any case, the need to inform the medical community of the finding is the same, whether or not new patients are still being enrolled and treated in the trial.

There are also practical reasons for carrying out periodic data analyses during the trial, even if the treatments are innocuous and pose no risks to those receiving them. The costs necessary to continue a trial are not justified once the accumulated results are adequate to make a judgment concerning the treatments. A trial that no longer has a chance of producing any more useful information should also be stopped. By the same token, use of a data collection procedure that entails risk, discomfort, or inconvenience to patients should be stopped once sufficient information has been obtained with it to answer the question it was designed to address, or once it becomes clear that no more useful information can be generated from its use.

22.4 ADVISORY–REVIEW FUNCTIONS

Most trials will require external reviews for various reasons over their course. The reviews will

be preparatory to the start of the trial or before implementation of a protocol change during the trial. Examples include:

- Review of patient recruitment experience in order to offer advice to the study leadership or sponsor on the need for additional clinics
- Review of the performance of a clinic in order to offer advice to the study leadership or sponsor on the desirability of continued funding for the clinic
- Review of a recommendation to add a new treatment to the trial or to terminate use of an existing treatment because of adverse effects

The advisory and review functions may be performed on an ad hoc basis by consultants selected by the study investigators or on a regular basis via a committee appointed by the investigators or sponsor of the trial. Such committees, especially when appointed by the sponsor, are usually intended to provide advice to both the sponsor and study investigators. Advice to the sponsor will focus on policy and fiscal issues, whereas advice to the study investigators will center on operational issues.

22.5 COMMITTEE PROCEDURES

The general rules to be followed when forming the committee structure in a trial are provided in Table 22–2. The next chapter provides details on committee structures for multicenter trials. However, such structures are not unique to multicenter trials. They are required in large single-center trials as well.

No committee should be created without a written specification of its charge and duties. It should indicate the composition of the committee, criteria for membership, and voting rights and rules. Some studies, such as MILIS, have actually written bylaws detailing the committee structure and governance of the trial (Multicenter Investigation of the Limitation of Infarct Size Research Group, 1983). Such documentation, whether or not formalized to the degree in MILIS, is essential in avoiding disputes among committees with overlapping or competing functions. Once created, a member of the study staff should be charged with the task of maintaining a running account of committee meetings and of additions or deletions to the charge of the committee and to its membership. A cumulative record of committee membership over the course of

Table 22-2 Guidelines for committee operations

A. General

- Create no more committees than necessary
- Provide a written charge for each committee that outlines the need for it and the function it is to perform
- Indicate the individual or group that has authority to appoint or dissolve committees
- Avoid overlap of responsibilities with other committees
- Outline the relationship of one committee to another and the communications structure for committee-to-committee interactions
- Specify whether or not a committee has decision-making authority; if so, indicate the issues for which it will serve as the final authority and those for which it will serve only in an advisory capacity

B. Chairmanship

- Specify the method of selection (e.g., election or appointment) and the term of office
- Designate a chairman for each committee created; a vice-chairman should also be designated for any committee that is to perform essential ongoing functions in the trial

C. Membership

- Specify the membership criteria for each committee

- Specify the methods to be used for rotation of members (if any), for filling vacancies, and for replacing nonfunctioning members
- Indicate ex officio committee positions (e.g., chairman of the study, director of the data center, etc.)
- Specify conditions that disqualify individuals from filling a committee position, including conflicts of interest

D. Voting

- Specify quorum requirement for conduct of committee business
- Identify voting and nonvoting committee members and ex-officio voting and nonvoting positions
- Specify committee voting rules

E. Documentation and maintenance

- Maintain an up-to-date list of committee members, their respective terms of office, and voting rights
- Designate an individual to serve as committee secretary
- Carry out periodic reviews in which committee charges are updated and committee-to-committee communication structures revised, where appropriate
- Dissolve committees that have completed their work or are no longer functional

the trial is useful when preparing credits for manuscripts.

The committee structure may require major revisions at intervals over the course of the trial. Revisions may be needed as patient recruitment is completed and again in preparation for closeout of patient follow-up and for final analysis of study data. Committees that are no longer needed should be disbanded.

22.6 PREFERRED SEPARATION OF RESPONSIBILITIES AND FUNCTIONS

Preferred separations inlcude:

- Separation of personnel responsible for treatment administration and data collection in unmasked trials
- Separation of personnel responsible for patient care from those responsible for safety monitoring
- Separation of the investigative and advisory-review roles
- Separation of sponsor and investigative roles

- Separation of the data collection and data processing functions
- Separation of centers in a multicenter trial

Some of the above separations are desirable simply for reasons of efficiency and proficiency, as suggested in Chapter 5. Others are required for scientific reasons as detailed below.

22.6.1 Separation of treatment administration and data collection personnel in unmasked trials

As noted in Chapter 8, masked administration of the study treatments offers the best safeguard against treatment-related biases in the data collection process. However, masked treatment administration is not always possible and therefore other designs must be used. One approach is to vest responsibilities for administering the study treatments with one group, and those for data collection with a different group (e.g., as was done to some degree in the Macular Photocoagulation Study, Sketch 4, Appendix B, and in the Hypertension Prevention Trial, Sketch 13, Appendix B). The need for separation is especially important when the outcome measure is subject to observer error. However, it is not always easy to achieve, particularly when the patients themselves may reveal the treatment they have received while outcome measurements are being made. It is much easier to ensure when the outcome measure is based on some reading or determination made by personnel who have no patient contact.

22.6.2 Separation of personnel responsible for patient care and safety monitoring

The ethical underpinnings for a trial rest on the fact that there is no reliable way to choose among the treatments being studied. A physician is willing to allow his patients to be randomized only so long as he remains uncertain regarding the relative merits of the study treatments. He is not, once he believes he knows which treatment is best. Exposure to data and emerging trends as the trial progresses may make him reluctant to enroll new patients or to continue treating those already enrolled once the data suggest one treatment is better than another. Separation of the type suggested avoids this dilemma by shielding the treating physicians from emerging trends and by transferring responsibility for dealing with them to a group not directly responsible for patient care (see Chapter 23). A second and perhaps more convincing argument has to do with the desire to reduce the possibility for feedback bias in the way in which patients are treated and in the data collection process. Biases can creep in if study physicians know the direction of emerging treatment trends.

22.6.3 Separation of investigative and advisory-review roles

The advisory-review process, by its very nature, should be performed by a group that is external to the trial (see Chapter 23). The reasons are obvious. Advice rendered by personnel in the study may be self-serving, especially if rendered by people who are emotionally involved in the trial and who are dependent on it for salary support. In addition, some of the issues requiring review may concern whether funding should be continued in a clinic with a poor patient recruitment or data collection record. Investiga-

tors from within the trial may find it hard to take an adverse action against a colleague.

22.6.4 Separation of sponsor and investigative roles

This separation is desirable whether funding is from government or industry. The preferred approach is one in which all of the essential scientific activities for the trial are located outside the sponsoring agency. This separation is particularly important whenever the sponsoring agency has a proprietary interest in the product being tested.

The best example of such separation for an industry-sponsored trial is provided by the Persantine Aspirin Reinfarction Study (PARIS). None of the investigative functions in that trial were associated with the sponsor (Persantine Aspirin Reinfarction Study Research Group, 1980a). The structure of the Anturane Reinfarction Trial (ART), another industry-sponsored trial, represents a step in the right direction, but it failed to provide complete separation. Data center operations were housed in the firm sponsoring the trial (Anturane Reinfarction Trial Research Group, 1980).

22.6.5 Separation of data collection and data processing functions

Every trial will have activities related to data collection as well as those concerned with data processing. These two activities should be carried out by different people under different administrative heads. Effective quality control procedures for the data collection process will be impossible to implement without this separation.

Data processing operations should be on a par with the data collection operations in the trial. The two activities should be provided with separate budgets via different awards direct from the sponsor or via agreements with the chairman of the study as to how funds are to be allocated for the two activities when they are funded out of the same budget.

Separation of these two activities is generally assured in the multicenter trial by creation of a dedicated data center with its own funding. It may be more difficult to achieve in the single-center trial. However, it can be accomplished if the clinic is able to establish a working relationship with another department willing to assume responsibility for the data intake and analyses processes.

22.6.6 Separation of centers in multicenter trials

Centers in a multicenter trial, in addition to being located outside the sponsoring agency, should be administratively distinct from one another. The separation is usually assured by virtue of geographic location. However, there are occasions when two or more centers are located in the same institution. For example, the University of Minnesota housed a clinical center, nutrition coding center, ECG coding center, and coordinating center for MRFIT (Multiple Risk Factor Intervention Trial Research Group, 1982).

The relationship of the data coordinating center to clinics in the trial is of special importance because of the key role it has in monitoring the data collection process (see Chapter 5). The ideal structure is one in which the center is both physically and administratively distinct from all other centers in the trial. It may be difficult for the center to maintain equity in the way in which it interacts with clinics if it is affiliated with one of the clinics in the trial. The actions of the data coordinating center in monitoring the performance of clinics must be viewed by personnel in the clinics as being fair and without prejudice if they are to be effective.

Structures that provide funding via a consortium award (see Glossary) to the lead clinic (see Glossary) should provide a separate budget for the data coordinating center, even if it is located in the same department as the lead clinic. The center should not be headed by the director of the lead clinic, or by any other clinic director in the trial for that matter. The budget and director separation is essential if the center is to have the independence it needs to operate effectively.

Ideally, all centers in a multicenter trial should have the same administrative relationship to the sponsor, and thereby to one another. The administrative equality of centers will help to create a collegial relationship among the investigators and facilitate interaction and communication. The potential for administrative equity is greater when each center is funded directly by the sponsoring agency, or by a board as in PARIS (Persantine Aspirin Reinfarction Study Research Group, 1980a), than when funding is provided via a consortium award.

22.7 SPECIAL MANAGEMENT ISSUES

22.7.1 Disclosure requirements for potential conflicts of interest

Participation in a trial as an investigator is a form of public trust. This trust is violated if the investigator has conflicts of interest that bias the data collection, analysis, or reporting processes of the trial. The mere suspicion of a financial conflict of interest can cause the public to view results and conclusions from the trial as suspect. A case in point, albeit outside the field of clinical trials, is the report of the Food and Nutrition Board (1980) of the National Academy of Sciences on dietary standards. The amount of credence given to the report has been diminished in the eyes of some because of relationships of Board members to segments of the food industry (Wade, 1980).

Some relationships and activities are clear conflicts of interest and should be avoided (e.g., working for a firm producing one of the drugs being tested while serving as a member of the treatment effects monitoring committee). Certainly, investigators involved in drug trials should be free of all consulting and retainer arrangements with any drug firms that stand to gain or lose depending on the results of the trials. The same is true for perquisites (e.g., travel to an exotic place for an investigator and his/her spouse ostensibly for a scientific meeting) offered by manufacturers standing to gain or lose from the trial.

It is prudent to establish mechanisms to monitor for potential conflicts of interest within the investigative group and related committees, including the treatment effects monitoring and advisory-review committees. Systems for disclosure of conflicts are of little value if the persons covered by the systems are insensitive to the issues or activities that can be perceived as constituting a conflict of interest. Any disclosure system, to be useful, should be updated at periodic intervals over the course of the trial. Further, the statements filed by members of the study and related committees must be reviewed by an appropriate body (e.g., the sponsor in government-supported trials or the advisory-review committee) as they are received to identify conflicts that are serious enough to disqualify a person from involvement in the trial. All statements filed should be open for public inspection once results have been published (e.g., as was done in the National Cooperative Gallstone Study, 1981b).

22.7.2   Level of compensation for committee members outside the trial

Members of committees, such as the treatment effects monitoring and advisory-review committees, who are not associated with any center in the trial, will usually be paid an honorarium or a consulting fee for meeting activities. Excessively large payments should be avoided since they themselves have the potential of creating a conflict of interest when members are required to decide whether or not a trial should continue. Governmental agencies, such as the National Institutes of Health and the Veterans Administration, typically pay only travel expenses and a standard fee of $100 or $150 per meeting day. Generally, these agencies do not pay members for time spent in travel to or from meetings or for time spent in preparing for them.

22.7.3   Review and approval of proposed ancillary studies

An ancillary study is defined as an investigation, stimulated by the trial and intended to generate information of interest to it. It is designed and carried out by investigators from one or more of the centers in the trial and utilizes resources of the trial, but is not a required part of the design or data collection protocol of the trial. A large-scale multicenter trial may spawn a number of such studies. In fact, the opportunity to engage in such investigations may represent an inducement for investigators to become involved in the trial in the first place and may help them to maintain their interest in the trial as it proceeds (see also Sections 6.3.4 and 6.4.5 and Section 15.2.1).

The leadership of the trial (usually the steering committee) is responsible for establishing the general guidelines and policies concerning the type of studies that may be undertaken, and for review of proposals before they are implemented. The review should focus on:

- Aim and rationale of the proposed investigation
- Type and amount of data to be collected

- Relevance in relation to the main aims of the trial
- Extent to which investigations are likely to interfere with patient enrollment and follow-up, or with established data collection procedures
- Possibilities of biasing the data collection or patient treatment procedures in the trial
- Amount of analytic help needed from the data center
- Amount of study resources needed to carry out the investigations

Investigations that have the potential of reducing a patient's willingness to be enrolled into the trial or to continue after enrollment should not be undertaken for obvious reasons. Patients approached for participation should be informed of the ancillary nature of the investigations being proposed and of their right to refuse without affecting their participation in the trial.

Investigations in masked trials that entail collection of data that have the potential of unmasking treatment assignments in the clinics should be proscribed, or should be done in such a way so as to preserve the mask. The same is true for analyses that have the potential for unmasking treatment assignments. Such analyses may have to wait until the trial is over and the treatment codes have been released.

Ancillary studies involving only modest time commitments from a few study personnel may be supported with funds from the trial. Large undertakings, involving major time commitments from existing study personnel or the recruitment of additional staff, should be done with independent funding.

One of the issues that should be covered during the review is the proposed authorship of papers arising from the investigation and the credit to be given to the trial in such publications. The arrangement proposed should be compatible with the general authorship guidelines established for the trial (see Chapter 24).

22.7.4   Publication and internal editorial review procedures

A key issue in any trial has to do with mechanisms for the review and authorship of study publications. The considerations related to this issue are discussed in Chapter 24.

22.7.5 Publicity and information access policy issues

The leadership of the study is responsible for guidelines concerning investigator-initiated publicity during the trial (see Chapter 24). Most publicity, whether contemplated on a local (e.g., in relation to patient recruitment at individual clinics in a multicenter trial) or national level should be cleared through a central body in the study. Similarly, as noted in Chapter 24, it is prudent to develop general guidelines to indicate how investigators are to deal with requests for information from the news media or from members of the scientific or lay community while the trial is under way.

23. Committee structures of multicenter trials

We shall have long sittings, much fighting is anticipated.

Sir Robert Christensen

23.1 INTRODUCTION

The three functions discussed in Chapter 22, leadership, safety monitoring, and advisory-review, are usually met through committees in the typical multicenter trial as considered in this book. The main organizational units are listed in Table 23-1. Table 23-2 provides a description of the principal duties of each unit listed.

Table 23-1 Key organizational units

Organizational unit	Function	Other designations*
A. Study chairman	• Head the investigative group and chair the SC	• Study director • Principal investigator
B. Steering committee (SC)	• Leadership body of the investigative group	• Director's committee • Executive committee
C. Executive committee (EC)	• Executor of SC	• Chairman's committee
D. Treatment effects monitoring committee (TEMC)	• Safety monitoring	• Data monitoring committee • Data and safety monitoring committee • Ethics review committee • Ethics committee
E. Advisory-review committee (ARC)	• Advise sponsor and/or investigators on conduct of trial	• Policy advisory board • Policy advisory committee • Advisory committee • Review committee
F. Advisory-review and treatment effects monitoring committee (ARTEMC)	• Advise sponsor and/or investigators on conduct of trial and perform safety monitoring	• Operations committee

*Not used in this book.

240

Table 23–2 Functions and responsibilities of the main organizational units of multicenter trials

A. Study chairman

- Serve as senior executive officer of the investigative group
- Chair steering committee
- Serve as principal spokesman for the study
- Maintain communications within the study and with the sponsor

B. Steering committee (SC)

- Assume responsibility for general design and conduct of the trial, including preparation of essential study documents, such as manual of operations, data forms, treatment protocol, etc.
- Review data collection practices and procedures, as summarized in performance monitoring reports, from visits to participating clinics, and other means, to identify and correct remediable deficiencies
- Consider and adopt changes in study procedures as necessary and desirable during the course of the trial
- Appoint and disband subcommittees needed for execution of the trial
- Make decisions on resource allocations and on priorities for meeting competing demands in the trial
- Review progress of study in achieving its main goal and take steps required to enhance likelihood o success in achieving them
- Review and implement recommendations from the ARC and TEMC (or ARTEMC) for a treatment protocol change, such as termination of a treatment because of lack of efficacy
- Review and react to other general advice or recommendations from the TEMC and ARC (or ARTEMC)

C. Executive committee (EC)

- Act as the administrative and executive arm of the SC
- Make decisions on behalf of the SC on day-to-day operational issues requiring immediate action
- Assign priorities for activities in the trial, consistent with the dictates of the SC

- Perform executive functions for the trial, including scheduling meetings, preparation of SC and other meeting agendas, etc.
- Coordinate preparation of progress reports requested by the sponsoring agency in conjunction with funding renewal requests and as needed at other times
- Perform other functions assigned by the SC

D. Treatment effects monitoring committee (TEMC)*

- Direct or carry out data analyses needed for assessing treatment effects during the trial
- Review interim reports prepared by the data coordinating center for evidence of adverse or beneficial treatment effects
- Recommend changes in the treatment protocol to the ARC
- Provide advice to the SC on operational procedures affecting the quality of the trial

E. Advisory-review committee (ARC)*

- Advise the sponsor on performance of the trial and whether funding for it should be continued
- Review and approve recommendations from the TEMC for changes in the treatment protocol
- Recommend termination of support of centers when warranted because of poor performance or for other reasons
- Advise the SC and sponsor on important policy issues
- Review performance monitoring reports prepared by the data coordinating center to detect deficiencies in the data collection or intake processes and recommend corrective action when necessary
- Assume responsibility for external review of the data coordinating center and other resource centers in the trial

F. Advisory-review and treatment effects monitoring committee (ARTEMC)

- Committee has the combined functions of the TEMC and ARC

---

*Functions assumed by the ARTEMC in structures not having a separate TEMC and ARC.

The chairman of the study,[1] in conjunction with the steering committee (SC), or SC and executive committee (EC) when the structure includes both committees, provides the general leadership for the trial. Membership on the committee(s) is generally limited to personnel associated with centers in the trial. Exceptions are cases in which membership is augmented to include consultants with expertise in areas not represented within the study.

1. In this book, the individual chairing the steering committee is considered to be chairman of the study.

The advisory-review functions will be provided through a specially constituted committee, herein referred to as the advisory-review committee (ARC). The same is true for the safety monitoring function; generally, it will be met through a committee herein referred to as the treatment effects monitoring committee (TEMC), or through a committee that fulfills both the advisory-review and safety monitoring functions, herein referred to as the advisory-review and treatment effects monitoring committee (ARTEMC). The ARC and TEMC or

ARTEMC are composed primarily of people not associated with any of the centers in the trial.

All 14 trials sketched in Appendix B included a SC. Several (5 of the 14) also included an EC. Six of the 14 had separate committees for meeting the safety monitoring and advisory-review functions. Four combined the functions into a single ARTEMC and the remaining 4 had only a TEMC or an ARC, but not both (line 27, Table B-4, Appendix B).

The committee structure of a trial is generally more complex than suggested above, as indicated in Table 23-3 for one of the trials sketched in Appendix B—the Coronary Drug Project (CDP; see citation 104 for details). See also citations 346, 375, and 476 for detailed listings of committee structures in the National Cooperative Gallstone Study (NCGS), Persantine Aspirin Reinfarction Trial (PARIS), and University Group Diabetes Program (UGDP). Other references pertinent to the topic of this chapter include citations 315, 318, and 479.

23.2 STUDY CHAIRMAN

The terms *principal investigator* and *chairman of the study* may be synonymous in a single-center trial, but not in a multicenter trial where there are, in effect, multiple "principal" investigators (see Glossary for comment). Someone must be chosen or designated to head the investigative group (IG) and to chair the steering

Table 23-3   Functioning committees of the Coronary Drug Project (Sketch 6, Appendix B)

CDP committee*	Function
• Steering Committee	• As described in Part B of Table 23-2
• Data and Safety Monitoring Committee	• As described in Part D of Table 23-2
• Policy Board	• As described in Part E of Table 23-2
• Criteria Committee	• Establish definitions and criteria used for determining patient eligibility in the trial
• Laboratory Committee	• Review procedures and results produced by the central laboratory for the trial
• Editorial Review Committee	• Review study manuscripts before presentation or submission for publication
• Statistical Committee	• Advise the Coordinating Center on methods of data analysis
• Natural History Committee	• Direct data analyses and paper writing activities concerned with the natural history of coronary heart disease, as based on results obtained from the placebo-treated group of patients
• Mortality Classification Committee	• Classify deaths by cause
• Hepatology Committee	• Plan analyses and review data relating to liver function tests
• Data Repository Committee	• Review ancillary study proposals requiring access to the main study file and establish special data collection procedures and respositories for results of ancillary studies that threaten treatment masking
• Arrangements Committee	• Select site of semiannual investigative group meetings and coordinate arrangements with host city
• Resources Committee	• Advise the SC on future studies and activities involving CDP patients
• Newsletter Committee	• Prepare patient newsletter

*Members of all committees, except those serving on the Data and Safety Monitoring Committee and Policy Board, were appointed by the Steering Committee. Members of the Data and Safety Monitoring Committee were appointed by the Steering Committee or Director of the NHLBI. Members of the Policy Board were appointed by the Director of the NHLBI.

committee in such trials. This individual is referred to as chairman of the study throughout this book. Desired qualities of this individual include:

- A keen intellect
- An understanding of and interest in the area of study
- Research experience, preferably in other clinical trials
- Experience in collaborative research
- A respected research record
- Strong leadership capabilities
- Self-assurance but not arrogance
- The ability to make decisions, but not capriciously
- Integrity
- An ability to listen to others and to modify a stand in the face of convincing arguments
- The ability to compromise
- Evenhandedness and fairness in dealing with others
- Respect for others and their ideas
- Sensitivity to the needs and feelings of others
- Patience and perseverance

Ideally, the individual selected should be chosen with this list in mind. However, in actual fact, there may be little room for choice, especially in an investigator-initiated trial, in which the individual who conceives the trial is the one who heads it. Room for choice is greater in sponsor-initiated trials. The approach used in the Aspirin Myocardial Infarction Study (AMIS) serves as a useful model. A temporary study chairman was appointed by the National Heart, Lung, and Blood Institute (NHLBI) shortly after selection of the clinics and the coordinating centers for the study. A permanent chairman was appointed by the Institute some months later, after input was received from the investigative group regarding possible choices.

The choice, when one exists, should be limited to persons who do not have a strong emotional commitment to any of the treatments being tested and who have open minds concerning their merits. For obvious reasons, the individual selected should be devoid of financial interests in the treatments under test.

The chairman is sometimes selected by a vote of the investigative group. In this case, the choice should be made from a slate of suitable candidates proposed by a nominating committee appointed by the investigative group, or that has been screened in some other way. A popular election, without any screening, can lead to an unwise choice (e.g., selection of a highly popular but poorly qualified individual).

All of the trials listed in Appendix B were headed by persons with M.D. degrees (line 28.a.i, Table B-4, Appendix B). However, only 5 of the 14 chairmen had responsibility for patients in the trials, although several others were located in institutions housing a study clinic. The association with a clinic has advantages and disadvantages. On the one hand, it helps to ensure that the chairman has firsthand knowledge of the data collection procedures in the trial. The knowledge is useful when chairing discussions concerning protocol changes or when writing papers containing results from the trial. On the other hand, the association may make it difficult for the chairman to maintain a balanced and evenhanded approach when dealing with other clinical investigators in the trial, especially if the clinic he is associated with is one of the more inept clinics in the trial. In addition, the need to treat study patients, if the chairman has such responsibilities, may conflict with some of his other responsibilities (e.g., see Section 23.6).

It is perhaps no accident that none of the chairmen for the 13 multicenter trials represented in Appendix B were from coordinating centers or sponsoring agencies. The addition of chairmanship responsibilities on top of those normally assumed by the coordinating center or sponsoring agency is unwise because of the separation requirements discussed in Chapter 22. In addition, the added concentration of power at the coordinating center or sponsoring agency, through the study chairmanship, may make it difficult to establish the checks and balances needed for a robust structure.

As a rule, the chairman will be appointed or elected to serve for the duration of the trial (see item 28.a.iv, Table B-4, Appendix B). The advantage of an appointment without term stems from the continuity of leadership provided when the same person presides over the trial from beginning to end. The main disadvantage is that difficulties can arise if the chairman proves to be an ineffective leader and must be replaced. A term appointment can provide a graceful way out in such cases.

Most of the above considerations pertain to the position of study vice-chairman as well. Ideally, the chairman and vice-chairman should be from different centers in the trial. Location of both individuals in the same center may concentrate too much power and influence in a single center and may restrict the range of ideas presented to the SC and investigative group.

23.3   STEERING COMMITTEE

The steering committee is the main leadership committee of the study. It is the body which is responsible for overall direction of the study.

Every multicenter trial must face two key issues in the formation of this committee. The first has to do with center representation on the committee. The issue is easily resolved when the total number of centers in the trial is small (say ten or less) and where, as a result, it is practical to have a position for each center on the committee. However, this form of representation is impractical if the number of centers is large. For example, this method of representation would have led to a steering committee of more than 60 members in the CDP. Clearly, a representative form of government is required in such cases to avoid the expense, to say nothing of the logistical difficulties, involved in convening the committee. The CDP operated with a steering committee of 15 members by providing for a mix of standing and elected members. The chairman and vice-chairman of the study, director of the coordinating center, project officer, and directors of the five clinical centers named in the initial funding application were designated as permanent standing members. In addition, there were four elected members, chosen by the IG from among directors of clinical centers not accorded permanent representation on the committee. Elected members served for a three-year term, with provision for re-election. Terms were staggered to allow for an orderly rotation of elected members.

The SC should not be created under the one-center-one-member rule if there is any likelihood of having to reconstitute the committee later on in the trial under a representative form of government. It is far better to anticipate the need for such a form of government from the outset than it is to attempt to switch to it once the trial is under way.

Several of the trials listed in Appendix B provided SC representation for each center director, even though it led, in some cases, to steering committees with 20 or more members. See item 28.c.iii, Table B–4, Appendix B and Table 23–4 for specifics.

A second issue has to do with the nature of representation on the committee for key professional groups involved in carrying out the study. Formation of the committee along center lines automatically leads to overrepresentation of some types of personnel (e.g., clinical investigators), underrepresentation of others (e.g., personnel concerned with data analysis), and exclusion of still others (e.g., junior personnel performing essential functions in the trial).

Some studies have attempted to rectify this problem by reserving positions on the committee for designated classes of personnel. The approach offers two general advantages. First, it helps to provide the SC with the expertise needed to discharge its leadership functions. Second, it avoids the obvious morale problems that can arise if an important group of personnel in the trial has no voice in the way it is run.

Four of the SCs sketched in Appendix B had clinic coordinators represented (see Glossary for definition). The advantages of such representation have been discussed by Overton (1980) from the perspective of the Aspirin Myocardial Infarction Study. It was the only position represented in the trials sketched in Appendix B, other than the study chairman, vice-chairman, center directors, and project officers. One reason for the lack of representation may have to do with the natural reluctance of any group of senior investigators to dilute their base of power through the addition of members not in key leadership positions in the study. A second reason may have to do with the potential for embarrassment if a second representative from a center speaks or votes against a position held by the center director.

Table 23–5 provides a list of some of the general rules for SC formation (see Table 22–2 for general committee rules). The term of office should be designated when positions are filled. When less than the duration of the trial, terms should be long enough to permit individuals to play meaningful roles on the committee. General rules for filling vacancies should be spelled out before any are encountered. In addition, it is wise to indicate conditions that will lead to cancellation of membership on the committee because of conflicts of interest, lack of interest in the study as expressed by attendance records at committee meetings or in other ways. Termination of inactive members, so that their positions can be filled with new and more active members, is important in maintaining the vitality of the committee.

Table 23-4 Characteristics of steering committees and committees responsible for safety monitoring in the 14 trials sketched in Appendix B

	Steering Committee	Safety Monitoring Committee*
A. Chairman		
● Primary degree		
M.D.	14	12
Ph.D.	0	4
● Term		
For duration of study	14	16
For specified number of years	0	0
● Patient care responsibilities		
Yes	6	1
No	8	15
B. Vice-chairman		
● Number of trials with vice-chairman	8	2
● Primary degree		
M.D.	7	2
non-M.D.	1	0
● Term		
For duration of study	8	2
For specified number of years	0	0
● Patient care responsibilities		
Yes	6	0
No	2	2
C. Number of members (voting plus nonvoting)		
≤10	2	7
11–15	5	5
16–20	5	1
≥20	2	1
D. Study positions represented		
Study chairman	14	13
Study vice-chairman	8	5
Director of coordinating center	14	13
Project officer	10	13
Clinic coordinator	4	0
Clinic director	13	6
Nonhealth professional or lay representative	0	3
E. Nonstudy members		
Yes	6	12
No	8	2

*Two studies had safety monitoring committees headed by co-chairmen.

23.4 EXECUTIVE COMMITTEE

Most steering committees, even for a trial involving as few as five or six clinics, will be too large to deal with the day-to-day decision making needed for efficient operation of the trial. A smaller, more compact committee will be needed for this purpose (see Part C of Table 23-2). The EC is usually headed by the study chairman and includes the study vice-chairman (if there is one), director of the coordinating center, project officer (in the case of trials funded by the National Institutes of Health), and perhaps a few other members of the IG as well. As a rule, it will meet more frequently than the SC (either face-to-face or via conference telephone).

The usefulness of the committee will be defeated if it has more than a half dozen members

Table 23–5　Do's and don'ts for formation of the steering committee

DO

- Provide for input from the investigative group when organizing the committee
- Consult with the sponsor about the functions and proposed membership of the SC
- Listen to suggestions made by the sponsor regarding organization and function of the SC
- Outline general membership criteria, methods for selecting members, and terms of office
- Provide for representation of all essential skills and disciplines needed for effective operation of the SC
- Set an upper membership limit on the SC and stick to it
- Provide for rotation of at least a portion of the SC members by appointment or election, especially for trials with large numbers of centers
- Designate the study chairman as chairman of the SC
- Designate the study vice-chairman, director of the coordinating center, and directors of other key resource centers as ex-officio voting members of the committee
- Make the project officer an ex officio (voting or non-voting) member of the committee
- Outline rules for filling vacancies on the committee
- Specify disqualifying conflicts of interest and other conditions (such as poor meeting attendance) that will lead to termination of SC membership

DON'T

- Limit membership on the SC to center directors or senior investigators
- Use appointment to the SC as a method of dispensing rewards or favors
- Include people on the SC known to have conflicts of interest in relation to the study treatments
- Limit voting rights for selection of elected members simply to senior members of the investigative group
- Permit the sponsor to dictate the organizing tenets of the trial

or so. The temptation to make the committee a "mini" steering committee, by including a number of elected representatives from the parent committee, should be resisted. The ability to convene the committee (by phone or in person) on short notice will become progressively more difficult the larger it is.

The concept of delegating executive responsibilities to the EC should be established before the SC is created. Members of the SC may resist creation of the EC once the SC has been established, especially if they view the move as one which lessens their influence in the study.

Only 5 of the 14 trials sketched in Appendix B had formally constituted executive committees (line 27, Table B–4, Appendix B). The number of members ranged from 7 to 10.

23.5　OTHER SUBCOMMITTEES OF THE STEERING COMMITTEE

The SC may commission a number of subcommittees, in addition to the EC, to perform defined tasks (see Table 23–3 for list of CDP standing committees). Care must be taken to avoid needless proliferation of subcommittees and overlap of functions among the committees commissioned. The larger the number of committees, the more cumbersome the organizational structure of the trial, and the greater the likelihood of overlap of functions among the committees.

Only committees that are commissioned to fulfill a continuing need over the course of the trial should be created on a standing basis. Committees that are commissioned to perform time-limited tasks should be designated as ad hoc committees and should be disbanded once the tasks are finished.

Each committee, whether created on a standing or ad hoc basis, should have a defined charge and should have sufficient authority and resources to carry out its charge. It should have a chairman who has responsibility for convening the committee and for reporting to the parent committee as needed. Its members should be derived from the entire IG, not simply from the parent committees, although each subcommittee should have at least one member from the parent committee. The overlap in membership helps to facilitate communications between the two committees.

23.6　TREATMENT EFFECTS MONITORING AND ADVISORY-REVIEW COMMITTEES

The discussion in this section assumes the trial is one that requires both safety monitoring and advisory-review (see Chapter 22). A key design question in this context has to do with whether to vest both functions in the same committee or in two separate committees. Table 23–6 provides an outline of the conditions under which a separate ARC and TEMC may be needed and where a single combined ARTEMC may do.

The main advantage of separate committees has to do with the separation of functions made

Table 23-6 Considerations leading to a separate ARC and TEMC or a combined ARTEMC

A. Considerations for separate ARC and TEMC

- When treatment monitoring activities require frequent meetings and where each meeting requires a half day or more to carry out the necessary data reviews
- When the TEMC meets other general analysis needs of the study (e.g., is responsible for developing analytic approaches for dealing with special analytic problems)
- When the trial is investigator-initiated and grant-supported
- When the sponsor and/or investigators desire separate committees

B. Considerations for combined ARTEMC

- When the time required for treatment monitoring is small relative to the time required to perform more general advisory and review functions normally assumed by the ARC
- When there is little or no need for advice or guidance concerning the analysis procedures used for assessing treatment effects
- .When the trial is sponsor-initiated
- When the sponsor and/or investigator desire a single combined committee

possible in this way. The separation, among other things, helps to ensure that adequate time will be spent on the safety monitoring process. This assurance is more difficult to achieve when the safety monitoring function is only one of a larger set of responsibilities assumed by an ARTEMC. The use of separate committees also makes it possible for one committee to serve as a check on the other for key decisions involving termination of a treatment because of adverse or beneficial effects. The main disadvantage is the added complexity involved in creating and staffing two committees rather than one.

Whatever structure is chosen should be designed to meet the advisory-review needs of the sponsor and of the investigative group. These needs, while overlapping, are different. Cooperation between the sponsor and investigators will be needed to develop a structure that satisfies both needs.

Appointments to the TEMC and ARC or ARTEMC may be made by the sponsor, or by the study chairman on behalf of the SC. They should be made by the study chairman in cases where the sponsor has a proprietary interest in the treatments being tested. However, it is important, regardless of how the appointments are made, to ensure that the appointments proposed are acceptable to both the IG and the sponsor.

Investigators may have no choice but to proceed with formation of their own treatment monitoring and advisory-review structure if the sponsor has no interest in establishing such a structure or sees no need for it (e.g., as in some investigator-initiated grant-supported trials). The lack of cooperation can lead to problems later on if the sponsor concludes that the structure is inadequate to serve its needs and therefore elects to superimpose its own structure on top of one already in place. This problem occurred in the Program on the Surgical Control of Hyperlipidemia (POSCH). The original structure provided for both a TEMC and ARC, with members of both committees appointed by the study chairman. Later on, as the study progressed and the need in the NHLBI for an advisory and review process independent of POSCH came to be recognized, the Institute requested POSCH investigators to accept an expansion of the two committees via the addition of members appointed by the Institute. This arrangement was sufficient to satisfy the needs of the Institute until well into the trial. However it ultimately moved to create its own ARC. This move required dissolution of the existing ARC and led to a series of discussions (involving the study chairman, chairman of the TEMC, and NHLBI staff) to define the domain and responsibilities of the new ARC in relation to the existing POSCH committee structure.

The typical TEMC and ARC, or ARTEMC, as seen through the sketches in Appendix B, for the most part, is made up of experts from specialty fields of medicine and biostatistics, although, a few included a professional from a nonhealth field (e.g., a lawyer or clergyman) or a lay representative as a means of broadening the perspective of the committee (see item 29.e, Table B-4, Appendix B). The virtues of membership for a nonhealth professional are discussed in a paper by Hamilton (1981).

Table 23-4 provides a summary of the information tabulated in Appendix B (item 29, Table B-4) for the committees that performed safety monitoring (TEMCs in nine trials, ARTEMCs in four trials, and the SC in one trial—the UGDP). All of the committees were chaired by persons with expertise in epidemiology or biostatistics and who had an M.D. or Ph.D. The number of members ranged from 5 to 27, counting voting as well as nonvoting members. Several of the committees restricted voting privileges to members not affiliated with any study center. This restriction is a good idea, especially in cases in which study members are dependent on the study for salary support. Most of the committees included the director of the coordinating center, either as a voting or nonvoting member. Representation from this center is essential in the monitoring process because of its key role in data analyses. All of the NIH-sponsored trials sketched included representation of the project office on the committee as well. The majority of the committees also included the study chairman or vice-chairman, again as either voting or nonvoting members.

Inclusion of the study chairman on the TEMC or ARTEMC is open to debate when that person has patient care responsibilities in the trial. The emotional commitment needed to treat can affect any person's scientific objectivity thereby reducing that person's effectiveness on the committee. Further, it can be argued that a study physician who has access to interim results of the trial will be affected by them, thereby increasing the risk of bias in the treatment and data collection processes performed by that person. In addition, having access to the results can create a dilemma for any study physician still involved in recruiting patients for the trial if they suggest one treatment is better than another, even if the trend is not large enough to justify stopping the trial. Shielding study physicians from the interim results protects them from the dilemma mentioned by transferring responsibility to the TEMC or ARTEMC.

The virtues of inclusion have to do with the special qualifications of the study chairman. This person may have the best perspective on the trial and its data collection and treatment processes—a perspective that may be invaluable when the TEMC or ARTEMC is faced with a major decision concerning the study. In addition, the chairman's presence on the committee can be reassuring to other clinical investigators in the trial. In fact, they may be reluctant to delegate responsibility for safety monitoring to any group without such representation.

The approach practiced in some studies has been to include both the chairman and vice-chairman of the study on the treatment effects monitoring committee, whether or not they have treatment responsibilities in the studies. For example, the CDP opted for this approach, even though the vice-chairman of the study had such responsibilities. The TEMC in the Hypertension Detection and Follow-Up Program

(HDFP) was reconstituted during the trial to include both the study chairman and vice-chairman.

Ideally, persons selected to serve on the TEMC, ARC, or ARTEMC should have prior experience with multicenter clinical trials. This is especially true for the chairmen of these committees.

All voting members should be screened for conflicts of interest before appointment. In addition, mechanisms should be established to alert the appointing authority to conflicts of interest that may develop during the trial (see Section 22.7 of Chapter 22).

Members of the treatment effects monitoring and advisory-review committees are usually appointed for the duration of the trial. None of the TEMCs, ARCs, or ARTEMCs listed in Appendix B made any provision for term appointments. Undoubtedly, this is due to the desire of the study leaders to maximize continuity of function in these committees via a stable membership. However, this approach, as suggested in Section 23.3, can cause difficulty if members lose interest in the trial. Hence, it is prudent to have some means of dismissing inactive members in the absence of term appointments in order to maintain a properly functioning committee.

23.7 COMMITTEE-SPONSOR INTERACTION

Smooth interaction of the SC with the TEMC and ARC, or with the ARTEMC in the case of a single committee with combined advisory-review and safety monitoring functions, is essential for operation of the trial. Figure 23–1 provides stylized diagrams of three types of interaction models, as viewed from the perspective of the sponsoring agency. It also outlines the main characteristics of each of the models.

Communications between the SC and the sponsor in the models are concerned with design and operation of the trial. Communications between the ARC or ARTEMC and the sponsor are concerned primarily with assessment of the adequacy of the study design, the nature of the treatment results, and with fiscal affairs. None of the models in Figure 23–1 provides for flow of treatment results to the SC during the trial. Information of this sort passes only in conjunction with a recommended treatment protocol change.

Each of the trials sketched in Appendix B has been classified (by the author) as to type of communication model using the criteria given in

Figure 23-1 Committee-sponsor interaction models

Model	Characteristics
Model A. *Sponsor Directive* 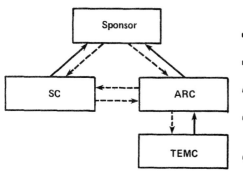	• Trial usually sponsor initiated • Members of ARTEMC appointed by sponsor, sometimes with little or no investigator input • Advisory and review functions provided by ARTEMC, as prescribed by the sponsor • Communication between SC and ARTEMC via the sponsor • Little or no direct communication between SC and ARTEMC • Recommendations for treatment change made by the ARTEMC. Those approved by the sponsor are passed, via the sponsor, to the SC for implementation
Model B. *Sponsor Nondirective* 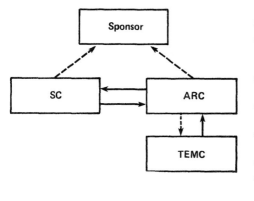	• Trial usually investigator initiated and grant supported, or initiated via a joint effort of the investigators and sponsor • Members of the ARC and TEMC may be appointed by the sponsor or chairman of the SC • Appointments made to the ARC and TEMC generally limited to individuals who are acceptable to both the sponsor and investigative group • Advisory and review functions provided by ARC, as prescribed by mutual consent of investigative group and sponsor • ARC provides advice and review for both the sponsor and investigators • Primary communications of the TEMC directed to ARC; limited communications from the ARC to TEMC • Recommendation for treatment change originates with TEMC, reviewed by ARC, and passed to SC, via the sponsor, for implementation • Primary communications from the ARC to sponsor and from SC to sponsor. Only limited communication from the sponsor to the SC, or from the sponsor to the ARC. No direct communication between TEMC and SC or between TEMC and the sponsor • Some direct communication between SC and ARC, but not with regard to treatment results
Model C. *Sponsor Passive*	• Trial usually small-scale, investigator initiated, and grant supported • Advisory and review function provided by ARC, as prescribed by the SC • ARC has no advisory-review role for the sponsor • Members of ARC and TEMC appointed by chairman of SC. Little or no interest expressed by the sponsor in the selection or appointment process • Virtually no communication from sponsor to SC or from sponsor to ARC • Limited communications from SC to sponsor and from ARC to sponsor • Same communication structure as for Model B regarding ARC and TEMC • Major communications between SC and ARC • Recommendation for treatment change originates with TEMC, reviewed by ARC, and passed by the ARC to the SC for implementation with knowledge of the sponsor, but without its approval

Note: Arrows indicate direction of communications. Solid lines indicate major communication pathways. Dashed lines indicate secondary communication pathways.

Figure 23–1. Four of the 14 trials were classified as sponsor-directive and the remaining 10 were classified as sponsor non-directive (see item 30, Table B–4, Appendix B for specifics).

23.8   CENTER-TO-CENTER COMMUNICATIONS

The coordinating center (or data coordinating center) is the primary communication channel in most multicenter structures. The center will require linkages with each clinic as well as with all other organizational units in the trial to perform its functions effectively. The volume of information flowing in other communications channels, such as those associated with the chairman's office, project office, and other resource centers in the trial, will depend on the way in which coordination responsibilities are divided (see Chapter 5). Generally, it will be small compared with that of the coordinating center or data coordinating center.

Information flowing from the clinics to the coordinating center (or data coordinating center) will consist primarily of data, either as contained on completed data forms or as tapes or disks of data already keyed at the clinics from the data forms. Information flowing from the coordinating center to the clinics will relate to:

- Edit queries concerning completed data forms
- Procedural memos concerning the data collection process
- Manuals of operation or parts or sections of manuals and related revisions
- Approved data forms and related revisions
- Progress reports and clinic performance monitoring reports
- Minutes of study meetings
- Miscellaneous study correspondence

The flow into and out of the clinics should be via a defined pathway. Multiple entry and exit points for the clinic will make it difficult, if not impossible, to control information leaving the clinic and to keep track of information flowing into it. The preferred structure is one in which a single person, usually the clinic coordinator, is designated to serve as the conduit through which correspondence and materials flow into the clinic and through whom data forms and related materials flow out of the clinic. One person who should not serve as a primary channel for routine information flow is the clinic direc-

tor. The likelihood of a smooth and continuous flow is low because of the multiple commitments and general lack of discipline and interest of such a person in handling routine flows.

The designation of a single individual in the clinic to receive and distribute important procedural information arriving from the coordinating center (or data coordinating center) simplifies the distribution task of the coordinating center. Mailings from the coordinating center to several persons in each clinic is expensive and may not, in any case, work as well as local distribution systems. However, some mailing redundancy is wise to protect against communication breakdowns if the primary channel fails. The HPT data coordinating center used a primary (clinic coordinator) and secondary (clinic director) mail contact for all communications concerning data collection and study procedures. The primary mail contact received originals and all accompanying attachments to mailings from the data coordinating center. The secondary contact received, via a separate mailing, copies of all numbered memos and a list of attachments received by the primary mail contact.

The address directory is an essential communications aid in the multicenter trial. To be useful, it must be up-to-date and should contain the names, mailing addresses, and phone numbers of all study personnel at each participating center. Other useful information in the document includes:

- An indication of the functions of each person listed, including areas of certification for data collection
- The name of the primary and secondary mail contacts at a center
- The deputy director of a center
- List of study committees and the names, addresses, and phone numbers of committee members

The information system of a trial will require a numbering scheme to facilitate the identification of the various documents in the study. The need for a form numbering scheme has already been addressed (Chapter 12). However, the need does not stop there. It extends to other documents as well, such as:

- Committee minutes
- Procedural memos, etc.

- Manuals of operation
- Materials used by clinic staff and patients for treatment administration

The ground rules for document numbering and communications should be established before data collection is begun. Rules should be written and reviewed by the SC before they are promulgated in the study. The rules should be reviewed and, when necessary, revised at intervals over the course of the trial.

Part VI. Reporting procedures

Chapters in This Part

Chapter 24 deals with general policy issues involved in the production and publication of study manuscripts. Chapter 25 outlines the content requirements of a finished report and the steps involved in the preparation of such reports. The last chapter contains a review of methods for locating reports of trials in the published literature. It also contains a list of points a reader should consider when reading a report. It closes with a discussion of the responsibilities of persons who critique study publications.

24. Study publication and information policies

Never be so brief as to become obscure.

Tyron Edwards

24.1 INFORMATION CONSTRAINTS

The types of trials described in this book typically require constraints on the flow of information while they are under way. Commonly imposed constraints relate to:

- Randomization (e.g., by withholding details concerning the randomization process from clinic personnel to keep them from predicting future assignments; see Chapter 10)
- Treatment masking (e.g., by constructing methods for assigning and administering treatments so that a patient and his doctor remain masked with regard to treatment assignment; see Chapters 8 and 10)
- Data collection and coding procedures (e.g., through separation of treatment and data collection responsibilities in the clinic so that observations are made and recorded by personnel who are kept ignorant of the treatment received by the study patients; see Chapter 8)
- Treatment monitoring where only selected members of the study organization are privy to interim treatment results (see Chapter 20)

All of the trials listed in Appendix B imposed constraints of these types. All of the coordinating centers withheld details concerning the method of randomization until recruitment was finished or until the end of the study. Most had structures that allowed only certain members of the study group to see interim treatment results. Clinic personnel, as a rule, were not allowed access to outcome data by treatment group until the study was concluded, or until a treatment was terminated.

Information constraints, whether limited to members of the community at large, or to selected study personnel as well, should not be imposed unless there is a good rationale for doing so. Further, they should be lifted as soon as the need for them no longer exists.

24.2   PUBLICATION QUESTIONS[1]

24.2.1   When to publish?

Any investigator who undertakes a trial has a responsibility to make the results obtained from it available for public scrutiny via a published manuscript. The manuscript should be prepared and made available as soon after the results have been obtained as possible. Normally, the manuscript (or manuscripts) describing the results will be produced after the trial has entered the termination stage (see Chapter 3 for stages). Exceptions are cases in which interim publications are needed to report results related to a treatment protocol change, as in the Coronary Drug Project (CDP), Macular Photocoagulation Study (MPS), and University Group Diabetes Program (UGDP). See reference citations 102, 103, 105, 291, 292, 293, 468, 470, 472 for publications of this type.

Investigators in long-term trials should decide whether or not to allow publication of interim results not related to a protocol change. The pros and cons of such publications are outlined in Table 24-1. The preferred policy is one proscribing publication or presentation of treatment results during the trial, except those related to protocol changes. A permissive policy has the potential of compromising the trial, especially in cases where the results can affect subsequent recruitment or treatment patterns in the trial. In addition, it can open the study to criticism if the schedule of publication is perceived as having been designed to maximize the impact of the study.

Pressures to relax the proscription can be expected during the course of most long-term trials. They are most likely to arise from publication of related studies, especially if the results of these studies are contrary to those observed in the trial. Investigators in the Coronary Artery Surgery Study (CASS) were exposed to such pressures because of interim publications coming from a European sister study (European Coronary Surgery Study Group, 1979, 1980, 1982a, 1982b). Ultimately, the proscription was upheld, but not without a considerable amount of debate.

Investigators in some of the larger trials have elected to summarize details of the design, meth-

Table 24-1   Pros and cons of interim publications not related to a treatment protocol change

Pros

- Provides access to study results as they emerge
- May simplify preparation of the final publication
- Helps to maintain investigator interest in the trial
- Keeps the study in the "public eye"

Cons

- Inconclusive and preliminary nature of the results may lead to confusion
- May reduce investigator enthusiasm for continued patient recruitment or treatment if the interim results are viewed as "discouraging"
- Knowledge of an emerging treatment difference, especially in the case of unmasked trials, may bias subsequent treatment and data collection
- Publicity accorded the interim results may reduce the amount of attention investigators are able to devote to the conduct of the trial, especially if resources needed to carry out the remainder of the trial have to be diverted to respond to criticisms
- Impact of the study and its final conclusions may be diminished because of the way data were presented and analyzed in earlier publications

ods, and baseline results in a separate paper. Such papers may be prepared any time after patient recruitment is completed. Ideally, they should be published before any results for the trial have appeared in print, as in CASS (Coronary Artery Surgery Study Research Group, 1981), or in conjunction with the first results publication, as in the UGDP (University Group Diabetes Program Research Group, 1970d). However, in some instances they may not appear until results have been published, as in the CDP (Coronary Drug Project Research Group, 1973a).

24.2.2.   Presentation or publication?[2]

A key issue to be addressed is the way in which results are announced to the medical community. Options include:

- Making an announcement of the results to the news media with subsequent publication in a medical journal
- Making a presentation of the results at a national meeting (may lead to media cover-

---

1. The term *publication*, as used throughout this chapter and in the next one, relates to a public document. Access may be via a published periodical, book, or the like, or via a public repository for unpublished manuscripts and documents, such as the one maintained by the National Technical Information Service (NTIS).

2. The term *presentation*, as used throughout this chapter and in the next one, relates to a paper concerning a trial that is prepared and read by study investigators before a national meeting of some medical group, but that has not been published (with the exception of an abstract summary appearing in the meeting program).

age), with subsequent publication in a medical journal

- Publication of the results in a medical journal, with no prior public presentations or announcements

Table 24-2 contains summary comments concerning each option.

A presentation should not be made if it precludes publication in the journal of choice. Some journals may regard certain kinds of presentations as tantamount to publication and, hence, may not be willing to publish the results. In addition, various journals, such as the *New England Journal of Medicine*, discourage author-initiated press coverage of results in papers under consideration for publication.

Publicity emanating from presentations may not be in the best interest of patients or members of the medical community responsible for their care, especially if the results presented are con-

Table 24-2 Options for initial communication of results

A. Announcement of results to news media with subsequent publication in a medical journal

- Approach should be avoided, except where the press release is timed to correspond with publication

- Particularly undesirable when there is a large time gap between initial publicity and publication

- Members of the medical community may resent the advance publicity, especially if they are called upon to respond to questions stimulated by the publicity without benefit of a published manuscript

B. Presentation of results at a national meeting with subsequent publication in a medical journal

- Presentations are often used for initial communication of results to the medical community

- Presentation may provide authors with useful feedback for preparation of the final manuscript

- Approach suffers from the same problems noted in Part A above if presentation leads to news media coverage

- Generally best to forego presentation unless it can be timed to correspond with publication

- Approach should be avoided if presentation precludes publication in the journal of choice

C. Publication of results in a medical journal with no advance presentation or publicity

- Preferred approach, especially for results that are likely to be controversial or that challenge the value of an existing treatment

- Publication may be accompanied or followed by a press release

troversial and there is a large time gap between presentation and publication. The five-month period between presentation and publication of the tolbutamide results in the UGDP caused difficulties for patients and diabetologists alike (see Chapter 7 for chronology of events). Publicity surrounding the presentation caused many patients on oral hypoglycemic agents to question their physicians regarding the usefulness and safety of the treatment. Physicians had difficulty dealing with their concerns in the absence of a published report detailing the results.

24.2.3 Where to publish?

The choice should be limited to refereed journals that are covered in *Index Medicus*. Unrefereed journals, proceedings of meetings, and monographs should be avoided both because of the absence of a critical review process as a prerequisite to publication and because of the difficulties involved in identifying and retrieving any paper that is not listed in *Index Medicus*.

The nature of the study will influence the choice of the journal. Results with general implications should be directed to a wide circulation journal. A specialty journal should be considered if the results are of primary interest to a medical subspecialty. Both kinds of journals may be used in some cases, as in the UGDP with the phenformin results. The initial report appeared in the *Journal of the American Medical Association* in 1971. A more extensive report appeared in *Diabetes* in 1975 (University Group Diabetes Program Research Group, 1971b, 1975).

24.2.4 What to publish?

The goal in any publication should be to provide a clear and concise description of the study results. This requires a manuscript that contains carefully constructed graphs and tables that describe the results, as well as a description of the design and methods used in the study. General content requirements are discussed in Chapter 25.

The typical trial may produce only one publication on results. It will come at the end of the study and should contain results on all treatments studied in the trial. The decision as to how much treatment data to include is not so obvious if the paper is generated in conjunction with a protocol change made during the trial. The paper should satisfy the same content requirements as a paper published at the end of a trial if it serves the same purpose as a final publication. This will be the case in trials involving just one test and control treatment where one of the two treatments is discontinued because of lack of efficacy. The same is true for trials involving multiple test treatments but where one test treatment is considered superior to all others and hence the use of all other treatments is terminated in favor of the superior treatment.

The decision as to what to publish is not so straightforward when the study involves multiple test treatments and when only one of those treatments is to be discontinued. In this case, investigators must decide whether to limit results presented to those for the control treatment and the particular test treatment in question, or to include results from all other test treatments as well. Investigators in the CDP elected to follow the former approach in each of the three papers detailing protocol changes in that study (Coronary Drug Project Research Group, 1970b, 1972, 1973b). They followed this approach even when summarizing results leading to discontinuation of the 5.0 mg dose of estrogen. Results for a sister treatment, involving just half this dosage, were not presented in the report even though they tended to support the decision reached for the high-dose treatment. In fact, the low-dose treatment was discontinued about three years later. UGDP investigators followed the latter approach. They elected to include results for the two insulin treatments in manuscripts concerning terminations of tolbutamide and phenformin, even though the insulin treatments were not affected by the terminations (University Group Diabetes Program Research Group, 1970e, 1971b, 1975).

A complementary decision process is required when preparing the final results for a publication in which some of the treatments were discontinued before the end of the trial. In this case, the investigators must decide whether to include an updated report on the discontinued treatment groups. The UGDP investigators did include summaries for both tolbutamide and phenformin treatments in their final report (University Group Diabetes Program Research Group, 1982). The CDP investigators did not provide such updates in their final report for the three treatments stopped during the trial (Coronary Drug Project Research Group, 1975). However, many of the patients affected by those changes were enrolled and followed in a sister study (Coronary Drug Project Research Group, 1976).

24.2.5 Journal supplements versus regular issues

Investigators in large trials will have to decide whether to concentrate their paper writing efforts at the end of the trial on a single large manuscript or on a series of short manuscripts. The pros and cons of the two approaches are outlined in Table 24–3.

The trouble with any large manuscript has to do with the time and effort to prepare it and get it published. It is easier and often more satisfy-

Table 24–3 Long versus short papers

A. Long papers requiring publication as a supplemental issue of a journal

Comments
- Generally not necessary except for large-scale trials with complicated data sets
- Usually feasible only if study is prepared to cover the page charges associated with journal supplements

Advantages
- Avoids the usual space restrictions imposed on papers contained in regular journal issues
- May provide a more coherent picture of the results

Disadvantages
- Choice of journals limited to those that are willing to publish supplemental issues
- Manuscript is more difficult and time-consuming to prepare
- May be harder to locate and retrieve published papers for reasons mentioned in Section 24.2.5 (see also Chapter 26)

B. Short papers suitable for inclusion in a regular journal issue

Comment
- Task of preparing a series of short manuscripts less onerous than that of preparing one long manuscript

Advantages
- Articles appearing in regular issues of a journal may receive more reader attention and may be easier to locate and retrieve than those appearing in a journal supplement
- Need to generate a number of short papers for submission to the same or various journals over an extended time period may help maintain investigator and public interest in the trial

Disadvantages
- Space limitations by journals may make it difficult to present a coherent picture of the study results in any one paper
- A series of short papers, scattered over time and perhaps journals as well, may make it difficult for readers to obtain a comprehensive view of the study results

ing to write a series of small papers than one large one. Further, many journals have limits on the length of papers they receive. Editors may be unwilling to consider papers that exceed those limits and those who do may assess page charges to cover the cost of publication. Moreover, they may place them in supplemental issues of their journals. An added disadvantage when publication is via a journal supplement is that there may be problems in locating the issue after it is published. Journal supplements may not be listed in *Index Medicus* and MEDLINE, and even if they are, they may be hard to find in the library if they are not bound and stored with regular issues of the journal.

The main virtue of a single large manuscript rests in its completeness. It is usually easier for a reader to grasp the significance of a study if all pertinent design details and results are contained in one journal issue than when they are scattered across various issues of the same journal or among issues of different journals. The best strategy may well be a mix of the two approaches, as mentioned in Section 24.2.3 in conjunction with the UGDP phenformin results.

24.3 AUTHORSHIP AND INTERNAL REVIEW PROCEDURES

24.3.1 Introduction

A key issue in any research effort has to do with authorship and writing responsibilities for the papers produced. Basic guidelines should be worked out well in advance of the start of any writing effort. The guidelines that are developed should be reviewed and discussed by the entire investigative body before they are adopted. A good deal of debate may be required before an acceptable policy is developed.

24.3.2 Individual versus corporate authorship

The conventional approach is to list contributing authors in the masthead of the paper. All but 2 of the 113 papers reviewed in Chapter 2 had listings of this type. One paper, citation 113 in Appendix C, did not list any authors. The other paper listed a committee as the author (Management Committee of the Australian Therapeutic Trial in Mild Hypertension, 1980).

A conventional author listing works best for studies that are carried out at a single center and that involve a relatively small number of investi-

gators. It does not work well for large trials, especially those involving multiple centers. It is common in such cases to resort to corporate authorship, for example, as reflected in citations 102 through 109, from the Coronary Drug Project and most of the other citations in this chapter. However, this method of citation is not without problems. It obscures the contribution of individual authors and may work to the disadvantage of young investigators seeking promotion in university settings (Relman, 1979; Remington, 1979). Table 24–4 summarizes the pros and cons of the two authorship approaches.

The list of papers appearing in Table B–3 of Appendix B can be used to assess the authorship policies associated with trials sketched in that appendix. The 130 citations can be classified as

Table 24–4 Pros and cons of individual versus corporate authorship

---

A. Conventional authorship listing

Advantages
- Commonly accepted form of authorship
- Provides explicit indication of individuals involved in manuscript writing effort

Disadvantages
- Can result in lengthy author listing in a large-scale trial
- Can be an unfair method of dispensing credit, especially if author listing is limited simply to those involved in writing the paper
- Increases the likelihood that the study will be identified with specific individuals rather than with the entire investigative group

B. Corporate authorship

Advantages
- Avoids the interpersonal problems that can arise when it is necessary to name specific authors for key study publications
- Avoids the inequities of the conventional approach to authorship when it is not practical or feasible to list all key study personnel
- Helps underscore the collaborative nature of the study; especially important for multicenter trials
- Makes it possible to retrieve all papers of a study, via MEDLINE, under a standard corporate name, provided that the name appears as part of the title of each paper (see Section 26.2)

Disadvantages
- Corporate authorship may discourage preparation of needed papers, especially by people interested in establishing their research credentials
- Absence of named authors makes it difficult for readers to identify individuals responsible for its preparation

follows: Those listing only a corporate author (55), those listing only individual authors (55), with the remainder containing both the study name and the names of individual authors. The classification is based on author listing as provided by the individual studies. As such, they may differ from the citations appearing in Appendix I (Combined Bibliography). Preference has been given to use of corporate listings in the body of this book to allow all citations for a given study to appear together under the same heading.

The listings in Table B–3 do not necessarily correspond to those appearing in *Index Medicus* or computerized versions of the Index. For example, the author listing for citation 346 (Combined Bibliography), as retrieved via MED-LINE, lists Lachin, Marks, Schoenfield, Tyor, Bennett, Grundy, Hardison, Shaw, Thistle, and Vlahcevic as authors. No mention is made of the NCGS Protocol Committee or the National Cooperative Gallstone Study Group in the author field. Only Schoenfield and Lachin are listed as authors for citation 347 in the MED-LINE file. The official study listing in Appendix B (citation 5.4 in Table B–3) lists 16 other authors and the National Cooperative Gallstone Study Group.

The authorship approach used for specific papers produced in a trial may vary depending on their relevance to the main aims of the trial. Most of the studies sketched in Appendix B that have published papers used a corporate listing (with or without mention of individual authors) for mainline papers, i.e., those containing original treatment results or basic information on the design and methods of the study. Papers of secondary importance to the trial, for example, those related to ancillary studies or to secondary aims of the trials, for the most part, were published using a conventional author format. However, even here exceptions can be noted, such as in the Coronary Drug Project. It used a corporate format for nearly all of its publications.

24.3.3   Writing responsibilities

The head of the investigative group, in conjunction with the leadership committee of the study, is responsible for stimulating the production of manuscripts. The first step in the process is to prepare a list of potential publications early in the course of the trial. The list should be as exhaustive as possible and may include papers that never get written. The entries on the list should be ranked in order of their importance in relation to the aims and needs of the trial. It is also useful to prepare a timetable indicating when work might begin for each paper on the list. The list should be reviewed at periodic intervals over the course of the trial to reflect changes in writing strategies as the trial proceeds.

Most writing efforts will involve a team approach. The team should be designated by the head of the investigative group (in conjunction with the leadership committee). Each team should have a designated chief and should be composed of members with the expertise and resolve needed to write the paper. Papers that involve analyses of study results should include a biostatistician. The number of papers commissioned for development at any one time should be controlled so as not to exceed the manpower and computing resources of the study.

The finished paper may or may not list the writing team. Team members may be included in the masthead of the paper, as in the NCGS papers discussed above, in a footnote to the title of the paper or on the credit page, as in the Coronary Drug Project paper on design, methods, and baseline results (citation 104), or may not be revealed at all, as in CDP results publications (citations 102, 103, 105, 107, and 108).

24.3.4   Credit rosters

Completed papers should contain a general credit roster that lists the centers in the study and their key personnel. The roster should also specify the membership of committees responsible for operation of the trial. The roster serves the dual purpose of documenting individual contributions to the study while at the same time providing readers with information concerning facilities and staff involved in the study. Exemplary credit rosters are contained in citations 104, 346, and 376.

24.3.5   Internal review procedures

The study investigators should subject manuscripts to rigorous review before they are submitted for publication. The review may be carried out by a standing committee of senior investigators from the study or by an ad hoc group appointed for the purpose of reviewing a given manuscript. The CDP used the former approach and had a standing committee of seven senior investigators that was responsible for all reviews. The chairman of the committee selected two or three persons from the committee to review any given manuscript.

It may be useful to supplement the review process by circulating the penultimate draft of a manuscript to the entire investigative group for comments. However, this step should not be used as a substitute for the review processes mentioned above.

The types of papers requiring internal review and the conditions that must be satisfied to clear them for submission to journals should be spelled out before any writing is done. The review and clearance processes will differ depending on the nature of the manuscript. The content and conclusions of papers containing key findings may have to be approved by the entire investigative group before submission. The investigative group may transfer approval authority to the chairman of the editorial review group for more technical papers dealing with results related to a secondary aim of the trial or with the design and methods of the trial. Papers concerning ancillary studies that are published under the names of individual authors may not go through any formal approval process.

24.4 INFORMATION ACCESS POLICY ISSUES

24.4.1 Access to study data during the trial by outside parties

Requests for study results by parties from outside the study can arise before any results have been published. The requests may be politely ignored in privately funded trials but they are not as easily disposed of in those that are federally funded, especially if the requests are made under the Freedom of Information Act (FOIA).[3] This Act has been used in a few instances to force investigators to release data against their will. For example, it was used by the *National Enquirer*, a weekly tabloid, to obtain treatment results from an ongoing trial sponsored by the Veterans Administration (Montgomery, 1979).

There is still a great deal of uncertainty regarding the limits of the Act as it relates to

---

3. See documents from the Ethics Advisory Board of the Department of Health and Human Services (1980) for a review of the Act and of testimony concerning the Act in relation to clinical trials.

ongoing federally funded trials. Proposals to amend the FOIA to exempt ongoing trials from requests under the Act have been introduced into Congress, but have not been enacted (personal communication with Office of the Director of the National Institutes of Health, July, 1983). There are obvious dangers in allowing any exemptions to the Act. However, unlimited public access to data before a trial is completed has dangers as well. The value of a trial can be compromised with a forced data release. The ensuing publicity may hamper the enrollment of additional patients and may make continued treatment of those already enrolled difficult, if not impossible. Other dangers may be more far-reaching. A pattern of forced releases would almost certainly render future investigators reluctant to undertake long-term trials. The end result would be even less adequate evaluation of treatments than that which exists at present.

Court rulings to date have not been of much help in defining the limits of the Act. Even the United States Supreme Court ruling concerning public access to UGDP data was limited to the specifics of that case (United States Supreme Court, 1980).

Requests for data or analyses not citing the FOIA should be considered on an individual basis. Most of the requests will arise from colleagues and researchers who are interested in some aspects of the disease or treatment being studied. Factors to be addressed in deciding how to respond to requests include assessments of the:

- Efforts involved in meeting the requests
- Medical and scientific importance of the data or analyses requested
- Willingness of the requesters to abide by constraints imposed by study investigators on the uses that can be made of the data or analyses requested

There should be an understanding of the way in which the data or analyses will be used before the request is filled. If the requested data or analyses are to be part of a publication, there should be an agreement as to how the trial will be acknowledged and the level of review authority retained in the trial over analyses or statements produced by the requester. No information should be released that reveals the identity of individual patients, nor should the release permit the requester to carry out analyses by treatment group if the trial is still under way.

24.4.2 Access to study data at the conclusion of the trial

Investigators involved in any trial have a responsibility to facilitate access to pertinent study data once the trial is completed. Part of this responsibility can be met with a publication policy that includes extensive data summaries and patient listings (devoid of personal identifiers) for key baseline and follow-up data, such as those provided in appendixes to several of the UGDP publications (University Group Diabetes Program Research Group, 1970e, 1975, 1982). A well-written paper will provide readers with sufficient detail to allow them to verify the accuracy of key analyses. Tables and listings that are too extensive to be published as part of the manuscript can be made available through other means, such as the National Technical Information Service (NTIS, see Glossary).

It is desirable to release the entire data file (except for patient identifying information) during the termination stage of the trial or sooner in trials involving treatment terminations. The usual approach is to prepare a paper listing or magnetic tape of pertinent baseline and follow-up data, which is deposited at a central facility, as was done in the UGDP (University Group Diabetes Program Research Group, 1977). The repository may be the sponsoring agency, the data center, or some other study center (provided it remains in operation after termination of the trial). The NTIS or some commercial repository should be used if there is no center in the study willing or able to assume the repository role.

24.4.3 Access to study forms and manuals

Copies of data forms, manuals, and other design documents used in the trial should be made available to the public once they have been approved for use in the trial, unless there are convincing arguments to the contrary. The arguments should indicate how the study would be harmed if the documents in question were released. Any release proscription should be lifted as soon as possible and always by the time the trial is completed. Multicenter trials should designate the access point for design documents. Publications from the trial should specify the types of documents that are available and where and how they may be obtained.

24.4.4 Inquiries from the press

Queries from the press can arise at any point in the course of the trial. However, they are most likely at the start and when results are presented or published. Press coverage can serve a useful purpose when done in a responsible manner. Publicity at the start of the trial can help with patient recruitment. That arising in conjunction with a presentation or publication of results can help familiarize physicians and patients alike with the key findings of the trial.

Requests for information should be handled as forthrightly and expeditiously as possible. A good reporter will indicate the purpose of his request and will provide respondents with the opportunity to review his copy for errors or misstatements before it is aired or printed. Requests for information having to do with the design and methods of the trial should be honored regardless of when they arise in the course of the trial, unless there are sound operational or scientific reasons for withholding the information. Requests for interim results or other details arising during the trial which, if honored, are likely to compromise patient care or have an adverse effect on the trial must of necessity be denied. Most reporters, once given the rationale for the denial, will appreciate the need for withholding the information.

There should be only one individual authorized to speak for a center in the trial (e.g., the center director or the public relations officer of his institution). All queries received by that center should be referred to that individual for response.

The chairman of the study, director of the coordinating center, project officer, or some other person designated by the investigative group should be chosen to respond to queries concerning the study design or results in multicenter trials. The choice should be made early in the course of the trial and should be made known to all personnel in the various centers in the trial. Investigators should agree on the types of queries that may be answered locally and those that must be referred for response.

Publicity concerning study results in preparation for presentation or publication should be avoided. Publicity arising from "leaks" at those times can serve to divert the energies of study personnel from the task at hand and may anger members of the medical and lay community if they read or hear of results in the news media before they have been presented or published in a scientific forum. Investigators need to avoid actions that may attract unwanted attention. Members of the study group, particularly those privy to interim results, such as members of the safety monitoring committee, need to be reminded of the importance of silence until results have been presented or published. This policy of restraint should be coupled with defensive measures that can be implemented if leaks occur. The measures may include preparation of a statement concerning the study results that can be released to the press if publicity occurs prior to the scheduled publication or presentation. Investigators in the Coronary Drug Project took this precautionary step with each of their mainline results papers (Coronary Drug Project Research Group, 1970b, 1972, 1973b, 1975). Fortunately none of the statements were needed.

Investigators should be mindful of the practices of the organizers of meetings and journals that may lead to unexpected press coverage. Some publishers provide members of the press with copies of selected papers in advance of publication. Others, such as the *New England Journal of Medicine*, while having policies against such practices, offer subscription packages that include provisions for express delivery of journals after they have been printed. Investigators should assume that major newspapers and wire services will have such subscriptions and that they will have their copies several days before they appear on the desks of regular subscribers. Further, it is wise to assume that the program and published abstracts of papers to be presented at national meetings will be available to members of the press before the actual meeting date. The advance publicity concerning the UGDP tolbutamide results arose from distribution of the program of the American Diabetes Association several weeks before the actual meeting date (see Section 7.4 for details).

24.4.5 Special analyses in response to criticisms

Once the results have been published, study investigators may be urged to carry out a number of special analyses by friends and foes of the study. They will have to decide how much time and effort they wish to devote to such activities. The approach taken will depend on the relevance of the requests in relation to the aims and needs of the trial. Certainly, any analysis that

has the potential of shedding additional light on the results should be pursued.

As a result, the cost of such analyses will have to be borne by the study, except in cases where they are done simply to satisfy the needs of the requesting party. An intangible benefit from deposit of a data listing or tape with an outside agency, as discussed in Section 24.4.2, has to do with outside requests for analyses. Once the deposit is made, any request can be dealt with by referring the requester to the repository for the data needed to perform his own analyses.

A particularly vexing question has to do with the resources that should be devoted to responding to published critiques of a trial. Some restraint is necessary because of the investment of effort required if the criticisms are extensive. In addition, the energy devoted to response may limit that available for other more essential activities. Investigators in the UGDP were concerned enough about energy dissipation that they limited their responses to criticisms which appeared in refereed journals. They declined to reply to editorials and critiques appearing in unrefereed publications such as the *Medical Tribune*.

There is another reason for restraint. Investigators run the risk of losing objectivity and damaging their credibility if they become too preoccupied with defending their own work. The philosophy needed for a sound investigation is at odds with that needed for advocacy of a position. For this reason, if none other, it is important that responses be thoughtful and devoid of emotion.

24.4.6 Outside audits

It may be necessary to provide for special audits of the study results if there are questions regarding their accuracy. The data records and analyses of the UGDP were subjected to two independent audits (Committee for the Assessment of Biometric Aspects of Controlled Trials of Hypoglycemic Agents, 1975; Food and Drug Administration, 1978). Special clearances will be required if auditors are to be provided access to the medical records of specific patients. To be of any value, the audits should be done by parties who are independent of the study, the sponsoring agency, and firms or groups that stand to gain or lose from the study results. The auditors should prepare a written report of the audit that is then published or placed on file for public access.

25. Preparation of the study publication

Revise and revise and revise—the best thought will come after the printer has snatched away the copy.

Michael Monahan

25.1 INTRODUCTION

This chapter focuses on the task of preparing the study findings for publication. The outline in Table 25–1 assumes a single publication that contains a summary of the main findings of the trial, as well as information on its design and operation. In fact, as noted in Chapter 24, a trial may produce a number of publications.

25.2 PREPARATORY STEPS

Most of the preparatory steps needed to write the paper have been alluded to in previous chapters. An essential first step involves preparation of the data for analysis by creation of an analysis tape, as discussed in Section 17.7.

There must be agreement among investigators as to how the paper will be authored and as to who will head the writing team (see Sections 24.3.2 and 24.3.3). The review steps that must be completed before the paper is submitted for publication should be delineated as well. In addition, there should be agreement among the investigators as to who in the study will have review authority over the paper and how conflicts between the authors and the review group will be resolved (see Section 24.3.5).

An essential step involves preparation of an outline of the paper. The outline should be as detailed as possible and should include a mockup of tables needed for the paper. It should be reviewed and approved by the leadership of the study before the writing starts and should be revised as needed during the writing effort.

25.3 CONTENT SUGGESTIONS

Table 25–1 outlines general content suggestions for the publication. The remainder of this section relates to this outline.

25.3.1 Title section

The title is one of the most important parts of any publication. It is the prime item used by readers to screen for publications of interest. A good title is neither cute nor cryptic. It conveys its message in a crisp and succinct manner. It should indicate the main thrust of the paper in as few words as possible. Superfluous words add to its length without making any contribution to content.

Examples of good and bad titles follow, as taken from citations listed in Appendix C. The number in parentheses following each title refers to the citation number in that Appendix.

Cryptic

- Blood pressure in the elderly (16). *What kind of blood pressure? High blood pressure? Low blood pressure? There is no way of knowing from the title if the paper contains data pertinent to the assessment of different forms of antihypertensive treatments in the elderly.*

- Event recording in a clinical trial of a new medicine (89). *What kind of event? What kind of new medicine?*
- Clinical metrology—A future career grade? (122). *Metrology in what area? What is meant by a career grade?*
- Evaluation of toxicity: Clinical issues (175). *What kind of toxicity? What clinical issues?*

Needlessly detailed

- High-dose methotrexate with "RESCUE" plus cyclophosphamide as initial chemotherapy in ovarian adenocarcinoma. A randomized trial with observations on the influence of C parvum immunotherapy (7). *Title could be shortened without much loss of information by deleting the phrase* with observations on the influence of C parvum immunotherapy.
- A clinical trial of alignment of teeth using a 0.019 inch thermal nitinol wire with a transition temperature range between 31 degrees C. and 45 degrees C. (115). *Too much methodological detail.*
- Medical, ethical and legal aspects of clinical trials in pediatrics. Summary of a forum discussion held at the 'International Workshop on Perinatal and Pediatric Aspects of Clinical Pharmacology,' Heidelberg, Federal Republic of Germany, February 27-29, 1980 (143). *Details regarding the meeting are not necessary.*

Good

- Controlled trial of cimetidine in reflux esophagitis (27).
- Amoxycillin versus ampicillin in treatment of exacerbations of chronic bronchitis (53).
- Cimetidine in the prophylaxis of migraine (69).
- Postoperative epilepsy: A double-blind trial of phenytoin after craniotomy (71).

Titles should be written to include the term *trial* to facilitate identification via title scans. One way this can be accomplished is to include the name of the study in the title if it includes the term. Unfortunately, investigators often use other less descriptive terms, such as *study, program,* or *project,* in place of *trial* (see Table B–6 of Appendix B for list of study names). The term *trial* should be added to the title of the paper when it is not part of the official title of the study.

A titling convention in which papers are sequentially numbered, for example, as in the University Group Diabetes Program (UGDP), is worth considering, especially if it is clear from the outset that the study will generate a number of publications. The numbering scheme alerts readers to the existence of other papers in the series.

Some journals require authors to list a few key words that characterize the content of the paper. The words usually appear below the title or abstract of the paper. Key words serve two purposes: They indicate the thrust of the paper to readers, and they help indexers classify it under the proper subject headings in *Index Medicus* and MEDLINE.

25.3.2 Abstract section

The abstract of the paper is second only to the title in importance. It provides a summary of the paper and, as a result, is usually the first and often the only part that is read, other than the title. In addition, inclusion of the abstract in the MEDLINE data file (the computerized version of *Index Medicus*) makes it possible for users of that file to identify the paper by searching the abstract for terms or phrases of interest. The abstract should include the items of information, listed in Part 2 of Table 25–1. A sample abstract, taken from the Persantine Aspirin Reinfarction Study (PARIS), meets most of the content requirements listed (Persantine Aspirin Reinfarction Study Research Group, 1980b).

Summary. In the Persantine-Aspirin Reinfarction Study (PARIS) trial, 2026 persons who had recovered from myocardial infarction (MI) were randomized into three groups: Persantine plus aspirin (PR/A) (n = 810); aspirin alone (ASA) (n = 810); placebo (PLBO) (n = 406). The average length of follow-up study was 41 months. Results for the three specified primary end points were: total mortality 16% lower in PR/A and 18% lower in ASA compared with PLBO; coronary mortality 24% and 21% lower; incidence of nonfatal MI plus fatal coronary disease 25% and 24% lower. These differences were not statistically significant by the study criterion (Z ≥ 2.6). By life-table analysis, the rates of coronary mortality and coronary incidence were about 50% lower in the PR/A group than in the PLBO group from 8-24 months, and for

Table 25-1 Content suggestions for the study publication

---

1. Title section
- Descriptive title
- List of author-selected key words indicating general content of paper (useful for readers and as an aid to NLM indexers)
- Author(s)
- Source(s) of financial support for the study
- Acknowledgments
- Credit roster (see Section 24.3.4)
- Address for reprint requests

2. Abstract section
- Purpose of study
- Primary outcome measure
- Test treatment(s)
- Control treatment(s)
- Level of treatment masking
- Number of patients enrolled
- Method of treatment allocation
- Conclusion(s)

3. Introduction section
- Historical background of trial
- Rationale for a trial
- Objective(s)
- Rationale for choice of test and control treatment(s)
- Literature review

4. Methods section
- Study population
  Eligibility and exclusion criteria
  Method of patient recruitment
- Treatments
  Study treatments used
  Method of treatment administration
  Level of treatment masking
  Treatment proscriptions
  Methods of measuring treatment adherence
- Outcome measures
  Primary and secondary outcome measures
  Diagnostic criteria for outcome measurements
  Methods for coding and classifying outcomes
- Design specifications
  Method of randomization
    Description of the safeguards used to ensure the integrity of the allocation process
    List of stratification variables
    Blocking specifications

Description of procedures for packaging and dispensing study medications in the case of masked drug trials
Primary outcome measure and rationale for choice
Planned length of patient follow-up and rationale for specification
Planned recruitment goal
Type I and II error protection level for planned recruitment goal
- Patient safeguards
  Outline of steps for obtaining patient consent
  Method of updating consent (especially for long-term follow-up trials)
  Measures taken to protect patient confidentiality
  Description of procedures used to monitor study results for evidence of treatment effects
- Data collection schedule
  Sequence of baseline and follow-up visits
  List of data items collected
  Definition of missed visits and dropouts
  Name of person or agency to contact for copies of data forms, study manuals, etc.
- Data processing
  Cut-off date for data included in manuscript
  Description of approach and supporting rationale for dealing with missing data and departures from the treatment protocol (statement especially important if analysis method departs from preferred approach described in Chapter 18)
  Literature references for methods used
  Description of any special analysis procedures not already described in existing literature
  Methods for judging statistical importance of differences observed (e.g., simple p-values, adjusted p-values, RBOs, etc.)
- Quality control procedures
  General data editing
  Quality control of laboratory tests and for special reading and coding procedures
  Checks on data entry, programming, and analysis
  Other quality controls, such as site visits to clinics, training and certification, etc.
- Performance monitoring
  Measures used for assessing performance of participating clinics and resource centers
  Frequency of performance assessments
  Methods used for reviewing performance monitoring reports and for implementing corrective action based on those reviews
- Treatment monitoring
  Frequency of interim analyses for treatment monitoring
  Methods used to carry out interim analyses

Table 25-1 Content suggestions for the study publication (*continued*)

Individual or group responsible for carrying out interim analyses

Procedures for implementing protocol changes based on results from interim analyses

- Organizational structure
  Number and location of participating centers
  Location of data center
  Location of other resource centers
  Standing committees and their membership
  Mode of funding (e.g., grant or contract, individual or consortium award)
  Policy on investigator conflicts of interests and method used to monitor for potential conflicts of interest

- Other items
  Notation and language conventions in manuscript
  Listing of special actions taken during the trial including:
    Addition or deletion of a treatment
    Data purges because of questions concerning data reliability or accuracy
    Major modifications of data collection forms or coding procedures during the course of the trial

5. Results section
- Number of patients enrolled by treatment group

- Number of deaths by treatment group

- Comparison of treatment groups for the primary and secondary outcome measures using various analytic techniques, including simple comparisons of proportions, as well as lifetable methods, etc.

- Indicators of the completeness of follow-up by treatment group, such as:
  Number of missed examinations
  Number of dropouts
  Number of patients lost to follow-up

- Indicators of treatment adherence, such as:
  Comparison of treatment groups using an adherence score or some laboratory test
  Count of number of patients in each treatment group who received none of the assigned treatment
  Count of number of patients in each treatment group who received an alternative treatment

- Assessment of the comparability of the treatment groups with regard to important baseline characteristics

- Treatment group comparisons for differences in:
  Occurrence of serious side effects
  Rate of hospitalization
  Other general health indicators

- Treatment comparisons by selected baseline characteristics

- Multiple regression analyses using baseline characteristics to provide adjusted treatment comparisons

- Treatment comparisons by level of adherence

- Treatment comparisons by clinic (in multicenter trials)

- Other special analyses relating follow-up data for one variable (e.g., cholesterol level) to a primary or secondary outcome measure (e.g., death)

6. Discussion section
- Discussion of how reported findings relate to previous studies, paying particular attention to those considered to be new and those that are not consistent with findings of previous studies

- Discussion of the implications of the findings

- Enumeration of questions or areas needing further analysis or research

7. Conclusion section
- Statement of conclusion

- Limits on generalization of the conclusions, including discussion of observed statistical power if no treatment difference is detected

8. Reference section
- List of literature references in required journal format

- Suitable reference citations for:
  References to previous work
  Data analysis methods
  Methods not described in the paper
  Laboratory methods
  Coding or reading procedures for abstracting information from special records or documents
  Treatment methods
  Study rationale
  Discussion of results

- List of study documents that may be obtained on request, such as study manual of operations, study data forms, data listings, data tapes, etc.

9. Appendix section*
- Descriptions of special procedures needed to understand results, but too detailed to be included in the body of the publication

- List of definitions, codes, diagnostic criteria, etc.

- Special analyses, tabulations, and data listings

- Sample data forms

---

*Not required if previous publications contain essential details or if authors have provided some other means of supplying them (e.g., by depositing documents containing details in a public repository or by supplying them upon written request).

coronary incidence all Z values were $\geq$ 2.6; ASA rates were about 30% lower than PLBO rates, and for coronary incidence, Z values were $\geq$ 2.6 at two points. For these end points, from 8-20 months, PR/A rates were about 30% lower than ASA rates, but all Z values were $<$ 2.0. PR/A and ASA patients entering within 6 months of last MI showed the largest percentage reductions in mortality; only the difference between PR/A and PLBO groups for 3-year coronary mortality yielded a Z value of 2.6.[1]

25.3.3 Introductory section

This section may be short or quite long depending on the nature of the literature review. Its prime purpose is to set the stage for the remainder of the paper. It should indicate why the paper is being written, describe the rationale for the study and its objectives, and should recap research that led to initiation of the study.

25.3.4 Methods section

The details contained in most reports of clinical trials are too sketchy to allow readers to make informed judgments concerning their quality, as noted in Chapter 2 and in Meinert et al. (1984). The absence of essential details is a reflection of the failure of authors and editors alike to recognize their importance in making these judgments.

The contents of the methods section must be checked against some predefined list, such as contained in Part 4 of Table 25-1, if reporting lapses are to be avoided. Information found to be missing when the check is made should be added before the paper is submitted for publication. Details that have to be omitted because of space constraints imposed by the journal should be provided via other means (e.g., in another paper devoted primarily to the design and methods of the trial, or by depositing essential design and operating documents from the trial in some repository for access by interested parties).

25.3.5 Results section

This section is usually the longest one in the paper. Suggestions for its content are outlined in Part 5 of Table 25-1. The essence of a paper

1. Reference citation 376. Reproduced with permission of the American Heart Association, Inc., Dallas, Texas.

should be captured in the tables, charts, and figures it contains. They should be interpretable without reference to supporting text in the body of the paper. The titles and legends accompanying them should be accurately and succinctly written.

25.3.6 Discussion section

This section (see Part 6 of Table 25-1) should highlight noteworthy findings appearing in the results section. It should be used to discuss the clinical implications of the findings and to indicate the extent to which they are considered to support or refute previous findings.

25.3.7 Conclusion section

This section (see Part 7 of Table 25-1) may appear at the beginning or end of the paper. It should contain a statement of the conclusions drawn from the trial and of the limitations on the generalizability of the findings. It should also contain a discussion of the statistical power of the study if the conclusion favors the null hypothesis (see Section 9.7).

25.3.8 Reference section

A well-written paper will contain a supporting bibliography. The papers included should be those that are needed to document data collection and analysis methods used in the trial, as well as those needed in the introduction and discussion sections of the paper. The citations should be listed at the end of the paper and should either be arranged alphabetically or in the order in which they are referenced in the text. Most journals will indicate the referencing style to be followed. A paper that is written before a decision is reached on the journal that is to receive it should be referenced using general methods, such as outlined by editors of medical journals (International Committee of Medical Journal Editors, 1982) or in a general desk reference, such as the *Chicago Manual of Style* (University of Chicago Press, 1982).

Only papers cited in the text should be listed in the reference section of the paper. Original articles should be referenced whenever possible. A secondary source, such as a textbook or review article, may be cited if the original article appeared in an obscure or foreign language journal, or if the secondary source helps to explain or expand upon information contained in the original article.

The listing should provide all the authors' names in the case of conventionally authored materials. The preferred approach is to list the last name, followed by the initials of each author. The author field should contain the appropriate corporate designation if the article in question was written on behalf of some research group, institute, agency, or committee. See reference citations 104, 375, 376, 467, 468, 472, and 476 in the Combined Bibliography (Appendix I) for examples.

The citations should include the full titles of the articles being cited. They are useful to readers when scanning the references for articles of interest. They should also include full journal names or accepted abbreviations, such as those used in *Index Medicus* and MEDLINE (National Library of Medicine, 1983). The volume number of the journal, date of publication, and beginning and ending page numbers of each article cited should be listed as well.

The citation listing should be checked for accuracy before the manuscript is submitted for publication. The checking should be done from the actual articles cited and not from MEDLINE printouts or citations listed in other bibliographies.

25.3.9 Appendix section

This section should contain materials that, while important in understanding the paper, are too technical or detailed to warrant inclusion in the main body of the paper. Items that appear in the appendixes of publications (see 104, 375, 467, 468, 472, and 476 cited above) include:

- Details of the sample size calculations
- Baseline frequency distributions
- Sample data forms
- Data collection schedules
- Derivation of analytic procedures
- Special charts or figures
- Data listings
- Special analyses or tabulations
- Descriptions of coding and classification schemes
- Consent statements
- Organizational and administrative documents

The use of appendixes is possible only if the journal in question allows them. Other avenues, such as discussed in Chapter 24 involving supplemental issues of a journal or deposit of key documents at a public repository, will have to be used when appendixes are ruled out by page limitations or other policies imposed by the journal.

25.4 INTERNAL REVIEW AND SUBMISSION

The manuscript should be subjected to a series of reviews and checks before it is submitted for publication. The first review should be done by the authors and should be designed to check for inconsistencies in format or style, for redundant statements, and for reporting deficiencies. The later review should be made using a checklist, such as represented in Table 25-1. The titles and legends of tables, charts, and figures should be checked for clarity of exposition and accuracy. The numerical information presented in tables and graphs should be checked for errors. The text of the paper should be checked to make certain that figures cited agree with the numbers appearing in the tables. Key analyses should be repeated, ideally by a second person, and the results of the two analyses should be compared. All discrepancies should be resolved before the paper is submitted for publication.

Information taken from published literature should be checked against the cited source. This checking process will be simplified if all cited documents are collected as the manuscript is developed. The resulting file will serve as a valuable resource for future papers on the same subject and for checking reference listings and other information contained in the manuscript.

The second round of reviews should be by colleagues selected by the authors or the study leadership (see Section 24.3.5). These reviews will help to identify areas of the paper that are confusing and that need additional work. Major changes proposed during this round of reviews or any of the other reviews outlined above may require a total revision of the paper and another round of checks and reviews.

It is a good idea to allow some time for "maturation" of the paper after it is drafted and before it is submitted for publication. The checking and review processes take time. They will lose much of their value if performed under duress because of the imposition of unrealistic deadlines.

The final draft of the paper should be checked to make certain that the format conforms to that specified by the journal selected to receive it. The instructions supplied by the journal should be reviewed to make certain that the correct number of copies is submitted and that glossy prints of all figures and charts are provided. The paper should contain the address and phone number of the corresponding (usually senior) author. A copy of the paper and accompanying glossy prints (if any) should be retained by the corresponding author. The cover page of the manuscript should indicate the date the paper was submitted for publication. All previous drafts of the paper should be removed from the author's file and stored elsewhere once it has been mailed to the journal to avoid mixups if the journal, a reviewer, or someone else requests copies of the manuscript before it is published.

25.5 ACCEPTANCE AND PUBLICATION

The journal will carry out its own reviews of the manuscript. They will be used by the editor to reach a decision as to whether to accept the paper. They may also serve as the basis for additional changes to the paper if it is accepted for publication. Publication may take place shortly after acceptance or months later, depending on the backlog of manuscripts awaiting publication and the publication schedule of the journal.

The corresponding author is responsible for ordering reprints. The number ordered should be sufficient to supply co-authors with an appropriate number, as well as all other people listed in the credit roster of the paper.

The corresponding author (or one of the other authors) should establish an archive that contains all documents related to the development and publication of the paper. The initial steps for this process should be taken long before publication. The last steps in the process should take place just after the paper has been published. The completed file should contain:

- Copies of data tapes and computer programs used for analyses included in the paper
- Copies of papers and other documents referenced in the paper
- Intermediate drafts of the paper, particularly those containing major revisions
- A copy of the manuscript submitted for publication
- Copies of written critiques of the paper, as provided by the journal, and correspondence relating to the critiques
- A copy of the manuscript as accepted for publication
- Page proofs
- The published manuscript

The archive should be kept in a safe place and maintained indefinitely. Key documents, such as data tapes and related materials, should be duplicated and stored in separate locations if they are considered irreplaceable.

Errors in the paper detected after publication should be noted by the corresponding author. The journal editor should be informed of those that are serious.

26. Locating and reading published reports

Be sparing of criticism, since the habit of trivial comment weakens the force of real protest.
Alan Gregg

26.1 INTRODUCTION

This chapter deals with a potpourri of topics related to the identification and evaluation of reports relevant to the design and conduct of clinical trials. Section 26.2 focuses on a review of methods for developing bibliographies of results from clinical trials. Section 26.3 is concerned with issues to be considered when reviewing a published report from a trial. The last two sections are written from the point of view of an individual who is responsible for preparing a written critique of a report from a clinical trial. Section 26.4 provides a discussion of what constitutes valid criticisms. The last section outlines the characteristics of a responsible critic.

26.2 BIBLIOGRAPHY DEVELOPMENT

The development of a bibliography is likely to include any of the following techniques:

- Review of selected journals for papers of interest
- Search of classes of journals, via *Current Contents* or some other means, for titles of interest
- Systematic search of papers or computerized indexes, such as contained in *Index Medicus* or MEDLINE
- Use of the *Science Citation Index* to identify authors who have cited a particular paper

(used to identify authors working in a particular field as an aid to building a bibliography of papers related to that field)
- Review of bibliographies of published papers for citations of interest
- Pursuit of leads offered by colleagues or from other sources, such as the news media, regarding specific papers or pieces of work

Table 26-1 contains a list of databases of published reports and work in progress (see also Roper and Boorkman, 1980; Sciotti et al., 1982). The list represents a selection of existing files considered by the authors to be useful in constructing bibliographies related to the design, conduct, and results of clinical trials.

Locating reports of clinical trials is complicated by the way in which they are titled (as discussed in Section 1.3 and in Section 25.3.1) and because of the absence of a subject heading for clinical trials in most existing indexes. A notable exception is *Index Medicus* and MEDLINE, starting with 1980 (see Chapter 2). The usefulness of title searches for identification of trials is limited without such headings. Only 21 of the 130 references (16%) in Table B-3, Appendix B, had the term *trial* in the title. Designers of trials appear to prefer terms such as *study, program,* or *project.* Only two of the 14 trials listed in Appendix B had names containing the term *trial* (see Table B-1, Appendix B). Among the 113 trials reviewed in Chapter 2, less than 40% (44 out of 113) of the titles contained the term *trial* or the design words *blind, randomized,* or *controlled.*

The difficulty in identifying work in progress extends to methodological work as well. The best that can be done at present is to rely on special annotated bibliographies, such as the one produced by Fletcher and co-workers (Research Development Committee, Society for Research and Education in Primary Care Internal Medicine, 1983) concerning clinical research methods, and by Hawkins (see citations 227 through 230), in her periodic reviews of literature related to clinical trials.

Papers concerned with statistical issues in the design, conduct, or analysis of clinical trials must be

271

Table 26-1   Selected printed and computerized databases of published literature and work in progress

Database	Comments
A. Published literature	
• *Index Medicus*	• Listings of titles, authors, and abstracts of papers appearing in some 2,700 medical journals and periodicals. Publication started in 1879. Published under the title *Index Medicus* beginning in 1960. Entries indexed by author and subject. Has subject heading for clinical trials starting in 1980. Before 1980, articles on clinical trials appeared under the more general heading *clinical research.*
• MEDLINE (Medical Literature Analysis Retrieval System: MEDLARS on Line)	• Computer file of *Index Medicus, International Nursing Index, Index to Dental Literature,* and part of *Hospital Index.* File contains titles, authors, and abstracts of papers appearing in some 3,000 biomedical journals. File may be searched by author or subject. Titles and abstracts can be searched with user-selected words. Introduced in 1966; with abstracts since 1975. Contains subject heading for clinical trials starting in 1980. Before 1980, articles on clinical trials appeared under the heading *clinical research.*
• SCI (*Science Citation Index*)	• Exists both as a paper and computer file (SCISEARCH). The computer file contains all entries published in the *Science Citation Index* plus additional entries from the *Current Contents* series of publications. SCI is unique in that it identifies papers cited in articles appearing in some 2,600 journals and periodicals. The Index allows users to identify articles that reference a particular paper. May be searched by author or title words. Started in 1961. Published on a continuing basis since 1964; computerized version since 1970.
• BIOSIS (*Biological Abstracts*)	• Exists both as a paper and computer file. Includes publications from journals, books, symposiums, reviews, notes, and research communications from the life sciences. Does not have subject headings, only broad headings called *concept headings.* First publication of printed version of the file: 1926; computerized version of file introduced in 1969. Contains citations for some statistical literature.
• CATLINE (Catalog on Line)	• Computer equivalent of *National Library of Medicine Current Catalog.* Includes listing of all serials, monographs, and books (all languages), collected by the National Library of Medicine, and published after 1801. The Catalog was first published in 1966. It has a subject heading for clinical trials beginning in 1980.
• CLINPROT (Clinical Protocols)	• Computer-based data file containing summaries of clinical investigations of new anticancer agents and treatments,

identified by screening statistical journals or methods journals, such as *Controlled Clinical Trials.* There are a number of indexes that contain citations to statistical and methods papers pertinent to clinical trials (e.g., *Biological Abstracts, Current Contents, Psychological Abstracts, Chemical Abstracts, Public Affairs Information Service* (PAIS), *Mathematical Reviews,* and *Excerpta Medica*), but they are not identified as such in the indexes.

26.3 QUESTIONS AND FACTORS TO CONSIDER WHEN READING A REPORT FROM A CLINICAL TRIAL

Table 26–2 lists questions to be considered when reading a published report. The greater the number of affirmative answers the better the reporting process.

The reader should form his own judgment on the

Table 26-1 Printed and computerized databases of published literature and work in progress (*continued*)

Database	Comments
	with emphasis on clinical trials. File may be searched using an index of 300 clinical terms or via user-selected words.
• CANCERLIT (Cancer Literature)	• Computer-based data file containing over 260,000 citations and abstracts of published literature relating to cancer. Created originally from *Cancer Therapy Abstracts* (started in 1967) and *Carcinogenesis Abstracts* (started in 1963). Both ceased publication in 1980. Titles or abstracts may be searched via user-selected words. Entries since 1980 have been indexed using NLM subject headings, including one for clinical trials.
• EMED (*Excerpta Medica*)	• Computer-based data file containing citations from over 3,500 biomedical journals. File consists of entries from 43 abstract journals and the two literature indexes that make up the printed *Excerpta Medica*, plus selected entries not appearing in the printed publications. Contains citations from June 1974 forward. Has subject headings for clinical trials and controlled clinical trials.
• MATHFILE (*Mathematical Reviews*)	• Computer-based data file of references to mathematical and statistical papers.
B. Unpublished work in progress	
• CRISP (Computer Retrieval of Information on Scientific Projects)	• Computer-based data file of information on research projects currently funded via the NIH and other agencies of the United States Public Health Service. File may be searched by subject, project, agency of support, or investigator. Introduced in 1971. Does not contain heading for clinical trials.
• RAI (*Research Award Index*)	• Paper listing of research grants and contracts awarded by the National Institutes of Health, by fiscal year. Produced from CRISP. Published in two volumes: Volume I is arranged by research subject; Volume II contains sections organized by project, by grant or contract number, and by investigator. Produced since 1962. Does not contain a subject heading for clinical trials.
• NTIS (National Technical Information Service)	• Both a paper-based and computerized data file of over 970,000 documents available through the NTIS. Documents stored at the NTIS are government-sponsored research reports prepared by federal agencies of the United States government or their grantees or contractors. NTIS has been in operation since 1964. The computer data file covers acquisitions at NTIS from 1975 forward.

basis of the merits of the study before considering opinions and critiques of others. Reviews supplied gratis by sales people from firms with a proprietary interest in the treatments should be ignored when making the judgment. The same is true for commentaries and editorials on the study appearing in throwaway medical journals.

The reader should be conscious of the motivating forces behind the study and of their possible influence on the conduct of and reports from the study. The conclusions in the paper should be questioned, if not ignored, if they appear to have been written to support the preconceived notions of the sponsor or investigators regarding the merits of the study treatments.

The role of the sponsor in the trial should be considered when reading the paper. Published reports of trials that are carried out by firms produc-

Table 26-2   Questions to consider when assessing a published report

---

1. General
- Does the manuscript indicate the purpose of the trial and rationale for the treatments studied?
- Does the trial address a relevant question?
- Is the paper in a peer review journal?

2. Investigators
- Have the investigators done any previous work related to the trial being reported? If so, do you consider the work to have been of good quality?
- Does the paper indicate the location and institutional affiliation of the various members of the team responsible for carrying out the trial?
- Does the team include people with appropriate training and expertise for conduct and analysis of the trial?

3. Sponsorship and structural
- Does the paper indicate how the trial was funded?
- Is the role of the sponsor in designing, directing, or analyzing the trial indicated? (Especially important in trials involving proprietary products.)
- Are the key investigators, especially those responsible for analyzing the results and for writing the paper, independent of the sponsor?
- Did responsibility for data collection and analysis in the trial reside with a group of people who were independent of the sponsor?
- Did the authors recognize the possibility of conflicts of interest for study members (especially important if the report concerns a proprietary product) and do they indicate steps taken to avoid such conflicts?
- If the trial involved multiple centers, does the paper list all affiliated centers and the functions performed by each?
- For multicenter trials, does the paper list committees, along with their membership and a brief description of their functions?

4. Study design

a. Outcome measure
- Is the primary outcome measure identified?
- Does it have clinical relevance?

- If multiple outcomes are used, is it clear which one is of primary importance in the trial?

b. Treatments
- Is there a defined test treatment?
- Is the test treatment of any interest and does the administration of it correspond roughly to the way it would be used in general practice?
- Is there an appropriate control treatment?

c. Study population and sample size
- Are the eligibility and exclusion criteria for patient entry into the trial stated?
- Is there a discussion of the type I and II error protection provided with the observed sample size?

d. Allocation
- Is the method of treatment allocation described?
- Does it appear to have been free of selection bias?
- Does it meet the general conditions specified in Section 8.4?

e. Data collection procedures
- Is the data collection schedule described?
- Are patients in the test and control-treated groups enrolled and followed over the same time frame?
- Does the design include adequate provisions to protect against bias in the administration of the treatment and in measurement of the outcome, as evidenced by the use of appropriate masking procedures or other safeguards?

5. Study performance
- Was a recruitment goal for the trial stated? Was it achieved?
- Was the missed examination rate low?
- Was the dropout rate low?
- Was the dropout rate among the treatment groups about the same?
- Was it possible to locate all patients, including dropouts, at the end of the study to update key morbidity and mortality data? If not, was the number who could not be located small and about the same for each treatment group?
- Did all the patients enrolled meet the eligibility criteria of the trial? If not, was the number who did not small?

---

ing the products being tested, or that fail to indicate the source of the funding, should be viewed with a healthy skepticism. The same is true for reports produced by private foundations that derive their funds from unnamed sources or from sources with interests that stand to gain or lose financially, depending on the conclusions stated in the reports. For example, the Kilo, Miller, and Williamson critique (1980) of the University Group Diabetes Program (UGDP) tolbutamide results, simply states that the analyses were supported by the Kilo Research Foundation. Evaluations of the authors' objectivity may very well be influenced by the extent to which support for the Foundation depends on money supplied by manufacturers of the oral hypoglycemic agents.

The reproducibility of the results and the generalizability of the findings reported should be care-

Table 26-2 Questions to consider when assessing a published report (*continued*)

- Was the proportion of patients who failed to receive their assigned treatment low?
- Was there a reasonably high level of adherence to the treatment regimens over the course of the study?
- Is there a description of the effort made to monitor for departures from the study protocol and for maintaining data quality? Do you consider the procedure to have been adequate, given the needs and goals of the trial?
- Does the paper indicate how laboratory analyses and readings from ECGs and other similar procedures were done?
- Does the paper contain a description of the quality control procedures used to monitor laboratory analyses and readings such as ECGs? Do you consider those procedures adequate, given the needs and goals of the trial?
- Did the laboratory or readers perform the indicated analyses or readings in a masked fashion (i.e., without knowledge of patient treatment)?

6. Data analysis procedures
- Does the methods section of the paper include descriptions of the data analysis procedures used, and are the descriptions supported with appropriate literature references?
- Are the methods of analysis appropriate?
- Is the paper based on data from all study patients? If not, does it contain a statement indicating the rationale for the data selection presented in the report? Is the rationale reasonable?
- Are the key analyses based on original treatment assignment and do they account for all patients enrolled in the trial? If not, is the number of patients not accounted for small and about the same for each treatment group?
- Are data presented to describe the baseline comparability of the study groups?
- Is there an analysis that summarizes primary outcome data by original treatment assignment?
- Are patients who failed to receive the prescribed treatment or who had low adherence to the assigned treatment counted in the treatment group to which they were randomized?

- Do the tables and graphs have intelligible headings and legends?
- Are treatment comparisons adjusted for baseline differences?
- Have the authors used a variety of analytic approaches to support their conclusions, and do they yield consistent results?
- Are there tabulations that describe the treatment trends over time, such as via the use of lifetables or cohort analyses?
- Are data presented in sufficient detail to permit the serious reader to carry out additional analyses?
- Are the results internally consistent?
- Is there a stated cutoff date for the data included in the report, and is there a stated rationale for the date used? (Especially important if the report is based on interim results.)
- Do the authors display statistical sophistication by minimizing the use of *p*-value and significance testing as a means of data interpretation?

7. Discussion
- Have the authors provided a discussion of their results?
- Are the authors familiar with other relevant findings for the treatments being evaluated?
- Do the authors support statements contained in the discussion section with appropriate literature references?

8. Conclusions
- Are the conclusions supported by the analyses presented?
- Have the authors exercised a sufficient degree of caution and conservatism in stating their conclusions?
- Have the authors refrained from overgeneralization of the findings?
- Do the authors limit their conclusions to the types of patients studied and to the treatments investigated?
- If the authors have concluded in favor of the null hypothesis, do they provide a discussion of the type II error possible with the sample size used?

---

fully examined. The reader should be skeptical of any results that pertain to a selected subset of the patients or outcomes observed. Unfortunately, it is not always easy to determine if this is the case. The fact that certain patients or outcomes have been excluded will be apparent only if the report contains statements to this effect and data for all patients randomized into the trial. Sometimes the only clue that some patients have been omitted is in

the use of a single word or phrase (e.g., as in the use of the term *evaluable patients* or the phrase *analysis by treatment received*).

In general, results from all clinics in a multicenter trial following a common study protocol should be presented in a single publication. However, another way selection can occur is when individual clinics in such trials have the option of analyzing and publishing independently of other clinics. An investigator at a clinic producing a "statistically significant" treatment difference is more likely to publish than his colleague at a clinic who failed to produce any noteworthy treatment differences. There is no easy way to know if this form of selection occurs unless the authors so indicate.

A judgment should be formed regarding the level of statistical sophistication of the authors. Slavish use of hypothesis testing should be seen as a mark of naivety in the authors. The same is true for simple characterizations of results as significant or nonsignificant, depending on whether or not associated *p*-values are below or above the magical 0.05 level.

The study design, particularly as it relates to safeguards against biases in the data collection process, should be examined. Some feeling for this may be obtained by observing the extent to which the investigators have attempted to mask data collectors in the trial. Vague statements concerning the method of patient selection and assignment to treatment should raise questions concerning the adequacy of the treatment allocation process. Any suggestion that the authors equate a haphazard (see Glossary) method of assignment to formal randomization (see Glossary for definition of random) should raise doubts regarding the validity of the study.

Part of the assessment should focus on questions concerning the quality and integrity of the data generated. The methods section of the paper should contain sufficient detail to answer questions concerning methods used to edit the data for errors or inadequacies. The absence of any discussion of this kind should raise questions concerning the adequacy of the data collection procedures used.

The reader must decide if the results observed can be explained by differences in the baseline composition of the treatment groups, by a differential dropout rate, or by major differences in treatment compliance. Failure to provide information that allows the reader to address these issues should be viewed as a deficiency in the report.

Finally, a good paper will indicate if the results presented are from interim or final analyses of the data, and if they are of the former type why they are being presented now as opposed to later when the trial is finished.

26.4   VALID AND INVALID CRITICISMS

There is no such thing as a perfect study, only varying degrees of imperfection. The professional critic can always cite one or more of the criticisms listed in Table 26-3 without fear of contradiction. For example, he can always argue that the results of the trial should be ignored because the investigators studied the "wrong" population. Or he can challenge the choice of treatments or the way in which they were administered. And it is always possible to chide investigators because they failed to collect "important" data—at least as viewed from the perspective of the critic. The problem is not coming up with criticisms, but in deciding whether or not they are valid. The trouble with the criticisms listed in Table 26-3 is that they are so broad and sweeping as to be beyond debate.

A criticism, to be valid, should:

- Have some basis in fact
- Be buttressed with supporting evidence
- Make a difference in the interpretation of the results

All three tests should be met. Among the three, the third is the most difficult one to satisfy. For example, it is fairly easy to criticize a trial because of differences in the baseline composition of the treatment groups. However, it is quite another thing to show how those differences might have accounted

Table 26–3   Universal criticisms

- Wrong study population (too old, too young, too sick, too healthy)
- Sample size not large enough
- Treatment groups not comparable with regard to some baseline characteristic
- Important data overlooked in the data collection or analysis processes (key baseline data missing, analysis of some secondary outcome not done)
- Wrong treatments studied (dosage too high, dosage too low, test treatment studied is not used in real life)
- Treatment protocol not followed in all cases
- Treatments not properly administered
- Amount of follow-up inadequate
- Clinical implications of findings questionable
- Design of the study flawed (wrong design, inadequate stratification, wrong method of randomization)
- Execution of the trial faulty
- Errors made in the data collection, coding, or classification processes
- Inappropriate data analysis
- Important subgroups of patients overlooked in the analysis
- Results cannot be generalized to ordinary clinical practice
- Results are inconsistent with previous experience
- Results not definitive

for the results observed. The variability has to be sizable and must occur in connection with an important predictor of outcome to make any real differences in the results.

26.5   DESIRABLE CHARACTERISTICS OF A CRITIC

A clinical trial is not designed to produce absolute truth. A good critic will recognize that its main strength is in the framework it provides for comparing one treatment with another and that comparisons among the treatment groups remain valid, given proper methods of treatment assignment, even if the populations studied are select. He will avoid criticism for the mere sake of criticism, and will recognize that criticism, to be useful, must be focused on specific issues concerning the design, execution, or analysis of the trial. He will avoid vague criticisms that are beyond debate. He will formulate his own list of criticisms after reading the original report and related documents and submit each of those criticisms to the tests discussed in the previous section before promulgating them. He will avoid parroting the criticisms offered by others unless he has carried out sufficient analyses of his own to support them.

A critic should recognize that his views may be colored by preconceived notions regarding the treatments studied or by his specific interests, scientific as well as financial, and hence will disclose those interests in his critique. Critiques that are commissioned and supported by a business firm with a proprietary interest in the treatments being evaluated should be so labeled. Feinstein (1971) took pains to disclose his interests in and incentives for doing the UGDP critique. His critique stands in marked contrast to those pre-

Table 26-4   Characteristics of a responsible critic

- Reserves judgment until he has personally reviewed and read all pertinent study reports and documents
- Avoids dogmatic pronouncements
- Appreciates the danger of subgroup analyses and the limitations of a straight significance testing approach to data interpretation
- Refrains from flamboyant statements designed more for effect than for enlightenment
- Persuades through the force of argument rather than via clever debating techniques and rhetoric
- Does not make unsubstantiated claims
- Does not impugn the integrity of others without factual data to support the charge
- Knows the general design strengths and weaknesses of clinical trials
- Understands the concept of randomization and its uses in a research setting
- Concentrates criticisms on weaknesses that could have been corrected by better design procedures, not on weaknesses common to any clinic trial
- Knows his own limitations and seeks the help of others for assessment of areas outside his domain of competence
- Reveals any motivations and incentives (including those of a financial nature) that may have influenced his judgment regarding the trial
- Voluntarily discloses any interests that have the potential of being viewed as a conflict of interest

pared by others concerning the study, such as those by Schor (1971) and Seltzer (1972). Disclosure of motivations and interests is important in that it permits readers to make their own judgment as to the degree to which they may have influenced the objectivity of the critic. Table 26–4 lists characteristics of a good critic.

Part VII. Appendixes

A. Glossary
B. Sketches of selected trials
C. Year 1980 clinical trial publications
D. Activities by stage of trial
E. Sample consent statements
F. Data items and forms illustrations
G. Sample manual of operations, handbook, and monitoring report
H. Budget summary for Hypertension Prevention Trial Data Coordinating Center
 I. Combined bibliography

Appendix A contains terms and acronyms used in this book plus terms considered to be common to the class of trials considered herein. Appendix B contains detailed design and operational information on 14 long-term trials. Appendix C provides the list of papers considered for review in Chapter 2. Appendix D relates to Chapter 3. It details the activities of a "typical" trial as it progresses from beginning to end. Appendix E relates to Chapter 14. It contains sample consent forms from the Hypertension Prevention Trial (HPT), Macular Photocoagulation Study (MPS), and the Persantine Aspirin Reinfarction Study (PARIS). Appendix F provides illustrative material related to the construction of data forms, as discussed in Chapter 12. Appendix G contains illustrative materials from a manual, handbook, and treatment monitoring report from the HPT, MPS, and PARIS. It relates to Chapters 16 and 20. Appendix H relates to Chapter 21 and the budgetary process for coordinating centers. Appendix I provides a combined bibliography of all references listed in the various chapters and appendixes of this book, except Appendixes B and C.

A. Glossary

A.1 PREFACE

This appendix sets forth terms and acronymns appearing in this book, plus other terms common to the class of clinical trials considered. Terms from other fields, most notably statistics and epidemiology, are covered, but only to a limited extent. Readers should see Last (1983); Kotz et al. (1982); Kruskal and Tanur (1978); Kendall and Buckland (1960); and James and James (1959) for more comprehensive glossaries of terms for these two fields.

Appendix I contains a list of reference sources used in the Glossary. Citations 69, 125, 128, 263, 272, 309, 330, 332, 343, 431, 438, 491, 495, and 502 represent general reference sources. Sources related to specific terms are cited in conjunction with those terms.

The impetus for this Glossary arose from work of the author in the Coordinating Centers Models Project (Coordinating Center Models Project Research Group, 1979a, 1979c). That work required a vocabulary to facilitate comparative analyses of the design, organizational, and operating features of the trials reviewed in that project.

Communication in clinical trials is confused by use of different terms to designate the same concept, detail, or practice. A case in point involves the term *outcome*, defined herein as a result, condition, or event associated with individual study patients and which is used to assess the efficacy of the study treatments. Other related or equivalent terms include *event, response variable*, and *endpoint*.

Practice in this book varies with regard to use of modifiers of base terms. They are frequently dropped when meanings are considered to be clear without their use. For example, the term *allocation* is often used as shorthand for treatment allocation, and *trial* is frequently used as a shorthand expression for clinical trial. Many of the more commonly used shorthand expressions appear in the Glossary.

Various terms in the Glossary are accompanied by usage notes (e.g., see *endpoint, cooperative clinical trial*, and *blind*). These notes are used to indicate the way in which a specific term is used in this book, or reasons for avoiding its

use. Terms with more than one definition, such as *sequential analysis* and *treatment effect*, may be used in different ways depending on the context. Italic print is used to denote terms that are defined elsewhere in the Glossary.

This Glossary, while extensive enough to cover usage conventions in this book, is not comprehensive enough to cover the entire scope of clinical trials. The hope is that it will serve to stimulate others to extend coverage to other classes of trials and that it will lead to greater uniformity of language conventions in the field of clinical trials (Meinert, 1980a).

A.2. GLOSSARY

A

AAW Ask as written.

achieved sample size Observed sample size.

ACTH Adrenocorticotrophic hormone.

active control *Active control treatment.*

active control treatment A *control treatment* that involves use of a pharmacologically or medically active substance. See *inactive control treatment* for opposing term.

ad hoc review group A *review group* that is created for the sole purpose of reviewing a specified application or set of applications. Also referred to as *ad hoc study section*, especially if the applications are for *grant* support.

ad hoc study section A *study section* created to review a specified application or set of applications, especially applications for *NIH grant* support.

ADA American Diabetes Association.

adaptive allocation A *treatment assignment process* in which the *treatment allocation ratio* is allowed to change as a function of the number of patients enrolled, observed *baseline data*, or observed *outcomes* (see Simon, 1977).

adaptive allocation design *Adaptive treatment allocation design.*

adaptive random allocation *Adaptive allocation* in which the *treatment assignments* are made via a *random process.*

adaptive randomization A *treatment assignment process* using *adaptive random allocation.*

adaptive treatment allocation design A *treatment allocation design* in which the *treatment allocation* *ratio* is allowed to change over the course of *patient enrollment.*

adaptive treatment allocation schedule   A *treatment allocation schedule* constructed using an *adaptive allocation* scheme.

adherence   *Treatment adherence.*

adverse drug reaction   Any *side effect* associated with use of a drug that has adverse health implications.

adverse side effect   Any *side effect* associated with a *treatment procedure* that produces an adverse effect or that has adverse health implications for the patient receiving the treatment.

advisory-review committee   (ARC) A committee in the organizational structure of a *trial* that is responsible for advising the *steering committee* and the *sponsor* on operation of the trial. Usually composed of individuals neither directly involved in the execution of the trial nor associated with any of the participating *centers* or *sponsor* of the trial. A *key committee* in the organizational structure of a *multicenter trial.* See *policy board* and *policy-advisory board.*

advisory-review and treatment effects monitoring committee   (ARTEMC) A committee that performs the functions of both the *advisory-review committee* and *treatment effects monitoring committee.* A *key committee* in the organizational structure of a *multicenter trial.*

allocation   The process of making a *treatment allocation.*

allocation ratio   *Treatment allocation ratio.*

allocation schedule   *Treatment allocation schedule.*

allocation strata   *Treatment allocation strata.*

alternative hypothesis   1. An alternative to the *null hypothesis* that specifies some true underlying difference or set of differences between two or more populations or groups with regard to some function, trait, characteristic, or effect. It may be stated in such a way so as to be concerned with a difference(s) in only one direction (*one-sided alternative hypothesis*) or in either direction (*two-sided alternative hypothesis*) relative to the null value. 2. *Alternative treatment hypothesis.*

alternative treatment hypothesis   A hypothesis that states that the true underlying effect of the *test treatment,* as expressed by a specified *outcome measure,* is different from that associated with the *control treatment.*

AMIS   Aspirin Myocardial Infarction Study.

analysis by intention to treat   A method of data analysis in which the primary tabulations and summaries of *outcome* data are by assigned treatment. See also *analysis by treatment administered.*

analysis by treatment administered   A method of data analysis in which the primary tabulations and summaries of outcome data are by treatment administered, not by treatment assigned (see Taylor et al., 1982, for usage example). See also *analysis by intention to treat.*

analysis database   The subset of data contained in the *study database* that can be accessed for data analysis. Generally limited to *data* from the study database that have been coded, keyed, and stored electronically for easy retrieval and manipulation.

ancillary study   An investigation, stimulated by the *trial* and intended to generate information of interest to the trial, that is designed and carried out by investigators from one or more of the centers in the trial and that utilizes resources of the trial (e.g., money, *study patients,* staff time, etc.), but that is not a required part of the design or data collection procedures of the trial.

applicant   Anyone who makes an application to carry out a designated research project, particularly under the *grant* mode of funding. See also *offeror* and *proposer.*

ARC   Advisory-review committee.

ART   Anturane Reinfarction Trial.

ARTEMC   *Advisory-review and treatment effects monitoring committee.*

assigned treatment   The *treatment* designated to be administered to a *patient,* as indicated at the time of his *enrollment* into the *trial.*

assignment probability   *Treatment assignment probability.*

assignment process   *Treatment assignment process.*

assignment unit   *Treatment assignment unit.*

award   *Funding award.*

B

balancing interval   *Treatment block.*

baseline   A time point or set of data that serves as a basis for gauging changes in subsequent measurements or observations.

baseline adaptive allocation   A *treatment assignment process* in which *assignment probabilities* are allowed to change over the course of the *trial* as a function of observed differences among the treatment groups for one or more *baseline variables.* Changes in the assignment probabilities are made so as to achieve comparable *study groups* with regard to the *variable*(s) used in the adaptive process.

baseline adaptive random allocation   *Adaptive random allocation* based on one or more observed *baseline characteristics* of enrolled patients.

baseline adaptive randomization   A *treatment assignment process* using *baseline adaptive random allocation.*

baseline characteristic   *Baseline variable.*

baseline data   1. The set of *data* collected on a specific *patient* or set of patients during the *prerandomization* and *randomization visits.* 2. The same as definition 1, except excluding data collected at the randomization visit. In this book, data collected at the randomization visit are considered to be part of the baseline data set.

baseline examination An examination that is carried out as part of a *baseline visit* and that is designed to assess a patient's eligibility for *enrollment* into the *trial* and to produce required *baseline data*.

baseline observation An observation or recording of a *baseline variable* made on the *observational unit*.

baseline variable A variable that is measured, observed, or assessed on a *patient* at or shortly before *treatment assignment* and the initiation of *treatment*.

baseline visit 1. A *visit* that takes place either before *randomization* or during the *randomization visit*. 2. Any *prerandomization visit*, excluding the randomization visit. Usage note: The visit at which randomization occurs is considered to be a baseline visit in this book. Reasonable, so long as there are no data collected after randomization, or so long as data collected after randomization are free of treatment effects.

Bayesian analysis A method of *data analysis* that provides a posterior probability distribution for some *parameter* which is a function of observed data and a prior probability distribution for the parameter (see Cornfield, 1966b, 1969).

Bernoulli random variable A *random variable* that is capable of assuming one of two values, e.g., 0 or 1, with fixed probabilities, P and 1-P, respectively (see Feller, 1968).

Bernoulli trial A single replication of an experimental procedure on a defined *observational unit* with a *Bernoulli random variable* as the *outcome*.

BHAT Beta Blocker Heart Attack Trial.

bias 1. A preconceived personal preference or inclination that influences the way in which a measurement, analysis, assessment, or procedure is performed or reported. From Old French *biais*, meaning oblique. From Old Provencal, perhaps from Greek *epikarsios*, meaning oblique. 2. A specified instance of a preconceived preference or inclination.

biased coin randomization A method of *randomization* in which *treatment assignment probabilities* are modified as a function of the observed difference in the number of *patients* already assigned to the *study treatment groups*.

BID Bureau, institute, or division.

binary outcome *Binary variable*.

binary outcome measure An *outcome measure* that can assume only one of two values, such as in a *trial* with death as the outcome measure.

binary variable A *variable* that is capable of assuming one of two possible values, 0 or 1, or more generally E_1 or E_2. The variable is equivalent to a *Bernoulli random variable* if the probabilities of E_1 and E_2 are fixed.

BIOSIS Biological Abstracts (a literature database; see Chapter 26).

blind *Masked*. (Usage note: Term not used because of potential for confusion, especially when used in conjunction with a *trial* where loss of vision is the *outcome measure*, or in a trial involving *patients* who have lost their vision.)

blinded *Masked*. (See *blind* for usage note.)

BLIPS Biometrics Laboratory Information Processing System.

block 1. A group, quantity, section, or segment that is considered as a unit for some purpose, procedure, process, or action. 2. (clinical trials) *Treatment block*.

block size 1. The number of individual elements making up a *block*. 2. *Treatment block size*.

blocking The process of establishing defined groups, as in a *treatment allocation schedule* designed to provide prespecified *treatment block sizes*.

BMDP Bio-Mathematics Data Processing.

business office The office in an investigator's institution with legal responsibility for receiving funds from the *sponsor* and for expenditure of those funds under specified ground rules.

C

CANCERLIT Cancer Literature (a literature database; see Chapter 26).

case-control study (epidemiology) A study that involves the identification of persons with the disease or condition of interest (cases) and a suitable group of persons without the disease or condition of interest (controls). Cases and controls are compared with respect to some existing or past attribute or exposure believed to be causally related to the disease or condition. Also referred to as a retrospective study because the research approach proceeds from effect to cause. The term applies even if cases and controls are accumulated in a prospective manner (Last, 1983, Schlesselman, 1982).

CASS Coronary Artery Surgery Study, including the Coronary Artery Surgery Trial (*CAST*).

CAST Coronary Artery Surgery Trial, see *CASS*.

CATLINE Catalog on Line (a literature database; see Chapter 26).

CC *Coordinating center*.

CCD Committee for the Care of the Diabetic.

CCMP Coordinating Center Models Project.

CCU Coronary care unit.

CDC Centers for Disease Control (a part of the United States Public Health Service), Atlanta, Georgia.

CDP Coronary Drug Project

center An autonomous unit in the structure of a *clinical trial* that is involved in the collection, determination, classification, assessment, or analysis of *data*, or that provides logistical support for the trial. To be counted as a center, the unit must have a defined function to perform, must be administratively distinct from other centers in the trial, and must function during one or more stages of a trial. Centers include *clinical center, data center, coordi-*

nating center, data coordinating center, treatment coordinating center, central laboratory, procurement and distribution center, project office, reading center*, and *quality control center*.

center director   The administrative head of a *center*.

central distribution of funds   A method for distribution of funds in which one *center* in a *multicenter trial* receives funds for execution of the trial and which, in turn, is responsible for distribution of funds to other centers in the trial.

central laboratory   A *center* in a *multicenter trial* responsible for performing specified laboratory determinations on specimens collected from *patients* enrolled or considered for *enrollment* into the trial. Not counted as a separate center if administered as part of another center in the trial.

centralized database   A *database* held and maintained in a central location, especially in a multicenter trial. See also *distributed database*.

centralized data entry   A system in which all *data* generated in a *trial* are received at a central point for keying.

chairman of the study   *Study chairman*.

CHD   Coronary heart disease.

check digit   A single digit that is used to reveal recording errors in some numeric identifier in a record, such as *patient identification number*. It is typically the last digit of the identifier and is assigned when the identifying number is issued. The assigned digit is compared with the one calculated using the identifying number (devoid of the check digit). The entire record is rejected for entry into an existing data file if the assigned digit does not agree with the calculated digit (see Selmer, 1967; Smythe, 1968; Fellegi and Sunter, 1969; and Anderson et al., 1974 for discussion of check digits).

clinic   *Study clinic*.

clinic coordinator   1. An individual in a *study clinic* responsible for coordinating the data collection activities for that clinic and who expedites the flow of data and related records from the clinic to the *data center, data coordinating center*, or *coordinating center*. 2. An individual in the data center, data coordinating center, or coordinating center who is responsible for coordinating the receipt of data from study clinics and for communicating with clinics regarding data flow. See *data coordinator*.

clinic director   The administrative head of a *study clinic*.

clinic monitor   1. An individual located in the *data center, data coordinating center, coordinating center*, or in the *sponsoring agency* who is responsible for receiving data from participating *clinics* and for initiating communications with those clinics regarding data collection and data flow procedures. 2. *Field monitor*.

clinic visit   Any patient visit to the *study clinic* during the *enrollment* or *follow-up* process that is related to the data collection, examination, treatment, or patient care procedures of the *trial*.

clinical center   1. A *center* in the organizational structure of a *clinical trial* that is responsible for recruiting, enrolling, treating, and following *patients* in order to generate required data for the trial. 2. *Study clinic*.

clinical coordinating center   *Treatment coordinating center*.

clinical event   A change in a patient's state of health characterized by the occurrence of some discrete *event* that is considered to have adverse health implications (e.g., diagnosis of cancer, hospitalization for an MI, initiation of treatment for hypertension, death).

clinical research associate   An individual, usually having an advanced degree, typically in medicine, employed by a drug firm to facilitate the initiation and direction of *clinical trials* sponsored by the firm.

clinical trial   A research activity that involves administration of a *test treatment* (e.g., a drug, surgical procedure, diagnostic test, or medical device) to some *experimental unit* in order to evaluate the *treatment*. The term is subject to wide variation in usage. In some cases it may refer to the first use of a new treatment in man without any *control treatment*. In other cases it may refer to a rigorously designed and executed experiment involving a test and control treatment and *randomization*. The experimental unit in most cases is man (or a larger unit involving man, such as a hospital ward), but can be some other experimental animal. (Usage note: In this book, the term *clinical trial* or simply *trial* always refers to a *controlled clinical trial* involving human beings.)

CLINPROT   Clinical Protocols (a cancer literature database; see Chapter 26).

close of trial   The point at which the *trial* is considered to be finished. Marked by completion of the *patient close-out* or *termination stage* of the trial, depending on whether the closing point is associated with completion of *regular follow-up visits* or with data analysis.

close-out   The process of separating a *patient* from the *trial* after completion of required *follow-up*.

close-out examination   The *final examination* or series of final examinations performed on *patients* just prior to termination of *regular follow-up* in the *trial*.

close-out follow-up visit   A *follow-up visit* made by a *study patient* to a *study clinic* that is used for data collection and to carry out specified procedures related to his separation from the *trial*.

close-out stage   *Patient close-out stage*.

closed sequential design   A *sequential design* that allows the experimenter to terminate the *trial* after a certain number of observations, even if the observed *treatment difference* is not large enough to allow the experimenter to conclude for or against the *test treatment*. Distinct from an *open sequential design*, which requires continuation of the trial until the difference is large enough to warrant a conclusion for or against the test treatment (see Chapter 9).

closed sequential trial A *trial* with a *closed sequential design* (see Chapter 9).

cohort A group of people defined by a common characteristic or set of characteristics. Middle English, from Old French *cohorte*, from Latin *cohors*, meaning enclosed yard, company of soldiers, multitude. One-tenth part of an ancient Roman legion.

common calendar date close-out A method of *patient close-out* in which all patients enrolled in the *trial* are separated from it at or about the same calendar date, regardless of when they were enrolled. See *common period of follow-up close-out* for opposing term. See also Chapter 15.

common period of follow-up close-out A method of *patient close-out* in which *patients* are separated from the *trial* after a specified period of *follow-up* (e.g., after two years). See *common calendar date close-out* for opposing term. See also Chapter 15.

comparative clinical trial Any *clinical trial* involving two or more *treatment groups*. See *controlled clinical trial*.

comparative study A *study* involving two or more defined groups of patients in which groups are compared, one with another, in order to make a judgment regarding the influence of some factor, condition, trait, or procedure that is present or applied to one group but not to the other(s). Synonymous with *controlled clinical trial* if the study entails comparison of different treatments involving patients enrolled and treated over the same period of time.

comparison group The group of *patients* designated or selected for comparison with all other groups in a *study*. The *control-treated group* of patients in a *controlled clinical trial*.

comparison treatment *Control treatment.*

compliance 1. To be in a *compliant* state. 2. A quantitative indication of the compliant state, as in the sentence: Compliance to the protocol was low.

compliant Willing to carry out a set of procedures or practices in accordance with established guidelines or standards.

composite event An *event* that is considered to have occurred if any one of several different *outcomes* are observed (e.g., occurrence of an attack of angina pectoris, a transient ischemic attack, or a myocardial infarction in a trial using a composite vascular event as the *outcome measure*).

computer A programmable electronic device that can be used to store and manipulate data in order to carry out some designated function.

computer terminal Any device (dumb or intelligent) that can be used for data input or output. It may be part of a network of terminals connected to a larger computing facility or may operate independently of all other facilities.

concurrent control A *control* that is based on *data* collected over the same period of time as that used to generate all other data in the study. See also *historical control*.

confounding variable 1. (epidemiology) A *variable* that is related to two factors of interest (e.g., disease state and degree of exposure to some agent in a *case-control study; treatment assignment* and *outcome* in a *clinical trial*) that falsely obscures or accentuates the relationship between the factors (see Breslow and Day, 1980; Last, 1983). 2. A *baseline variable* in a clinical trial that influences the outcome and that has a different distribution in the *treatment groups* being compared.

consortium agreement An agreement between the *sponsor* and one of the *centers* in a *multicenter study* in which the center agrees to receive funds for its own operations and that of other centers in the study and to disperse funds among the centers on an as-needed basis or as specified in the agreement.

consortium award 1. A *grant* or *contract* awarded by the *sponsor* to a *center* for execution of a *study* involving multiple *centers*. The center receiving the *award* assumes responsibility for allocation of funds to all other participating centers in the study. 2. Same as definition 1 except that the award is for support of only certain other centers in the study. Remaining centers are funded in other ways.

continuous variable A *variable* that is capable of assuming any value over a specified range.

contract A legally binding written agreement between the *sponsor* and the *business office* of the investigator's place of employment that outlines the nature and schedule of work to be performed and terms of payment for said work.

contract office The office in the *sponsoring agency* or *lead center* whose members are responsible for negotiating, awarding, and funding contracts.

contract officer The individual in the *sponsoring agency* or *lead center* who is responsible for negotiating, awarding, and funding contracts for specified projects.

control A standard of comparison for testing, verifying, or evaluating some observation or result.

control group *Comparison group, control-treated group.*

control patient A *patient* assigned to the *control treatment*.

control-treated group 1. The group of *patients* in a *trial* assigned to the *control treatment*. 2. The group of patients in a trial who received the control treatment, whether or not originally assigned to that treatment (not used this way in this book).

control treatment The drug, device, test, or procedure administered in a *clinical trial* that serves as the standard against which *test treatments* are evaluated. The control treatment may consist of a placebo medication, sham procedure, a standard treatment regimen, or no treatment of any kind, depending on the study design.

control trial *Controlled clinical trial.* (See *randomized control clinical trial* for comment.)

controlled 1. Constrained, monitored, or watched. 2. A system of observation and data collection that provides a basis for comparison, as with a *comparison group.*

controlled clinical trial A *clinical trial* involving one or more *test treatments*, at least one *control treatment*, and concurrent *enrollment, treatment,* and *follow-up* of all *patients* in the trial.

controlled trial *Controlled clinical trial.*

conventional author citation A method of citation in which specific individuals are designated on the title page or elsewhere in a manuscript as its authors. See *corporate author citation* for opposing term.

cooperative agreement 1. An agreement between an institute in the National Institutes of Health and a set of investigators that provides a defined structure for sponsor-investigator cooperation in the design and execution of a research project. 2. Any written agreement between a *sponsor* and *investigator*(s) that provides a defined role for both parties in the design and conduct of a specified research project.

cooperative clinical trial Term frequently used to denote a *multicenter trial.* The term is avoided in this book. Cooperation is required for execution of any trial, whether or not it involves multiple clinics.

coordinating center A *center* in the structure of a study that is responsible for receiving, editing, processing, analyzing, and storing *data* generated in a study and that, in addition, has responsibility for coordination of activities required for execution of the study. See also *data center, data coordinating center,* and *treatment coordinating center.*

coordinating center director The administrative head of the *coordinating center.*

coordinator 1. The individual in the *data center, data coordinating center,* or *coordinating center* who is responsible for coordinating the receipt of *data* from *study clinics* and for communicating with clinics regarding data flow. *clinic coordinator, data coordinator.* 2. The *director* of the *coordinating center.* (Usage note: Term not used in either definition 1 or 2 context in this book.)

corporate author citation A method of citation in which authorship of a given manuscript is ascribed to a corporate entity (e.g., as in a paper listed as having been authored by the Coronary Drug Project Research Group).

cost-reimbursement contract A *contract* in which the amount of money paid to the contractor by the *sponsor* is dictated by reasonable and allowable expenses for the work performed.

Cox proportional hazards regression model A method of analysis developed by D. R. Cox (1972) involving *regression analysis* which is used to adjust observed *event rates*, such as those obtained in

a *clinical trial* where *patients* are enrolled over a period of time and followed to a common calendar date, for *variables* (usually observed at *baseline*) which are believed to influence the rates.

CPHA Commission on Professional and Hospital Activities.

CPPT Coronary Primary Prevention Trial, a trial conducted by the Lipid Research Clinics.

CPU Central processing unit (of a computer).

CRISP Computer Retrieval of Information on Scientific Projects (a database of ongoing work; see Chapter 26).

cross contamination *Treatment cross contamination.*

crossed treatment design 1. *Crossover treatment design.* 2. *Factorial treatment structure.*

crossed treatments Two or more *study treatments* that are used in sequence (e.g., as in a *crossover design*) or in combination (e.g., as in a *factorial treatment structure*).

crossover *Treatment crossover.*

crossover design *Crossover treatment design.*

crossover treatment design A *treatment design* that calls for the administration of two or more of the *study treatments* in a specified order to *experimental units* in the *trial.*

crossover trial *Crossover clinical trial.*

crossover clinical trial A *clinical trial* involving a *crossover treatment design.*

CRT Cathode ray tube.

cut-point 1. The point or value in an ordered sequence of values that is used to separate those values into two subparts. 2. *Subgrouping cut-point.*

CV Curriculum vitae.

D

data (pl. of *datum*) Factual information, such as measurements, observations, or statistics, which is used as a basis for reasoning, discussion, or calculation. (Usage note: In this book, the term refers to information collected and recorded on *patients* considered for *enrollment* or actually enrolled in a *trial.*)

data audit The comparison of specific items of information contained in an original *data form* (or some other kind of record) with that produced for some transcribed version of that form or record (e.g., as contained on a listing of the computer data file of the form or record) as a check for discrepancies.

data center 1. A *center* in a study structure that is responsible for receiving, editing, processing, analyzing, and storing data generated in the *study*, but that has few if any of the other general coordination responsibilities assumed by a *data coordinating center* or *coordinating center.* 2. A center in a study structure that is responsible for receiving, editing, processing, analyzing, and storing data generated in the study, regardless of whether or not the center has other more general coordination responsibilities. Used in this sense in this book where there is no need to distinguish between a data center, data coordinating center, or coordinating center, and where the emphasis is on data intake and processing functions.

data collection visit Any *visit* by a *patient* to the *study clinic* that is used for data collection in the *trial*.

data coordinating center A *center* that has the duties of a *data center* as well as general coordination duties for data collection. The modifier *data* is sometimes used in structures having two or more centers with specified coordination responsibilities (e.g., in a structure with both a *treatment coordinating center* and a *data coordinating center*).

data coordinator An individual in the *data center, data coordinating center,* or *coordinating center* who is responsible for coordinating the receipt of data from *study clinics* and for communicating with clinics regarding data flow. Sometimes also *clinic coordinator,* but not in this book.

data dredging A term used to characterize analyses that are done on an ad hoc basis, without benefit of prestated hypotheses, as a means of identifying noteworthy differences.

data editing 1. The process of reviewing *data* for the purpose of detecting deficiencies or errors in the way they are collected or recorded. 2. The process of detecting deficient or erroneous values on completed *data forms*.

data entry 1. The process of keying *data*, as contained on completed *data forms*, in order to render information into an arrangement more suitable for storage and subsequent use, usually for tabulations and analyses, especially on a *computer*. 2. The process of filling out a *data form*.

data field 1. A space on a *data form* or in an electronic *record* designated to contain, or that actually contains, alphabetic or numeric characters of information recorded in response to a specific *data item* on the form. 2. The actual collection of alphabetic or numeric characters used to denote information recorded in response to a specified question or statement on a data form.

data file A collection of *data records*. The collection may be of paper records or of electronic records that are arrayed in some way.

data form A collection of *data items* all arrayed on the same paper *record*.

data item 1. A question or statement and related area to be used by the respondent in answering the question or completing the statement appearing on a *data form*. 2. *Data field*.

data monitoring committee 1. *Treatment effects monitoring committee*. 2. A committee with *treatment effects monitoring* responsibilities plus other monitoring responsibilities, such as those needed for assessing data quality or for assessing the performance of clinics participating in a *trial*. 3. A committee that is responsible simply for monitoring data quality and the performance of *centers* in a trial (i.e., has no treatment effects monitoring responsibilities).

data record A collection of *data items* that is treated as a unit for some purpose or function.

data reduction 1. The process of taking *raw data*, as recorded on *study forms*, and of codifying and classifying them in such a way so as to condense them into a form suitable for data entry and electronic storage. 2. The process of taking data already contained in an electronic record and summarizing them, through the use of various classification schemes and arithmetic manipulations, so as to condense them into a form suitable for tabulations, analyses, listings, etc.

data and safety monitoring committee *Treatment effects monitoring committee*.

data system A package of interrelated procedures or routines that are performed by hand or computer to carry out some function or set of functions (e.g., data management or data analysis).

database A collection of data files that are organized in a specified manner and that are accessed by designated personnel for designated purposes.

datum Singular of *data*.

DCC *Data coordinating center*.

DCCT Diabetes Control and Complications Trial.

dedicated computer A *computer* that is under the exclusive control of a single user (or group of users) and that is used for a specified project, function, or activity.

DESI Drug Efficacy Study Implementation.

design unit The *observational unit* used for sample size calculations in a *trial*. Usually a *patient*, but may be some larger unit in special cases, such as in trials using hospital wards, families, or the like as the *treatment unit*. Always a patient in this book.

DHEW Department of Health, Education and Welfare (a department in the executive arm of the United States government until May 1980; its functions are now met by the Department of Health and Human Services and the Department of Education).

DHHS Department of Health and Human Services (a department in the executive arm of the United States government).

diagnostic clinical trial A *clinical trial* designed to evaluate the usefulness of some diagnostic procedure, tool, or device.

diagnostic trial *Diagnostic clinical trial*.

dichotomous variable A *discrete variable* that has only two possible values. *Binary variable*.

direct award An award of funds (*grant* or *contract*) made directly from the *sponsor* to a study *center*. See also *indirect award*.

direct distribution of funds Distribution of funds to *centers* in a *study* directly from the *sponsor*, as in *direct awards*.

direct patient contact Patient contacts that are initiated by the *study clinic* for the purpose of patient recruitment and that are directed at specified patients without any reliance on interviewing persons, agencies, institutions, or generalized advertising campaigns to make the contacts. See also *indirect patient contact* and Chapter 14.

direct patient recruitment Any method of patient recruitment that involves *direct patient contact.*

direct research cost The cost for salaries, equipment, supplies, and the like associated with the actual design, conduct, and analysis of a research project. See also *indirect research cost.*

director *Center director.*

discrete variable A *variable* that is capable of assuming only certain values over a defined range, as for *dichotomous* (binary) or *polychotomous variables.* See also *continuous variable.*

distributed data analysis Any arrangement in a *multicenter trial* whereby investigators in the various *centers* have access to the *analysis database*, or portions of it, for the purpose of carrying out data analyses.

distributed data entry A method of *data entry* in *multicenter trials* where data generated at the *clinics* are keyed on site.

distributed data system A *data system* that is established and maintained at the various *clinics* in a *multicenter trial* in order to perform functions normally carried out at the *data coordinating center.*

distributed database A *database* that is made up of component parts which reside at geographically diverse locations (e.g., in clinics in a *multicenter trial*).

distribution center *Procurement and distribution center.*

DMSO Dimethyl sulfoxide.

double-blind *Double-masked* in this book. See *blind* for usage comment.

double-blinded *Double-masked* in this book. See *blind* for usage comment.

double-blinded clinical trial *Double-masked clinical trial.*

double-mask *Double-masked.*

double-masked 1. A procedure in a *clinical trial* for issuing and administering *treatment assignments* by code number in order to keep *study patients* and all members of the clinic staff, especially those responsible for patient treatment and data collection, from knowing the assigned treatments. 2. Any condition in which two different groups of people are purposely denied access to a piece of information in order to keep that information from influencing some measurement, observation, or process.

double-masked clinical trial A *clinical trial* with *double-masked* administration of the *study treatments.*

DRG Division of Research Grants of the *National Institutes of Health.*

drop-in A term sometimes used (not in this book) to denote a *patient* in a *clinical trial* who, although assigned to one *study treatment*, receives one of the other study treatments in place of, or in addition to, the *assigned treatment.* See *treatment crossover* for related term.

dropout A patient enrolled in a *clinical trial* who is either unwilling or unable to return to the *study clinic* for *regular follow-up visits.*

DRS Diabetic Retinopathy Study.

drug trial A *clinical trial* in which the *test treatments* are drugs.

dumb terminal A *computer terminal* that can act as an input or output device, but that does not have independent processing capabilities (as opposed to an *intelligent terminal*).

dynamic allocation *Adaptive allocation.*

dynamic randomization *Adaptive randomization.*

dynamic treatment allocation schedule *Adaptive treatment allocation schedule.*

E

early stopping 1. A condition or provision incorporated into the design of a *clinical trial* that enables investigators to terminate *patient recruitment* or *treatment* if data accumulated during the trial suggest an adverse or beneficial *treatment effect.* 2. A term used to characterize an action involving termination of a *study treatment* in a trial because of adverse or beneficial treatment effects.

early stopping rule *Stopping rule.*

EC *Executive committee.*

ECG *Electrocardiogram.*

ECOG Eastern Cooperative Oncology Group.

edit check The process of reviewing a *data item* on a completed *data form* for deficiencies in the way it is completed or in the value reported.

edit query A statement generated from a review of a completed *data form* that draws attention to a suspected deficiency in an item of information on the form and that requires some action by personnel responsible for generation of the data to clear the query.

editorial review committee A committee created in the organizational structure of an *investigative body* that has responsibility for reviewing manuscripts produced by that body.

effective sample size *Sample size* after reductions due to *dropouts* and *treatment noncompliance.* See *expected effective sample size* and *observed effective sample size.*

EFM Electronic fetal monitoring.

EMED Excerpta Medica (a literature database; see Chapter 26).

endpoint 1. A *primary* or *secondary event* that, when observed in a *patient*, leads to termination or alteration of *treatment* or *follow-up.* 2. A primary or secondary event observed in a patient during the course of treatment or follow-up. 3. *Outcome.*

4. *Early stopping.* 5. *Stopping rule.* (Usage note: The term, *endpoint* is not used in this book because of the potential for confusion. Use of the term in the sense of definitions 1, 2, or 3 can mean that patients are no longer eligible for treatment or follow-up once they experience a specified event. This is obviously true where the event is death, but need not be so for nonfatal events. In fact, the design of the *trial* may require continued treatment and follow-up of patients over the entire course of the trial, regardless of the number of nonfatal "endpoints" observed. See *event, clinical event, primary outcome,* and *primary event* for preferred terms.)

enrollment *Patient enrollment.*

enrollment process *Patient enrollment process.*

equal allocation *Equal treatment allocation.*

equal treatment allocation A scheme in which the *assignment probability* in the *randomization process* for any one *treatment* is the same as for every other treatment in the *trial.* See *uniform treatment allocation.*

estimated sample size The number of *patients* required for a *study,* as derived from a *sample size calculation* or in some other way.

ETDRS Early Treatment of Diabetic Retinopathy Study.

ethics committee 1. *Treatment effects monitoring committee.* 2. *Institutional review board.*

ethics review committee 1. *Treatment effects monitoring committee.* 2. *Institutional review board.*

evaluable patient *Evaluable study patient.*

evaluable patients *Evaluable study patients.*

evaluable study patient A *study patient* who is regarded by investigators in the *trial* as having satisfied certain conditions (e.g., developed a tumor of a certain size during the trial, followed the assigned treatment) and, as a result, is retained for analysis purposes (a patient not satisfying the conditions is not so retained).

evaluable study patients The subgroup of *study patients* considered by investigators in the *trial* to satisfy certain conditions and, as a result, are retained for analysis purposes. Patients not satisfying the conditions are not so retained.

event 1. An occurrence, incident, or experience, especially one of some significance. 2. *Binary outcome measure.* 3. *Clinical event.* 4. The actual occurrence of a condition, trait, or characteristic that is defined by a binary outcome measure.

event rate The number of events experienced by a specified number of *patients* in a specified unit of time.

examination *Patient examination.*

executive committee (EC) One of the *key committees* in the organizational structure of a *trial.* Responsible for direction of the day-to-day affairs of the trial. Usually consists of the *officers of the study* and perhaps others selected from the *steering committee.* Headed by the chairman or vice-chair-man of the steering committee and reports to that committee.

expected allocation ratio The *allocation ratio* expected using a given set of *treatment assignment probabilities.* See *specific allocation ratio.*

expected effective sample size The number of *randomization units* (usually *patients*) specified when the *trial* was planned, less reductions due to anticipated losses from *dropout* and treatment *noncompliance.*

expected power The *power* computed for a given *treatment comparison* when the *trial* was planned (see Chapter 9).

experimental unit *Treatment assignment unit.*

explanatory trial Term used to characterize *trials* that are designed to explain how a treatment works (see Schwartz and Lellouch, 1967; Sackett and Gent, 1979; Sackett, 1980). Term not used in this book. See also *management trial.*

F

factorial structure *Factorial treatment structure.*

factorial treatment structure A *treatment structure* in which one *study treatment* is used in combination with at least one other study treatment in a *trial,* or where multiples of a defined dose of a specified treatment are used in the same trial. See *partial* and *full factorial treatment structure.*

FDA Food and Drug Administration (a regulatory agency of the United States government, located in Rockville, Maryland).

feasibility study A preliminary study designed to determine the practicality of a larger study. See *pilot study.*

field monitor An individual employed by the *sponsor* or a *center* of a *trial* (e.g., *coordinating center*) to visit participating *clinics* to monitor data collection procedures. See *clinic monitor.*

final data analysis The term given to data analyses carried out at the end of the *trial,* normally in the *termination stage,* for characterizing results obtained from the trial.

final examination *Final patient examination.*

final patient examination 1. The last *examination* of a *patient* prior to *close-out.* 2. The last examination of a patient prior to *enrollment.*

fixed allocation Any method of *treatment assignment* involving a *fixed treatment allocation ratio.*

fixed allocation design *Fixed treatment allocation design.*

fixed allocation ratio *Fixed treatment allocation ratio.*

fixed allocation schedule *Fixed treatment allocation schedule.*

fixed-cost contract A *contract* in which there is a prior agreement between the *sponsor* and the investigator's institution on the amount to be paid for work to be performed, regardless of the actual costs incurred.

fixed sample size design   A design in which the number of *patients* to be enrolled is considered to be fixed in advance of the start of *patient enrollment* for the *study*. The number may be determined from a *sample size calculation*, or via other considerations (e.g., cost, patient availability). It is conventional to consider any study that does not involve a *sequential design* as involving a fixed sample size design, even if the number is not determined before the start of the trial. See *sequential design* for opposing term.

fixed treatment allocation design   A *treatment allocation design* in which the *treatment allocation ratio* is fixed.

fixed treatment allocation ratio   An *allocation ratio* that remains fixed.

fixed treatment allocation schedule   A *treatment allocation schedule* based on fixed *treatment assignment probabilities*.

fixed treatment randomization   A *treatment assignment process* in which the *treatment assignment probabilities* remain fixed.

FOIA   Freedom of Information Act (see Chapter 24).

follow-up   *Patient follow-up.*

follow-up cohort   1. A group of *patients* enrolled into a *trial* during the same time period. 2. A group of patients enrolled at different time points, but who are followed for the same length of time (e.g., each patient for two years).

follow-up data   *Data* collected on a *patient*, or a set of patients, after *enrollment* into a *trial*.

follow-up data collection visit   Any *data collection visit* that takes place after a patient is enrolled into the *trial*.

follow-up examination   A *patient examination* made at a *follow-up visit*.

follow-up observation   An item of data collected on a *patient* (or larger *treatment unit*) after *enrollment* in a *trial*.

follow-up study   *Prospective follow-up study.*

follow-up variable   A *variable* observed on individual patients (*treatment units*) after *enrollment* into a *trial*.

follow-up visit   Any *patient clinic visit* that takes place after the *randomization visit* for study-related purposes. See *required* and *nonrequired follow-up visit* for classes of follow-up visits. See also *treatment adjustment, regular, interim, close-out, post-close-out,* and *post-trial follow-up visit* for specific types.

free treatment arm   1. A *treatment* that is selected by the *study physician* or *study patient*. 2. A *study group* that receives the *treatment* selected by study physicians or study patients.

FTE   Full-time equivalent.

full factorial structure   *Full factorial treatment structure.*

full factorial treatment structure   A *treatment structure* in which each *study treatment* is used in com-

bination with every other study treatment. The treatments may involve different drugs or procedures, or different levels or doses of the same treatment.

funding agency   The institution, organization, or foundation that provides fiscal support for a given study. *Sponsoring agency.*

funding award   A *grant* or *contract* awarded to an institution for a designated project.

funding office   The office responsible for fiscal negotiations with the *centers* of a *study* and for the disbursement and administration of funds for use in the study. *Grants management office, contract office.*

funding officer   The head of the *funding office*. *Grants management officer, contract officer.*

FY   Fiscal year.

G

general-use computer   A computer that is used by a variety of users working on unrelated tasks or studies.

grant   A *funding award* from the *sponsor* to an investigator, via his institution, to support designated work. A grant, as opposed to a *cooperative agreement* or *contract*, is generally made in anticipation of relatively little involvement in the work by the sponsor.

grants management office   The office in the *sponsoring agency* whose members are responsible for negotiating and awarding *grants* and for disbursement of funds for execution of grant-funded projects. See *contract office* for corresponding term in contract-funded work.

grants management officer   The individual in the *sponsoring agency* with legal authority to negotiate grant *awards* and to disburse funds in connection with those awards. See *contract officer* for corresponding terms for contract-funded projects.

group sequential analysis   A method of *interim data analysis* that is carried out after *enrollment* of a specified number of patients, as discussed by Pocock (1977) and DeMets and Ware (1980).

H

handbook   *Study handbook.*

haphazard   A process occurring without any apparent order or pattern. Distinct from random, as used in this book, in that there is no mathematical basis for characterizing a haphazard process.

hard endpoint   *Hard outcome.*

hard outcome   Any *outcome measure* that is not subject to serious errors of interpretation or measurement. Usually death or some other explicit *clinical event.*

HDFP   Hypertension Detection and Follow-Up Program.

health scientist administrator An individual at the *National Institutes of Health* who is responsible for providing technical and scientific assistance to investigators in a grant-funded study.

HEW (Department of) Health, Education and Welfare, *DHEW.*

HEX Committee Human experimentation committee. See *institutional review board.*

HHS (Department of) Health and Human Services, *DHHS.*

historical control A *control* that is based on *data* collected in a period of time previous to that used for generation of data on the *test-treated* group of patients. See *concurrent control* for opposing term.

historical control group A group of patients (may be loosely or explicitly defined) considered to have the same disease or condition as the *study group,* but who were diagnosed and treated in a period of time prior to that of the study group and who received the conventional form of therapy for that time. Historical control groups are generally only useful for evaluations of treatments involving rare diseases with highly predictable *outcomes* and where it is considered impractical or unethical to carry out a *controlled clinical trial.*

historical controls A collection of *patients* used as a *comparison group* who were diagnosed and treated for the disease or condition of interest in the past and in a period of time that predates the period of time covered for other *study groups.*

HPT Hypertension Prevention Trial.

human experimentation committee *Institutional review board.*

human volunteers committee *Institutional review board.*

I

ID Identification.

ID check digit A digit that is part of the *identification number* of a record and that is used as a check for transcription errors in that number. See *check digit.*

IDE *Investigational Device Exemption* (see IND for corresponding term for drugs).

IDEA *Investigational Device Exemption Application* (see INDA for corresponding term for drugs).

identification number *Patient identification number.*

IG *Investigative group.*

IMPACT International Mexiletine Placebo Antiarrhythmic Coronary Trial.

inactive control treatment A *control treatment* that is not considered to have any pharmacological or physiological effect. A *placebo treatment* or *sham procedure.* See also *active control treatment.*

IND Investigational New Drug (see IDE for corresponding term for medical devices).

INDA *Investigational New Drug Application.*

indirect award A *funding award* made to one *center* via another using funds received from the *sponsor,* as in a *consortium award.*

indirect patient contact Methods of patient contact that are initiated by the *patient,* his own physician, or some other intervening person, agency, or institution, for the purpose of patient recruitment. See *direct patient contact* for opposing term and Chapter 14.

indirect patient recruitment Any method of *patient recruitment* that involves *indirect patient contact.*

indirect research cost The cost incurred by the institution housing a research project for general administrative support and for providing space, heat, light, and the like in connection with the project. See *direct research cost* for opposing term.

informed consent The voluntary consent given by a patient to participate in a *study* after being informed of its purpose, method of treatment, procedure for assignment to treatment, benefits and risks associated with participation, and required data collection procedures and schedule.

initial design stage The first stage of a *trial.* Concerned with design and planning (see Chapter 3 and Appendix D).

institutional review board A committee or board, as set forth in United States Public Health Service guidelines for research involving humans and appointed by authorities in a research institution, constituted to review and approve studies to be carried out on humans in that institution. The review focuses on the ethics of the proposed research and on the adequacy of the proposed patient *informed consent* process.

intelligent terminal A *computer terminal* that can be used to perform data processing independent of the computer to which it is connected (as opposed to a *dumb terminal*).

interaction 1. (statistics, James and James, 1959) A case in which one *variable, y,* is a function of another, *x,* and in which variation in *x* associated with a given change in *y* is affected by the value assumed by a third variable, *z.* Interaction is said to exist between *y* and *z.* 2. (clinical trials) A situation in which the magnitude of the *test-control treatment difference* for the *outcome* of interest depends upon the value assumed by a third factor, such as age or prior disease state of the *study patients.*

interaction effect *Treatment interaction effect.*

interim analysis *Interim data analysis.*

interim data analysis 1. Any data analysis carried out during the *trial* for the purpose of *treatment effects monitoring.* 2. Any data analysis done before the trial is finished, for whatever reason, but usually concerned with assessments of *treatment effects.* (Usage note: Strictly speaking, the term applies to any fixed sample size or sequential trial where such analyses are done. However, it is conventional to reserve the term for use with *fixed* *sample size designs*. That convention is followed herein.)

interim follow-up visit In this book, any *visit* by a study patient to the *clinic* after *randomization* that is not part of the required sequence of *follow-up visits* and that is initiated by the *study patient* or *study physician* because of some medical or treatment problem. Not counted as a *required follow-up visit* unless it takes place within the specified time period for a required visit and all the required procedures for that visit are carried out as part of the interim visit. See *nonrequired follow-up visit*.

interim result 1. Any *test-control treatment difference* observed during the *trial*. 2. A test-control treatment difference observed during the trial that results in a treatment protocol change.

interim visit *Interim follow-up visit*.

intervention study A study in which there is an effort to change the natural course of a disease or condition by attempting to alter the risk factors or precursors associated with that disease or condition.

intervention trial Technically, any *clinical trial*, since administration of any *treatment* in a trial setting is a form of intervention. However, the term is usually reserved for trials in which the test treatment entails life-style changes.

Investigational Device Exemption Application (IDEA) An application directed to the Food and Drug Administration by the manufacturer of a *medical device* or independent investigator for permission to evaluate the device in humans (Food and Drug Administration, 1983). See *Investigational New Drug Application* for corresponding term for drugs.

Investigational New Drug Application (*INDA*, also *IND*) An application directed to the Food and Drug Administration (made by submitting a *Notice of Claimed Investigational Exemption for a New Drug*) for permission to evaluate a drug (new or old) for a new indication in humans. See *Investigational Device Exemption* for corresponding term for *medical devices*.

investigative body *Investigative group*.

investigative group The entire staff involved in a *study*. Includes *center directors*, representatives from the *sponsoring agency*, members of all study committees and key support staff.

investigative team *investigative group*.

investigator *Study investigator*.

I/O Input/output.

IRB *Institutional review board*.

IRSC International Reflux Study in Children.

IUD Intra-uterine device.

K

Kaplan-Meier product limit A nonparametric method developed by Kaplan and Meier (1958) for estimating *follow-up event rates* using conditional probabilities. The method is especially well suited to situations, such as encountered in clinical trials, where *patients* are enrolled over a period of time and followed to a common calendar time point.

key committee In this book any of the following: *steering committee, executive committee, advisory-review committee, treatment effects monitoring committee*, or alternatively, the steering committee, executive committee, and *advisory-review and treatment effects monitoring committee*. Also *major committee*.

L

label insert *Package insert*.

landscape-style page orientation A form of orientation in which printed and visual information is arrayed on the long axis of a page. See also *portrait-style page orientation*.

lay representative A member of a committee, usually the *advisory review* or *advisory-review and treatment effects monitoring committee*, who is chosen to represent *patients* in the *trial* and who has no recognized research credentials.

lead center 1. A *center* designated in a *multicenter* study to take the lead in testing or performing certain procedures in a study or that is designated to assume a leadership role in the direction of the study. 2. The center responsible for disbursing funds to other centers in a study funded under a *consortium agreement*.

lead clinic 1. The *clinic* in a *multicenter trial* that is responsible for testing patient examination and data collection procedures to be used in a trial. 2. The first clinic funded, especially when that clinic is responsible for developing and testing data collection procedures to be used in a *study*.

lifetable An assembly of *data* in table or graph form that summarizes the survival (or mortality) experience of the *observational units* (*patients* in this book) from some specified starting point. The starting point may be based on age, as in most lifetables compiled by demographers, or on some event, such as diagnosis of disease, or *enrollment* into a *study*, in the case of a *clinical trial*.

lifetable analysis A method of analysis that relies on a count of the number of *events* observed and the time points at which those events occurred, relative to some zero point. The event may be death or some other event. In *clinical trials*, the time to an event for a *patient* is usually measured from the *time of enrollment*. *Treatment effects* are assessed by comparing *event rates* in the different *treatment groups*.

likelihood principle (statistics) A principle that implies that the magnitude of the probability associated with a given outcome of an experiment under hypothesis A relative to the magnitude of the probability associated with that outcome under hypothesis B contains all the information provided by the data from the experiment in choosing between the two hypotheses (Cornfield, 1966b; Dupont, 1983a).

log rank test statistic A *test statistic* used to compare the distribution of event times among different groups (usually with some censoring) in a clinical trial. See *Mantel-Haenszel test statistic* and Chapter 18.

loss to follow-up Any loss of *follow-up data* on a *study patient* after *enrollment* into a *trial*. The loss may occur because of the patient's refusal or inability to return to the *study clinic* for follow-up *data collection visits*, or because of the inability of clinic staff to locate the patient for collection of information not requiring a *clinic visit*.

losses to follow-up The sum total of information lost because of *loss to follow-up*.

lost to follow-up A patient who can no longer be followed for the *outcome* of interest, e.g., a patient who is unwilling or unable to return to the *clinic* for *follow-up examinations* in the case of a *clinical trial* using an outcome measured at the clinic, or a patient who cannot be located for subsequent *follow-up* in the case of a trial involving mortality or some other outcome that can be measured outside the clinic setting.

lost to mortality follow-up A person whose vital status cannot be determined, either because the person cannot be traced or because of insufficient identifiers to query data files such as the *National Death Index*. Losses to mortality follow-up in a *clinical trial* arise from *patients* who drop out and who cannot be located for subsequent contacts.

LRC Lipid Research Clinics.

LRC-CPPT Lipid Research Clinics-Coronary Primary Prevention Trial.

M

mainline paper Paper detailing the design, methods, or baseline results of the *trial* or containing original results related to the primary objective of the trial and written by study personnel commissioned by the *investigative group* or their representative.

major committee *Key committee.*

management trial Term used by some to characterize a trial that is designed primarily to provide information on the value of a treatment in normal usage (see Schwartz and Lellouch, 1967; Sackett and Gent, 1979; Sackett, 1980). Term not used in this book. See also *explanatory trial*.

Mantel-Haenszel test statistic A *test statistic* developed by Mantel and Haenszel (1959) to test for the equality of proportions in two groups over a series of independent 2×2 tables. In the case of comparing the probability of failure at different points in time, the statistic is equivalent to the *log rank test statistic* (see Chapter 18).

manual of operations *Study manual of operations.*

mask A condition imposed on an individual (or group of individuals) for the purpose of keeping that individual or group of individuals from knowing or learning of some fact or observation, such as *treatment* assignment. (Usage note: Term used in place of *blind* in this book. See entry for *blind* for reasons.)

masked The condition of having a *mask* in place, e.g., as in a *single-*, *double-*, or *triple-masked* trial.

matching placebo A pill (capsule or tablet) that is designed to resemble in shape, texture, size, taste, etc., a therapeutically active drug and that is used as the *control treatment*.

MATHFILE Mathematical Reviews (a literature database; see Chapter 26).

mean priority score The mean of the *priority scores* assigned by individual members of a *review group*.

medical device A diagnostic or therapeutic contrivance that does not interact chemically with a person's body. Includes diagnostic tests, kits, pacemakers, arterial grafts, intraocular lens and orthopedic pins (Food and Drug Administration, 1983).

medical liaison office *Project office.*

medical liaison officer *Project officer.*

medical research associate *Clinical research associate.*

MEDLARS Medical Literature Analysis Retrieval System.

MEDLINE Medical Literature Analysis Retrieval System on Line.

MeSH Medical subject heading.

MI Myocardial infarction.

MILIS Multicenter Investigation for Limiting Infarct Size.

monitoring Ongoing evaluation of a continuing process to determine when and if changes in that process are necessary for reasons of efficiency, data quality, safety, etc.

Monte Carlo simulation A method of simulating some stocastic process or procedure using random or pseudo-random numbers.

MPS Macular Photocoagulation Study.

MRFIT Multiple Risk Factor Intervention Trial.

multicenter Having more than one *center*.

multicenter clinical trial 1. A *clinical trial* involving two or more *clinical centers*, a common *study protocol*, and a *data center, data coordinating center*, or *coordinating center* to receive, process, and analyze *study data*. 2. A clinical trial involving two or more *clinics*. 3. A clinical trial involving at least one clinical center and one or more *resource centers*. (Usage note: A trial, to qualify as multicenter in this book, must satisfy definition 1. Trials simply involving two or more clinical centers, as specified in definition 2, do not qualify as multicenter unless they have a common study protocol and a center to receive and process *data* from the study. A trial involving a single clinic, whether or not supported by other resource centers, is classified as a single-center trial in this book.)

multicenter trial   *Multicenter clinical trial.*

multiple comparisons   In this book, a term used to refer to the fact that two or more *treatment comparisons*, each involving the same *outcome measure*, are made or are to be made at a designated time point in the course of the trial. The comparison may involve all members of the treatment groups or subsets (e.g., as in analyses involving subgroups of patients defined by the presence or absence of some *baseline characteristic*.)

multiple linear regression analysis   (statistics) A method of data analysis using a *multiple linear regression model*. Often used in *clinical trials* to adjust treatment results for differences in the baseline composition of the *treatment groups*.

multiple linear regression model   (statistics) A mathematical model in which the *outcome variable*, y_i for the ith *patient* is written as a function of a series of independent observations, $X_{1i}, \ldots, X_{ki}$, *parameters*, $\beta_0, \ldots, \beta_k$, and an error term, ϵ_i. The usual form of the model, when no *interaction* terms are required, is:
$$y_i = \beta_0 + \beta_1 X_{1i} + \beta_2 X_{2i} + \cdots + \beta_k X_{ki} + \epsilon_i$$
The model derives its name from the fact that all parameters enter as linear terms (i.e., all raised to unit power). The independent variables, X_{ji}, for $j = 1, \cdots, k$, in the *clinical trial* setting are usually *baseline characteristics*. The outcome variable may be a continuous measure or a *binary outcome*, such as life-death.

multiple logistic regression analysis   (statistics) A method of data analysis using a *multiple logistic regression model*. Often used in *clinical trials* to adjust observed treatment results for differences in the baseline composition of the *treatment groups*.

multiple logistic regression model   (statistics) A mathematical model in which an *outcome variable*, y_i for the ith patient, is written as:
$$y_i = 1/(1 + e^{\tau_i})$$
where e is the natural constant, the quality τ_i, is a function of a series of observations, $X_{1i}, \cdots, X_{ki}$, made on the ith patient and that are independent of y_i, the model *parameters*, and the error term ϵ_i. The usual form for τ_i, when no interaction terms are required, is:
$$\tau_i = \beta_0 + \beta_1 X_{1i} + \beta_2 X_{2i} + \cdots + \beta_k X_{ki} + \epsilon_i$$
The model is especially well suited for analyses of event data since probability estimates derived from it lie between 0 and 1.

multiple looks   In this book, a term used to refer to the fact that *treatment comparisons* are made or are to be made at various time points over the course of a *trial*.

multiple outcomes   In this book, a term used to refer to the fact that a *trial* involves several different *outcome measures*, each of which is used or is to be used to make *treatment comparisons*.

N

National Death Index   (NDI) A central registry of deaths, started in 1979 and operated by the National Center for Health Statistics of the United States Public Health Services (see reference citation 345).

National Institutes of Health (NIH)   A group of institutes and related support structures located in Bethesda, Maryland, that is part of the United States Public Health Service. Responsible for funding basic and applied research in the health field. Also initiates and carries out medical research on an intramural and extramural basis.

natural history of disease   1. The course of a disease when left untreated. 2. The course of a disease when treated with standard modes of therapy.

natural history study   A *prospective follow-up study* designed to yield information on the natural course of a disease or condition. Such studies generally focus on the *control-treated group* in a *clinical trial* (especially one in which the *control treatment* is a *placebo* or standard medical care).

NCDS   National Cooperative Dialysis Study.

NCGS   National Cooperative Gallstone Study.

NCI   National Cancer Institute (part of the NIH).

NCR   No carbon required (a type of paper).

NDA   *New Drug Application.*

NDI   *National Death Index.*

negative control   *Inactive control treatment.*

negative control treatment   *Inactive control treatment.*

NEI   National Eye Institute (part of the NIH).

New Drug Application   (NDA) An application submitted by the manufacturer of a drug to the Food and Drug Administration for a license to market the drug for a specified indication (see *Pre Market Approval Application* for corresponding term for *medical devices*).

NHLBI   National Heart, Lung, and Blood Institute (part of the NIH and previously the National Heart Institute).

NIADDK   National Institute of Arthritis, Diabetes, and Digestive and Kidney Diseases (part of the NIH and previously the National Institute of Arthritis, Metabolism, and Digestive Diseases).

NIAID   National Institute of Allergy and Infectious Diseases (part of the NIH).

NIAMDD   National Institute of Arthritis, Metabolism, and Digestive Diseases (now the National Institute of Arthritis, Diabetes, and Digestive and Kidney Diseases).

NICHD   National Institute of Child Health and Human Development (part of the NIH).

NIDR   National Institute of Dental Research (part of the NIH).

NIGMS National Institute of General Medical Sciences (part of the NIH).

NIH *National Institutes of Health.*

NINCDS National Institute of Neurological and Communicative Disorders and Stroke (part of the NIH).

NLM National Library of Medicine (part of the NIH).

noncompliance Not in *compliance* with a designated procedure. Usually in reference to some treatment or data collection procedure in this book.

noncompliant 1. The absence of a *compliant* state in relation to a designated procedure. 2. Term used to describe a patient who is unable or unwilling to follow the *assigned treatment* regimen.

noncrossover design A design for a *clinical trial* in which a *patient* is assigned to receive only one of the *study treatments*. See also *crossover design.*

noncfactorial treatment structure A *treatment structure* that has no factorial structuring.

nonhealth professional A member of a committee, usually the *advisory-review* or *advisory-review and treatment effects monitoring committee*, chosen for expertise in an area outside the health field (e.g., philosophy, theology, law).

nonmasked clinical trial A *clinical trial* that does not involve any *treatment masking.*

nonmasked trial *Nonmasked clinical trial.*

nonrandom Any method that does not conform to the statistical definition of *random*. Used primarily in this book in contexts where there is a need to emphasize the nonrandom nature of a haphazard or systematic process.

nonrandom clinical trial A *clinical trial* that uses a *nonrandom* method of *treatment assignment.*

nonrandom trial *Nonrandom clinical trial.*

nonrequired follow-up visit Any *visit* by the *patient* to the *clinic* after the *randomization visit* that is not part of the required sequence of *follow-up visits.* The visit may be initiated by the patient or by study personnel, and includes *interim follow-up visits*, nonrequired *post-close-out follow-up visit*, as well as *post-trial follow-up visits.* Data generated at such visits are not generally used to satisfy data collection needs for *required follow-up visits*, unless they take place within the *time windows* for those visits and all necessary procedures are carried out during the visits.

nonsequential design A design that does not involve a *sequential design. Fixed sample size design.*

nonuniform treatment allocation A *treatment allocation* scheme in which the *assignment probabilities* for the various *study treatments* differ.

Notice of Claimed Investigational Exemption for New Drug A notice filed with the Food and Drug Administration by a drug sponsor or independent investigator requesting permission to test a new drug, or an existing one for a new indication, in humans. See *Investigational New Drug Application* and *phase I, II, III,* and *IV trials.*

NTIS National Technical Information Service, located in Springfield, Virginia, and affiliated with the United States Department of Commerce.

null hypothesis 1. (statistics) A hypothesis that postulates no underlying difference in the populations or groups being compared with regard to the factor, trait, characteristic, or condition of interest. 2. *Null treatment hypothesis.*

null treatment hypothesis A hypothesis that states that the true underlying effect of the *test treatment*, as expressed by a specified *outcome measure*, is no more or less than for the *control treatment.*

number adaptive allocation *Adaptive allocation* using the difference in the number of *patients* assigned to the various *treatment groups* as the basis for adapting the *treatment allocation ratio.*

number adaptive random allocation *Adaptive random allocation* using the difference in the number of *patients* assigned to the various *treatment groups* as the basis for change of the *treatment allocation ratio.*

number adaptive randomization A *treatment assignment process* using *number adaptive random allocation.*

O

observation variable A condition or characteristic associated with individual *patients* (e.g., age, history of myocardial infarction, blood glucose level) that may assume different values and that is observed and recorded at one or more time points over the course of data collection.

observational unit An identifiable unit, always a *patient* in this book but may be a collection of individuals in other contexts (e.g., as characterized by household members, a hospital ward, or an entire community), that forms the basis for data collection and analyses. Usually synonymous with *treatment assignment unit* in a *clinical trial.*

observed allocation ratio The actual *allocation ratio* in a completed *trial.*

observed effective sample size The *observed sample size* after reduction due to *dropouts* and treatment *noncompliance.*

observed power The actual *power* for detecting a specified *treatment difference*, given an *observed sample size*, observed outcome *event rate*, and observed *losses to follow-up* due to *dropout* and *noncompliance.*

observed sample size The number of *patients* enrolled in a *study.*

observed treatment difference The actual *treatment difference* observed either at the end of the *trial* or at some designated time point during the trial.

offeror The party or individual who offers or proposes to carry out a designated research project, normally indicated via submission of a formal proposal to the *sponsoring agency.* Term normally reserved in the *National Institutes of Health* language for proposals received in response to a *request for proposal* (RFP) and funded via the contract mechanism. See *applicant* and *proposer*.

officers of the study   In this book, generally taken as the chairman and vice-chairman of the *steering committee*, the *director* of the *data center*, *data coordinating center*, or *coordinating center*, and *project officer*.

OMB   Office of Management and Budget (office in the executive arm of the United States government).

one-sided alternative hypothesis   *One-tailed alternative hypothesis*.

one-sided test   (statistics) *One-tailed test*.

one-tailed alternative hypothesis   An alternative to the *null hypothesis* that specifies a range of permissible values of all which lie to one side of the null value (e.g., $H_o : \mu_1 = \mu_2$ versus $H_A : \mu_1 > \mu_2$). See also *two-tailed alternative hypothesis*.

one-tailed test   (statistics) A statistical *test of significance* based on the null value of no difference versus the set of all alternative values that are either to the right or to the left of the null value (e.g., the set indicating a positive treatment effect in a *clinical trial*. See also *two-tailed test*.

open clinical trial   1. A *clinical trial* in which a *study physician* or *study patient* decides on the treatment to be administered. *Nonrandom clinical trial*. 2. A *nonmasked clinical trial*. 3. A clinical trial with an open sequential design. (Usage note: Term not used in this book. Trials satisfying definition 1 are referred to as nonrandom trials. Trials satisfying defintion 2 are referred to as nonmasked trials.)

open label trial   1. *Nonmasked drug trial*. 2. Any *nonmasked trial*. (Usage note: The term *open label* not used in this book because of potential for confusion, e.g., with *open clinical trial*, and because nonmasked is considered to be more descriptive.)

open sequential design   A *sequential design* in which *enrollment* of *patients* continues until the *test treatment* is shown, in a statistical sense, to be either better or worse than the *control treatment*. Distinct from a *closed sequential design*, which allows for termination of enrollment after observation of a specified number of *outcomes*, even if it is not possible to draw a conclusion for or against the test treatment.

open sequential trial   A *trial* with an *open sequential design*.

operations committee   The term used in Veterans Administration sponsored *multicenter trials* to designate the standing committee that performs the functions of the *treatment effects monitoring committee* and some of the functions of the *advisory-review committee*.

outcome   1. A result, condition, or *event* associated with individual *study patients* that is used to assess the efficacy of the *study treatments*. 2. *Primary* or *secondary outcome, event*. 3. An observed event in a particular patient.

outcome adaptive allocation   *Adaptive allocation* based on *outcomes* observed for enrolled *patients*.

outcome adaptive random allocation   *Adaptive random allocation* based on *outcomes* observed for enrolled *patients*.

outcome adaptive randomization   A *treatment assignment process* using *outcome adaptive random allocation*.

outcome event   The *event* of primary interest in a *trial*, e.g., the one used for *sample size calculations* and for key data analyses in the trial.

outcome measure   An *observation variable* recorded for *patients* in the *trial* at one or more time points after *enrollment* for the purpose of assessing the effects of the *study treatments*. See *outcome variable*.

outcome variable   An *observation variable* recorded for *patients* in the *trial* at one or more time points after *enrollment* for the purpose of assessing the effects of the *study treatments*. See *outcome measure*.

outlier   Any value, reading, or measurement that is outside established limits and, for this reason, is questioned or considered to be in error.

P

***p*-value**   (statistics) A value associated with an observed *test statistic* that indicates the probability that a value as extreme or more extreme than the one observed will arise by chance alone in repeated replications of a study.

package insert   A document approved by the Food and Drug Administration and furnished by the manufacturer of a drug for use when dispensing the drug, which indicates approved uses, contraindications, and potential *side effects*. See *label insert*.

PAHO   Pan American Health Organization.

PAIS   Public Affairs Information Service (a literature database; see Chapter 26).

parallel design   *Parallel treatment design*.

parallel treatment design   A term sometimes used (but not in this book) to refer to *treatment designs* involving *uncrossed treatments*. See *noncrossover design*.

parameter   1. (statistics) A constant appearing in a mathematical expression that characterizes some population, process, or the like, whose true value is generally unknown but that can be estimated. 2. (clinical medicine) *Observation variable*. (Usage note: Not used in the latter context in this book.)

parent center   1. The *center* to which *satellite centers* report. 2. *Lead center*.

parent clinic   1. The *clinic* to which *satellite clinics* report. 2. *Lead clinic*.

parent institution   1. The institution that has administrative responsibilities for a specified *study cen-*

ter and associated investigators. 2. The center responsible for disbursing funds to other centers in a study funded under a *consortium agreement*.

PARIS Persantine Aspirin Reinfarction Study.

partial factorial structure *Partial factorial treatment structure*.

partial factorial treatment structure A *treatment structure* involving some but not all possible combinations of the treatments used in the *trial*.

partially masked clinical trial 1. A *clinical trial* in which some, but not all, of the *study treatments* are administered in a *single-* or *double-masked* fashion. 2. A clinical trial in which some, but not all, of the staff in a *clinic* are masked to *treatment assignment*.

participant *Study participant*.

patient Shorthand for study patient in this book. From Middle English *pacient*, from Old French *patient*, from Latin *patiens*, from the present participle of *pati*, to suffer.

patient close-out The process of separating patients from a *clinical trial* at the end of the *treatment and follow-up stage* (see Chapter 3 and Appendix D).

patient close-out stage The stage of a *trial* in which patients are separated from the trial at the end of the *treatment and follow-up stage* (see Chapter 3 and Appendix D). The fifth stage of a *trial* in this book.

patient compliance The degree to which a *patient* follows a prescribed set of procedures or routines. Synonymous with *treatment adherence* when the procedures or routines in question are those concerned with administration of a patient's *assigned treatment*.

patient enrollment The act of enrolling a *patient* (*treatment unit*) into a *trial*. In this book, considered to occur when the *treatment assignment* for the patient is revealed to clinic staff, or when *treatment* is initiated when assignments are known in advance of *enrollment*.

patient enrollment process The process of enrolling *patients* into a *clinical trial*. The process includes all the examinations and data collection procedures associated with the *prerandomization* and *randomization visits*.

patient examination Any *examination* done to evaluate a *patient* to determine eligibility for *enrollment* into a *trial* or to provide *follow-up data*.

patient follow-up A process involving periodic contact with *patients* enrolled in a *clinical trial* for the purpose of administering the *assigned treatment*(s), observing the effects of treatment(s), modifying the course of treatment(s), or for collecting required *data*.

patient identification number A unique sequence of numbers, or numbers and letters, that are used to identify a *patient*.

patient monitoring *Patient safety monitoring*.

patient population *Study population*.

patient recruitment The process of identifying suitable patients for *enrollment* into a *clinical trial*.

patient recruitment goal The number of *patients* scheduled to be enrolled into the trial. Usually set before the trial starts, or shortly thereafter, via a *sample size calculation* or via practical considerations.

patient recruitment quota A specification, usually set before *patient recruitment* is started or shortly thereafter, that indicates the mix of patients to be enrolled with regard to some characteristic, trait, or condition (e.g., the number of males versus females).

patient recruitment stage The stage of a *clinical trial* concerned primarily with *patient recruitment* (see Chapter 3 and Appendix D). The third stage of a trial in this book.

patient safety monitoring 1. Any ongoing process of reviewing accumulated outcome data for groups of *patients* in a *trial* to determine if a designated treatment procedure should be altered or stopped. *Treatment effects monitoring*. 2. The process of watching for treatment effects in an individual patient (term not ordinarily used in this context in this book).

payline A term used in connection with National Institutes of Health *grants* to indicate the *priority score* required on an approved application to permit payment. The payline is a function of the number of approved applications received by an institute, the distribution of priority scores across applications, and the amount of money available for new research initiatives by the institute.

performance monitoring An ongoing process carried out over the course of a *trial* to assess the performance of some *center*, group of centers, or some other task-oriented group in the structure of a trial.

phase I trial The first stage in testing a new drug in man. Performed as part of an approved *Investigational New Drug Application* under Food and Drug Administration guidelines. The studies are usually done to generate preliminary information on the chemical action and safety of the drug using normal healthy volunteers. Usually done without a *comparison group* (see Food and Drug Administration, 1977c; Pines, 1980).

phase II trial The second stage in testing a new drug in man. Performed as part of an approved *Investigational New Drug Application* under Food and Drug Administration guidelines. Generally carried out on patients with the disease or condition of interest. The main purpose is to provide preliminary information on treatment efficacy and to supplement information on safety obtained from *phase I trials*. Usually, but not always, designed to include a *control treatment* and *random allocation* of patients to treatment (see Food and Drug Administration, 1977c; Pines, 1980).

phase III trial　The third and usually final stage in testing a new drug in man. Performed as part of an approved *Investigational New Drug Application* under Food and Drug Administration guidelines. Concerned primarily with assessment of dosage effects and efficacy and safety. Usually designed to include a *control treatment* and *random allocation* to treatment. Once this phase is completed the drug manufacturers may request permission to market the drug by submission of a *New Drug Application* to the Food and Drug Administration, assuming the results of the *phase I, II* and *III trials* are consistent with such a request (see Food and Drug Administration, 1977c; Pines, 1980).

phase IV trial　Generally, a *randomized controlled trial* that is designed to evaluate the long-term safety and efficacy of a drug for a given indication and that is done with Food and Drug Administration approval. Usually carried out after licensure of the drug for that indication (see Food and Drug Administration, 1977c).

PHS　Physicians' Health Study.

PI　Principal investigator.

pilot study　A preliminary study designed to indicate whether a larger study is practical. See *feasibility study.*

placebo　A pharmacologically inactive agent given to a patient as a substitute for an active agent and where the patient is not informed whether he is receiving the active or inactive agent.

placebo-controlled clinical trial　A *clinical trial* in which *patients* assigned to the *control treatment* receive a *placebo.*

placebo effect　The effect produced by a *placebo.* The effect in *placebo-controlled clinical trials* is generally measured by comparison of the effect observed in *patients* receiving the placebo treatment with the effect observed in patients receiving the *active treatment.*

placebo reactor　A *patient* who reports *side effects* normally associated with the *test treatment* while receiving a *placebo.*

placebo treatment　1. A treatment involving the use of a *placebo.* 2. A treatment that is harmless.

play the winner treatment allocation scheme　An *outcome adaptive allocation* scheme based on work of Robbins (1952, 1956) in which the next *treatment assignment* is a function of the success or failure of the *test treatment,* as assessed in the last *patient* enrolled. A success would cause the next assignment to be made to the test treatment. A failure would cause the next assignment to be made to the *control treatment.* Modified by Zelen (1969) so as not to require complete dependence on the outcome observed in the last patient enrolled. The goal is to minimize the number of patients assigned to the inferior treatment.

PMA　Pre-Market Approval (PMA) application (for a new *medical device*; see *New Drug Application* for corresponding term for drugs).

PO　1. *Project office.* 2. *Project officer.*

policy-advisory board　*Advisory-review committee.*

policy board　*Advisory-review committee.*

polychotomous variable　A *discrete variable* that may assume two or more different values.

portrait-style page orientation　A form of orientation in which printed and visual information is arrayed on the short axis of a page (e.g., as the pages in this book). See *landscape-style page orientation* for opposing term.

POSCH　Program on the Surgical Control of Hyperlipidemia.

positive control　*Active control treatment.*

positive control treatment　*Active control treatment.*

post-close-out follow-up visit　1. Any *follow-up visit* of a *patient* that takes place after his separation from the *trial,* as indicated by completion of the *close-out follow-up visit.* 2. Any follow-up visit which takes place after completion of the *close-out stage* of a trial. 3. *Post-trial follow-up visit.*

post-close-out visit　*Post-close-out follow-up visit.*

post-marketing surveillance　Term used by the Food and Drug Administration to characterize any procedure, implemented after licensure of a drug for a given indication, that is designed to provide information on the actual use of the drug for that indication and on the occurrence of related *side effects.* The surveillance usually involves survey techniques rather than *controlled trials.*

post-randomization examination　Any *patient examination* made by *clinic* personnel during a *post-randomization follow-up visit* for *data collection.*

post-randomization follow-up visit　Any *visit* by a patient to the *clinic* after the *randomization visit,* *required* as well as *nonrequired* follow-up visits. The former class includes *treatment application and adjustment, regular, close-out,* and *post-close-out follow-up visits.*

post-randomization visit　*Post-randomization follow-up visit.*

post-stratification　The process of classifying *patients* into *strata* after they have been enrolled in the *study*—usually for data analysis purposes.

post-treatment follow-up　1. Any *patient follow-up* after the first application of the *assigned treatment,* especially in *clinical trials* involving a single application of the treatment, e.g., as in most surgery trials. 2. *Post-trial follow-up.*

post-trial follow-up　A term used to refer to any form of *patient follow-up* after completion of the *close-out stage* of a *trial.*

post-trial follow-up stage　One of the seven stages of a trial in this book (see Chapter 3 and Appendix D). Defined as an optional stage that occurs during or after completion of the *termination stage* of the trial and that is designed to provide *follow-up data* on mortality or some other *outcome measure.*

post-trial follow-up visit　1. Any *follow-up visit* that takes place after the *close of the trial,* the main purpose of which is to enable clinic personnel to collect *data* on a *primary* or *secondary outcome measure* to assess *treatment effects*. 2. The same as 1 except that the visit may take place any time after the *close-out follow-up visit*. See *post-close-out follow-up visit*.

power The probability of rejecting the *null hypothesis* when it is false.

Pre-Market Approval (PMA) application An application to the Food and Drug Administration for permission to market a specified *medical device* (Food and Drug Administration, 1983). See *New Drug Application* for corresponding term for drugs.

prerandomization examination Any *examination* that is part of the evaluation process of a *patient* for *enrollment* into a *trial* and that is carried out before the *randomization examination*.

prerandomization visit Any *visit* made to the *clinic* by a potential *study patient* for the purpose of evaluation for *enrollment* into the *trial* and that takes place prior to the *randomization visit*.

pretreatment examination Any *examination* done on a *patient* before the initiation of *treatment* and that is a required part of the procedures for the *trial*. Synonymous with *prerandomization examination* if *randomization* and initiation of treatment take place during the same visit.

prevention trial *Prophylactic trial*.

primary event 1. A *primary outcome variable* that is binary. 2. The actual occurrence of a *primary outcome*.

primary outcome 1. The *event* or condition the *trial* is designed to ameliorate, delay, or prevent. 2. The actual occurrence of a *primary event* in a *study patient*.

primary outcome variable The *outcome variable* that is designated or regarded as key in the design or analysis of the results of a *trial*. Generally, the variable used for *sample size calculations* in the design of the trial or, when no sample size calculation is made, for the main avenue of data analyses.

primary prevention trial A *prophylactic trial* that involves *patients* selected for the absence of a specified disease or condition and a *test treatment* that is being used ostensibly to prevent or delay the onset of that disease or condition.

principal investigator 1. The designation used by the *National Institutes of Health* to denote the individual named on a *grant* application who is responsible for directing the proposed research. 2. The lead scientist in a research project. (Usage note: It is best to avoid use of the term to designate the head of a *center* in a *multicenter trial*. It should be used in such settings only when there is a single individual, such as the *chairman of the study*, who is regarded by everyone in the trial as the principal investigator. Otherwise some other term, such as *center director*, should be used.)

priority score 1. The score assigned to a research

application by an individual member of a *review group* that reflects that individual's judgment regarding the scientific merit of the proposal. In *National Institutes of Health* grant reviews the score may range from 1 (high scientific merit) to 5 (low scientific merit). 2. The score assigned to a research application as computed from the scores assigned by individual reviewers of the application.

procurement center *Procurement and distribution center*.

procurement and distribution center A facility in the structure of a *clinical trial* that is responsible for procuring, packaging, and distributing a needed supply or product (e.g., drugs, laboratory supplies, forms) to selected *centers* in the trial.

program director 1. The individual who heads a research project. 2. *Principal investigator*. (Usage note: Term not used in the context of a *multicenter trial* in this book. See usage note appearing under *principal investigator* for reason.)

program office 1. *Project office*. 2. An office containing a *project office* for several different but related studies.

program officer *Project officer*.

project director 1. The individual who heads a research project. 2. *Principal investigator*. (Usage note: Term not used in the context of a *multicenter trial* in this book. See usage note appearing under principal investigator for reason.)

project office 1. The office, located in the *sponsoring agency* and usually staffed with one or more individuals trained in a medical or research field, that is responsible for dealing with technical, scientific, and programmatic aspects of a *grant*- or *contract*-funded project. 2. *Program office*.

project officer 1. The individual in the *sponsoring agency* who is responsible for dealing with technical, scientific, and programmatic aspects of a *grant* or *contract*-funded project. 2. *Health scientist administrator* in *National Institutes of Health* grant-funded projects. See also *program officer*.

prophylactic trial A *trial* that is designed to assess the efficacy of a treatment procedure aimed at preventing the development or progression of a specific disease or condition.

proposer The party or individual who proposes, normally via submission of a written proposal, to carry out a designated research project. See also *offeror* and *applicant*.

prospective follow-up study A study in which people with a specific attribute or characteristic are identified and then observed for some period of time thereafter for the occurrence of the outcome or condition of interest, usually disease or death. The study may or may not involve a *comparison group*. *Clinical trials* represent a special subset of prospective follow-up studies.

prospective study *Prospective follow-up study*.

protocol *Study protocol*.

protocol development stage The second stage of a

clinical trial in this book. Usually undertaken after the initiation of funding and characterized by work involving development of the *protocol* and procedures needed to carry out the trial (see Chapter 3 and Appendix D).

pseudo random number   A number that has been generated via a deterministic process, that has, or appears to have, the properties of a *random number*, e.g., as with some computer-generated "random" numbers (see Knuth, 1969).

PSRO   Professional Standards Review Organization.

Q

quality assurance   Any procedure, method, or philosophy for collecting, processing, or analyzing data that is aimed at maintaining or improving the reliability or validity of the data and the associated procedures used to generate them.

quality control center   One of the possible *resource centers* in a *trial*. Defined as the *center* with responsibility for quality assurance for one or more aspects of the data collection or analysis processes. (Usage note: Term not used in this book except where there is a specified center with designated quality control functions that are over and above those normally assumed by the *data center, data coordinating center*, or *coordinating center*.)

quasi random number   *Pseudo random number.*

R

R and D   Research and development.

RAI   Research Award Index (a database of research funded by the United States Public Health Service; see Chapter 26).

random   (general) 1. Having no specific pattern or objective. Of or designating a chance process in which the occurrence of previous events is of no value in predicting future events. From Old French, *random*, meaning force, violence, impetuosity. 2. Sometimes used as a synonym for haphazard, but never in this book. Usage in this book always refers to a formal process meeting, or believed to meet, the conditions specified under the statistical definition of random.

random   1. (statistics) A term used to refer to a sequence of observations, activities, assignments, etc., that is the result of a chance process in which the probability of any given sequence is known or can be determined. 2. The term used to refer to a process that meets the probability conditions outlined above.

random allocation   A method for assigning *patients* to *treatment* using a *random process.*

random number   A number generated or drawn via some defined *random process.*

random process   Any method or procedure that

yields output that has the defined mathematical properties of a *random variable.*

random variable   A *variable* that may assume any one of a number of different values, where the set of possible values is determined by a probability distribution, such as Bernoulli or normal.

randomization   1. The process of assigning patients (*treatment units*) to treatment using a *random process*, such as via use of a table of random numbers. 2. The process of deriving an order or sequence of items, determinations, specimens, readings, or the like using a *random process.*

randomization examination   A *patient examination* that is done during the *randomization visit.*

randomization unit   *Treatment assignment unit.* Usually *patient*, but may be a larger unit, as in studies involving families, hospital wards, or the like.

randomization visit   The *clinic visit* at which the *patient* is *randomized.*

randomized   The condition of having been assigned to a *treatment* via a *random process*. Normally considered to have occurred when the *treatment assignment* is revealed to any member of the clinic staff, e.g., when the envelope containing the treatment is opened at the *clinic.*

randomized control clinical trial   Term sometimes used (e.g., Chalmers et al., 1981) to emphasize the nature of the *randomization process* in relation to the *control treatment* (i.e., that patients are randomly assigned to the control treatment). (Usage note: Phrase not used in this book. The preferred term is *randomized controlled clinical trial*).

randomized control trial   *Randomized controlled clinical trial.* (See *randomized control clinical trial* for usage note.)

randomized controlled clinical trial   A *clinical trial* (always in man in this book) that involves at least one *test treatment* and one *control treatment*, concurrent *enrollment* and *follow-up* of the *test-* and *control-treated groups*, and in which the treatments to be administered are selected by a *random process*, such that neither the patients nor the persons responsible for their selection or treatment can influence the assignments, and where the assignments remain unknown to the patients and clinic staff until the patients have been determined to be eligible for *enrollment* into the trial (and then may be revealed to patients and clinic personnel only by letter or number codes in *masked trials*).

randomized controlled trial   *Randomized controlled clinical trial.*

raw data   1. Measurements and observations recorded on study *data forms*. 2. Unedited computer-generated listings of data from study data forms, prior to use of reduction and summary procedures needed for data analysis.

RBO   *Relative betting odds.*

RCT   1. *Randomized clinical trial.* 2. *Randomized controlled trial.*

reading center   A *center* that is responsible for interpreting and codifying information from a specified set of materials, records, or documents (e.g., ECGs, fundus photographs, chest X rays, biopsy or autopsy specimens, death certificates) provided by the *clinical center*(s) in the *study*.

record (n). A paper or electronic document that contains or is designed to contain a set of facts related to some occurrence, transaction, or the like.

recruitment goal *Patient recruitment goal.*

recruitment log A log maintained by a *clinic* that lists each *patient* considered for *enrollment* into a *study*. Usually maintained to provide a description of the characteristics of the population screened for enrollment. See *screening log.*

recruitment quota *Patient recruitment quota.*

regression to the mean A phenomenon that occurs when a second determination or measurement is made only on those individuals with an extreme initial determination or measurement. On average, the second determination or measurement tends to be less extreme than the initial one. Term originally coined by Sir Francis Galton (1886) to characterize the tendency for tall parents to produce shorter offspring and vice versa.

regular follow-up visit A *required follow-up visit*, the main purpose of which is to enable clinic personnel to carry out treatment assessment and data collection procedures, as specified in the study protocol. Called regular because such visits are normally required at fixed periods over the course of *follow-up*. Does not include visits done simply for treatment application or treatment adjustment.

relative betting odds A method of analysis developed by Cornfield (1966b) involving the ratio of two likelihood functions computed under the *null hypothesis* and a specified alternative.

request for application (RFA) A document prepared and distributed by a *sponsoring agency* to solicit applications for *grant* support to perform work described in the request.

request for proposal (RFP) A document prepared and distributed by a *sponsoring agency* to solicit proposals for execution of specific work. Normally used in conjunction with *contract* funding.

required follow-up visit Any *follow-up visit* that is a required part of the *study protocol* and that is to be done at a specified time after the *randomization visit*. Visits include *treatment application and adjustment, regular, close-out,* and *post-close-out,* and *post-trial follow-up visits.*

research group *Investigative group.*

resource center Any *center*, other than a *clinical center*, identified in the structure of a *trial*, that is involved in performing a specified set of support functions. The term includes *data center, data coordinating center, treatment coordinating center, coordinating center, central laboratory, reading center, quality control center, project office,* and *procurement and distribution center.*

response variable *Outcome variable.*

restricted allocation scheme Any allocation scheme in which the *treatment allocation schedule* is designed to satisfy certain preset constraints, as in *blocking* in a *fixed allocation schedule.*

restricted random allocation *Restricted allocation scheme* involving use of a *random process* to make *treatment assignments.*

restricted randomization The process of generating or issuing *treatment assignments* via a *restricted random allocation* treatment schedule.

restricted treatment allocation schedule A *treatment allocation schedule* that is constrained to yield the *expected allocation* ratio, as with *blocking* in a *fixed allocation schedule.*

review group A group of individuals, normally recruited by the *sponsoring agency* or its representative, charged with the review of a specific research proposal or set of research proposals for scientific merit. *study section.*

RFA *Request for application.*

RFP *Request for proposal.*

risk factor Any environmental exposure, personal characteristic, or event that affects the probability of developing a given disease or experiencing a change in health status (Morgenstern and Bursic, 1982).

risk factor analysis (epidemiology) Any analysis, usually involving regression or *subgroup analyses*, that is aimed at identifying *risk factors* for a given disease or condition.

RJE Remote job entry (via a *computer terminal*).

routine follow-up visit *Regular follow-up visit.*

S

safety committee *Treatment effects monitoring committee.*

safety monitoring *Treatment effects monitoring.*

safety monitoring committee *Treatment effects monitoring committee.*

sample size 1. The actual number of *patients* enrolled in a *study*. 2. The anticipated number of patients to be enrolled in a study, or the *patient recruitment goal.*

sample size calculation A mathematical calculation, usually carried out when a *trial* is planned, that indicates the number of patients to be enrolled in order to provide a specified degree of statistical precision for a specified *type I* and *type II* error protection (see Chapter 9).

sample size requirement The sample size yielded by a *sample size calculation*. See *recruitment goal.*

SAS Statistical Analysis System (a package of data analysis programs).

satellite center A *center* that is subservient to the *parent center* and that is organized to perform a designated set of functions considered to be part of the workscope of the parent center.

satellite clinic A *clinic* that is subservient to the *parent clinic* and that is organized and operated to screen, identify, enroll, treat, or follow a segment of the *study population* that cannot, for matters of convenience or other reasons, be seen at the parent clinic.

SAW   Show as written.

SC   Steering committee.

scheduled follow-up visit   *Required follow-up visit.*

SCI   Science Citation Index.

screening log   *Recruitment log.*

secondary event   1. A *secondary outcome variable* that is binary. 2. The actual occurrence of a *secondary outcome.*

secondary outcome   1. An *event* or condition related to the *primary outcome* but of less clinical or medical importance than the primary outcome. 2. The actual occurrence of a *secondary event* in a *study patient.*

secondary outcome variable   An *outcome variable* that is known or believed to be related to the *primary outcome variable* and that is used, in addition to the primary outcome variable, for evaluation of treatments in the trial (e.g., observation of patients for the occurrence of nonfatal myocardial infarctions in a *clinical trial* using death as the *primary outcome* measure). 2. Any other outcome variable, regardless of its relationship to the primary outcome variable, that is used for treatment evaluation.

secondary paper   Paper dealing with a secondary objective of the *trial* and written by study personnel commissioned by the *investigative group* or their representative.

secondary prevention trial   A *prevention trial* involving *patients* with a history of some disease or condition in which the *test treatment* is administered to prevent or delay further development or progression of that disease or condition. For example, a *drug trial* involving use of a daily dose of aspirin over a period of years for prevention of myocardial infarction in patients with a prior history of myocardial infarction.

secular trend   A trend or pattern that is time related; temporal trend.

self-checking digit   *Check digit.*

sequential analysis   1. The analysis done after *enrollment* of a *patient*, pair of patients, or larger *block* of *patients*, in a *sequential trial* to determine whether additional patients should be enrolled. The decision is made by observing the *test-control difference* in observed *outcomes*. Enrollment of the next patient, pair of patients, or block of patients is carried out if the difference does not exceed prespecified boundary limits. 2. Periodic analyses carried out for *treatment monitoring* in trials with *fixed sample size designs*. (Usage note: Use in the context of definition 2 is avoided in this book. See *interim analysis* for preferred term.)

sequential design   Any design in which the decision as to whether to enroll the next patient, pair of patients, or *block* of *patients* is determined by whether the cumulative *treatment difference* for all previous patients is within specified limits. *Enrollment* is continued if the difference does not exceed the limits. It is terminated if it does.

sequential trial   1. A trial involving a *sequential design*. 2. Term sometimes used (but not in this book) in conjunction with a *fixed sample size design* in which decisions concerning the *enrollment* of additional *patients*, or the continued *treatment* and observation of patients already enrolled, is dependent on accumulated *data* in the *trial*.

sham   Something false presented to be genuine; a spurious imitation. Derived from the word *shame*, meaning trick or fraud.

sham procedure   A procedure designed to resemble the real one and that is performed on a *patient* for the purpose of masking the patient or the patient's *study physician* as to whether the patient has received the real procedure.

side effect   A secondary by-product of an action or procedure. Usually *treatment side effect* in this book.

significance level   (statistics) 1. The permissible *type I error* level for a test of the *null hypothesis* with a specified *test statistic*. The null hypothesis is accepted if the test statistic yields a *p-value* which is larger than the specified level and is rejected if it is equal to or less than this value. 2. *p-value.*

significance test   *Test of significance.*

significance testing   (statistics) The act of carrying out a *test of significance.*

simple randomization   *Unrestricted randomization.*

simple treatment structure   *Nonfactorial treatment structure.*

single-blind   *Single-masked* in this book. See *blind* for usage comment.

single-blinded   *Single-masked* in this book. See *blind* for usage comment.

single-blinded clinical trial   *Single-masked clinical trial.*

single-center trial   1. A *clinical trial* involving only one *clinic* (with or without *satellite clinics*) and no other *resource center*. 2. A trial involving only one clinic and a *center* to receive and process data. 3. A trial involving only one clinic and one or more resource centers. 4. A trial with no clinical centers, but one or more resource centers, as in the Physicians' Health Study sketched in Appendix B. 5. A *clinical trial* involving two or more clinical centers, but no center to receive and process *study data*. 6. A trial with multiple clinics not having a common *study protocol* (see usage note under *multicenter clinical trial*).

single-mask   *Single-masked.*

single-masked   A condition where certain persons (e.g., *study physicians*) are informed of some fact or condition whereas other persons (e.g., *patients*) are purposefully denied information regarding that fact or condition.

single-masked clinical trial   1. A *clinical trial* in

which treatments are administered in such a manner that patients in the trial are not informed of whether they have been assigned to the *test* or *control treatment*, but clinic staff are. 2. A clinical trial in which the patient knows the treatment assigned, but the treating physician, examiner, or observer does not. (Usage note: Term not used in the context of definition 2 in this book.)

site visit A visit to a *center* or prospective center in a *trial* by personnel from outside that center for the purpose of assessing its performance or performance potential in the trial.

soft endpoint *Soft outcome.* (See usage note for *endpoint*.)

soft outcome Any *outcome measure* that is subject to major errors of interpretation or measurement. Usually, a measurement or assessment that depends on clinical judgment.

software Computer programs and related manuals and documents needed to operate them.

specified allocation ratio The particular *allocation ratio* used in constructing the *allocation schedule*.

sponsor *Sponsoring agency.*

sponsoring agency The institution, organization, or foundation that provides fiscal support, and often administrative and scientific support as well, for a given project. See *funding agency*.

SPSS Statistical Package for the Social Sciences.

SSIE Smithsonian Scientific Information Exchange.

stages of a clinical trial An arbitrary classification to characterize the stages of a trial. The stages used in this book are: Initial design, protocol development, patient recruitment, treatment and follow-up, patient close-out, termination, and (optional) post-trial follow-up (see Chapter 3 and Appendix D).

standard treatment The accepted mode of treatment for a given disease or condition. Equivalent to the *control treatment* in *clinical trials* when chosen to mimic standard medical practice.

statistical significance (statistics) *p-value*.

steering committee (*SC*) 1. A committee responsible for directing the activities of a designated project. 2. One of the *key committees* in the organizational structure of a *multicenter clinical trial*. Committee responsible for conduct of the *trial* and to which all other committees report, except the *treatment effects monitoring committee* and *advisory-review committee* or *advisory-review and treatment effects monitoring committee*.

stop condition 1. A condition encountered when carrying out a procedure (e.g., completing a *data form*, performing a *patient examination*) that requires the person performing the procedure to terminate the procedure until or unless the condition can be removed. 2. A defined condition that, when encountered for a *patient* enrolled in a *trial*, requires or permits clinic personnel to take some action related to that patient, such as instituting a

change in treatment or terminating *follow-up* of that patient.

stop item An item or response category on a *data form* that when used or checked indicates the presence of a *stop condition* (see Chapter 12).

stopping boundary The set of values formed by a line or set of lines (or curves), usually specified before or shortly after the start of patient recruitment, which, if exceeded, indicates the existence of a *test-control treatment difference* that satisfies certain statistical properties (e.g., has a *p-value* of less than a certain size). The boundaries will be used as a basis for stopping the *trial* when developed in conjunction with a *sequential design*, but not necessarily when used in conjunction with a *fixed sample size design*.

stopping rule A rule, usually set before or shortly after the start of patient recruitment, that specifies a limit for the observed *test-control treatment difference* for the *primary outcome*, which, if exceeded, automatically leads to termination of the *test* or *control treatment*, depending on the direction of the observed difference.

strata (pl. of stratum) A series of distinct levels or layers. In this book, generally *subgroups* of patients formed by classification on some *variable* or set of variables, usually *baseline variables*.

stratification 1. The process of classifying *observation units* into *strata*. 2. The process of classifying *patients* into strata as part of the *randomization* process or for purposes of data analysis.

stratification variable A *variable* used to classify the *observational units* into *strata*.

stratified allocation A method of *treatment assignment* in which *patients* are first classified into defined *subgroups* based on one or more *baseline variables* and then assigned to *treatment* within the defined subgroups.

stratified random allocation *Random allocation* within defined *allocation strata*.

stratified randomization A *treatment assignment process* using *stratified random allocation*.

stratum (sing. of *strata*) A layer, level, or defined *subgroup*.

study 1. A general term used to refer to any one of a variety of research activities involving the collection, analysis, or interpretation of data. 2. Often used in this book as a synonym for *clinical trial*. 3. A project involving multiple types of investigations, only one of which is a clinical trial (e.g., as in the Coronary Artery Surgery Study since it includes both a clinical trial and an uncontrolled *prospective follow-up study*.

study chairman Chairman of the *steering committee*.

study clinic A facility with defined responsibilities for recruiting, enrolling, treating, and following *patients* in a *trial*.

study database The entire set of *data*, whether or not codified and keyed for storage in a *computer*, collected on study *patients*, as contained on official *data forms* of the *trial*. Note: Data contained in patients' charts, unless transcribed onto official study data forms, are not considered part of the study database.

study group   1. Any defined group of patients on whom specified data are collected. 2. The entire group of patients included in a *study*. 3. Often synonymous with *treatment group*, as used in this book. 4. The group of investigators carrying out a study, especially a *multicenter* study. (Usage note: Term not used in the sense of definition 4 in this book.)

study handbook   A book that contains a series of tables, charts, figures, and specification pages that detail the main design and operating features of a *study*, largely without use of written narrative.

study investigator   General term used in this book to designate any individual who has a key role in the design, conduct, or analysis of a *study*.

study manual of operations   A document or collection of documents that describes the procedures used in a *center* or set of centers in a *clinical trial* (e.g., manual of operations for *study clinics, coordinating center* manual of operations, ECG *reading center* manual of operations).

study participant   1. A term sometimes used in place of *study patient* when there is a desire to avoid the connotation of illness, as in *trials* involving well people. 2. *Study investigator* (but not in this book).

study patient   Term used in this book to characterize an individual considered for *enrollment* or actually enrolled into a *trial* regardless of whether or not there is a perceived need for medical care. See *study subject* and *study participant*.

study physician   Any physician associated with a *study clinic* who is responsible for administering the *study treatments* to *patients* in the *trial* or who is responsible for patient care, as dictated by the *study protocol*.

study population   1. The set of patients enrolled in a *trial*. 2. The entire set of patients considered for *enrollment* into the trial (not used in this context in this book).

study protocol   A narrative document that describes the general design and operating features of a *trial*. Distinguished from the *study manual of operations* by its generality and absence of specific details needed for day-to-day execution of the trial.

study section   1. Any *review group* of the *National Institutes of Health*, especially one that is chartered to carry out reviews of research applications in a general area of research and that meets at regular intervals during the calendar year to perform those reviews. 2. A group of individuals, normally recruited by the *sponsoring agency* as its representatives, charged with the review of a specific research proposal or set of research proposals to assess scientific merit. See *review group*.

study subject   General term used to denote an individual enrolled in a study. Not used in this book. The advantage of the term, as opposed to *study patient*, is that it avoids the connotation of illness—useful in cases where well people are being studied. The disadvantage is that it carries a connotation of subjugation—a notion that is at variance with the concept of informed consent and a patient-investigator partnership.

study treatment   General term used throughout this book to refer to either a *test* or *control treatment*.

study vice-chairman   The individual elected or designed to perform the functions of *study chairman* in his absence.

subgroup   A subpart of the *study population* distinguished by a particular characteristic or set of characteristics (e.g., males under age 45 at entry).

subgroup analysis   Any data analysis that focuses on a selected *subgroup* or *patients*. Generally in this book, any analysis that is aimed at elucidating *treatment differences* within a defined subgroup of patients.

subgrouping cut-point   The value of a *subgrouping variable* used to separate patients (*treatment units*) into *subgroups*. For example, formation of subgroups of patients less than 35 years of age, 35 through 54 years of age, and 55 years of age or older requires use of cut-points at 35 and 55 years of age.

subgrouping variable   A *variable*, such as age, used to classify *patients* (*treatment units*) into *subgroups*. Usually a *baseline characteristic* for most *subgroup analyses* in *clinical trials*.

subject   *Study subject*.

support center   *Resource center*.

surgical trial   A *trial* in which the *test treatment* is a surgical procedure.

surrogate outcome   An *outcome*, based on some test or measurement, that is used instead of a *clinical event* in the design or analysis of *clinical trial*.

surrogate outcome variable   A test, measurement, score, or some other similar *variable* that is used in place of a *clinical event* (e.g., use of blood pressure change in place of clinical hypertension) in the design of a *trial*, or in summarizing results from it. Used because the variable is believed to be correlated with the clinical event of interest and because of its perceived utility in yielding detectable *treatment differences*.

survival analysis   1. Any method of data analysis that focuses on the length of survival of the *observational units*. 2. *Lifetable analysis*.

T

technical group   *Investigative group*.

TEMC   *Treatment effects monitoring committee*.

terminal   *Computer terminal*.

termination stage   The sixth and usually last stage of a *clinical trial* as used in this book. Concerned primarily with analysis of the study results (see Chapter 3 and Appendix D).

test-control difference   *Test-control treatment difference.*

test-control treatment difference   The postulated or observed difference between the *test-* and *control-treated groups* of *patients* with regard to a specified *outcome measure.*

test group   A group of *patients* defined by the study design—patients assigned to the *test treatment* in a *clinical trial*—who are contrasted with the *control group* of patients to reach a conclusion regarding some factor, condition, or treatment.

test of significance   (statistics) 1. The evaluation of observed data by calculating a specified test statistic and then deriving the associated *p-value.* 2. *Test statistic.*

test statistic   1. The formula or computing algorithm used to carry out a *test of significance.* 2. The numerical value provided by the formula or computing algorithm for a specified test of significance using a defined data set.

test-treated group   1. The group of *patients* assigned to the *test treatment.* 2. The group of patients who receive the test treatment. (Usage note: Use of the term in this book is always from the point of view of the *assignment process*, regardless of the treatment actually administered.)

test treatment   The drug, device, or procedure to be evaluated in a particular *trial.*

therapeutic trial   A *trial* designed to test the safety and efficacy of a particular drug, device, or procedure that is considered to have therapeutic value.

throwaway medical journal   A pejorative term used to characterize a medical periodical that is distributed by a profit-making firm to a segment of the medical community free of charge.

time of enrollment   The time point at which a patient (*treatment unit*) is regarded as having officially entered the *trial* and after which is regarded as a part of the *study population.* Operationally, the time point at which the *treatment assignment* is revealed to clinic staff, or when *treatment* is initiated when assignments are known in advance of *enrollment.*

time window   The permissible time interval for performing a specified *baseline* or *follow-up examination.*

toxic drug reaction   An *adverse drug reaction* that results in morbidity or mortality.

toxic side effect   An *adverse side effect* that results in morbidity or mortality.

treatment   1. The act of treating, as in caring for a *patient.* 2. The specific regimen, method, or procedure being tested in a *clinical trial.*

treatment adjustment follow-up visit   *Treatment application and adjustment follow-up visit.*

treatment adjustment visit   *Treatment application and adjustment follow-up visit.*

treatment adherence   The degree to which a *patient* follows his assigned treatment regimen. See *treatment compliance.*

treatment allocation   1. The process of assigning *pa-tients* to *treatment.* 2. The *treatment assignment* of a particular patient.

treatment allocation design   The plan for assigning *patients* to *treatment.*

treatment allocation ratio   The ratio of the number of *patients* assigned or to be assigned to the *test-treated group* to those assigned or to be assigned to the *control-treated group* (e.g., an allocation ratio of 1:2 in a completed trial is one in which twice as many patients were assigned to the *control treatment* as were assigned to the *test treatment*).

treatment allocation schedule   The schedule used for issuing *treatment assignments.*

treatment allocation strata   *Strata*, designated before the start of *patient enrollment* and defined by *baseline characteristics*(s) or clinic, that are used to define subsets of *patients* who are assigned to *treatment* using *allocation schedules* constructed for the individual strata.

treatment application and adjustment follow-up visit   A *follow-up visit*, the main purpose of which is to enable clinic staff to apply or adjust treatment, depending on patient needs and study specifications.

treatment application and adjustment visit   *Treatment application and adjustment follow-up visit.*

treatment application follow-up visit   *Treatment application and adjustment follow-up visit.*

treatment application visit   *Treatment application and adjustment follow-up visit.*

treatment arm   Term sometimes used in place of *study treatment*, or *study group*, especially in cancer *trials* (but not in this book).

treatment assignment   The *treatment* to be administered to the *assignment unit* (usually a *patient*, but may be some other larger unit such as all members of a family or members of a hospital ward) as indicated in the *treatment allocation schedule.*

treatment assignment probability   The probability associated with a specified *treatment assignment.* The value is fixed over the course of *patient enrollment* in *trials* with *fixed allocation designs.* It changes in trials using *adaptive allocation designs.*

treatment assignment process   The process of assigning *patients* to treatment in a *clinical trial.*

treatment assignment unit   The unit used in the *treatment assignment process*, usually *patient*, but the unit may be made up of multiple individuals in special cases such as in a *trial* involving treatment of a family unit or an entire hospital ward. Equivalent to *randomization unit* in trials involving *random allocation.*

treatment block   A *block* consisting of a prespecified number of *patients*, all enrolled in reasonably close proximity to one another and assigned to the various *study treatments* in such a way so as to satisfy a preset *allocation ratio.* See also *treatment block size.*

treatment block size   The number of allocations required for a specified *treatment block.* For example, a random allocation schedule for a *trial* involving two treatments, constructed using blocks of size 8 and an allocation ratio of 1:1, would require constraints on the *assignment process* such that the *specified allocation ratio* is satisfied after every eighth assignment.

treatment comparison   Any comparison involving two or more of the study *treatment groups* for a designated *outcome* or *follow-up variable*.

treatment compliance   The degree to which a *patient* follows his *assigned treatment* regimen. See *treatment adherence*.

treatment coordinating center   A *center* in a *clinical trial* that is responsible for coordinating the development and administration of the *treatment protocol*, but that has few or no other responsibilities for coordinating other aspects of the trial. Usually present only in *multicenter trials* involving a complicated treatment protocol. See also *coordinating center* and *data coordinating center*.

treatment cross contamination   Any instance in which a *patient*, who was assigned to receive one *treatment* in a *trial*, is exposed to one of the other *study treatments* during the course of *treatment* or *follow-up*.

treatment crossover   Any change of *treatment* for a *patient* in a *clinical trial* involving a switch of *study treatments*. The switch may be planned, as in a *crossover trial*, or may be unplanned, as in the case of a *noncrossover trial* in which a patient assigned to one treatment is exposed to one of the other study treatments sometime during the *trial*. Unplanned crossovers are said to result in *treatment cross contamination*.

treatment design   The portion of the study design that specifies the *treatments* to be evaluated, the nature of the *treatment structure*, and the way in which the treatments are to be administered.

treatment difference   1. A difference observed between the *test-* and *control-treated* groups of *patients* for some specified *outcome measure*. 2. Any specified or observed difference for a designated *outcome* or *follow-up variable* involving two or more *treatment groups* in the *trial*.

treatment effect   1. An effect attributed to the *test treatment*. Usually in *clinical trials* inferred from a comparison of the *test-* and *control-treated groups* of *patients* using observed results for a specified *outcome measure*. 2. The effect produced or assumed to be produced by a treatment in an individual patient. Usually assessed by measurements made before and after administration of the treatment in that individual.

treatment effects monitoring   1. Any process of reviewing accumulated *outcome data* for groups of *patients* in a *trial* as it proceeds to determine whether a designated treatment procedure should be altered or stopped. 2. The process of watching for *treatment effects* in an individual patient (term not ordinarily used in this context in this book).

treatment effects monitoring committee (TEMC) 1. A standing committee responsible for periodi-

cally reviewing accumulated data for evidence of adverse or beneficial *treatment effects* during the *trial* and for initiating recommendations for modification of a *study treatment*, including termination of the treatment when appropriate. 2. One of the *key committees* in the organizational structure of a *multicenter trial*. Usually composed primarily, if not exclusively, of individuals not directly involved in patient care or data collection in the trial.

treatment failure   1. Term sometimes used to characterize a *study patient* whose *study physician* has found it necessary to alter his *assigned treatment* because of the "failure" of the treatment to produce a desired effect. 2. A patient in a *clinical trial* who is no longer maintained on his assigned treatment, whether or not he continues under *follow-up*. (Usage note: Term not used in either context in this book.)

treatment and follow-up stage   The fifth stage of a *clinical trial* in this book. Concerned with patient *treatment* and *follow-up* (see Chapter 3 and Appendix D).

treatment group   The group of patients assigned to receive a specified *treatment*. See *study group*.

treatment interaction   A situation in which the effect exerted by a *treatment* is influenced by the level, or presence or absence, of some other factor or condition not related to treatment (e.g., one would say there is a treatment-sex interaction if the *test-control treatment difference* is in one direction for males and in the other direction, or is of a different order of magnitude, for females).

treatment interaction effect   The observed effect associated with a *treatment interaction*.

treatment lag   The time required, or presumed to be required, for a treatment to exert its full effect.

treatment mask   A condition or procedure that is imposed to keep someone from knowing the true identity of the *treatment assignment*.

treatment masking   1. A process in which *treatments* are administered so as to be *single-* or *double-masked*. 2. Any process that is designed to withhold information on *treatment assignment* from some individual or group of individuals in a *clinical trial*.

treatment monitoring   *Treatment effects monitoring*.

treatment procedure   The method of applying a particular *treatment* in a *clinical trial*.

treatment protocol   A document that describes the *treatment procedures* used in a *clinical trial*.

treatment related bias   A condition in which the nature of a reading, measurement, or classification recorded on a particular *patient* is influenced by the fact that the individual responsible for making the reading, measurement, or classification has knowledge of the patient's *treatment assignment*.

treatment side effect   A by-product of treatment, either expected or unexpected, desired or undesired.

treatment structure   The interrelationship of *treat-*

ments used in a *clinical trial*, e.g., as characterized by treatments that are arranged in a *factorial structure*.

treatment trial A *trial* in which the *test treatment* consists of a procedure used for *treatment* of a specific disease or health condition. *Therapeutic trial*.

treatment unit The unit to which treatment is administered in a *clinical trial*. Usually *patient*, but the unit may be composed of multiple individuals, such as a family unit.

trial 1. *Clinical trial*. 2. Any tentative or experimental action done in order to obtain data for some judgment or conclusion.

triple-blind *Triple-masked* in this book. See *blind* for usage comment.

triple-blinded 1. *Triple-masked* in this book. See *blind* for usage comment. 2. Sometimes used in a jocular fashion (not in this book) to characterize a situation in which neither the patient, physician, nor statistician knows how the *trial* is designed or operated.

triple-blinded clinical trial *Triple-masked clinical trial*.

triple-mask *Triple-masked*.

triple-masked *Double-masked* plus masking for the individual (or group of individuals) who are responsible for *treatment monitoring*.

triple-masked clinical trial A *double-masked clinical trial* in which data analyses done for *treatment monitoring* are presented to the individual or group responsible for such monitoring in a way that conceals the identity of the *treatment groups*.

two-armed bandit A method of *outcome adaptive allocation* in which the *treatment assignment probability* for a particular treatment is a function of the observed *treatment difference* in *outcomes* of *patients* already *enrolled* in the *trial*. The motivation being to minimize the number of patients assigned to the inferior treatment (Robbins, 1952, 1956; Smith and Pyke, 1965; Zelen, 1969).

two-sided alternative hypothesis *Two-tailed alternative hypothesis*.

two-sided test (statistics) *Two-tailed test*.

two-tailed alternative hypothesis An alternative to the *null hypothesis* that specifies a range of permissible values that are symmetrically distributed about the null value (e.g., $H_0: \mu_1 = \mu_2$ versus $H_A: \mu_1 \neq \mu_2$). See *one-tailed alternative hypothesis* for opposing term.

two-tailed test (statistics) A statistical *test of significance* based on the null value of no difference versus the set of all alternative values (i.e., those that lie to the right and left of the null value).

type I error (statistics) The probability of rejecting the *null hypothesis* when it is true, usually denoted by the Greek letter α.

type II error (statistics) The probability of accepting the *null hypothesis* when it is false, usually denoted by the Greek letter β.

U

UGDP University Group Diabetes Program.

uncontrolled Not *controlled*.

uncontrolled clinical trial A *clinical trial* that does not involve a *control treatment*. In this book, any study that does not have a *control group* made up of patients treated and followed over the same time period as those in a *test-treated group*.

uncrossed treatments 1. A *treatment structure* not involving a *crossover design*. 2. *Nonfactorial treatment structure*.

uniform treatment allocation A scheme in which the *assignment probability* of any one *treatment group* is the same as for every other treatment group in a *trial*. See *equal treatment allocation*.

unmask To reveal the *treatment assignment* of an individual *patient* or group of patients to an individual or group of individuals associated with the *trial* (e.g., patients, *study physicians, treatment effects monitoring committee*) who have heretofore been denied this information.

unmasked trial *Nonmasked trial*.

unmasking The process of revealing a previously masked item of information, such as *treatment assignment*, to an individual or group of individuals in a *clinical trial*.

unrestricted allocation 1. Any system of *treatment allocation* that does not require the imposition of any restriction on the *assignment process*, over and above those implied with the *adaptive* or *fixed allocation* scheme used. 2. Use of *allocation schedules* within *clinics* in a multicenter trial, or *strata* within a clinic, but where there is no blocking within clinic or strata within clinic.

unrestricted allocation schedule An *allocation schedule* constructed using *unrestricted allocation*.

unrestricted random allocation Any *unrestricted allocation* scheme that uses a *random process* for generating *treatment assignments*.

unrestricted randomization The process of generating or issuing *treatment assignments* via an *unrestricted allocation schedule*.

unscheduled interim follow-up visit *Interim follow-up visit*.

USPHS United States Public Health Service.

V

VA Veterans Administration.

VA 43 *VACSP No. 43*.

VACSP Veterans Administration Cooperative Studies Program.

VACSP No. 43 Veterans Administration Cooperative Studies Program Number 43.

variable In this book, any trait, characteristic, test, measurement, or assessment that is recorded, or scheduled to be recorded, on *patients* enrolled, or to be enrolled, in a *clinical trial*.

VDT Video display terminal.

verification   A process that is carried out to *verify* an item of information.

verify   To confirm or substantiate an item of information recorded in a *data file* or keyed for entry into the *analysis database*.

visit   *Clinic visit.*

W

WHO   World Health Organization.

withdrawal   1. A technical term used to refer to the process of removing a specific individual from a *lifetable analysis* because of termination of *follow-up*, or because of the occurrence of an *event* that precludes further follow-up. 2. *Dropout* (not used in this context in this book).

writing team   A team of *study investigators* who are appointed or designated to write a specified manuscript for presentation or publication.

B. Sketches of selected trials

B.1 INTRODUCTION

Table B–1 provides a list of the trials sketched in this Appendix. They are all multicenter trials, except the Physicians' Health Study (Sketch 1), and they all involve periods of follow-up of a year or longer. They represent seven different disease areas. The majority of the trials involve cardiovascular disease. The National Institutes of Health (NIH) serve as the sole source of support for 11 of the 14 trials, and they share funding responsibilities with a European foundation in the case of the International Reflux Study in Children. One of the other two trials was funded by the Veterans Administration and the other was funded by a pharmaceutical firm.

Eight of the trials involved tests of drugs, four involved surgical procedures, and one, the Hypertension Prevention Trial (HPT), involved testing diet modifications as preventive measures for hypertension. The remaining trial, the Multiple Risk Factor Intervention Trial (MRFIT), involved testing several different forms of intervention, all aimed at reducing known risk factors for heart disease.

The sketches are designed to:

- Acquaint readers with the design and operating features of some typical long-term trials
- Supplement information contained in the body of this book on some of the more frequently cited trials
- Provide a data resource for tabulations presented in chapters throughout the book

B.2 METHODS

The initial draft of each sketch was prepared by the senior author using:

- Published manuscripts produced from the trial (see Table B–3 for publication list)
- Basic design documents, such as original funding applications or requests for proposals
- Operational documents, such as manuals of operations, treatment protocols, data forms, etc.
- Personal communications with study personnel

Each sketch consisted of:

- An abstract summary of the trial
- A list of study publications
- Enumeration of the operating features of the trial

A copy of the draft sketch was sent to the chairman or vice-chairman of the study, director of the coordinating center or data coordinating center, or project officer for review. The date the review was completed (see item 33, Table B–4) was used as the cutoff date for information contained in the sketch and is considered the completion date for the sketch. Committee listing and membership information (items 27, 28, and 29, Table B–4) are as of this date for trials that had not yet entered the patient close-out stage. The committee structure is characterized as of the start of the close-out stage for trials that were already in this or in a later stage when the sketch was reviewed. Information on the steering committee and the committee responsible for treatment monitoring, as represented in items 28 and 29 of Table B–4, is based on data in the sketch (see Table B–5 for sample) and was collected on a supplementary form that was completed by the individual chosen to review the sketch.

B.3 RESULTS

Table B–2 contains the abstract summary of each trial sketched. Table B–3 lists official papers of the 14 study groups. Only papers appearing in peer review journals or periodicals are listed. The list does not include:

- Papers published after the date in item 33, Table B–4
- Papers in preparation, submitted for publication but still under review, or accepted for publication but not yet published as of the date in item 33, Table B–4
- Abstracts or editorials concerning the study
- Papers published as part of a book, monograph, or the like, except where papers so published are part of a periodical indexed by the National Library of Medicine
- Reports published by the federal government
- Reports and documents placed on deposit at the National Technical Information Service or other similar repositories

The full list of publications is much more extensive than is shown in Table B–3 for some of the trials sketched, such as NCGS and CASS.

The author citations in Table B–3 are reproduced as supplied from the study, via the individual who reviewed the sketch, except for the exclusions listed above and minor editing. A comparison of citations in the table with those appearing in the body of the book will reveal differences. For example, named authors appear in the author field of citation 5.2 in Table B–3.

The author designation in the body of the book for this citation is simply the National Cooperative Gallstone Study Group.

There are several reasons for the differences in the citations. First, it is not always clear how a paper should be listed from the arrangement of information in the masthead of the paper. Second, preference was given to corporate author designations when there was a choice between a conventional or corporate format in the body of the book. Use of corporate designations yielded shorter citations and made for a more logical grouping of related publications appearing in the combined bibliography (Appendix I) at the end of this book. Third, the listings in Table B–3 as supplied by the individuals selected to review the sketches were used to answer item 31.b in Table B–4. This was considered to provide the best basis for making the counts needed for that item.

Table B–4 contains summary tabulations derived from the sketches (See Table B–5 for sample sketch). The notes below relate to those tabulations. Table B–6 contains the name of the director of the data coordinating center or coordinating center and address of the center for all trials sketched, as well as the other multicenter trials referenced in this book.

Item number in Table B–4	Comment
1	• See Glossary for definition of type of trial.
2	• See Chapter 9 or Glossary for definition of fixed sample size design. All trials were of this type. None involved a sequential design.
3	• See Chapter 3 or Glossary for definitions of stages. The category *Completed* was checked if all funding for the trial had terminated by the date recorded in item 33.
5	• See Glossary for definitions.
6	• See Chapter 21.
7	• See Glossary for definitions of direct, indirect, and consortium awards.
8	• Start of funding taken as date of first award to any center in the trial. Awards issued simply for planning purposes were not counted in fixing the date. The ending date is the projected date for termination of all financial support for the trial. It is the termination date for completed trials.
9	• Number of clinics as of sketch completion for trials in the treatment and follow-up stage or earlier stage. Number of clinics entering the patient close-out stage for trials in that stage or beyond as of the sketch completion date given in item 33.
10	• See Glossary for definitions.
11.b	• Degree of coordinating center or data coordinating center director. Indicated as Bio (biostatistics), Epi (epidemiology), or Med (medicine).

Item number in Table B–4	Comment
11.c	• Answered *No* if the coordinating center or data coordinating center was financially and administratively independent of all other centers in the trial. Answered *Yes* if the center was funded through a clinical center in the trial or if it was under the administrative control of a clinic center director.
12, 13, 17	• See Glossary for definitions.
19.a	• See Chapter 14. Direct checked when potential study patients were identified and approached by study personnel, such as when patients are recruited from a primary care facility under the control of clinic investigators, or when patients are identified through special screening or direct mailings initiated by clinic personnel. Indirect checked if the initial contact is through some other agent or party outside the clinic, such as a referring physician, through review of records held by nonstudy physicians or at nonstudy hospitals, or via mass advertising compaigns initiated from the study and aimed at the general public.
19.b	• Month and year first patient was randomized.
19.c	• Month and year last patient was randomized. Projected date for trials still in the patient recruitment stage.
19.d	• Total number of patients enrolled (all treatment groups combined). Count at or before the date given in item 33.
20.a	• All 14 trials involved formal methods of randomization, as opposed to informal, nonrandom, or quasi-random methods, such as discussed in Chapter 8. All trials used patients as the randomization unit except one, the Macular Photocoagulation Study in which eyes served as the randomization unit.
20.b	• See Glossary for defninitions.
20.d	• The total number of allocation strata. Given by the product of the number of subgroups formed with each stratification variable. For example, a trial involving stratification by clinic (10 clinics), age (three levels), and sex would have $10 \times 3 \times 2 = 60$ allocation strata.
20.e	• See Chapter 10 and Glossary for definitions. Characterized as uniform if the allocation scheme was designed to yield equal numbers of assignments to the study treatments within a strata. Classified as nonuniform (denoted as *Nonuni* in the table) if this condition does not apply.
20.f	• Answered *Yes* if the allocations are blocked (see Chapter 10) to force the treatment assignments to satisfy a specified allocation ratio at various points during the patient enrollment process.
20.g	• Locus of control for the randomization classified as *Central* if release of individual assignments was triggered by written or telephone contact of clinic staff with staff of the coordinating center or data coordinating center (or staff of some other control center), or release was controlled via an on-site computer under the control of the coordinating center or data coordinating center. Control considered *Local* if clinic staff could obtain an allocation without use of an on-site computer controlled by the coordinating center or data coordinating center or without any contact with a coordinating center or other control facility.
21	• See Chapter 12 and Glossary for definitions. Regular follow-up visits do not include visits done simply for treatment application or adjustment.
22.a	• Recorded as the average length of follow-up or as a range. Anticipated values for trials that had not yet entered the patient close-out stage. Ranges recorded for trials in the close-out stage or beyond based on actual times of enrollment of the first and last patients entered into the study.
22.b	• Indicated as *NA* (not applicable) for trials still in the patient close-out stage or an earlier stage. Indicated as *None done* if trial is completed and no post-trial follow-up was done. The average length of follow-up provided or anticipated if post-trial follow-up was done or is under way.
24	• See Chapters 8 and 15.
26.a	• Original recruitment goal: That set when the trial was planned. Value recorded is as stated in the original design documents of the trial (e.g., original grant application, RFP, or RFA), or as reported in a study publication.

Item number in Table B-4	Comment
26.b	• The category *Sample size calculation* was checked if the goal was based on a sample size calculation with a specified level of type I and II error protection. The category *Pragmatic* was checked if a recruitment goal was set, but was based on practical considerations rather than on a formal sample size calculation.
26.c	• The number of patients recruited (all treatments combined). Listed as *NA* (not applicable) if recruitment not yet completed as of date in item 33.
26.d	• Answer based on information in published reports of results from the listed trials (see Table B-3 for list). The category *Not applicable* checked for trials that have yet to publish any results. The category *None required* checked for trials that produced a significant effect before patient recruitment was completed. The category *None stated* checked if the treatment effect observed was not considered to be significant by the authors of the report and the report contains no discussion of the rationale for the achieved sample size, or of the power provided to detect a specified treatment difference with the observed sample size and control event rate. The category *Sample size calculation* checked if the original recruitment goal was achieved and if the goal was the result of a sample size calculation made during or prior to the close of the patient recruitment stage. The category *Pragmatic* checked if recruitment was completed and the report contains a statement indicating the achieved sample was the result of practical considerations (i.e., was not the result of a formal sample size calculation). A check in both categories *Power calculation* and *Sample size calculation* indicates the report satisfied the requirements for both categories.
27	• See Chapter 23 and Glossary for definitions.
28.a, ii	• Patient care responsibilities? Answered *Yes* if chairman was responsible for treatment or care of any patients in the trial.
28.a, iii	• Recorded as *Self-appt* (self-appointed) in investigator-initiated trials where the chairman was designated on the initial application. Recorded as *E* (elected) if chairman was chosen by the investigative group after the trial was funded, either by acclamation or through a formal election. Recorded as *Appt* (appointed) if chairman was selected by the sponsor or the advisory-review committee of the trial.
28.a, iv	• Recorded as $\overline{WT}$ (without term) if the chairman, regardless of whether self-appointed, elected, or appointed, serves without term. Recorded as *Term* if chairman selected or appointed for a specified term less than the expected duration of the trial.
28.b, ii through iv	• See comments for 28.a, ii through iv.
28.c, i	• The study centers referred to in this item and in item 28.c, ii include clinical centers, as well as all resource centers. The number of members and their voting status is based on information supplied in study publications and as supplied from the study on a special form completed by the individual selected to review the sketch, as described in Section B.2.
28.d	• See Glossary for definitions of the positions listed. The positions denoted by items i through vi that were represented on the steering committee (SC) are marked *Yes. No* indicates that the position exists in the study, but that it is not represented on the SC. Positions that do not exist in the study are marked *NA* (not applicable). The positions represented by items vii and viii were marked *Yes* if individuals of the type indicated were on the SC, and were marked *No* if not.
28.e	• This item indicates the number of individuals elected to membership on the SC by some body of the study—generally the entire investigative body. The letter *T* following the number indicates election for a specified term. The letters $\overline{WT}$ indicate election without term.
29.a	• The committee scheduled to perform the treatment effects monitoring function for trials where monitoring is not yet under way. The actual committee performing that function for all other trials. See Glossary and Chapter 23.
29.b through f	• See comments for 28.a through e.
29.g	• The actual or planned number of meetings per year of the committee listed in item 29.a.

Item number in Table B-4	Comment
30	• See Chapter 23 for distinguishing features of communication models. Classifications made by author.
31.a	• Number from Table B–3.
31.b	• A paper was counted in the first category (corporate format) if the author field, as displayed in Table B–3, only contained the study name. It was counted in the second category (conventional format) if the author field only contained names of individual authors. It was counted in the third category (both formats) if the author field contained both the study name and the name of one or more authors.
32	• Item used to indicate the degree of involvement of the senior author of this book in the particular trials sketched.
33	• Taken as the date of review, as discussed in Section B.2.

Table B-1   List of trials sketched

Sketch number	Study name	Acronym	Disease	Sponsor
1	Physicians' Health Study	PHS	Cancer, cardiovascular	NIH
2	University Group Diabetes Program	UGDP	Diabetes	NIH
3	VA Cooperative Studies Program Number 43	VA 43	Diabetes	VA
4	Macular Photocoagulation Study	MPS	Eye	NIH
5	National Cooperative Gallstone Study	NCGS	Gallbladder	NIH
6	Coronary Drug Project	CDP	Cardiovascular	NIH
7	Aspirin Myocardial Infarction Study	AMIS	Cardiovascular	NIH
8	Persantine Aspirin Reinfarction Study	PARIS	Cardiovascular	Industry
9	Hypertension Detection and Follow-Up Program	HDFP	Cardiovascular	NIH
10	Multiple Risk Factor Intervention Trial	MRFIT	Cardiovascular	NIH
11	Coronary Artery Surgery Study	CASS	Cardiovascular	NIH
12	Program on the Surgical Control of Hyperlipidemia	POSCH	Cardiovascular	NIH
13	Hypertension Prevention Trial	HPT	Cardiovascular	NIH
14	International Reflux Study in Children	IRSC	Kidney	NIH and foundation

Table B-2   Abstract summaries of trials sketched

1. Physicians' Health Study (PHS)

The PHS is a randomized, double-masked, placebo-controlled clinical trial designed to test the value of regular use of aspirin on all cause and cardiovascular mortality after 4.5 years of follow-up, as well as beta-carotene on total cancer incidence in the last 2.5 years of the trial. Patients are randomly assigned to one of the four treatments listed below.

Treatment	Dosage
• Aspirin + beta-carotene: ASA + β	• One (325 mg) aspirin tablet every other day. One (30 mg) beta-carotene capsule on alternate days.
• Aspirin + beta-carotene placebo: ASA + $\bar\beta$	• One aspirin tablet every other day. One beta-carotene placebo capsule on alternate days.
• Aspirin placebo + beta-carotene: $\overline{ASA}$ + β	• One aspirin placebo tablet every other day. One beta-carotene capsule on alternate days.
• Aspirin and beta-carotene placebos: $\overline{ASA}$ + $\bar\beta$	• One aspirin placebo tablet every other day. One beta-carotene placebo capsule on alternate days.

Over 21,500 male physicians, 40 to 84 years of age at entry, are to be enrolled. Physicians volunteering to participate will receive their assigned medication via mail and will be asked to complete a short questionnaire first at 6-month and later at 1-year intervals after enrollment. The questionnaires will be collected by mail and will be used to assemble information on treatment adherence, treatment side effects, and morbidity. Participants are not required to make any clinic visits.

2. University Group Diabetes Program (UGDP)

The UGDP was a randomized, controlled, multicenter clinical trial designed to evaluate the effectiveness of long-term hypoglycemic drug therapy in preventing or delaying the vascular complications of diabetes. Only newly diagnosed, noninsulin dependent, adult-onset diabetics were eligible for enrollment. The study started patient enrollment in early 1961. All patient follow-up terminated in 1975. A total of 1,027 patients were enrolled and randomly assigned to one of the treatments listed below.

Treatment	Dosage
• Insulin variable: IVAR	• As much insulin (U-80 Lente Iletin or other insulins) per day as required to maintain "normal" blood glucose levels. Administered via subcutaneous injections.
• Insulin standard: ISTD	• 10, 12, 14, or 16 units of insulin (U-80 Lente Iletin) per day, depending on patient body surface. Administered via subcutaneous injections.
• Tolbutamide: TOLB	• 3 tablets per day, each containing 0.5 gms of tolbutamide.
• Phenformin: PHEN	• 1 capsule per day during first week of treatment, thereafter 2 capsules per day; 50 mg of phenformin per capsule.
• Lactose placebo: PLBO	• Number of tablets or capsules similar to those used for tolbutamide or phenformin treatments.

The tolbutamide and phenformin treatments were terminated in 1969 and 1971, respectively, because of lack of efficacy. The two insulin treatments were continued to the end of planned patient follow-up (1975), but were not judged to be any more effective than placebo medications in prolonging life or in delaying the onset and development of vascular complications.

3. VA Cooperative Studies Program Number 43 (VA 43)

The study is a long-term, randomized, double-masked, placebo-controlled clinical trial of aspirin and dipyridamole in diabetics with advanced vascular disease. The test treatment is a combination of aspirin and dipyrida-

Table B-2 Abstract summaries of trials sketched (*continued*)

mole (one 325 mg tablet of aspirin and one 75 mg tablet of dipyridamole, three times per day). Patients assigned to placebo treatment received a prescription for a tablet schedule identical to that of the test-treated group. Patients in the trial had to have gangrene of the feet at enrollment or had to have had an amputation on one or both of their feet for gangrene in the last 12 months prior to enrollment. The study enrolled 231 patients. Recruitment was completed in May 1980. The study investigators plan to announce the results of the trial sometime in 1984.

4. Macular Photocoagulation Study (MPS)

The MPS is a multicenter study designed to assess the value of photocoagulation in eyes with choroidal neovascularization. The study consists of two sets of trials. The first was started in 1979 and focuses on the assessment of argon laser photocoagulation in eyes with leaking choroidal neovascular membranes that are between 200 and 2,500 microns from the center of the foveal avascular zone (FAZ). The second set of trials, started in 1982, involves use of krypton laser photocoagulation. This mode of treatment is restricted to eyes that were judged ineligible for argon laser photocoagulation because the choroidal neovascular membranes to be treated fell within 200 microns of the FAZ. Both studies involve three different types of eye diseases, as outlined below.

Type of eye disease	Eligibility criteria
• Senile macular degeneration (SMD)	• Neovascularization; visible drusen bodies as large or larger than those defined by standard MPS fundus photographs; age $\geq$ 50 at entry.
• Presumed ocular histoplasmosis (HISTO)	• Neovascularization; at least one atrophic scar (histo spot) in either eye; age $\geq$ 18 at entry.
• Idiopathic neovascular membrane (INVM)	• Neovascularization; no evidence of SMD or any other cause for neovascularization; no drusen bodies greater than those defined by standard MPS fundus photographs; no histo spots in either eye.

Eligible eyes in both sets of trials are randomly assigned to receive photocoagulation or no treatment. All patients are followed for changes in vision. The only results available from the trial through the date listed in item 33, Table B-4, relate to argon-treated SMD patients. Patient recruitment for that trial was terminated because of the apparent superiority of argon treatment. Of the SMD untreated eyes, 60% had reduced visual capacity by the eighteenth month of follow-up, compared with only 25% of the argon-treated SMD eyes.

5. National Cooperative Gallstone Study (NCGS)

The NCGS was a double-masked, randomized, controlled, trial designed to assess the efficacy and safety of chenodiol (chenodeoxycholic acid) for dissolution of radiolucent gallstones. The treatments are outlined below.

Treatment	Dosage
• High dose chenodiol: H	• 6 capsules per day, each containing 125 mg of chenodiol.
• Low dose chenodiol: L	• 6 capsules per day, each containing 62.5 mg of chenodiol.
• Placebo: P	• 6 capsules per day, each containing 3 mg of sodium cholate.

Nine hundred sixteen patients (not counting the 128 patients enrolled in a preliminary biopsy study) were enrolled, treated, and followed by the ten clinical centers participating in the trial. The percentages of patients with complete gallstone dissolution, after two years of treatment, as determined by radiographic metrology, were 13.5 for H, 5.2 for L, and 0.8 for P. Partial (over 50% dissolution) or complete dissolution occurred in 40.8% of H-treated patients, 23.6% of the L-treated patients, and 11.0% of the P-treated patients. Clinically significant hepatotoxicity requiring termination of the assigned treatment occurred in 3% of the H-treated patients and in 0.4% of the L-treated and P-treated patients.

Table B–2   Abstract summaries of trials sketched (*continued*)

6. Coronary Drug Project (CDP)

The CDP was a double-masked, randomized, controlled clinical trial designed to evaluate the efficacy of several different lipid-influencing drugs in prolonging the lives of men (aged 30 through 64 at entry) with a prior history of myocardial infarction. The treatments investigated are listed below.

Treatment	Dosage per day*
• Low dose estrogen: ESG1	• 2.5 mg of mixed conjugated equine estrogen (Premarin®)
• High dose estrogen: ESG2	• 5.0 mg of mixed conjugated equine estrogen (Premarin®)
• Clofibrate: CPIB	• 1.8g of ethyl alpha parachlorophenoxy-isobutyrate (Atromid-S®)
• Dextrothyroxine: DT4	• 6.0 mg of dextrothyroxine (Choloxin®)
• Nicotinic acid: NICA	• 3.0 mg of nicotinic acid
• Placebo: PLBO	• 3.8g of lactose (placebo)

*Patients were required to take 9 capsules per day (3 capsules 3 times a day) to receive the specified dosage. They were started on 3 capsules per day. They were stepped to 6 capsules per day 1 month later and then to 9 capsules per day 1 month thereafter. They were then maintained on 9 capsules per day, except where contraindicated.

The study involved 55 clinics, a coordinating center, project office, central laboratory, ECG reading center, and drug procurement and distribution center. A total of 8,341 patients were enrolled. All patients were followed for a minimum of 5 years.

The two estrogen and dextrothyroxine treatments were discontinued during the course of the trial because of lack of efficacy. In addition, the clofibrate and nicotinic acid treatments, while continued to the end of the trial, did not show any evidence of efficacy. The 5-year mortality rates were 20.0, 21.2, and 20.9 per 100 population for CPIB, NICA, and PLBO, respectively.

7. Aspirin Myocardial Infarction Study (AMIS)

AMIS was designed to test the efficacy of aspirin in prolonging life in patients with a prior history of myocardial infarction. A total of 4,524 patients were enrolled and followed through the efforts of 30 clinical centers, a coordinating center, project office, central laboratory, ECG reading center, and drug procurement and distribution center. Patients assigned to aspirin treatment (ASA) received 1.0g of aspirin per day (two capsules per day, each containing 0.5g of aspirin). Patients assigned to the placebo treatment (PLBO) received a capsule schedule similar to that for aspirin-treated patients. Patients were followed for a minimum of 3 years.

The study failed to show any benefit for ASA treatment. In fact, the 3-year mortality rate for the ASA treatment group was higher than that for the PLBO treatment group (9.6 versus 8.8 per 100 population).

8. Persantine Aspirin Reinfarction Study (PARIS)

PARIS was an industry-sponsored randomized, controlled, clinical trial designed to test the efficacy of Persantine® (dipyridamole) and aspirin in prolonging lives of patients with an ECG-documented history of myocardial infarction (MI). The trial involved 2,026 patients. Clinics from both the United States and the United Kingdom participated. Patients were treated and followed for a minimum of 3 years. The treatments were as outlined below.

Treatment	Dosage
• Persantine® + Aspirin: PR + ASA	• 2 tablets, 3 times per day. 1 containing 75 mg of Persantine® and the other containing 324 mg of aspirin.
• Persantine® placebo + Aspirin: $\overline{PR}$ + ASA	• 2 tablets, 3 times per day. 1 containing 324 mg of aspirin and the other containing placebo medication.
• Persantine® placebo + Aspirin placebo: $\overline{PR}$ + $\overline{ASA}$	• 2 tablets, 3 times per day. Both containing placebo medication (starch, calcium phosphate, and microcrystalline cellulose).

There was no significant difference among the treatment groups in mortality. The percentages dead at the end of the study were 10.7, 10.5, and 12.8 for the PR + ASA, $\overline{PR}$ + ASA, and $\overline{PR}$ + $\overline{ASA}$ treatment groups, respectively. However, subgroup analyses of the data suggested the combination of Persantine® and aspirin may be beneficial in prolonging life, if used within a few months following an MI. This finding led to initiation of PARIS, Part II (not sketched).

9. Hypertension Detection and Follow-Up Program (HDFP)

The HDFP was a randomized, controlled, clinical trial of stepped care versus referred care for patients with hypertension. The study involved 14 clinics, a coordinating center, project office, central laboratory, ECG reading center, and a drug procurement and distribution center. A total of 10,940 men and women with a qualifying diastolic blood pressure (DBP) of 90 mmHg or higher were enrolled. Patients assigned to stepped care were treated at the study clinics by clinic personnel using a treatment protocol calling for stepped increases in the dosage of a prescribed medication or in the number of antihypertensive agents used in order to achieve desired BP reductions. Patients assigned to the referred care group were referred to their usual source of medical care for treatment.

Five-year mortality (all cause) was 17% lower for the stepped care group than for the referred care group (6.4 per 100 population for stepped care versus 7.7 per 100 population for referred care). The investigators concluded that the findings "indicate that the systematic effective management of hypertension has a great potential for reducing mortality for the large number of people with high BP in the population, including those with 'mild' hypertension."

10. Multiple Risk Factor Intervention Trial (MRFIT)

MRFIT was a randomized, controlled, clinical trial designed to assess the value of a multifactor intervention program aimed at reducing known risk factors for coronary heart disease (CHD). The three risk factors were elevated serum cholesterol, high blood pressure, and cigarette smoking. Only men aged 35 through 57 at entry, with no overt evidence of CHD, were eligible for enrollment. The 12,866 men enrolled were randomly assigned to either special intervention (SI) or usual care (UC). Those assigned to SI were placed on specific treatments for the risk factors present. A dietary approach was used for cholesterol reduction, antihypertensive drugs (plus weight reduction where appropriate) were used for blood pressure reduction, and a behavioral approach was used to achieve cessation or reduction of cigarette smoking. Participants assigned to UC were not given any care via study clinics for elevated blood pressure or advice on how to reduce cholesterol or cigarette consumption. However, hypertensives diagnosed via the study were referred to their usual source of care for treatment.

The trial completed participant recruitment in early 1976. Participants assigned to SI continued to be exposed to the required interventions until termination of follow-up in early 1982. The first report of findings appeared in late 1982. The report showed the interventions practiced on the SI-treated group to be effective in lowering blood pressure, cholesterol, and cigarette consumption. However, these reductions had virtually no effect on mortality. There was a slight but nonsignificant reduction in deaths from coronary heart disease (17.9 versus 19.3 per 100 population for the SI-treated versus the UC-treated groups). However, all cause mortality was slightly higher in the SI-treated group than in the UC-treated group (4.1 versus 4.0 per 100 population). Subgroup analyses presented in the 1982 publication raise the possibility that SI-treated men with hypertension and resting ECG abnormalities at entry may have fared worse than the corresponding UC-treated group of men.

11. Coronary Artery Surgery Study (CASS)

CASS is a multicenter study consisting of two components: A trial designed to assess the efficacy of coronary artery surgery in patients with proven coronary artery disease and a registry of consecutive patients undergoing coronary arteriography. The trial component involved 780 patients assigned to coronary bypass surgery or conventional medical therapy. The registry is made up of 24,959 patients, including randomized patients. Patients in both components are followed for mortality, as well as for various nonfatal cardiovascular events. The study involves 15 clinical centers, a coordinating center, project office, and ECG reading center. Results comparing surgical and medical treatment in the randomized portion of the study had not been published, as of the completion date for this sketch.

12. Program on the Surgical Control of Hyperlipidemia (POSCH)

POSCH is a randomized clinical trial designed to determine whether reducing cholesterol levels via partial ileal bypass, in patients with high cholesterol levels and a prior history of myocardial infarction (MI), is useful in prolonging life and mitigating atherosclerosis. Patients in the trial are randomly assigned to bypass surgery or regular medical care. Patient recruitment is scheduled to continue through May 1983 with the goal being to enroll 800+ patients. Follow-up is expected to continue for a minimum of 5 years after completion of recruitment. There are no publications containing treatment results, as of the date in item 33, Table B-4.

Table B-2   Abstract summaries of trials sketched (*continued*)

13. Hypertension Prevention Trial (HPT)

The HPT is a randomized, controlled, multicenter trial designed to assess the efficacy of different forms of dietary intervention in preventing the development of hypertension. Current funding is for the first stage of a possible two-stage effort. The first stage is designed to develop and test methods and procedures needed for the second stage and will involve 800 participants randomly assigned to the treatment groups indicated below. The second stage, if warranted by results from the first stage, may involve as many as 6,000 participants and is expected to start in 1985 or 1986.

Treatment	Dietary goal
High weight strata	
• Sodium restriction: Na	• Reduce sodium intake to ≤ 70 mEq per day.
• Sodium restriction and potassium supplementation: NaK	• Reduce sodium intake to ≤ 70 mEq per day and increase potassium intake to ≥ 100 mEq per day.
• Sodium restriction plus caloric restriction for weight reduction: NaCal	• Reduce sodium intake to ≤ 70 mEq per day and restrict calorie intake to bring body weight within normal limits.
• Caloric restriction for weight reduction: Cal	• Reduce calorie intake to bring body weight within normal limits.
• Control: Ct	• None.
Normal weight strata	
• Sodium restriction: Na	• Reduce sodium intake to ≤ 70 mEq per day.
• Sodium restriction and potassium supplementation: NaK	• Reduce sodium intake to ≤ 70 mEq per day and increase potassium intake to ≥ 100 mEq per day.
• Control: Ct	• None.

Only nonhypertensive individuals with diastolic blood pressures ≥ 78 mm Hg but < 90 mm Hg are eligible for enrollment in the first stage. Individuals who fall in the high weight strata, as determined by Quetelet's Index, are assigned to any one of the five treatments listed above. Individuals who are not considered to be overweight by this index are assigned either to the control treatment or to one of the two dietary treatments not involving caloric restriction.

The dietary goals stated above are pursued via a series of group counseling sessions in which individuals are shown how to shop, cook, and eat to achieve the desired goals. The counseling process will be maintained over the course of the trial. All participants will be followed for a period of 2 to 3 years for blood pressure changes.

14. International Reflux Study in Children (IRSC)

The IRSC is a randomized, controlled, clinical trial of surgical versus conventional medical treatment of vesicoureteral reflux (VUR) in children under the age of ten at entry. The study involves a multinational set of clinics directed by a steering committee with representatives from Europe and the United States. Data collection in the United States is supervised by a data center based in New York. Data collection in Europe is supervised by a data center based in Essen. The German data center will serve as the analysis center for the combined United States–European data set.

Grade III (European clinics only) and IV reflux patients are being enrolled and followed for evidence of renal scarring and measurement of renal growth. The trial has been under way for 3 years and is scheduled to continue for several more years. No results have been published as of the date in item 33, Table B-4.

Table B-3 Publication list of sketched trials

1. Physicians' Health Study (PHS)

None

2. University Group Diabetes Program (UGDP)

2.1 University Group Diabetes Program: A study of the effects of hypoglycemic agents on vascular complications in patients with adult-onset diabetes. I: Design, methods and baseline characteristics. *Diabetes* 19(suppl 2): 747–783, 1970.

2.2 University Group Diabetes Program: A study of the effects of hypoglycemic agents on vascular complications in patients with adult-onset diabetes. II: Mortality results. *Diabetes* 19(suppl 2): 785–830, 1970.

2.3 University Group Diabetes Program: Effects of hypoglycemic agents on vascular complications in patients with adult-onset diabetes. III: Clinical implications of UGDP results. *JAMA* 218:1400–1410, 1971.

2.4 University Group Diabetes Program: Effects of hypoglycemic agents on vascular complications in patients with adult-onset diabetes. IV: A preliminary report on phenformin results. *JAMA* 217:777–784, 1971.

2.5 Prout TE, Knatterud GL, Meinert CL, Klimt CR: The University Group Diabetes Program: The UGDP Controversy: Clinical trials versus clinical impressions. *Diabetes* 21:1035–1040, 1972.

2.6 University Group Diabetes Program: A study of the effects of hypoglycemic agents on vascular complications in patients with adult-onset diabetes. V: Evaluation of phenformin therapy. *Diabetes* 24(suppl 1):65–184, 1975.

2.7 University Group Diabetes Program: A study of the effects of hypoglycemic agents on vascular complications in patients with adult-onset diabetes. VI: Supplementary report on nonfatal events in patients treated with tolbutamide. *Diabetes* 25:1129–1153, 1976.

2.8 University Group Diabetes Program: Effects of hypoglycemic agents on vascular complications in patients with adult-onset diabetes. VII: Mortality and selected nonfatal events with insulin treatment. *JAMA* 240:37–42, 1978.

2.9 Prout T, Knatterud G, Meinert C: The University Group Diabetes Program: Diabetes drugs: Clinical trial (letter). *Science* 204:362–363, 1979.

2.10 University Group Diabetes Program: Effects of hypoglycemic agents on vascular complications in patients with adult-onset diabetes. VIII: Evaluation of insulin therapy: Final report. *Diabetes* 31(suppl 5):1–78, 1982.

3. VA Cooperative Studies Program Number 43 (VA 43)

None

4. Macular Photocoagulation Study (MPS)

4.1 Macular Photocoagulation Study Group: Argon laser photocoagulation for senile macular degeneration. *Arch Ophthalmol* 100:912–918, 1982.

5. National Cooperative Gallstone Study (NCGS)

5.1 Croke G: Recruitment for the National Cooperative Gallstone Study. *Clin Pharmacol and Ther* 25:691–694, 1979.

5.2 Lachin JM, Marks JW, Schoenfield LJ; the NCGS Protocol Committee (Malcolm P. Tyor, Chairman, Peter H. Bennett, Scott M. Grundy, William G. M. Hardison, Lawrence W. Shaw, Johnson L. Thistle, Z. R. Vlahcevic) and the National Cooperative Gallstone Study Group: Design & methodological considerations in the National Cooperative Gallstone Study: A multicenter clinical trial. *Controlled Clin Trials* 2:177–229, 1981.

5.3 Lasser EC, Amberg JR, Baily NA, Varady P, Lachin J, Okun R, Schoenfield L: Validation of a computer-assisted method for estimating the number and volume of gallstones visualized by cholecystography. *Invest Radiol* 16:342–347, 1981.

5.4 Schoenfield LJ, Lachin JM, the Steering Committee (Baum RA, Habig RL, Hanson RF, Hersh T, Hightower NC, Jr., Hofmann AF, Lasser EC, Marks JW, Mekhjian H, Okun R, Schaefer RA, Shaw L, Soloway RD, Thistle JL, Thomas FB, Tyor MP), and the National Cooperative

Gallstone Study Group: Chenodial (chenodeoxycholic acid) for dissolution of gallstones: The National Cooperative Gallstone Study. A controlled trial of efficacy and safety. *Ann Intern Med* 95:257–282, 1981.

5.5   Albers JJ, Grundy SM, Cleary PA, Small DM, Lachin JM, Schoenfield LJ, and the National Cooperative Gallstone Study Group: National Cooperative Gallstone Study: The effect of chenodeoxycholic acid on lipoproteins and apolipoproteins. *Gastroenterology* 82:638–646, 1982.

5.6   Fisher RL, Anderson DW, Boyer JL, Ishak K, Klatskin G, Lachin JM, Phillips MJ, and the Steering Committee for the National Cooperative Gallstone Study Group: A prospective morphologic evaluation of hepatic toxicity of chenodeoxycholic acid in patients with cholelithiasis: The National Cooperative Gallstone Study (NCGS). *Hepatology* 2:187–201, 1982.

5.7   Hofmann AF, Grundy SM, Lachin JM, Lan SP, Baum RA, Hanson RF, Hersh T, Hightower NC, Jr., Marks JW, Mekhjian H, Schaefer RA, Soloway RD, Thistle JL, Thomas FB, Tyor MP, and the National Cooperative Gallstone Study Group: Pretreatment biliary lipid composition in white patients with radiolucent gallstones in the National Cooperative Gallstone Study (NCGS). *Gastroenterology* 83:738–752, 1982.

5.8   Habig RL, Thomas P, Lippel K, Anderson D, Lachin J: Central laboratory quality control in the National Cooperative Gallstone Study. *Controlled Clin Trials* 4:101–123, 1983.

5.9   Lachin JM, Schoenfield LJ, and the National Cooperative Gallstone Study Group: Effects of dose relative to body weight in the National Cooperative Gallstone Study: A fixed-dose trial. *Controlled Clin Trials* 4:125–131, 1983.

5.10   Phillips MJ, Fisher RL, Anderson DW, Lan SP, Lachin JM, Boyer JL and the Steering Committee for the National Cooperative Gallstone Study Group. Ultrastructural evidence of intrahepatic cholestasis before and after chenodeoxycholic acid (CDCA) therapy in patients with cholelithiasis: The National Cooperative Gallstone Study (NCGS). *Hepatology* 3:209–220, 1983.

5.11   Schoenfield LJ, Grundy SM, Hofmann AF, Lachin JM, Thistle JL, Tyor MP, for the National Cooperative Gallstone Study: The National Cooperative Gallstone Study viewed by its investigators. *Gastroenterology* 84:644–648, 1983.

6. Coronary Drug Project (CDP)

6.1   Coronary Drug Project Research Group: The Coronary Drug Project: Initial findings leading to modifications of its research protocol. *JAMA* 214:1303–1313, 1970.

6.2   Coronary Drug Project Research Group: The Coronary Drug Project: Findings leading to further modifications of its protocol with respect to dextrothyroxine. *JAMA* 220:996–1008, 1972.

6.3   Coronary Drug Project Research Group: The prognostic importance of the electrocardiogram after myocardial infarction: Experience in the Coronary Drug Project. *Ann Intern Med* 77:677–689, 1972.

6.4   Coronary Drug Project Research Group: The Coronary Drug Project: Design, methods and baseline results. *Circulation* 47(suppl I): 1-1—1-50 (plus appendixes), 1973.

6.5   Coronary Drug Project Research Group: The Coronary Drug Project: Findings leading to discontinuation of the 2.5-mg/day estrogen group. *JAMA* 226:652–657, 1973.

6.6   Coronary Drug Project Research Group: Prognostic importance of premature beats following myocardial infarction: Experience in the Coronary Drug Project. *JAMA* 223:1116–1124, 1973.

6.7   Coronary Drug Project Research Group: Factors influencing long-term prognosis after recovery from myocardial infarction: Three-year findings of the Coronary Drug Project. *J Chronic Dis* 27:267–285, 1974.

6.8   Coronary Drug Project Research Group: Left ventricular hypertrophy patterns and prognosis: Experience post-infarction in the Coronary Drug Project. *Circulation* 49:862–869, 1974.

6.9   Coronary Drug Project Research Group: The prognostic importance of premature ventricular complexes in the late post-infarction period: Experience in the Coronary Drug Project. *Acta Cardiol* (suppl 18):33–53, 1974.

6.10   Coronary Drug Project Research Group: The Coronary Drug Project. Clofibrate and niacin in coronary heart disease. *JAMA* 231:360–381, 1975.

6.11   Coronary Drug Project Research Group: Reply to letter from D. J. Gans. *JAMA* 234:22–23, 1975.

6.12 Coronary Drug Project Research Group: Aspirin in coronary heart disease. *J Chronic Dis* 29:625–642, 1976.

6.13 Coronary Drug Project Research Group: Serum uric acid: Its association with other risk factors and with mortality in coronary heart disease. *J Chronic Dis* 29:557–569, 1976.

6.14 Coronary Drug Project Research Group: The prognostic importance of plasma glucose levels and of the use of oral hypoglycemic drugs after myocardial infarction in men. *Diabetes* 26:453–465, 1977.

6.15 Coronary Drug Project Research Group: Gallbladder disease as a side-effect of drugs influencing lipid metabolism: Experience in the Coronary Drug Project. *N Engl J Med* 296:1185–1190, 1977.

6.16 Coronary Drug Project Research Group: The Coronary Drug Project: Implications for clinical care. *Primary Care* 4:247–253, 1977.

6.17 Coronary Drug Project Research Group: The Coronary Drug Project Aspirin Study: Implications for clinical care. *Primary Care* 5:91–95, 1978.

6.18 Coronary Drug Project Research Group: The natural history of myocardial infarction in the Coronary Drug Project: Long-term prognostic importance of serum lipid level. *Am J Cardiol* 42:489–498, 1978.

6.19 Coronary Drug Project Research Group: Clofibrate and gallbladder disease (letter). *N Engl J Med* 298:461, 1978.

6.20 Coronary Drug Project Research Group: Estrogens and cancer (letter). *JAMA* 239:2758–2759, 1978.

6.21 Coronary Drug Project Research Group: Reply to editorial by L. Carlson (letter). *Atherosclerosis* 30:239–241, 1978.

6.22 Coronary Drug Project Research Group: Reply to letter from C. A. Caceres and K. Enslein. *JAMA* 240:1483–1484, 1978.

6.23 Coronary Drug Project Research Group: Cigarette smoking as a risk factor in men with a prior history of myocardial infarction. *J Chronic Dis* 32:415–425, 1979.

6.24 Coronary Drug Project Research Group: Influence of adherence to treatment and response of cholesterol on mortality in the Coronary Drug Project. *N Engl J Med* 303:1038–1041, 1980.

6.25 Coronary Drug Project Research Group: Treatable risk factors—hypercholesterolemia, smoking, and hypertension—after myocardial infarction: Implications of the Coronary Drug Project data for clinical management. *Primary Care* 7:175–179, 1980.

6.26 Coronary Drug Project Research Group: Practical aspects of decision making in clinical trials: The Coronary Drug Project as a case study. *Controlled Clin Trials* 1:363–376, 1981.

6.27 Coronary Drug Project Research Group: Implications of findings in the Coronary Drug Project for secondary prevention trials in coronary heart disease. *Circulation* 63:1342–1350, 1981.

6.28 Coronary Drug Project Research Group: The natural history of coronary heart disease: Prognostic factors after recovery from myocardial infarction in 2789 men. The 5-year findings of the Coronary Drug Project. *Circulation* 66: 401–414, 1982.

6.29 Coronary Drug Project Research Group: High-density lipoprotein cholesterol and prognosis after myocardial infarction. *Circulation* 66:1176–1178, 1982.

7. Aspirin Myocardial Infarction Study (AMIS)

7.1 Aspirin Myocardial Infarction Study Research Group: A randomized, controlled trial of aspirin in persons recovered from myocardial infarction. *JAMA* 243:661–669, 1980.

7.2 Howard J, Whittemore AS, Hoover JJ, Panos M, and the Aspirin Myocardial Infarction Study Research Group: Commentary: How blind was the patient blind in AMIS? *Clin Pharmacol Ther* 32:543–553, 1982.

7.3 Wasserman AG, Bren GB, Ross AM, Richardson DW, Hutchinson RG, Rios JC: Prognostic implications of diagnostic Q waves after myocardial infarction. *Circulation* 65:1451–1455, 1982.

8. Persantine Aspirin Reinfarction Study (PARIS)

8.1 Persantine Aspirin Reinfarction Study Research Group: Persantine Aspirin Reinfarction Study: Design, methods, and baseline results. *Circulation* 62(suppl II):II-1—II-42, 1980.

Table B-3 Publication list of sketched trials (*continued*)

8.2   Persantine Aspirin Reinfarction Study Research Group: Persantine and aspirin in coronary heart disease. *Circulation* 62:449–461, 1980.

9. Hypertension Detection and Follow-Up Program (HDFP)

9.1   Labarthe DR, Hawkins CM, Remington RD: Evaluation of performance of selected devices for measuring blood pressure. *Am J Cardiol* 32:546–553, 1973.

9.2   Remington RD: The Hypertension Detection and Follow-Up Program. Institut National de la Santé et de la Recherche Medicale (INSERM) 21:185–194, 1973.

9.3   Hypertension Detection and Follow-Up Program Cooperative Group (Borhani NO, Kass EH, Langford HG, Payne GH, Remington RD, Stamler J): The Hypertension Detection and Follow-Up Program. *Prev Med* 5:207–215, 1976.

9.4   Hypertension Detection and Follow-Up Program Cooperative Group: The Hypertension Detection and Follow-Up Program: A progress report. *Circ Res* 40(suppl I):I–106—I–109, 1977.

9.5   Hypertension Detection and Follow-Up Program Cooperative Group (Castle CH, Daugherty S, Detels R, Hawkins CM, Krishan I, Oberman A, Wassertheil-Smoller S): Blood pressure studies in 14 communities: A two-stage screen for hypertension. *JAMA* 237:2385–2391, 1977.

9.6   Hypertension Detection and Follow-Up Program Cooperative Group (Heymsfield S, Kraus J, Lee ES, McDill M, Stamler R, Watson R): Race, education and prevalence of hypertension. *Am J Epidemiol* 106:351–361, 1977.

9.7   Hypertension Detection and Follow-Up Program Cooperative Group (Apostolides A, Schnaper H, Stamler R, Taylor J, Tyler M, Wassertheil-Smoller S): Patient participation in a hypertension control program. *JAMA* 239:1507–1514, 1978.

9.8   Hypertension Detection and Follow-Up Program Cooperative Group (Apostolides A, Blaufox MD, Borhani NO, Cutter G, Daughtery S, Lewin AJ, Polk BF): Mild hypertensives in the Hypertension Detection and Follow-Up Program. *Ann NY Acad Sci* 304:254–266, 1978.

9.9   Hypertension Detection and Follow-Up Program Cooperative Group (Cutter G, Hebel JR, Labarthe D, Oberman A, Prineas R, Varady P): Variability of blood pressure and the results of screening in the Hypertension Detection and Follow-Up Program. *J Chronic Dis* 31:651–667, 1978.

9.10   Hypertension Detection and Follow-Up Program Cooperative Group (Blaufox MD, Curb D, Kralios A, Polk BF, Tyler M): Therapeutic control of blood pressure in the Hypertension Detection and Follow-Up Program. *Prev Med* 8:2–13, 1979.

9.11   Hypertension Detection and Follow-Up Program Cooperative Group: Five-year findings of the Hypertension Detection and Follow-Up Program: I. Reduction in mortality of persons with high blood pressure, including mild hypertension. *JAMA* 242:2562–2571, 1979.

9.12   Hypertension Detection and Follow-Up Program Cooperative Group: Five-year findings of the Hypertension Detection and Follow-Up Program: II. Mortality by race-sex, and age. *JAMA* 242:2572–2577, 1979.

9.13   Wassertheil-Smoller S, Apostolides A, Miller M, Oberman A, Thom T (on behalf of the Hypertension Detection and Follow-Up Program): Recent status of detection, treatment, and control of hypertension in the community. *J Community Health* 5:82–93, 1979.

9.14   Cowan L, Detels R, Farber M, Lee ES, McCray G, O'Flynn S, Parnell MJ (on behalf of the Hypertension Detection and Follow-Up Program): Residential mobility and long-term treatment of hypertension. *J Community Health* 5:159–166, 1980.

9.15   Cutter G, Heyden S, Kasteler J, Kraus JF, Lee ES, Shipley T, Stromer M (on behalf of the Hypertension Detection and Follow-Up Program): Mortality surveillance in collaborative trials. *Am J Public Health* 70:394–400, 1980.

9.16   Apostolides A, Cutter G, Daugherty SA, Detels R, Kraus J, Wassertheil-Smoller S, Ware J: Three-year incidence of hypertension in thirteen U.S. communities. *Prev Med* 11:487–499, 1982.

9.17   Curb JD, Hardy RJ, Labarthe DR, Borhani NO, Taylor JO: Reserpine and breast cancer in the Hypertension Detection and Follow-Up Program. *Hypertension* 4:307–311, 1982.

9.18   Hypertension Detection and Follow-Up Program Cooperative Group: Five-year findings of the Hypertension Detection and Follow-Up Program: III. Reduction in stroke incidence among persons with high blood pressure. *JAMA* 247:633–638, 1982.

Table B-3 Publication list of sketched trials (*continued*)

9.19   Hypertension Detection and Follow-Up Program Cooperative Group: The effect of treatment on mortality in "mild" hypertension—Results of the Hypertension Detection and Follow-Up Program. *N Engl J Med* 307:976–980, 1982.

9.20   Kraus JF, Conley A, Hardy R, Sexton M, Sweezey Z: Relationship of demographic characteristics of interviewers to blood pressure measurements. *J Community Health* 8:3–12, 1982.

9.21   Shulman N, Cutter G, Daugherty R, Sexton M, Pauk G, Taylor MJ, Tyler M: Correlates of attendance and compliance in the Hypertension Detection and Follow-Up Program. *Controlled Clin Trials* 3:13–27, 1982.

9.22   Smith EO, Curb JD, Hardy RJ, Hawkins CM, Tyroler HA: Clinic attendance in the Hypertension Detection and Follow-UP Program. *Hypertension* 4:710–715, 1982.

9.23   Hardy RJ, Hawkins CM: The impact of selected indices of antihypertensive treatment on all-cause mortality. *Am J Epidemiol* 117:566–574, 1983.

9.24   Hypertension Detection and Follow-Up Program Cooperative Group (SA Daugherty, G Entwisle, JD Curb, BF Polk, JO Taylor, editors): Hypertension Detection and Follow-Up Program: Baseline characteristics of the enumerated, screened, and hypertensive participants. *Hypertension* 5(suppl IV):IV-1—IV-205, 1983.

10. Multiple Risk Factor Intervention Trial (MRFIT)

10.1   Multiple Risk Factor Intervention Trial Group: Statistical design considerations in the NHLBI Multiple Risk Factor Intervention Trial (MRFIT). *J Chronic Dis* 30:261–275, 1977.

10.2   Zukel WJ, Paul O, Schnaper HW: The Multiple Risk Factor Intervention Trial (MRFIT): I. Historical perspective. *Prev Med* 10:387–401, 1981.

10.3   Sherwin R, Kaelber CT, Kezdi P, Kjelsberg MO, Thomas HE, Jr.: The Multiple Risk Factor Intervention Trial (MRFIT): II. The development of the protocol. *Prev Med* 10:402–425, 1981.

10.4   Benfari RC: The Multiple Risk Factor Intervention Trial (MRFIT): III. The model for intervention. *Prev Med* 10:426–442, 1981.

10.5   Caggiula AW, Christakis G, Farrand M, Hulley SB, Johnson R, Lasser NL, Stamler J, Widdowson G: The Multiple Risk Factor Intervention Trial (MRFIT): IV. Intervention on blood lipids. *Prev Med* 10:443–475, 1981.

10.6   Hughes GH, Hymowitz N, Ockene JK, Simon N, Vogt TM: The Multiple Risk Factor Intervention Trial (MRFIT): V. Intervention on smoking. *Prev Med* 10:476–500, 1981.

10.7   Cohen JD, Grimm RH, Jr., Smith WM: Multiple Risk Factor Intervention Trial (MRFIT): VI. Intervention on blood pressure. *Prev Med* 10:501–518, 1981.

10.8   Neaton JD, Broste S, Cohen L. Fishman EL, Kjelsberg MO, Schoenberger J: The Multiple Risk Factor Intervention Trial (MRFIT): VII. A comparison of risk factor changes between the two study groups. *Prev Med* 10:519–543, 1981.

10.9   Benfari RC, Sherwin R: The Multiple Risk Factor Intervention Trial after 4 years: A summing-up. *Prev Med* 10:544–546, 1981.

10.10   Multiple Risk Factor Intervention Trial Research Group: Multiple Risk Factor Intervention Trial: Risk factor changes and mortality results. *JAMA* 248:1465–1477, 1982.

11. Coronary Artery Surgery Study (CASS)

11.1   Kronmal RA, Davis K, Fisher LD, Jones RA, Gillespie MJ: Data management for a large collaborative clinical trial (CASS: Coronary Artery Surgery Study). *Comput Biomed Res* 11:553–566, 1978.

11.2   Davis K, Kennedy JW, Kemp HG, Jr., Judkins MP, Gosselin AJ, Killip T: Complications of coronary arteriography from the Collaborative Study of Coronary Artery Surgery (CASS). *Circulation* 59:1105–1112, 1979.

11.3   Weiner DA, Ryan TJ, McCabe CH, Kennedy JW, Schloss M, Tristani F, Chaitman BR, Fisher LD: Exercise stress testing: Correlations among history of angina, ST-segment response and prevalence of coronary artery disease in the Coronary Artery Surgery Study (CASS). *N Engl J Med* 301:230–235, 1979.

Table B-3   Publication list of sketched trials (*continued*)

11.4   Chaitman BR, Rogers WJ, Davis K, Tyras DH, Berger R, Bourassa MG, Fisher L, Hertzberg VS, Judkins MP, Mock MB, Killip T: Operative risk factors in patients with left main coronary artery disease. *N Engl J Med* 303:953–957, 1980.

11.5   Kennedy JW, Kaiser GC, Fisher LD, Maynard C, Fritz JK, Myers W, Mudd JG, Ryan TJ, Coggin J: Multivariate discriminant analysis of the clinical and angiographic predictors of operative mortality from the Collaborative Study in Coronary Artery Surgery (CASS). *J Thorac Cardiovasc Surg* 80:876–887, 1980.

11.6   Vlietstra RE, Frye RL, Kronmal RA, Sim DA, Tristani FE, Killip T III, and participants in the Coronary Artery Surgery Study: Risk factors and angiographic coronary artery disease: A report from the Coronary Artery Surgery Study (CASS). *Circulation* 62:254–261, 1980.

11.7   Chaitman BR, Bourassa MG, Davis K, Rogers WJ, Tyras DH, Berger R, Kennedy JW, Fisher LD, Judkins MP, Mock MB, Killip T: Angiographic prevalence of high-risk coronary artery disease in patient subsets (CASS). *Circulation* 64:360–367, 1981.

11.8   Chaitman BR, Fisher L, Bourassa MG, Davis K, Rogers WJ, Maynard C, Tyras DH, Berger RL, Judkins MP, Ringqvist I, Mock MB, Killip T: Effect of coronary bypass surgery on survival patterns in subsets of patients with left main coronary artery disease. Report of the Collaborative Study in Coronary Artery Surgery (CASS). *Am J Cardiol* 48:765–777, 1981.

11.9   Fisher LD, Kennedy JW, Chaitman BR, Ryan TJ, McCabe C, Weiner D, Tristani F, Schloss M, Warner HR: Diagnostic quantification of CASS (Coronary Artery Surgery Study) clinical and exercise test results in determining presence and extent of coronary artery disease. *Circulation* 63:987–1000, 1981.

11.10   Berger RL, Davis KB, Kaiser GC, Foster ED, Hammond GL, Tong TGL, Kennedy JW, Scheffield T, Ringqvist I, Wiens RD, Chaitman BR, Mock M: Preservation of the myocardium during coronary artery bypass grafting. *Circulation* 64(suppl II):II-61—II-66, 1981.

11.11   Kennedy JW, Kaiser GC, Fisher LD, Fritz JB, Myers W, Mudd JG, Ryan TJ: Clinical and angiographic predictors of operative mortality from the Collaborative Study in Coronary Artery Surgery (CASS). *Circulation* 63:793–802, 1981.

11.12   Principal Investigators of CASS and their associates, T Killip (editor), LD Fisher, MB Mock (associate editors): The National Heart, Lung, and Blood Institute Coronary Artery Surgery Study (CASS). *Circulation* 63(suppl I):I-1—I-81, 1981.

11.13   Alderman EL, Fisher L, Maynard C, Mock MB, Ringqvist I, Bourassa MG, Kaiser GC, Gillespie MJ: Determinants of coronary surgery in a consecutive patient series from geographically dispersed medical centers: The Coronary Artery Surgery Study. *Circulation* 66(suppl I): I-6—I-15, 1982.

11.14   Faxon DP, Ryan TJ, Davis KB, McCabe CH, Myers W, Lesperance J, Shaw R, Tong TGL: Prognostic significance of angiographically documented left ventricular aneurysm from the Coronary Artery Surgery Study (CASS). *Am J Cardiol* 50:157–164, 1982.

11.15   Fisher LD, Judkins MP, Lesperance J, Cameron A, Swaye P, Ryan T, Maynard C, Bourassa M, Kennedy JW, Gosselin A, Kemp H, Faxon D, Wexler L, Davis KB: Reproducibility of coronary arteriographic reading in the Coronary Artery Surgery Study (CASS). *Cathet Cardiovasc Diagn* 8:565–575, 1982.

11.16   Fisher LD, Kennedy JW, Davis KB, Maynard C, Fritz JK, Kaiser G, Myers WO: The association of sex, physical size, and operative mortality after coronary artery bypass in the Coronary Artery Surgery Study (CASS). *J Thorac Cardiovasc Surg* 84:334–341, 1982.

11.17   Kemp H, Davis K, Judkins MP, Gosselin A, Kennedy JW, Cameron A, Swaye PS, Maynard C, Fisher LD: Intrareader variability in the interpretation of coronary arteriograms from the Coronary Artery Surgery Study (CASS). Ischemic heart disease: Second USA-USSR Symposium, Seattle, Washington, March 20, 1981. *Kardiologiia* 22:37–42, 1982.*

11.18   Kennedy JW, Killip T, Fisher LD, Alderman EL, Gillespie MJ, Mock MB: The clinical spectrum of coronary artery disease and its surgical and medical management, 1974–1979: The Coronary Artery Surgery Study. *Circulation* 66(suppl III):III-16—III-23, 1982.

11.19   Killip T: Indications for coronary arteriography. Ischemic heart disease: Second USA-USSR Symposium, Seattle, Washington, March 20, 1981. *Kardiologiia* 22:33–37, 1982.*

Table B-3 Publication list of sketched trials (*continued*)

11.20 Lundberg ED, McBride R, Rawson TE, Mauritsen R, Ormond TH, Fisher LD, Kronmal RA, Gillespie MJ: C2: A data base management system developed for the Coronary Artery Surgery Study (CASS) and other clinical studies. *J Med Systems* 6:501–518, 1982.

11.21 Mock MB, Ringqvist I, Fisher LD, Davis KB, Chaitman BO, Kouchoukos NT, Kaiser GC, Alderman E, Ryan TJ, Russell RO Jr, Mullin S, Fray D, Killip T III, Participants in the Coronary Artery Surgery Study: Survival of medically treated patients in the Coronary Artery Surgery Study (CASS) Registry. *Circulation* 66:562–568, 1982.

11.22 Rogers WJ, Chaitman BR, Fisher LD, Bourassa MG, Davis K, Maynard CL, Tyras DH, Berger RL, Judkins MP, Ringqvist I, Mock MB, Killip T: Comparison of the cumulative survival of medically and surgically treated patients with left main coronary artery disease: The CASS experience. Ischemic heart disease: Second USA-USSR Symposium, Seattle, Washington, March 20, 1981. *Kardiologiia* 22:53–57, 1982.*

11.23 Ryan TJ, Fisher LD, Weiner DA, McCabe CH, Chaitman B, Kennedy JW, Ferguson J, Tristani F: Experience with electrocardiographic exercise testing in the Coronary Artery Surgery Study (CASS). Ischemic heart disease, Second USA-USSR Symposium, Seattle, Washington, March 20, 1981. *Kardiologiia* 22:22–26, 1982.*

11.24 Vlietstra RE, Kronmal RA, Seth A, Frye RL: Correlation of risk factors for coronary artery disease with coronary angiographic findings. Ischemic heart disease: Second USA-USSR Symposium, Seattle, Washington, March 20, 1981. *Kardiologiia* 22:67–72, 1982.*

11.25 Vlietstra RE, Kronmal RA, Frye RL, Seth AK, Tristani FE, Killip T III: Factors affecting the extent and severity of coronary artery disease in patients enrolled in the Coronary Artery Surgery Study. *Arteriosclerosis* 2:208–215, 1982.

11.26 Weiner DA, McCabe CH, Ryan TJ, Chaitman BR, Sheffield LT, Ferguson J, Fisher LD: Assessment of the negative exercise test in 4373 patients from the Coronary Artery Surgery Study (CASS). *J Cardiac Rehab* 2:562–568, 1982.

11.27 Wexler LF, Lesperance J, Ryan TJ, Bourassa MG, Fisher LD, Maynard C, Kemp HG, Cameron A, Gosselin AJ, Judkins MP: Interobserver variability in interpreting contrast left ventriculograms (CASS). *Cathet Cardiovasc Diagn* 8:341–355, 1982.

11.28 Zimmern SH, Rogers WJ, Bream PR, Chaitman BR, Bourassa MG, Davis KA, Tyras DH, Berger R, Fisher L, Judkins MP, Mock MB, Killip TA: Total occlusion of the left main coronary artery: The Coronary Artery Surgery Study (CASS) experience. *Am J Cardiol* 49:2003–2010, 1982.

11.29 Chaitman BR, Alderman FL, Sheffield LT, Tong T, Fisher LD, Mock MB, Wiens RD, Kaiser GC, Roitman D, Berger R, Gersh B, Schaff H, Bourassa MG, Killip T: Use of survival analysis to determine the clinical significance of new Q waves after coronary bypass surgery. *Circulation* 67:302–309, 1983.

11.30 Gersh BJ, Kronmal RA, Frye RL, Schaff HV, Ryan TJ, Gosselin AJ, Kaiser GC, Killip T: Coronary arteriography and coronary artery bypass surgery: Morbidity and mortality in patients 65 or older. A report from the Coronary Artery Surgery Study. *Circulation* 67:483–491, 1983.

11.31 Swaye PS, Fisher LD, Litwin P, Vignola PA, Judkins MP, Kemp HG, Mudd JG, Gosselin AJ: Aneurysmal coronary artery disease. *Circulation* 67:134–138, 1983.

12. Program on the Surgical Control of Hyperlipidemia (POSCH)

12.1 Buchwald H, Moore RB, Varco RL: Maximum lipid reduction by partial ileal bypass: A test of the lipid-atherosclerosis hypothesis. *Lipids* 12:53–58, 1977.

12.2 Moore RB, Long JM, Matts JP, Amplatz K, Varco RL, Buchwald H, and the POSCH Group: Plasma lipoproteins and coronary arteriography in subjects in the Program on the Surgical Control of the Hyperlipidemias. *Atherosclerosis* 32:101–119, 1979.

12.3 Long JM, Brashear JR, Matts JP, Bearman JE, and the POSCH Group: The POSCH information management system: Experience with alternative approaches. *J Med Syst* 4:355–366, 1980.

12.4 Moore RB, Buchwald H, Varco RL, and the Participants in the Program on the Surgical Control of the Hyperlipidemias: The effect of partial ileal bypass on plasma lipoproteins. *Circulation* 62:469–476, 1980.

12.5 Buchwald H, Fitch L, Moore RB: Overview of randomized clinical trials of lipid intervention for atherosclerotic cardiovascular disease. *Controlled Clin Trials* 3:271–283, 1982.

Table B-3   Publication list of sketched trials (*continued*)

12.6   Buchwald H, Moore RB, Matts JP, Long JM, Varco RL, Campbell GS, Pearce MB, Yellin AE, Blankenhorn CH, Holmes WL, Smink RD Jr, Sawin HS Jr and the participants in the Program on the Surgical Control of the Hyperlipidemias: A status report. *Surgery* 92:654–662, 1982.

12.7   Buchwald H, Moore RB, Rucker RD Jr, Amplatz K, Castaneda WR, Francoz RA, Pasternak RC, Varco RL, and the POSCH Arteriography Review Panel: Clinical angiographic regression of atherosclerosis after partial ileal bypass. *Atherosclerosis* 46:117–128, 1983.

13. Hypertension Prevention Trial (HPT)

None

14. International Reflux Study in Children (IRSC)

14.1   International Reflux Study Committee: Medical versus surgical treatment of primary vesicoureteral reflux: A prospective International Reflux Study in Children. *J Urol* 125:227–283, 1981.

14.2   International Reflux Study Committee: Medical versus surgical treatment of primary vesicoureteral reflux. *Pediatrics* 67:392–400, 1981.

*Also in National Institutes of Health publication 82-1965, United States Department of Health and Human Services, Bethesda, Maryland.

Table B-4 Summary tabulations from sketches

Item	PHS 1	UGDP 2	VA43 3	MPS 4	NCGS 5	CDP 6	AMIS 7	PARIS 8	HDFP 9	MRFIT 10	CASS 11	POSCH 12	HPT 13	IRSC 14	Freq.
1. Type of trial															
Therapeutic		✓	✓	✓	✓	✓	✓	✓	✓		✓	✓		✓	11
Prophylactic	✓									✓			✓		3
2. Type of design															
Fixed sample	✓	✓	✓	✓	✓	✓	✓	✓	✓	✓	✓	✓	✓	✓	14
3. Stage															
Initial design															0
Protocol development															0
Patient recruitment	✓			✓									✓		3
Treatment and follow–up											✓	✓		✓	3
Patient close–out															0
Termination			✓		✓					✓					3
Post–trial follow–up							✓	✓							2
Completed		✓				✓			✓						3

Table B-4 Summary tabulations from sketches (*continued*)

Item	PHS	UGDP	VA43	MPS	NCGS	CDP	AMIS	PARIS	HDFP	MRFIT	CASS	POSCH	HPT	IRSC	Freq.
	1	2	3	4	5	6	7	8	9	10	11	12	13	14	
4. Funding source															
NIH	✓	✓		✓	✓	✓	✓		✓	✓	✓	✓	✓	✓	12
VA			✓												1
Industry								✓							1
Private foundation														✓	1
5. Funding type															
Grant	✓	✓		✓		✓		✓				✓	✓	✓	8
Contract					✓		✓		✓	✓	✓				5
Neither			✓*												1
6. Mode of initiation															
Investigator	✓	✓	✓	✓								✓	✓	✓	7
Sponsor							✓	✓	✓	✓	✓				5
Sponsor–investigator					✓	✓									2

Table B-4 Summary tabulations from sketches (*continued*)

Item		PHS	UGDP	VA43	MPS	NCGS	CDP	AMIS	PARIS	HDFP	MRFIT	CASS	POSCH	HPT	IRSC	Freq.
		1	2	3	4	5	6	7	8	9	10	11	12	13	14	

7. Mode of fund dispersal

	PHS	UGDP	VA43	MPS	NCGS	CDP	AMIS	PARIS	HDFP	MRFIT	CASS	POSCH	HPT	IRSC	Freq.
Direct to individual centers	NA	✓	✓	✓		✓	✓			✓	✓				7
Indirect via a consortium award	NA				✓				✓				✓		✓	4
Direct to some centers indirect to others	NA									✓				✓		2

8. Funding date

	PHS	UGDP	VA43	MPS	NCGS	CDP	AMIS	PARIS	HDFP	MRFIT	CASS	POSCH	HPT	IRSC	Freq.
Start	Sept 1981	Sept 1960	Oct 1976	Jan 1979	June 1973	Mar 1965	Oct 1974	April 1974	June 1971	June 1972	May 1973	June 1973	Sept 1981	July 1979	–
End	Dec 1986	April 1982	Oct 1983	Dec 1986	Oct 1983	April 1984	Nov 1979	Sept 1980	June 1985	June 1985	May 1988	Not set	Aug 1986	Not set	–

9. Clinics

	PHS	UGDP	VA43	MPS	NCGS	CDP	AMIS	PARIS	HDFP	MRFIT	CASS	POSCH	HPT	IRSC	Freq.
No. in U.S. (incl P.R.)	NA	12	11	12	10	53	30	16	14	22	13	4	4	18	–
No. outside U.S.	NA	0	0	0	0	0	0	4	0	0	1	0	0	8	–
Total no.	NA	12	11	12	10	53	30	20	14	22	14*	4	4	26	–

Table B-4 Summary tabulations from sketches (*continued*)

							Acronym and sketch no.								
Item	PHS	UGDP	VA43	MPS	NCGS	CDP	AMIS	PARIS	HDFP	MRFIT	CASS	POSCH	HPT	IRSC	Freq.
	1	2	3	4	5	6	7	8	9	10	11	12	13	14	
10. Resource centers															
Data coord. center	NA	NA	1	NA	1	NA	NA	NA	NA	NA	NA	NA	1	NA	3
Trt. coord. center	NA	NA	1	NA	1	NA	NA	NA	NA	NA	NA	NA	1	NA	3
Coord. center	1	1	NA	1	NA	1	1	1	1	1	1	1	NA	1*	11
Project office	1	1	1	1	1	1	1	0	1	1	1	1	1	1*	13
Central laboratories	1	2	2	0	2	1	1	1	1	1	0	1	1	0	11
Reading centers	0	1	0	1	3	1	1	1	1	2	1	2	1	2*	12
Quality control center	0	0	0	0	0	0	0	1	0	1	0	0	0	0	2
Procurement and distribution center	0	0	1	0	0	1	1	1	1	1	0	0	0	0	6
Total no.	3	4	6	3	8	5	5	5	5	7	3	5	5	4*	14
11. Coord. center or data coord. center															
a. Location															
School of public health	✓								✓	✓			✓		4
School of medicine		✓		✓		✓	✓				✓	✓		✓	7
Other teaching inst.					✓										1
Nonteaching inst.			✓					✓							2

Table B-4 Summary tabulations from sketches (*continued*)

Item		PHS	UGDP	VA43	MPS	NCGS	CDP	AMIS	PARIS	HDFP	MRFIT	CASS	POSCH	HPT	IRSC	Freq.
		1	2	3	4	5	6	7	8	9	10	11	12	13	14	
11. CC or data CC (cont'd)																
b. Primary degree of director		MD (Epi)	PhD (Bio)	PhD (Bio)	MSc (Bio)	ScD (Bio)	PhD (Bio)	PhD (Bio)	MD (Epi)	ScD (Bio)	PhD (Bio)	PhD (Bio)	EdD (Bio)	PhD (Bio)	MD (Med)	11 Bio
c. Affiliation with other study centers																
Yes		NA				√*			√*				√*	√*	√*	5
No		NA	√	√	√		√	√		√	√	√				8
12. Type of treatment design																
Noncrossover		√	√	√	√	√	√	√	√	√	√	√	√	√	√	14
13. Type of treatment structure																
Simple			√	√	√	√	√	√		√	√	√	√		√	11
Partial factorial									√					√		2
Full factorial		√														1

Table B-4 Summary tabulations from sketches (*continued*)

Item	Acronym and sketch no.														
	PHS	UGDP	VA43	MPS	NCGS	CDP	AMIS	PARIS	HDFP	MRFIT	CASS	POSCH	HPT	IRSC	Freq.
	1	2	3	4	5	6	7	8	9	10	11	12	13	14	
14. Study treatments															
No. of test treatments........	3	3	1	2	2	5	1	2	1	1	1	1	4	1	--
No. of control treatments....	1	2	1	1	1	1	1	1	1	1	1	1	1	1	--
Total no. of study trts.	4	5	2	3	3	6	2	3	2	2	2	2	5	2	--
15. Type of test treatment															
Drug.............................	✓	✓	✓		✓	✓	✓	✓	✓	✓					9
Surgery..........................				✓							✓	✓		✓	4
Behavior change................										✓			✓		2
16. Type of control treatment															
Placebo pills....................	✓	✓	✓		✓	✓	✓	✓							7
Standard med. trt.		✓							✓	✓	✓	✓		✓	6
No treatment....................				✓									✓		3

332

Table B-4 Summary tabulations from sketches (*continued*)

Item	PHS	UGDP	VA43	MPS	NCGS	CDP	AMIS	PARIS	HDFP	MRFIT	CASS	POSCH	HPT	IRSC	Freq.
	1	2	3	4	5	6	7	8	9	10	11	12	13	14	
17. Level of trt. masking															
None		✓		✓					✓	✓	✓	✓	✓	✓	8
Single-masked															0
Double-masked	✓		✓		✓	✓	✓	✓							7
18. Patients studied															
Males	✓	✓	✓	✓	✓	✓	✓	✓	✓	✓	✓	✓	✓	✓	14
Females		✓	✓	✓	✓	✓	✓	✓	✓		✓			✓	10
Children														✓	1
Adults	✓		✓	✓	✓	✓	✓	✓	✓	✓	✓	✓	✓		13
19. Patient recruitment															
a. Primary mode of contact															
Direct	✓	✓	✓	✓	✓		✓	✓	✓	✓		✓	✓		10
Indirect		✓	✓	✓		✓				✓	✓	✓		✓	7

Acronym and sketch no.

Table B–4 Summary tabulations from sketches (*continued*)

Item	PHS 1	UGDP 2	VA43 3	MPS 4	NCGS 5	CDP 6	AMIS 7	PARIS 8	HDFP 9	MRFIT 10	CASS 11	POSCH 12	HPT 13	IRSC 14	Freq.
19. Patient recruitment (cont'd)															
b. Start of enrollment	Mid 1982	Feb 1961	Mar 1977	Mar 1979	Sept 1976	Mar 1966	May 1975	April 1975	Feb 1973	Nov 1973	Aug 1975	Sept 1975	Sept 1982	Jan 1980	–
c. End of enrollment	Mid 1983	Feb 1966	May 1980	Not set	June 1978	Oct 1969	Aug 1976	Sept 1976	May 1974	Feb 1976	May 1979	June 1983	Oct 1983	Not set	–
d. Total no. enrolled	17,350	1,027	231	756	916	8,341	4,524	2,026	10,940	12,866	780	838	235	260*	–
20. Method of randomization															
a. Type															
Fixed allocation ratio	✓	✓	✓	✓		✓	✓	✓	✓	✓	✓	✓	✓	✓	13
Number adaptive					✓										1
b. Stratification variables															
Clinic	Na	Yes	Yes	Yes	Yes	Yes	Yes	Yes	Yes	Yes	Yes	Yes	Yes	Yes	13 Yes
Disease state or type	No	No	Yes	Yes	No	Yes	No	No	Yes	No	Yes	Yes	No	Yes	7 Yes
Demographic characteristics	Yes Age	No	No	No	No	No	No	No	No	No	No	No	No	Yes Age,sex	2 Yes
Other	No	No	No	No	No	No	No	No	No	No	No	Yes*	Yes Wt	No	2 Yes
c. Total no. of variables controlled	1	1	2	2	1	2	1	1	2	1	3	4	2	4*	–

Table B-4 Summary tabulations from sketches (*continued*)

Item	Acronym and sketch no. PHS 1	UGDP 2	VA43 3	MPS 4	NCGS 5	CDP 6	AMIS 7	PARIS 8	HDFP 9	MRFIT 10	CASS 11	POSCH 12	HPT 13	IRSC 14	Freq.
20. Randomization (cont'd)															
d. Total no. of allocation strata	7	12	20	36	10	106	30	20	42	22	66	48	8	216*	--
e. Allocation ratio	Uni-form	Non-uni	Uni-form	Uni-form	Uni-form	Non-uni	Uni-form	Non-uni	Uni-form	Uni-form	Uni-form	Uni-form	Uni-form	Uni-form	11 Uni
f. Blocking in strata															
Yes	✓		✓	✓		✓	✓	✓	✓	✓	✓	✓	✓	✓	13
No					✓										1
g. Locus of control															
Central	✓		✓	✓	✓	✓	✓	✓		✓	✓	✓	✓	✓	13
Local									✓						1
h. Method of release															
From control center to clinic via phone		✓		✓	✓					✓	✓	✓		✓*	7
From control center to clinic via sealed schedule			✓			✓	✓	✓						✓*	5
From clinic via self-administered schedule									✓						1
From clinic via on-site micro-computer													✓		1
From control center direct to patient	✓														1

335

Table B-4 Summary tabulations from sketches (*continued*)

Item		PHS	UGDP	VA43	MPS	NCGS	CDP	AMIS	PARIS	HDFP	MRFIT	CASS	POSCH	HPT	IRSC	Freq.
	Acronym and sketch no.	1	2	3	4	5	6	7	8	9	10	11	12	13	14	
21. Data collection schedule																
a. Baseline clinic visits		NA*	2	2	1	2	3	3	2	2	3	1	2	3	1–2	-
b. Regular follow-up clinic visits/year		NA*	4	4	2	3–6*	3	3	3	0–3*	1*	2	1	2	1	-
22. Length of follow-up (yrs.)																
a. During trial		4.5	9.5–14.5	3–6	2+	2	5–8	3–4+	3–4+	5–6.5	6–8	4–8	≥5	≥2	Not set	-
b. Post-trial		NA	2	NA	NA	NA	6+	None done	None done	3	2–4	NA	NA	NA	NA	-
23. Primary outcome																
Deaths all causes		√	√				√	√	√	√		√	√			8
Deaths from specified cause				√							√					2
Other					√*	√*								√*	√*	4

Table B-4 Summary tabulations from sketches (*continued*)

Item	PHS 1	UGDP 2	VA43 3	MPS 4	NCGS 5	CDP 6	AMIS 7	PARIS 8	HDFP 9	MRFIT 10	CASS 11	POSCH 12	HPT 13	IRSC 14	Freq.
24. Method of follow–up close–out															
Common calendar date..........		√	√			√	√	√	√	√	√	√	√		10
Common period of follow–up..........					√										1
Not yet specified..........	√			√										√	3
25. Data entry															
a. Primary entry site															
CC or data CC..........	√	√	√	√	√	√	√	√	√	√		√		√	12
Clinic..........											√		√		2
b. Primary mode of entry															
Direct from forms..........	√	√	√	√	√	√	√	√	√	√	√	√	√	√	14
Indirect from code sheets prepared from forms..........															0
26. Sample size specification															
a. Original recruitment goal (all trts. combined)..........	21,500	1,000	456	522*	900	8,379	4,250	2,000	10,500	11,000	1,500	1,000	800	250*	—

Table B-4 Summary tabulations from sketches (*continued*)

Item		PHS	UGDP	VA43	MPS	NCGS	CDP	AMIS	PARIS	HDFP	MRFIT	CASS	POSCH	HPT	IRSC	
		1	2	3	4	5	6	7	8	9	10	11	12	13	14	Freq.

26. Sample size (cont'd)

b. Rationale for original recruitment goal

	PHS	UGDP	VA43	MPS	NCGS	CDP	AMIS	PARIS	HDFP	MRFIT	CASS	POSCH	HPT	IRSC	Freq.
Sample size calculation	✓		✓	✓	✓	✓	✓		✓	✓	✓	✓		✓	11
Pragmatic		✓						✓					✓		3

c. Achieved sample size

	PHS	UGDP	VA43	MPS	NCGS	CDP	AMIS	PARIS	HDFP	MRFIT	CASS	POSCH	HPT	IRSC	Freq.
All trts. combined	NA	1,027	231	236*	916	8,341	4,524	2,026	10,940	12,866	780	NA	NA	NA	–

d. Published rationale for achieved sample size

	PHS	UGDP	VA43	MPS	NCGS	CDP	AMIS	PARIS	HDFP	MRFIT	CASS	POSCH	HPT	IRSC	Freq.
Not applicable	✓		✓								✓	✓	✓	✓	6
None required				✓											1
None stated															0
Power calculation		✓			✓			✓		✓					4
Sample size calculation						✓	✓		✓	✓					4
Pragmatic		✓													1

Table B–4 Summary tabulations from sketches (*continued*)

Item		PHS	UGDP	VA43	MPS	NCGS	CDP	AMIS	PARIS	HDFP	MRFIT	CASS	POSCH	HPT	IRSC	Freq.
	Acronym and sketch no.	1	2	3	4	5	6	7	8	9	10	11	12	13	14	
27. Committees represented																
Steering committee		Yes	Yes	Yes	Yes	Yes	Yes	Yes	Yes	Yes	Yes	Yes	Yes	Yes	Yes	14 Yes
Executive committee		No	Yes	Yes	No	No	No	No	No	No	Yes	Yes	No	Yes	No	5 Yes
Treatment effects monitoring committee		Yes	No	NA	Yes	Yes	Yes	NA	Yes	Yes	NA	NA	Yes	Yes	Yes	9 Yes
Advisory review committee		No	Yes	NA	No	Yes	Yes	NA	Yes	Yes	NA	NA	Yes	Yes	No	7 Yes
Advisory review & treatment effects monitoring comm.		NA	NA	Yes	NA	NA	NA	Yes	NA	NA	Yes	Yes	NA	NA	NA	4 Yes
No. of other committees		2	10	2	1	7	11	8	1	8	8	4	3	3	0	–
Total no. of committees		4	13	5	3	10	14	10	4	11	11	7	6	6	2	–
28. Steering committee																
a. Chairman																
i. Primary degree		MD	MD	MD	MD	MD	MD	MD	MD	MD	MD	MD	MD	MD	MD	14 MD
ii. Patient care responsibilities		No	Yes	No	Yes	No	No	No	No	Yes	No	No	Yes	Yes	Yes	6 Yes
iii. Elected or appointed		Self-appt	E	E	Self-appt	Self-appt	Appt	Appt	Appt	E	Appt	Appt	Self-appt	E	E	5 E
iv. Term of office		WT	WT	WT	WT	WT	WT	WT	WT	WT	WT	WT	WT	WT	WT	14 WT

Table B–4 Summary tabulations from sketches (*continued*)

28. Steering committee (*cont'd*)

b. Vice-chairman

Item	PHS	UGDP	VA43	MPS	NCGS	CDP	AMIS	PARIS	HDFP	MRFIT	CASS	POSCH	HPT	IRSC	Freq.
	1	*2*	*3*	*4*	*5*	*6*	*7*	*8*	*9*	*10*	*11*	*12*	*13*	*14*	
i. Primary degree	MPH	NA	NA	NA	NA	MD	MD	MD	MD	MD	NA	NA	MD	MD	7 MD
ii. Patient care responsibilities	No	NA	NA	NA	NA	Yes	Yes	Yes	No	No	NA	NA	Yes	Yes	6 Yes
iii. Elected or appointed	Appt	NA	NA	NA	NA	Appt	Appt	E	E	Appt	NA	NA	E	E	4 E
iv. Term of office	W̄T̄	NA	NA	NA	NA	W̄T̄	W̄T̄	W̄T̄	W̄T̄	W̄T̄	NA	NA	W̄T̄	W̄T̄	8 W̄T̄

c. Membership

i. From study centers

	PHS	UGDP	VA43	MPS	NCGS	CDP	AMIS	PARIS	HDFP	MRFIT	CASS	POSCH	HPT	IRSC	Freq.
Voting	7	26	14	12	14	14	11	9	19	39	17	6	10	10	–
Nonvoting	4	1	0	0	1	0	7	0	0	0	2	0	2	0	–
Total	11	27	14	12	15	14	18	9	19	39	19	6	12	10	–

ii. From outside study centers

	PHS	UGDP	VA43	MPS	NCGS	CDP	AMIS	PARIS	HDFP	MRFIT	CASS	POSCH	HPT	IRSC	Freq.
Voting	5	0	0	1	2	1	0	2	0	0	0	0	0	0	–
Nonvoting	0	0	0	0	0	0	0	1	0	0	0	0	1	0	–
Total	5	0	0	1	2	1	0	3	0	0	0	0	1	0	–

Acronym and sketch no.

Table B-4 Summary tabulations from sketches (*continued*)

Item		Acronym and sketch no.														
		PHS	UGDP	VA43	MPS	NCGS	CDP	AMIS	PARIS	HDFP	MRFIT	CASS	POSCH	HPT	IRSC	Freq.
		1	2	3	4	5	6	7	8	9	10	11	12	13	14	
28. Steering committee (cont'd)																
c. Membership (cont'd)																
iii. Total																
Voting		12	26	14	12	16	15	11	11	19	39	17	6	10	10	–
Nonvoting		4	1	0	1	1	0	7	1	0	0	2	0	3	0	–
Total		16	27	14	13	17	15	18	12	19	39	19	6	13	10	–
d. Positions represented on committee																
i. Study chairman		Yes	Yes	Yes	Yes	Yes	Yes	Yes	Yes	Yes	Yes	Yes	Yes	Yes	Yes	14 Yes
ii. Vice-chairman		Yes	NA	NA	NA	NA	Yes	Yes	Yes	Yes	Yes	NA	NA	Yes	Yes	8 Yes
iii. CC or data CC director		Yes	Yes	Yes	Yes	Yes	Yes	Yes	Yes	Yes	Yes	Yes	Yes	Yes	Yes	14 Yes
iv. Clinic directors		NA	Yes	Yes	Yes	Yes	Yes	Yes	NA	Yes	Yes	Yes	Yes*	Yes	Yes	13 Yes
v. Project officer		Yes	Yes	No	Yes	No	Yes	Yes	No	Yes	Yes	Yes	No	Yes	No	10 Yes
vi. Clinic coordinators		NA	No	No	Yes	No	No	Yes	No	No	Yes	No	Yes	No	No	4 Yes
vii. Nonhealth professional		No	No	No	No	No	No	No	No	No	No	No	No	No	No	0 Yes
viii. Lay representative		No	No	No	No	No	No	No	No	No	No	No	No	No	No	0 Yes

341

Table B-4 Summary tabulations from sketches (*continued*)

Item	PHS 1	UGDP 2	VA43 3	MPS 4	NCGS 5	CDP 6	AMIS 7	PARIS 8	HDFP 9	MRFIT 10	CASS 11	POSCH 12	HPT 13	IRSC 14	Freq.
28. *Steering committee (cont'd)*															
e. No. of members elected	0	0	0	0	0	4,T	5,T	0	0	4,$\overline{WT}$	0	0	0	0	–
29. *Treatment effects monitoring committee*															
a. Responsible group															
Trt. effects monitoring comm.	✓			✓	✓	✓		✓	✓			✓	✓	✓	9
Advisory review & trt. effects monitoring comm.			✓				✓			✓*	✓				4
Steering committee.		✓													1
b. Chairman															
i. Primary degree.	MD (Epi)	MD (Med)	MD (Med)	PhD (Bio)	MD (Med)	PhD* (Bio)	MD (Med)	MD* (Epi)	MD (Epi)	MD (Med)	MD (Med)	MD (Epi)	PhD (Bio)	PhD (Bio)	10 MD
ii. Patient care responsibilities	No	Yes	No	No	No	No*	No	No*	No	No	No	No	No	No	1 Yes
iii. Elected or appointed	Appt	E	E	Appt	Appt	Appt*	Appt	Appt*	E	Appt	Appt	Appt	E	Appt	10 Appt
iv. Term of office	$\overline{WT}$	$\overline{WT}$	$\overline{WT}$	$\overline{WT}$	$\overline{WT}$	$\overline{WT}$*	$\overline{WT}$	$\overline{WT}$*	$\overline{WT}$	$\overline{WT}$	$\overline{WT}$	$\overline{WT}$	$\overline{WT}$	$\overline{WT}$	14 $\overline{WT}$

Table B-4 Summary tabulations from sketches (*continued*)

Item		PHS	UGDP	VA43	MPS	NCGS	CDP	AMIS	PARIS	HDFP	MRFIT	CASS	POSCH	HPT	IRSC	*Freq.*
	Acronym and sketch no.	*1*	*2*	*3*	*4*	*5*	*6*	*7*	*8*	*9*	*10*	*11*	*12*	*13*	*14*	
29. Treatment effects monitoring committee (*cont'd*)																
c. Vice-chairman																
Primary degree		NA	NA	NA	NA	NA	MD*(Epi)	NA	MD*(Epi)	NA	NA	NA	NA	NA	NA	2/MD
Patient care responsibilities		NA	NA	NA	NA	NA	No*	NA	No*	NA	NA	NA	NA	NA	NA	2/No
Elected or appointed		NA	NA	NA	NA	NA	Appt*	NA	Appt*	NA	NA	NA	NA	NA	NA	2/Appt
Term of office		NA	NA	NA	NA	NA	WT*	NA	WT*	NA	NA	NA	NA	NA	NA	2/WT
d. Membership																
i. From study centers																
Voting		1	26	0	0	0	11	0	5	5	0	2	0	7	0	-
Nonvoting		1	1	4	6	7	0	1	0	2	2	0	2	0	4	-
Total		2	27	4	6	7	11	1	5	7	2	2	2	7	4	-
ii. From outside study																
Voting		3	0	4	5	5	5	7	3	6	7	11	8	0	4	-
Nonvoting		0	0	0	0	0	0	0	1	0	0	0	1	0	0	-
Total		3	0	4	5	5	5	7	4	6	7	11	9	0	4	-

Table B-4 Summary tabulations from sketches (*continued*)

29. *Treatment effects monitoring committee (cont'd)*
   d. *Membership (cont'd)*
   iii. Total

   e. *Positions represented on committee*

Item		Acronym and sketch no.													
	PHS	UGDP	VA43	MPS	NCGS	CDP	AMIS	PARIS	HDFP	MRFIT	CASS	POSCH	HPT	IRSC	Freq.
	1	2	3	4	5	6	7	8	9	10	11	12	13	14	
Voting	4	26	4	5	5	16	7	8	11	7	13	8	7	4	–
Nonvoting	1	1	4	6	7	0	1	1	2	2	0	3	0	4	–
Total	5	27	8	11	12	16	8	9	13	9	13	11	7	8	–
i. Study chairman	No	Yes	Yes	Yes	Yes	Yes	Yes*	Yes	Yes	Yes*	Yes	Yes	Yes	Yes	13 Yes
ii. Vice-chairman	No	NA	NA	NA	NA	Yes	No	No	Yes	Yes*	NA	NA	Yes	Yes	5 Yes
iii. CC or data CC director	No	Yes	Yes	Yes	Yes	Yes	Yes*	Yes	Yes	Yes*	Yes	Yes	Yes	Yes	13 Yes
iv. Clinic directors	NA	Yes	No	Yes*	No	Yes*	No	No	Yes	No	No	No	Yes	Yes	6 Yes
v. Project officer	Yes	Yes	Yes	Yes	Yes	Yes	Yes	NA	Yes	Yes	Yes*	Yes	Yes	Yes	13 Yes
vi. Clinic coordinator	NA	No	No	No	No	No	No	No	No	No	Yes	No	No	No	0 Yes
vii. Nonhealth professional	No	No	No	Yes	No	No	No	No	Yes	No	No	No	No	No	2 Yes
viii. Lay representative	No	No	No	NA	No	No	No	No	Yes	No	No	No	No	No	1 Yes

Table B-4 Summary tabulations from sketches (*continued*)

Item	Acronym and Sketch no.														
	PHS	UGDP	VA43	MPS	NCGS	CDP	AMIS	PARIS	HDFP	MRFIT	CASS	POSCH	HPT	IRSC	Freq.
	1	*2*	*3*	*4*	*5*	*6*	*7*	*8*	*9*	*10*	*11*	*12*	*13*	*14*	
29. Treatment effects monitoring committee (cont'd)															
f. No. of members elected.........	0	0	0	0	0	0	0	0	0	0	0	0	0	0	--
g. Meetings per year................	2	2	2	2	2	2	2	2	2	2	2	3	2	2	--
30. Type of communications model															
Sponsor directive............	✓	✓	✓	✓	✓	✓	✓		✓	✓	✓				4
Sponsor nondirective........								✓				✓	✓	✓	10
31. Study publications															
a. No. of publications............	0	10	0	1	11	29	3	2	24	10	31	7	0	2	130
b. Method of authorship															
Papers with corporate format alone	0	8	0	1	0	29	1	2	6	2	0	0	0	2	51
Papers with conventional format alone	0	2	0	0	3	0	1	0	8	8	29	3	0	0	55
Papers with both formats	0	0	0	0	8	0	1	0	10	0	2	4	0	0	24

Table B-4 Summary tabulations from sketches (*continued*)

Item	Acronym and sketch no.														
	PHS	UGDP	VA43	MPS	NCGS	CDP	AMIS	PARIS	HDFP	MRFIT	CASS	POSCH	HPT	IRSC	Freq.
	1	2	3	4	5	6	7	8	9	10	11	12	13	14	
32. Author participation in trial															
None...........	✓						✓	✓		✓					4
Member of CC...........		✓				✓							✓		3
Member of trt. monitoring or advisory review committee			✓	✓	✓				✓		✓	✓		✓	7
33. Date sketch completed........	Mar 1983	April 1983	April 1983	May 1983	Mar 1983	April 1983	Mar 1983	Mar 1983	May 1983	May 1983	Mar 1983	May 1983	Mar 1983	Mar 1983	–

Notes for Table B-4

Item 5
- (VA 43) Technically, VA Cooperative studies are part of the VA intramural research program.

Item 9
- (CASS) Fourteen clinics participated in the registry component of the study. However, only 10 of the clinics randomized patients.

Item 10
- (IRSC) The structure involves separate data centers for the United States and European portions of the study. The two centers feed results to the study coordinating center located in Germany. The project office noted is for the United States portion of the study. The European portion has no corresponding office. The two reading centers are for X-ray determination of reflux grade and renal scarring. One center reads films generated by U.S. clinics and the other center reads films generated by the European clinics.

Item 11.c
- (NCGS) The data coordinating center receives its funding via a consortium award to the institution housing the study chairman.
- (PARIS) Coordinating center also responsible for dispersing funding to participating clinics.
- (POSCH) Coordinating center receives its funding via consortium award to the chairman of the study (also director of the Minnesota clinic).
- (HPT) Data coordinating center funds the central laboratory and food coding center of the HPT.
- (IRSC) Institution housing the coordinating center also houses a clinic in the study.

Item 19.d
- (IRSC) Grade IV reflux patients.

Item 20.b
- (POSCH) Cholesterol level and plasma lipoprotein type was used for stratification, in addition to clinic and level of coronary vessel disease.

Item 20.c and 20.d
- (IRSC) The two halves of the study used different stratification procedures. The number recorded is for the U.S. portion of the study. It used clinic (18), age (3 levels), sex, and renal scarring (2 levels), creating a potential for 216 allocation strata.

Item 20.h
- (IRSC) Method of release via phone for U.S. portion and via sealed envelope for European portion.

Item 21.a and 21.b
- (PHS) No clinic visits required (see abstract summary in Table B-2).

Item 21.b
- (NCGS) Visits at 1, 2, and 3 months after randomization for dosage adjustment and data collection and at 6, 9, 12, 16, 20, and 24 months after randomization for regular follow-up visits.
- (HDFP) Stepped care patients seen at least once every four months. Referred care patients seen at the end of 1, 2, 4, and 5 years of follow-up.
- (MRFIT) Participants assigned to special intervention visited the clinic on a regular basis for administration of the required interventions. All participants seen once per year for outcome assessment.

Item 23
- (MPS) Vision change using a standard visual acuity test.
- (NCGS) Gallstone dissolution.

- (HPT) Blood pressure change.
- (IRSC) Renal growth and scarring.

Item 26.a

- (MPS) Stated recruitment goals: 522 in SMD argon trial, 736 in HISTO argon trial, and 212 in SMD krypton trial. No goal set for INVM in the argon trial or for INVM or HISTO in the krypton trial.
- (IRSC) Goal for reflux grade IV patients. No goal set for grade III.

Item 26.c

- (MPS) The only trial with published results at the time the sketch was completed.

Item 28.d.iv

- (POSCH) The chairman of the study is the only clinic director represented.

Item 29.a

- (MRFIT) Originally the study had separate advisory-review and treatment effects monitoring committees. The latter committee was disbanded in 1977. Its functions were assumed by the advisory-review committee at that time.

Item 29.b and 29.c

- (CDP) The treatment effects monitoring committee was headed by co-chairmen. See items 29.b and 29.c for information on the two individuals.
- (PARIS) The treatment effects monitoring committee was headed by co-chairmen. See items 29.b and 29.c for information on the two individuals.

Item 29.e

- (MPS) The clinic director represented on the committee was also chairman of the study.
- (CDP) The only clinic director represented on the committee was also the vice-chairman of the study.
- (AMIS) The study chairman and director of the coordinating center attended meetings of the committee, but were not official members of the committee.
- (MRFIT) The chairman and vice-chairman of the study and the director of the coordinating center were present at meetings of the committee, but were not official members of the committee.
- (CASS) The project officer was present at meetings of the committee, but was not an official member of the committee.

Table B-5 Sample sketch for the UGDP

---

1. **General**
   a. *Official name:* University Group Diabetes Program
   b. *Official acronym:* UGDP
   c. *Sketch number:* 2
   d. *Type of trial:* Therapeutic
   e. *Type of design:* Fixed sample size design
   f. *Stage:* Completed

2. **Funding**
   a. *Source:* Public: National Institute of Arthritis, Metabolism and Digestive Diseases (now the National Institute of Arthritis, Diabetes, Digestive and Kidney Diseases), Bethesda, Maryland
   b. *Type:* Grant
   c. *Mode of initiation:* Investigator-initiated
   d. *Mode of fund dispersal to centers:* Direct
   e. *Start of funding:* September 1960
   f. *End of funding:* April 1982

3. **Clinics: 12 (including one in Puerto Rico)**

4. **Resource centers**
   a. *Types of centers represented*
      - Coordinating center
      - Reading center
      - Central laboratories (2)
   b. *Coordinating center*
      - *Study name:* Coordinating Center (Baltimore)
      - *Director:* Genell Knatterud, Ph.D. (Christian R. Klimt, M.D., Dr. P.H., through 1977)
      - *Affiliations with other centers:* None
      - *Address:* University of Maryland, School of Medicine, Baltimore, Maryland
   c. *Reading center*
      - *Study name:* ECG Reading Center
      - *Director:* Henry Blackburn, M.D. (Cardiology)
      - *Affiliations with other centers:* Lipid Laboratory and ECG Reading Center both under the direction of Henry Blackburn. There was a clinic at Minnesota as well, but it was organizationally and administratively independent of these two resource centers.
      - *Address:* University of Minnesota, School of Public Health, Minneapolis, Minnesota
   d. *Central Laboratory*
      - *Study name:* Lipid Laboratory (Minnesota)
      - *Director:* Henry Blackburn, M.D. (Cardiology)
      - *Affiliations with other centers:* Lipid Laboratory and ECG Reading Center both under the direction of Henry Blackburn. There was a clinic at Minnesota as well, but it was organizationally and administratively independent of the two resource centers.
      - *Address:* University of Minnesota, School of Public Health, Minneapolis, Minnesota
   e. *Central laboratory*
      - *Study name:* Lipid Laboratory (Morgantown)
      - *Director:* Margaret J. Albrink, M.D. (Medicine)
      - *Affiliations with other centers:* None
      - *Address:* West Virginia University Medical Center, Morgantown, West Virginia

5. **Project office**
      - *Study name:* Liaison Office
      - *Project Officer:* Keatha K. Krueger, Ph.D.

Table B-5   Sample sketch for the UGDP (*continued*)

- *Affiliations with other centers:* None
- *Address:* National Institute of Arthritis, Metabolism, and Digestive Diseases (now the National Institute of Arthritis, Diabetes, Digestive, and Kidney Diseases), Bethesda, Maryland

6. Treatments

a. *Type of treatment design:* Noncrossover

b. *Type of treatment structure:* Simple

c. *Test treatments*

   i. Number: 3

   ii. Mode of intervention: Drug

   iii. Treatment description: See abstract summary

d. *Control treatments*

   i. Number: 2

   ii. Type of treatment administered: Placebo pills or capsules, or standard dose of insulin via injections

   iii. Treatment description: See abstract summary

e. *Level of masking:* Oral hypoglycemic agents administered double-masked. Two insulin treatments administered in unmasked fashion.

7. Patient characteristics

a. *Eligibility criteria:* Adult-onset diabetes diagnosed within 12 months prior to enrollment.

b. *Demographic characteristics:* 20–79 years of age at entry. Mean age: 52.7, 71% female, 54% white.

8. Patient recruitment

a. *Mode of initial patient contact:* Direct from primary care clinics

b. *Start of patient enrollment:* February 1961

c. *End of patient enrollment:* February 1966

d. *Total number of patients randomized:* 1,027

9. Method of randomization

a. *Type:* Fixed allocation ratio

b. *Stratification variable:* Clinic

c. *Total number of allocation strata:* 12 (1 per clinic)

d. *Allocation ratio:* 1:0:1:1:1 for TOLB, PHEN, ISTD, IVAR, and PLBO, respectively, for 6 clinics not administering phenformin and for first 32 patients in the Boston clinic. Ratio of 1:3:1:1:1 was used in the 5 clinics using phenformin and after enrollment of the 32nd patient in the Boston clinic.

d. *Blocking constraints:* After every 16th allocation for the 1:0:1:1:1 allocation ratio and after every 14th allocation for the 1:3:1:1:1 allocation ratio.

f. *Locus of control:* Central

g. *Method of release:* Coordinating center, usually via telephone. By letter if time permitted.

10. Data collection schedule

a. *Baseline:* 2 examinations about 1 month apart

b. *Follow-up:* Examinations at 3-month intervals after enrollment

c. *Post-trial follow-up:* Some by individual clinics (see reference citation 2.10, Table B-3, for details)

11. Length of patient follow-up

a. *During the trial:* Minimum: 9.5 years. Maximum: 14.5 years.

b. *Post-trial:* 2 years. See comment for item 10.c.

12. Outcome

a. *Primary:* Death

b. *Secondary:* Nonfatal vascular complications, especially those affecting the eyes, heart, kidney, or peripheral vascular system.

13. Treatment effects monitoring

a. *Frequency:* Twice a year in conjunction with semiannual investigator meetings.

b. *Approach:* Data reports prepared by the coordinating center; reviewed by investigative group.

14. Method of close-out:

Common close-out date. Close-out examinations performed over a 3-month period, with separation completed by August 1975.

15. Data entry

a. *Site of entry:* At the coordinating center

b. *Primary mode of entry:* Direct from the data forms

16. Sample size specification

a. *Original recruitment goal:* 200 per treatment group

b. *Rationale for the original recruitment goal:* Pragmatic

c. *Achieved sample size:* 200+ per treatment group. Total of 1,027 patients assigned to the 5 treatment groups.

d. *Published rationale for achieved sample size:* Power argument as stated in reference citation 2.10, Table B-3.

17. Organizational structure

a. *Committees*

  i. *Key committees*

   • Steering Committee
   • Executive Committee
   • Advisory-Review Committee

  ii. *Standing subcommittees of the Steering Committee*

   • Analysis Coordination Committee
   • Eye Committee
   • Heart Committee
   • Kidney Committee
   • Medical Technology and Quality Control Committee
   • Mortality Committee
   • Peripheral Vascular and Neurological Committee
   • Statistical Committee
   • Clinic Review Committee
   • Editorial Review Committee

b. *Steering Committee*

  • *Name:* Investigative Group

  • *Chairman:* Max Miller, M.D., Case–Western Reserve University, Cleveland, Ohio

  • *Affiliations with other centers:* Director of one of the clinics in the trial.

  • *Number of members:* 26

  • *Membership representation:* 2 voting members from each of the 12 clinics and the coordinating center.

c. *Executive Committee*

  • *Name:* Executive Committee

  • *Chairman:* Max Miller, M.D., Case–Western Reserve University, Cleveland, Ohio

  • *Affiliations with other centers:* Director of one of the clinics in the trial.

  • *Number of members:* 9

  • *Membership representation:* Study chairman, director of the coordinating center, plus 2 other coordinating center representatives, plus 3 elected members from the study clinics (3-year terms), the project officer, and the chairman of the advisory-review committee.

d. *Advisory-Review Committee*

  • *Name:* Advisory-Review Board (appointed in 1971)

  • *Chairman:* Thomas Chalmers, M.D., Mount Sinai School of Medicine, New York, New York

  • *Affiliations with other centers:* None

  • *Number of members:* 9

  • *Membership representation:* Members appointed by the National Institute of Arthritis, Metabolism, and Digestive Diseases without term. Members included study chairman and director of the coordinating center. No other member had any affiliation with the trial.

Table B-5   Sample sketch for the UGDP (*continued*)

18. **Study publications**
    a. *Number of papers published:* 10 (See Table B–3)
    b. *General method of authorship:* Corporate, with writing committee indicated.

19. **Information sources used for completion of sketch**
    - Published papers
    - UGDP manual of operations

20. **Author's involvement in trial**
    - Deputy director of coordinating center from start of study to mid-1979

21. **Person reviewing sketch**
    - *Name:* Genell L. Knatterud, Ph.D.
    - *Position in study:* Director of Coordinating Center

22. **Date sketch completed**
    April 12, 1983

Table B-6 Data coordinating centers for multicenter trials referenced in this book

Study name and acronym	Data coordinating center director	Address
1. Anturane Reinfarction Trial (ART)	Sidney H. Kane, M.D.	Ciba-Geigy Corporation Pharmaceutical Division Summit, New Jersey 07901
2. Aspirin Myocardial Infarction Study (AMIS)	William F. Krol, Ph.D.	Maryland Medical Research Institute 600 Wyndhurst Avenue Baltimore, Maryland 21210
3. Beta Blocker Heart Attack Trial (BHAT)	C. Morton Hawkins, Sc.D.	School of Public Health University of Texas 1100 Holcombe Blvd. Houston, Texas 77025
4. Coronary Artery Surgery Study (CASS)	Lloyd D. Fisher, Ph.D.	School of Public Health University of Washington 1107 NE 45th Street Seattle, Washington 98105
5. Coronary Drug Project (CDP)	Paul L. Canner, Ph.D.	School of Medicine University of Maryland 600 Wyndhurst Avenue Baltimore, Maryland 21210
6. Diabetes Control and Complications Trial (DCCT)	John M. Lachin, Sc.D.	Department of Statistics The George Washington University 7979 Old Georgetown Road Bethesda, Maryland 20814
7. Diabetic Retinopathy Study (DRS)	Genell L. Knatterud, Ph.D.	School of Medicine University of Maryland 600 Wyndhurst Avenue Baltimore, Maryland 21210
8. Early Treatment of Diabetic Retinopathy Study (ETDRS)	Genell L. Knatterud, Ph.D.	School of Medicine University of Maryland 600 Wyndhurst Avenue Baltimore, Maryland 21210
9. Eastern Cooperative Oncology Group (ECOG)	Marvin Zelen, Ph.D.	School of Public Health Harvard University 44 Binney Street Boston, Massachusetts 02115
10. Hypertension Detection and Follow-Up Program (HDFP)	C. Morton Hawkins, Sc.D.	School of Public Health University of Texas 1100 Holcombe Blvd. Houston, Texas 77025
11. Hypertension Prevention Trial (HPT)	Curtis L. Meinert, Ph.D.	School of Hygiene and Public Health The Johns Hopkins University 615 North Wolfe Street Baltimore, Maryland 21205
12. International Mexilitene Placebo Antiarrhythmic Coronary Trial (IMPACT)	Jean-Pierre Boissel, M.D.	Dept. Unite de Pharmacologie Clinique Hopital Cardiologique B.P. Lyon Montchat 69394 Lyon Cedex 3 France
	Christian R. Klimt, M.D.	Maryland Medical Research Institute 600 Wyndhurst Avenue Baltimore, Maryland 21210

Table B-6   Data coordinating centers for multicenter trials referenced in this book (*continued*)

Study name and acronym	Data coordinating center director	Address
13. International Reflux Study in Children (IRSC)	Tytti Tamminen, M.D.	University Children's Hospital Hufelandstrabe 55 Essen, West Germany D-4300
	Robert Weiss, M.D.	Albert Einstein College of Medicine 1825 Eastchester Road New York, New York 10461
14. Lipid Research Clinics Coronary Primary Prevention Trial (LRC-CPPT)	O. Dale Williams, Ph.D.	School of Public Health University of North Carolina Chapel Hill, North Carolina 27514
15. Macular Photocoagulation Study (MPS)	Barbara S. Hawkins, M.Sc.	The Wilmer Ophthalmology Institute The Johns Hopkins University 550 North Broadway Baltimore, Maryland 21205
16. Multicenter Investigation for Limiting Infarction Size (MILIS)	W. Kenneth Poole, Ph.D.	Research Triangle Institute Research Triangle Park, North Carolina 27709
17. Multiple Risk Factor Intervention Trial (MRFIT)	Marcus O. Kjelsberg, Ph.D.	School of Public Health University of Minnesota Minneapolis, Minnesota 55455
18. National Cooperative Dialysis Study (NCDS)	Edmund G. Lowrie, M.D.	School of Public Health Harvard University 721 Huntington Avenue Boston, Massachusetts 02115
19. National Cooperative Gallstone Study (NCGS)	John M. Lachin, Sc.D.	Department of Statistics The George Washington University 7979 Old Georgetown Road Bethesda, Maryland 20814
20. Persantine Aspirin Reinfarction Study (PARIS)	Christian R. Klimt, M.D., Dr. P.H.	Maryland Medical Research Institute 600 Wyndhurst Avenue Baltimore, Md 21210
21. Physicians' Health Study (PHS)	Charles Hennekens, M.D.	Department of Medicine Harvard Medical School 55 Pond Avenue Boston, Massachusetts 02146
22. Program on the Surgical Control of Hyperlipidemia (POSCH)	John M. Long, Ed.D.	School of Medicine University of Minnesota Minneapolis, Minnesota 55455
23. University Group Diabetes Program (UGDP)	Genell L. Knatterud, Ph.D.	School of Medicine University of Maryland 600 Wyndhurst Avenue Baltimore, Maryland 21210
24. Veterans Administration Cooperative Studies Program No. 43 (VA 43)	Stephen F. Bingham, Ph.D.	Veterans Administration Medical Center Perry Point, Maryland 20801

C. Year 1980 clinical trial publications[1]

C.1 PAPERS REVIEWED (113)

1. Aktulga E, Altac M, Muftuoglu A, Ozyazgan Y, Pazarli H, Tuzun Y, Yalcin B, Yazici H, Yurdakul S: A double blind study of colchicine in Behcet's disease. *Haematologica* 65:399–402, 1980.

2. Alacron-Segovia D: Long-term treatment of symptomatic osteoarthritis with benoxaprofen. Double-blind comparison with aspirin and ibuprofen. *J Rheumatol* 7(suppl 6):89–99, 1980.

3. Antarkar DS, Vaidya AB, Doshi JC, Athavale AV, Vinchoo KS, Natekar MR, Tathed PS, Ramesh V, Kale N: A double-blind clinical trial of Arogya-wardhani—an Ayurvedic drug—in acute viral hepatitis. *Indian J Med Res* 72:588–593, 1980.

4. Australian Therapeutic Trial in Mild Hypertension Management Committee: Australian Therapeutic Trial in Mild Hypertension. *Lancet* 1:1261–1267, 1980.

5. Bain J, Rachlis V, Robert E, Khait Z: The combined use of oral medroxyprogesterone acetate and methyltestosterone in a male contraceptive trial programme. *Contraception* 21:365–379, 1980.

6. Banham SW, Moran F: A clinical trial of oxatomide in asthma. *Br J Clin Pract* 34:323–326, 1980.

7. Barlow JJ, Piver MS, Lele SB: High-dose methotrexate with "rescue" plus cyclophosphamide as initial chemotherapy in ovarian adenocarcinoma. A randomized trial with observations on the influence of C parvum immunotherapy. *Cancer* 46:1333–1338, 1980.

8. Blechman WJ: Crossover comparison of benoxaprofen and naproxen in osteoarthritis. *J Rheumatol* 7(suppl 6):116-124, 1980.

9. Bone GE, Pomajzl MJ: Prospective comparison of polytetrafluorethylene and bovine grafts for dialysis. *J Surg Res* 29:223–227, 1980.

10. Brewer C: Prevention of infection after abortion with a supervised single dose of oral doxycycline. *Br Med J* 281:780–781, 1980.

11. Brooks PM, Hill W, Geddes R: Diclofenac and ibuprofen in rheumatoid arthritis and osteoarthritis. *Med J Aust* 1:29–30, 1980.

12. Cardozo LD, Stanton SL, Robinson H, Hole D: Evaluation of flurbiprofen in detrusor instability. *Br Med J* 280:281–282, 1980.

13. Carmichael J, Bloomfield P, Crompton GK: Comparison of fenoterol and terbutaline administered by intermittent positive pressure breathing. *Br J Dis Chest* 74:268–272, 1980.

14. Cohen MM, Cheung G, Lyster DM: Prevention of aspirin-induced fecal blood loss in men with prostaglandin E_2. *Adv Prostaglandin Thromboxane Res* 8:1525–1528, 1980.

15. Collum LM, Benedict-Smith A, Hillary IB: Randomised double-blind trial of acyclovir and idoxuridine in dendritic corneal ulceration. *Br J Ophthalmol* 64:766–769, 1980.

16. Coope J: Blood pressure in the elderly. *J R Coll Gen Pract* (*Occas Pap*) 12:35–37, 1980.

17. Cooper SA, Precheur H, Rauch D, Rosenheck A, Ladov M, Engel J: Evaluation of oxycodone and acetaminophen in treatment of postoperative dental pain. *Oral Surg* 50:496–501, 1980.

18. Cooper SA, Reynolds DC, Kruger GO, Gottlieb S: An analgesic relative potency assay comparing zomepirac sodium and aspirin. *J Clin Pharmacol* 20:98–106, 1980.

19. Cross FS, Long MW, Banner AS, Snider DE, Jr: Rifampin-isoniazid therapy of alcoholic and nonalcoholic tuberculosis patients in a U.S. Public Health Service cooperative therapy trial. *Am Rev Respir Dis* 122:349–353, 1980.

---

1. Reprinted with permission of Elsevier Science Publishing Co., Inc., New York (from reference 321 in Appendix I). See Chapter 2.

20. D'Angelo LJ, Sokol RJ: Short- versus long-course prophylactic antibiotic treatment in cesarean section patients. *Obstet Gynecol* 55:583–586, 1980.

21. Davidson ED, Hersh T, Perkel MS, Moore C, Fajman WA: The effects of coherin on patients with idiopathic delayed gastric emptying. *Am J Gastroenterology* 74:419–422, 1980.

22. Davies J, Dixon AS, Steele CE: Tolmetin sodium and indomethacin in the treatment of osteoarthrosis of the hip: A double-blind crossover study. *Curr Med Res Opin* 7:115–120, 1980.

23. DeAndrade JR, Honig S, Ciccone WJ, Leffall L: Clinical comparison of zomepirac with pentazocine in the treatment of postoperative pain. *J Clin Pharmacol* 20:292–297, 1980.

24. Depew W, Boyer T, Omata M, Redeker A, Reynolds T: Double-blind controlled trial of prednisolone therapy in patients with severe acute alcoholic hepatitis and spontaneous encephalopathy. *Gastroenterology* 78:524–529, 1980.

25. Dyson AJ, Mackay AD: Two oral beta-adrenergic stimulant drugs, pirbuterol and salbutamol, in reversible airway obstruction. *Br J Dis Chest* 74:70–74, 1980.

26. Fairfax AJ, McNabb WR, Davies HJ, Spiro SG: Slow-release oral salbutamol and aminophylline in nocturnal asthma: Relation of overnight changes in lung function and plasma drug levels. *Thorax* 35:526–530, 1980.

27. Fiasse R, Hanin C, Lepot A, Descamps C, Lamy F, Dive C: Controlled trial of cimetidine in reflux esophagitis. *Dig Dis Sci* 25:750–755, 1980.

28. Forbes JA, White RW, White EH, Hughes MK: An evaluation of the analgesic efficacy of proquazone and aspirin in postoperative dental pain. *J Clin Pharmacol* 7:465–474, 1980.

29. Foster CS, Duncan J: Randomized clinical trial of topically administered cromolyn sodium for vernal keratoconjunctivitis. *Am J Ophthalmol* 90:175–181, 1980.

30. Gairola RL, Gupta PK, Pandley K: Antagonists of morphine-induced respiratory depression: A study in postoperative patients. *Anaesthesia* 35:17–21, 1980.

31. Groggins RC, Lenney W, Milner AD, Stokes GM: Efficacy of orally administered salbutamol and theophylline in pre-school children with asthma. *Arch Dis Child* 55:204–206, 1980.

32. Guinan ME, MacCalman J, Kern ER, Overall JC, Jr, Spruance SL: Topical ether and herpes simplex labialis. *JAMA* 243:1059–1061, 1980.

33. Henkin RE, Woodruff A, Chang W, Green AM: The effect of radiopharmaceutical incubation time on bone scan quality. *Radiology* 135:463–466, 1980.

34. Hill JF: Clinical comparison of the (polymacon) spin-cast hydrogel contact lens to the (polymacon) lathe-cut hydrogel lenses. *Am J Optom Physiol Opt* 57:523–527, 1980.

35. Hillas JL, Somerfield SD, Wilson JD, Aman MG: Azatadine maleate in perennial allergic rhinitis: Effects on clinical symptoms and choice reaction time. *Br J Clin Pharmacol* 10:573–577, 1980.

36. Hillson RM, Boyd E, Cunningham J: Prophylactic disopyramide: Its clinical effects related to plasma concentration in myocardial infarction. *J Int Med Res* 8:314–320, 1980.

37. Hortobagyi GN, Yap HY, Wiseman CL, Blumenschein GR, Buzdar AU, Legha SS, Gutterman JU, Hersh EM, Bodey GP: Chemoimmunotherapy for metastatic breast cancer with 5-fluorouracil, adriamycin, cyclophosphamide, methotrexate, L-asparaginase, corynebacterium parvum and pseudomonas vaccine. *Cancer Treat Rep* 64:157–159, 1980.

38. Hubay CA, Pearson OH, Marshall JS, Rhodes RS, DeBanne SM, Rosenblatt J, Mansour EG, Hermann RE, Jones JC, Flynn WJ, Eckert C, McGuire WL: Adjuvant chemotherapy, antiestrogen therapy and immunotherapy for stage II breast cancer: 45-month follow-up of a prospective, randomized clinical trial. *Cancer* 46(suppl 12):2805–2808, 1980.

39. Iles JD: Relief of postoperative pain by ibuprofen: A report of two studies. *Can J Surg* 23:288–290, 1980.

40. Jacobi GH, Altwein JE, Kurth KH, Basting R, Hohenfellner R: Treatment of advanced prostatic cancer with parenteral cyproterone acetate: A phase III randomized trial. *Br J Urol* 52:208–215, 1980.

41. Joos C, Kewitz H, Reinhold-Kourniati D: Effects of diuretics on plasma lipoproteins in healthy men. *Eur J Clin Pharmacol* 17:251–257, 1980.

42. Kayasseh L, Gyr K, Keller U, Stalder GA, Wall M: Somotostatin and cimetidine in peptic-ulcer hemorrhage: A randomised controlled trial. *Lancet* 1:844–846, 1980.

43. Khan AKA, Akhtar S, Mahtab H: Treatment of diabetes mellitus with Coccinia indica. *Br Med J* 28:1044, 1980.

44. Kim KK, Sirman A, Trainor FS, Lee BY: Anxiolytic efficacy and safety of ketazolam compared with diazepam and placebo. *Clin Ther* 3:9–14, 1980.

45. Kobayashi K, Nakaoka K, Tsuji H, Shohmori T: Effects of thyrotropin-releasing hormone in chronic schizophrenic patients. *Acta Med Okayama* 34:263–273, 1980.

46. Koyama H, Wada T, Takahashi Y, Nishizawa Y, Iwanaga T, Aoki Y, Terasawa T, Kosaki G, Kajita A, Wada A: Surgical adjuvant chemotherapy with mitomycin C and cyclophosphamide in Japanese patients with breast cancer. *Cancer* 46:2373–2379, 1980.

47. Lambert WG, Mullinger BM: Single-dose cefuroxime in the prophylaxis of abdominal wound sepsis. *Curr Med Res Opin* 6:404–406, 1980.

48. Lassus A: Systemic treatment of psoriasis with an oral retinoic acid derivative (Ro 10-9359). *Br J Dermatol* 102:195–202, 1980.

49. Lawrence CM, Millac P, Stout GS, Ward JW: The use of choline chloride in ataxic disorders. *J Neurol Neurosurg Psychiatry* 43:452–454, 1980.

50. Levitt NS, Vinik AI, Sive AA, Laff LJ, Phillips C: Synthetic luteinizing hormone-releasing hormone in impotent male diabetics: A double-blind cross-over trial. *S Afr Med J* 57:701–704, 1980.

51. Lutterodt A, Nattel S, McLeod PJ: Duration of antihypertensive effect of a single daily dose of hydrochlorothiazide. *Clin Pharmacol Ther* 27:324–327, 1980.

52. MacGregor AJ, Addy A: Value of penicillin in the prevention of pain, swelling and trismus following the removal of ectopic mandibular third molars. *Int J Oral Surg* 9:166–172, 1980.

53. Mackay AD: Amoxycillin versus ampicillin in treatment of exacerbations of chronic bronchitis. *Br J Dis Chest* 74:379–384, 1980.

54. Manyam NV, Hare TA, Katz L: Effect of isoniazid on cerebrospinal fluid and plasma gaba levels in Huntington's disease. *Life Sci* 26:1303–1308, 1980.

55. Marcial VA, Hanley JA, Chang C, Davis LW, Moscol JA: Split-course radiation therapy of carcinoma of the nasopharynx: Results of a national collaborative clinical trial of the Radiation Therapy Oncology Group. *Int J Radiat Oncol Biol Phys* 6:409–414, 1980.

56. Marks IN, Wright JP, Denyer M, Garisch JA, Lucke W: Comparison of sucralfate with cimetidine in the short-term treatment of chronic peptic ulcers. *S Afr Med J* 57:567–573, 1980.

57. Mendlewicz J, Linkowski P, Rees JA: A double-blind comparison of dothiepin and amitriptyline in patients with primary affective disorder: Serum levels and clinical response. *Br J Psychiatry* 136:154–160, 1980.

58. Merkatz IR, Peter JB, Barden TP: Ritodrine hydrochloride: A betamimetic agent for use in preterm labor: II. Evidence of efficacy. *Obstet Gynecol* 56:7–12, 1980.

59. Meyhoff HH, Hess J, Olesen KP: Pulmonary atelectasis following upper urinary tract surgery on patients in the 25° and 45° "jack-knife" position: A sequential analysis. *Scand J Urol Nephrol* 14:107–109, 1980.

60. Milman N, Scheibel J, Jessen O: Lysine prophylaxis in recurrent herpes simplex labialis: A double-blind, controlled crossover study. *Acta Derm Venereol* 60:85–87, 1980.

61. Mishra PC, Agarwal VK, Rahman H: Therapeutic trial of amitryptiline in the treatment of nocturnal enuresis—a controlled study. *Indian Pediatr* 17:279–285, 1980.

62. Moertel CG, Hanley JA, Johnson LA: Streptozocin alone compared with streptozocin plus fluorouracil in the treatment of advanced islet-cell carcinoma. *N Engl J Med* 303:1189–1194, 1980.

63. Mogg GA, Arabi Y, Youngs D, Johnson M, Bentley S, Burdon DW, Keighley MR: Therapeutic trials of antibiotic associated colitis. *Scand J Infec Dis Suppl* 22:41–45, 1980.

64. Moncloa F, Hwang IK, Muccilli AC: Multiclinic evaluation of the antihypertensive effect of a methyldopa, hydrochlorothiazine, and amiloride combination. *Clin Ther* 3:168–175, 1980.

65. Morisky DE, Levine DM, Green LW, Russell RP, Smith C, Benson P, Finlay J: The relative impact of health education for low- and high-risk patients with hypertension. *Prev Med* 9:550–558, 1980.

66. Muller-Lissner SA, Sonnenberg A, Eichenberger P, Blum AL: Ranitidine inhibits gastric acid and pepsin secretion following sham feeding. *Hepatogastroenterology* 27:377–380, 1980.

67. Munzenberg J, Tachibana S: Preliminary double-blind evaluation of a new, non-steroidal anti-inflammatory drug: proctacine. *Pharmatherapeutica* 2:279–284, 1980.

68. Mussche RA, Kluyskens P: Prognosis of primarily treated localized laryngeal carcinoma ameliorated through levamisole treatment: A randomized pilot study. *Oncology* 37:329–335, 1980.

69. Nanda RN, Arthur GP, Johnson RH, Lambie DG: Cimetidine in the prophylaxis of migraine. *Acta Neurol Scand* 62:90–95, 1980.

70. Norberg A, Norberg B, Parkhede U, Gippert H, Lundbeck K: Randomized double-blind study of prophylactic methenamine hippurate treatment of patients with indwelling catheters. *Eur J Clin Pharmacol* 18:497–500, 1980.

71. North JB, Penhall RK, Hanieh A, Hann CS, Challen RG, Frewin DB: Postoperative epilepsy: A double-blind trial of phenytoin after craniotomy. *Lancet* 1:384–386, 1980.

72. Paavonen J, Kousa M, Saikku P, Vartiainen E, Kanerva L, Lassus A: Treatment of nongonococcal urethritis with trimethoprim-sulphadiazine and with placebo. A double-blind partner-controlled study. *Br J Vener Dis* 56:101–104, 1980.

73. Pack AR, Thomson ME: Effects of topical and systemic folic acid supplementation on gingivitis in pregnancy. *J Clin Periodontol* 7:402–414, 1980.

74. Pegram V, Hyde P, Linton P: Chronic use of triazolam: The effects on the sleep patterns of insomniacs. *J Int Med Res* 8:224–231, 1980.

75. Petrie WM, McEvoy JP, Wilson WH, Ban TA, Guy W: Viloxazine in the treatment of depressive neurosis: A placebo and standard (imipramine) controlled clinical study. *Int Pharmacopsychiatry* 15:193–196, 1980.

76. Pettersson RF, Hellstrom PE, Penttinen K, Pyhala R, Tokola O, Vartio T, Visakorpi R: Evaluation of amantadine in the prophylaxis of influenza A(H1N1) virus infection: A controlled field trial among young adults and high-risk patients. *J Infect Dis* 142:377–383, 1980.

77. Prins D, Mandelkorn T, Cerf FA: Principal and differential effects of haloperidol and placebo treatments upon speech disfluencies in stutterers. *J Speech Hear Res* 23:614–629, 1980.

78. Reiling RB, Reiling WA Jr., Bernie WA, Huffer AB, Perkins NC, Elliott DW: Prospective controlled study of gastrointestinal stapled anastomoses. *Am J Surg* 139:147–152, 1980.

79. Ritchie JA, Truelove SC: Comparison of various treatments for irritable bowel syndrome. *Br Med J* 281:1317–1319, 1980.

80. Rivkin L, Rapaport M: Clinical evaluation of a new erythromycin solution for acne vulgaris. *Cutis* 25:552–555, 1980.

81. Rofman BA, Kulaga SF, Gabriel MA, Thiyagarajan B, Nancarrow JF, Abrams WB: Multiclinic evaluation of timolol in the treatment of mild-to-moderate essential hypertension. *Hypertension* 2:643–648, 1980.

82. Rosenthal AL: Clocortolone pivalate: A paired comparison clinical trial of a new topical steroid in eczema/atopic dermatitis. *Cutis* 25:96–98, 1980.

83. Rune SJ, Zachariassen A: Acute relief of epigastric pain by antacid in duodenal ulcer patients. *Scand J Gastroenterol* Suppl 15:41–45, 1980.

84. Ruoff GE, Andelman SY, Cannella JJ: Long-term safety zomepirac: A double-blind comparison with aspirin in patients with osteoarthritis. *J Clin Pharmacol* 20:377–384, 1980.

85. Santini A: The clinical assessment of the pulpotomy technique on teeth of various post-eruptive age groups: A four year assessment using standardized clinical methods (II). *Quintessence Int* 12:77–80, 1980.

86. Schroeder JS, Rosenthal S, Ginsburg R, Lamb I: Medical therapy of Prinzmetal's variant angina. *Chest* 78:231–233, 1980.

87. Scott DH, Arthur GR, Scott DB: Haemodynamic changes following buprenorphine and morphine. *Anaesthesia* 35(suppl 1): 957–961, 1980.

88. Seedat YK: Trial of atenolol and chlorthalidone for hypertension in black South Africans. *Br Med J* 281:1241–1243, 1980.

89. Simpson RJ, Tiplady B, Skegg DC: Event recording in a clinical trial of a new medicine. *Br Med J* 280:1133–1134, 1980.

90. Sleijfer DT, Mulder NH, DeVries-Hospers HG, Fidler V, Nieweg HO, Van Der Waaij D, Van Saene HK: Infection prevention in granulocytopenic patients by selective decontamination of the digestive tract. *Eur J Cancer* 16:859–869, 1980.

91. Smith JA, Skidmore AG, Forward AD, Clarke AM, Sutherland E: Prospective randomized, double-blind comparison of metronidazole and tobramycin with clindamycin and tobramycin in the treatment of intra-abdominal sepsis. *Ann Surg* 192:213–220, 1980.

92. Souka AR, Osman M, Sibaie F, Einen MA: Therapeutic value of indomethacin in threatened abortion. *Prostaglandins* 19:457–460, 1980.

93. Stuart RK, Braine HG, Lietman PS, Saral R, Fuller DJ: Carbenicillin-trimethoprim/sulfamethoxazole versus carbenicillin-gentamicin as empiric therapy of infection in granulocytopenic patients: A prospective, randomized, double-blind study. *Am J Med* 68:876–885, 1980.

94. Stunkard AJ, Craighead LW, O'Brien R: Controlled trial of behaviour therapy, pharmacotherapy, and their combination in the treatment of obesity. *Lancet* 2:1045–1047, 1980.

95. Svennevig JL, Bugge-Asperheim B, Bjorgo S, Kleppe H, Birkeland S: Methyl-prednisolone in the treatment of lung contusion following blunt chest trauma. *Scan J Thorac Cardiovasc Surg* 14:301–305, 1980.

96. Svensson G, Hegardt B, Lofkvist T: Effects of topical use of beta-adrenoceptor stimulants on nasal mucosa: Rhinomanometric evaluations in experiments with terbutaline and KWD 2131. *Acta Otolaryngol* 90:297–303, 1980.

97. Szmuness W, Stevens CE, Harley EJ, Zang EA, Oleszko WR, William DC, Sadovsky R, Morrison JM, Kellner A: Hepatitis B vaccine: Demonstration of efficacy in a controlled clinical trial in a high-risk population in the United States. *N Engl J Med* 303:833–841, 1980.

98. Theroux P, Waters DD, Debaisieux JC, Szlachcic J, Mizgala HF, Bourassa MG: Hemodynamic effects of calcium ion antagonists after acute myocardial infarction. *Clin Invest Med* 3:81–85, 1980.

99. Turkington RW: Depression masquerading as diabetic neuropathy. *JAMA* 243:1147–1150, 1980.

100. Vedin A, Wikstrand J, Wilhelmsson C, Wallentin I: Left ventricular function and beta-blockade in chronic ischaemic heart failure: Double-blind cross-over study of propranolol and penbutolol using non-invasive techniques. *Br Heart J* 44:101–107, 1980.

101. Velasco M, Guevara J, Morillo J, Ramirez A, Urbina-Quintana A, Hernandez-Pieretti O: Antihypertensive effect of atenolol alone or combined with chlorthalidone in patients with essential hypertension. *Br J Clin Pharmacol* 9:499–504, 1980.

102. Von Knorring L: A double-blind trial: Vivalan against placebo in depressed elderly patients. *J Int Med Res* 8:18–21, 1980.

103. Walinder J, Carlsson A, Persson R, Wallin L: Potentiation of the effect of antidepressant drugs by tryptophan. *Acta Psychiatr Scand Suppl* 61:243–249, 1980.

104. Washton AM, Resnick RB: Clonidine versus methadone for opiate detoxification: Double-blind out-patient trials. *Natl Inst Drug Abuse Res Monogr Ser* 34:89–94, 1980.

105. Weibel RE, Villarejos VM, Klein EB, Buynak EB, McLean AA, Hilleman MR: Clinical and laboratory studies of live attenuated RA 27/3 and HPV77-DE rubella virus vaccines (40931). *Proc Soc Exp Biol Med* 165:44–49, 1980.

106. White PF, Ham J, Way WL, Trevor AJ: Pharmacology of ketamine isomers in surgical patients. *Anesthesiology* 52:231–239, 1980.

107. Whittington J, Raftery EB: A controlled comparison of oxyfedrine, isosorbide dinitrate and placebo in the treatment of patients suffering attacks of angina pectoris. *Br J Clin Pharmacol* 10:211–215, 1980.

108. Williams KA, Ting A, French ME, Oliver D: Peroperative blood transfusions improve cadaveric renal-allograft survival in non-transfused recipients. *Lancet* 1:1104–1106, 1980.

109. Wilson EA: Diazepam and local anaesthetic spray versus general anaesthesia for gastroduodenoscopy. *S Afr Med J* 57:111–113, 1980.

110. Wilson WR, Byl FM, Laird N: The efficacy of steroids in the treatment of idiopathic sudden hearing loss: A double-blind clinical study. *Arch Otolaryngol* 106:772–776, 1980.

111. Wordsworth BP, Ebringer RW, Coggins E, Smith S: A double-blind crossover trial of fenoprofen and phenylbutazone in ankylosing spondylitis. *Rheumatol Rehabil* 19:260–263, 1980.

112. Zykov MP, Rudenko LG, Zoshchenkova NY, Rafael'Skaya TI: Subunit influenza vaccine and its testing in clinical immunology. *J Hyg Epidemiol Microbiol Immunol* 24:212–218, 1980.

113. (No author listed): The treatment of dyspepsia in general practice: A multicentre trial. *Practitioner* 224:105–107, 1980.

C.2 PAPERS EXCLUDED (67)

114. Adams FG, Horton PW, Selim SM: Clinical comparison of three liver scanning agents. *Eur J Nucl Med* 5:237–239, 1980.

115. Andreasen G: A clinical trial of alignment of teeth using a 0.019 inch thermal nitinol wire with a transition temperature range between 31° C. and 45° C. *Am J Orthod* 78:528–537, 1980.

116. Anturan: New use for an old drug. *Can Med Assoc J* 120:714–716, 1980.

117. Baker HW, Pepperell RJ: Lack of effect of bromocriptine on semen quality in men with normal or slightly elevated prolactin levels. *Aust NZ J Obstet Gynaecol* 20:158–161, 1980.

118. Banta HD, Thacker SB: More fetal monitoring debate (letter). *Pediatrics* 65:366–368, 1980.

119. Bedikian AY, Valdivieso M, Heilbrun LK, Withers RH, Bodey GP, Freireich EJ: Glycerol: An alternative to dexamethasone for patients receiving brain irradiation for metastatic disease. *South Med J* 73:1210–1214, 1980.

120. Beutler E, Dale GL, Kuhl W: Replacement therapy in Gaucher disease. *Birth Defects* 16:369–381, 1980.

121. Bicher HI, Sandhu TS, Hetzel FW: Hyperthermia and radiation in combination: A clinical fractionation regime. *Int J Radiat Oncol Biol Phys* 6:867–870, 1980.

122. Bird HA, Wright V, Galloway D: Clinical metrology—a future career grade? *Lancet* 2:138–140, 1980.

123. Borden EC, Hawkins MJ: Interferons for human neoplastic and viral diseases. *Compr Ther* 6:6–15, 1980.

124. Bruni J, Wilder BJ, Bauman AW, Willmore LJ: Clinical efficacy and long-term effects of valproic acid therapy on spike-and-wave discharges. *Neurology* 30:42–46, 1980.

125. Calne RY: Immunosuppression for organ grafting. *Transplant Proc* 12:239–243, 1980.

126. Cantell K: Interferon: The state of the art. *Triangle* 19:47–51, 1980.

127. Carter SK: Clinical chemotherapy: Its correlation with experimental models. *Recent Results Cancer Res* 75:31–36, 1980.

128. Chastang C, Auquier A, Gremy F: Prognostic knowledge: Interest and methods. *Bull Cancer* 67:430–436, 1980.

129. Chew CY, Brown BG, Singh BN, Hecht HS, Schnugg SJ, Wong M, Shah PM, Dodge HT: Mechanism of action of verapamil in ischemic heart disease: Observations on changes in systemic and coronary hemodynamics and coronary vasomobility. *Clin Invest Med* 3:151–158, 1980.

130. Conti CR: Management of stable and unstable angina with observations on lessons learned from the prospective controlled studies. *Adv Cardiol* 27:191–198, 1980.

131. Crowe JP, Phelan JJ, Cleere WF, Fottrell PF, McNicholl B, McCarthy CF: The lymphocyte transformation test in coeliac disease: Effect of gliadin and detoxified gliadin. *Digestion* 20:95–99, 1980.

132. Cunliffe WJ: Techniques in the investigation of acne. *Acta Derm Venereol Suppl* 89:39–46, 1980.

133. Davis TG, Pickett DL, Schlosser JH: Evaluation of a worldwide spontaneous reporting system with cimetidine. *JAMA* 243:1912–1914, 1980.

134. Donald JF, Rimmer DM: An open evaluation of a 3-day course of pivmecillinam (ten 200 mg tablets) in women with acute uncomplicated cystitis. *J Int Med Res* 8:112–117, 1980.

135. Emanueli A, Sacchetti G: An algorithm for the classification of untoward events in large scale clinical trials. *Agents Actions Suppl* 7:318–322, 1980.

136. Epstein M: Sounding boards. The LeVeen shunt for ascites and hepatorenal syndrome. *N Engl J Med* 302:628–630, 1980.

137. Fink M, Irwin P: EEG and behavioral profile of flutroline (CP-36, 584): A novel antipsychotic drug. *Psychopharmacology* 72:67–71, 1980.

138. Freeman H, Soni SD: Oxypertine for tardive dyskinesia (letter). *Br J Psychiatry* 136:522–523, 1980.

139. Friedman LM: Summary of design features: Clinical trials of platelet-active drugs in cerebrovascular disease. *Circulation* 62 (suppl V): V-88—V-89, 1980.

140. Furberg CD: Principles of clinical trials: U.S. viewpoint. *Triangle* 19:99–102, 1980.

141. George SL: Sequential clinical trials in cancer research. *Cancer Treat Rep* 64:393–397, 1980.

142. Gonzalez ER: Study to begin on whether aspirin can delay senile cataract formation. *JAMA* 244:2593–2594, 1980.

143. Gross F: Medical, ethical and legal aspects of clinical trials in pediatrics. Summary of a forum discussion held at the International Workshop on Perinatal and Pediatric Aspects of Clinical Pharmacology, Heidelberg, Federal Republic of Germany, February 27–29, 1980. *Eur J Clin Pharmacol* 18:121–127, 1980.

144. Hansen M, Hansen HH, Dombernowsky P: Long-term survival in small cell carcinoma of the lung. *JAMA* 244:247–250, 1980.

145. Herting RL, Lane AZ, Lorber RR, Wright JJ: Netilmicin: Chemical development and overview of clinical research. *Scand J Infec Dis Suppl* 23:20–29, 1980.

146. Hildebrand H, Berg NO, Hoevels J, Ursing B: Treatment of Crohn's Disease with metronidazole in childhood and adolescence: Evaluation of a six months trial. *Gastroenterol Clin Biol* 4:19–25, 1980.

147. Holt JA: Microwave adjuvant to radiotherapy and chemotherapy for advanced lymphoma (letter). *Med J Aust* 2:159–160, 1980.

148. Jerie P: Clinical experience with guanfacine in long-term treatment of hypertension. *Br J Clin Pharmacol* Suppl 10:37S–47S, 1980.

149. Lazzara R, Scherlag B: Treatment of arrhythmias by blocking slow current. *Ann Inter Med* 93:919–921, 1980.

150. Lewison EF: Changing concepts in breast cancer. *Cancer* 46(suppl 4):859–864, 1980.

151. Lorenz W, Fischer M, Rohde H, Triodl H, Reimann HJ, Ohmann C: Histamine and stress ulcer: New components in organizing a sequential trial on cimetidine prophylaxis in seriously ill patients and definition of a special group at risk (severe polytrauma). *Klin Wochenschr* 58:653–665, 1980.

152. Marcus P. Clinical trial or promotional exercise? (letter). *Lancet* 1:827, 1980.

153. McConkey B, Amos RS, Billingham ME, Constable TJ, Crockson RA, Crockson AP, Forster PJ: Rheumatoid arthritis: Effects of a new agent (ICI 55 897) on serum acute phase proteins and the erythrocyte sedimentation rate. *Ann Rheum Dis* 39:18–21, 1980.

154. Measham AR, Khan AR, Huber DH: Dizziness associated with discontinuation of oral contraceptives in Bangladesh. *Int J Gynaecol Obstet* 18:109–112, 1980.

155. Menken MM: Evaluation of surgical therapy (letter). *N Engl J Med* 303: 399, 1980.

156. Meyer BH, Hugo JM: Etomidate as anaesthetic induction agent in open-heart surgery. *S Afr Med J* 58:759–761, 1980.

157. Muser RK: Design of clinical trials for new drugs in animals. *J Am Vet Med Assoc* 176:1148–1150, 1980.

158. Norton A: Psychosurgery—why not ban it? *J R Soc Med* 73:526–528, 1980.

159. Oswald I: Sleep studies in clinical pharmacology. *Br J Clin Pharmacol* 10:317–326, 1980.

160. Owen M, Hills LJ: How safe is dextropropoxyphene? (letter). *Med J Aust* 1:617–618, 1980.

161. Pavelka K, Vojtisek O, Kankova D: The occurrence of adverse side-effects during controlled clinical trials of nonsteroidal antirheumatic agents. *Rheumatol Rehabil* 19:109–112, 1980.

162. Pethybridge RJ: Data Analysis: I. Some statistical tests for small related samples. *J R Nav Med Serv* 66:135–139, 1980.

163. Piver MS, Barlow JJ, Dunbar J: Doxorubicin, cyclophosphamide, and 5-fluorouracil in patients with carcinoma of the cervix or vagina. *Cancer Treat Rep* 64:549–551, 1980.

164. Poster DS, Penta J, Marsoni S, Bruno S, Macdonald JS: Bis-diketopiperazine derivatives in clinical oncology: ICRF-159. *Cancer Clin Trials* 3:315–320, 1980.

165. Redaksie VD: Sulphinpyrazone in the prevention of cardiac death after myocardial infarction (editorial). *S Afr Med J* 57:301–302, 1980.

166. Relman AS: Sulfinpyrazone after myocardial infarction: No decision yet (editorial). *N Engl J Med* 303:1476–1477, 1980.

167. Sauerbruch T, Kaess H: The Anturane Reinfarction Trial (letter). *N Engl J Med* 303:49–50, 1980.

168. Schultz RM: Less empirical interferon trials in cancer (letter). *Lancet* 2:1362, 1980.

169. Sebille A, Hugelin A: Muscle reinnervation enhanced by isaxonine in man. *Br J Clin Pharmacol* 9:275–276, 1980.

170. Sklaroff RB, Yagoda A: Methotrexate in the treatment of penile carcinoma. *Cancer* 45:214–216, 1980.

171. Spiers AS, Kasimis BS, Janis MG: High-dose intravenous infusions of 5-fluorouracil for refractory solid tumours—the HI-FU regimen. *Clin Oncol* 6:63–69, 1980.

172. Svedmyr N: General aspects on evaluation of drug effects on cough and expectoration. *Eur J Respir Dis* 110(suppl 61):81–92, 1980.

173. Van Durme JP: Evaluation of the antiarrhythmic efficacy of mexiletine in patients with chronic ventricular arrhythmias. *Acta Cardiol Suppl* 25:121–125, 1980.

174. Verstraete M: Registry of prospective clinical trials: Fourth report. *Thromb Haemost* 43:176–181, 1980.

175. Vietti TJ: Evaluation of toxicity: Clinical issues. *Cancer Treat Rep* 64:457–461, 1980.

176. (no author listed): Ethical and legal considerations associated with clinical field trials: Discussion. *J Dent Res* 59(special Issue C): 1267–1270, 1980.

177. (no author listed): Experimental evaluation of antitumor drugs in the USA and USSR and clinical correlations: *Natl Cancer Inst Monogr* 55:1–179, 1980.

178. (no author listed): Radial keratotomy—an operation for myopia. *Med Lett Drugs Ther* 22:97–98, 1980.

179. (no author listed): Small cell carcinoma of the bronchus—real progress is hard to come by (editorial). *Lancet* 1:77–78, 1980.

180. (no author listed): Trifluridine (Viroptic) for herpetic keratitis. *Med Lett Drugs Ther* 22:46–48, 1980.

D. Activities by stage of trial

This appendix lists the activities and functions required for each stage of a trial. The stages are (see Chapter 3):

I.   Initial design stage
II. Protocol development stage
III. Patient recruitment stage
IV. Treatment and follow-up stage
V.   Patient close-out stage
VI. Termination stage
VII. Post-trial follow-up stage (optional)

The time at which certain activities are started will vary from trial to trial. This should be recognized if this outline is used as a management tool in planning activities for a specific trial. Activities listed in one stage in this schedule may not begin until the following stage in an actual trial.

I. INITIAL DESIGN STAGE

A. Design specifications

Specify the initial design features concerning:

1. Purpose and rationale of trial
2. Number and type of test treatments
3. Number and type of control treatments
4. Level and method of masking
5. Primary and secondary outcomes
6. Type and frequency of observations
7. Required number of patients based on a sample size calculation for a specified outcome, type I and II error, length of follow-up, and projected treatment differences to be detected
8. Estimate of number of clinical centers required based on the sample size calculation
9. Number and type of other centers, e.g., coordinating center(s), central laboratory, and reading center(s)
10. Patient eligibility and exclusion criteria

11. Population(s) from which patients are to be selected
12. Stratification varibles to be used in randomization
13. Patient safeguard procedures
14. Projected timetable for the trial
15. Approach to patient close-out, i.e., fixed closing date versus fixed follow-up interval

B. Organizational structure

1. Develop general guidelines concerning:

   a. Desired qualities of the study chairman and members of the steering, advisory-review, and treatment effects monitoring committees
   b. Terms of office of study chairman and members of key committees
   c. Method of selection of study chairman and members of key committees
   d. Voting rules for key committees

2. Outline responsibilities of the steering, advisory-review, and treatment effects monitoring committees
3. Establish key elements of overall organizational structure of the trial
4. Outline meeting schedule for key committees
5. Specify functions/duties of the co-ordinating center(s)
6. Outline general plans for paper writing and authorship procedures

C. Patient recruitment, treatment, and data collection procedures

1. Develop methods for patient recruitment and procedures for randomization

2. Outline data collection procedures

3. Develop a timetable for testing and finalization of data collection forms

4. Determine specifications for drugs to be evaluated, including methods for bottling, labeling, and distributing drugs (if a drug trial)

5. Outline main elements of the treatment protocol

D. Data processing and analysis

1. Outline data processing and database management procedures

2. Develop a timetable for implementation of database management procedures

3. Outline general data analysis plans

4. Outline plans for quality control of data collection and processing activities

E. Other activities

1. Perform literature review to identify pertinent background information on the study treatment, including review of safety and efficacy data

2. Prepare and submit funding proposal

3. Submit research plan and draft consent statement to local institutional review boards (IRBs) for preliminary approvals

II. PROTOCOL DEVELOPMENT STAGE

A. Patient recruitment and care

1. Identify source of patients

2. Write treatment protocol

3. Determine recruitment goals for individual clinics

4. Develop detailed patient eligibility and exclusion criteria

5. Establish permissible time windows for prerandomization and follow-up examinations

6. Establish protocol for management of clinical conditions

known or suspected to be related to the disease or therapy under study

7. Establish procedures for monitoring the clinical management of individual patients

8. Develop patient information and consent procedures

9. Generate the treatment allocation schedule and write description of the methods used to generate the schedule

10. Develop publicity schemes needed to facilitate patient recruitment

B. Data processing and analysis

1. Develop procedures for data interface between clinics and the data center

2. Specify contents of data collection forms

3. Draft and test data collection forms

4. Submit forms to appropriate study body for review and approval

5. Develop data management systems, including data collection, processing, editing, and correction procedures

6. Initiate development of data system and test computer programs required for:
   a. Verifying patient eligibility
   b. Issuing treatment allocations
   c. Keying, inventorying, editing, and updating study data

7. Write study handbook and manual of operations. Include sections on:
   a. Informed consent procedures and methods for safeguarding patient rights
   b. Recruitment and randomization procedures
   c. Patient follow-up procedures
   d. Procedures for data collection and processing
   e. Study organizational structure

8. Outline procedures for monitoring the randomization process

9. Review data storage, backup, and security procedures

C. Training and communication

1. Develop and implement training and certification procedures for key study staff, especially staff at the clinical centers responsible for data collection
2. Acquaint staff of all participating centers with the following:
   a. Design and methods of the trial
   b. Importance of integrity in data collection
   c. Need for data security
   d. Study organization
   e. Performance and treatment monitoring procedures to be employed
3. Initiate regularly scheduled meetings of:
   a. Study investigative group
   b. Steering committee
   c. Other study committees
4. Consider distribution of newsletters at periodic intervals to inform staff of participating centers of study progress and procedural changes
5. Develop study address directory and procedures for maintaining same
6. Outline communication channels and ground rules for center-to-center communication
7. Identify center(s) responsible for coordinating study communications
8. Develop and initiate clinic site visiting procedures in order to:
   a. Identify and correct problems in patient recruitment
   b. Review administration of study procedures
   c. Identify and correct possible deficiencies in data collection methods
9. Develop procedures for dealing with requests for study information originating outside the study

D. Quality assurance

1. Develop procedures for monitoring and reviewing performance of participating centers in the trial
2. Outline content of performance monitoring reports concerning data collection and data quality
3. Mock up data tables needed for performance monitoring
4. Develop documentation procedures for:
   a. Treatment allocation
   b. Reporting primary and secondary outcomes
   c. Classification of primary outcome
   d. Modification of data collection instruments and procedures
   e. Data management and forms revision
   f. Informed consent
   g. Modifications of study handbooks and manuals of operations
5. Specify mechanisms for monitoring adequacy of documentation

E. Treatment monitoring

1. Outline content of treatment effects monitoring reports
2. Establish timetable for treatment monitoring and generation of treatment monitoring reports

F. Authorship

1. Establish authorship policies for study papers and for ancillary studies
2. Establish review procedures for study papers
3. Establish methods for review and approval of presentations made by members of the investigative group on behalf of the study

G. Management

1. Outline study policy concerning:
   a. Informed consent, including minimum standards for the

consent process and mechanisms to be used to monitor clinics for adherence to those standards

  b. Responsibilities for patient care

  c. Data security, including specification of mechanisms to be used to protect computer data files against loss or destruction

  d. Access to study data by investigators in the study; by people outside the study

  e. Rights of patients to privacy and confidentiality

  f. Collection and storage of study records

  g. Review and approval of ancillary studies performed by study investigators

  h. Communications with persons outside the study, including the news media, regarding study design and results

  i. National and local publicity

  j. Dissemination of study results to study patients; to study staff

  k. Acquisition of liability insurance for participating centers and investigators

  l. Nature and extent of follow-up of dropouts

2. Develop guidelines and procedures required to:

  a. Decide when to terminate a treatment because of adverse or beneficial effects

  b. Modify the general design specifications of the trial

3. Create treatment effects monitoring committee or some other body to monitor for treatment effects

4. Establish system for making work priority assignments for the data center and other resource centers in the trial

5. Designate the group responsible for dissemination of study information and results to the lay and scientific communities

6. Develop safeguards to protect against premature disclosure of study results to parties outside the study

H. Other activities

1. Develop projected budget and staffing requirements for the trial

2. Order study drugs and initiate packaging, labeling, and distribution procedures (if a drug trial)

3. Recruit staff at participating centers

4. Develop informational brochures, official study name, logo, etc.

5. Obtain Investigational New Drug Application (INDA) if required by the Food and Drug Administration (FDA)

6. Negotiate specialized contracts or agreements, such as study liability insurance, equipment contracts, etc.

7. Designate official repository for study documents, i.e., minutes of meetings, performance and treatment effects monitoring reports, completed data collection forms, etc.

8. Print and distribute essential materials, such as recruitment materials, forms, study handbooks and other manuals

9. Create necessary committees, beginning with the steering committee

10. Review and refine general design specifications

11. Evaluate preparedness of all centers to initiate patient recruitment and follow-up

III. PATIENT RECRUITMENT STAGE

A. Treatment and patient care

1. Establish liaison with appropriate medical and lay societies to facilitate patient recruitment

2. Establish channels for patient referral

3. Initiate local and national publicity campaigns for patient recruitment when appropriate

4. Inform local referring physicians of aims of study and of limits of study responsibility regarding patient care

5. Provide clinical centers with patient information brochures

6. Review progress in patient recruitment

7. Project time requirements for completion of patient recruitment based on recruitment performance

8. Establish date for termination of patient recruitment and inform patient referral sources of date

B. Data processing and analysis

1. Implement procedures for monitoring the treatment allocation process

2. Initiate and maintain procedures for collecting and processing study data and related materials (e.g., ECGs and fundus photographs)

3. Verify that incoming baseline data forms document patient eligibility for the trial

4. Initiate data editing procedures to provide checks for accuracy and consistency within and across forms

5. Establish and maintain monitoring procedures to identify deficiencies in data collection and data processing

6. Establish procedures to be followed in maintaining adherence to the examination schedule

7. Define responsibilities of clinical centers and of data center for locating patients lost to follow-up

8. Define responsibility of clinical centers in maintaining contact with dropouts

9. Review data storage, backup, security, and integrity procedures in all participating centers

10. Identify topics for analysis and methods to be used for analysis

11. Outline quality control procedures for data analyses

12. Complete final editing of recruitment and entry data

C. Training and communication

1. Maintain training and certification procedures for staff of participating centers

2. Continue site visits to participating centers

3. Initiate regular meetings of the treatment effects monitoring committee

4. Continue to hold regularly scheduled meetings of:
   a. Study investigative group
   b. Steering committee
   c. Other study committees

5. Initiate, if appropriate, preparation of a newsletter to inform staff of study progress and procedural changes

6. Consider central preparation and local distribution of newsletter for study patients

7. Update and distribute study address directory at periodic intervals

D. Quality assurance

1. Initiate external monitoring and review procedures for all centers in the trial, e.g., clinical centers, data center, central laboratory, reading centers, etc.

2. Review adequacy of the randomization procedure

3. Prepare periodic reports summarizing performance of clinical centers with regard to patient recruitment

4. Prepare reports summarizing:
   a. Adherence to study protocol
   b. Adherence to data collection and patient examination schedule
   c. Data quality

d. Data collection activities at clinical centers
e. Data processing activities at the data center
f. Activities at other resource centers

5. Review documentation standards and monitor adequacy of documentation for:

a. Treatment allocation procedures
b. Reporting of major events
c. Classification of cause of death or other major events
d. Informed consent procedures
e. Modification of data collection forms
f. Modification of study protocol
g. Data management and data analysis procedures

E. Treatment monitoring

1. Develop analytic techniques and computer programs needed to monitor study data for evidence of adverse or beneficial treatment effects
2. Begin generating treatment monitoring reports

F. Authorship and publications

1. Establish paper writing teams and schedules
2. Review and, if necessary, revise guidelines for authorship
3. Write paper(s) on design and methods of the study
4. Establish procedures for distribution of published papers to the study group
5. Distribute at periodic intervals updated listings of study publications and presentations to all participating investigators

G. Management

1. Review and, if necessary, revise:

a. Informed consent procedures
b. Guidelines on patient care
c. Guidelines on study publicity

d. Guidelines on data access, security, backup, and storage

2. Continue to review and assign priorities to activities carried out by the data center and other key resource centers in the trial
3. Initiate periodic review of study committee structure; dissolve nonfunctional committees
4. Develop patient close-out strategy

H. Other activities

1. Print and distribute data collection forms and related materials needed for follow-up examinations
2. Initiate reporting procedures with FDA (if trial involves INDA)
3. Establish a central resource of data slides on study design and findings for use by study investigators in making presentations concerning the trial
4. Implement procedures for documenting important events in the trial that may effect data quality

IV. TREATMENT AND FOLLOW-UP STAGE

A. Treatment and patient care

1. Monitor and report adverse treatment effects
2. Review procedures for monitoring and evaluating the clinical management of individual patients

B. Data processing and analysis

1. Continue procedures for maintaining adherence to follow-up visit schedule, including special procedures for patients classifed as inactive or lost to follow-up
2. Review and expand data edit procedures to provide checks for consistency within and across forms, including forms used for prerandomization visits
3. Review and expand, if necessary, monitoring procedures to iden-

tify deficiencies in data collection and processing

4. Initiate central coding procedures, if required, for cause of death or other primary outcome variables

5. Revise data collection forms as necessary

6. Reproduce and distribute data collection forms as needed

7. Develop and test data collection forms and data management systems required for patient close-out stage

8. Prepare to process data collected at close-out visit(s)

9. Revise data management procedures as appropriate

10. Monitor patient adherence to assigned treatment

C. **Training and communications**

1. Continue site visits to participating centers to:
   a. Review administration of study procedures
   b. Identify and correct the problems in data collection and processing

2. Continue to hold regularly scheduled meetings of:
   a. Study investigative group
   b. Steering committee
   c. Treatment effects monitoring committee
   d. Other study committees

3. Continue to publish newsletter (if initiated):
   a. To inform study investigators of study progress and procedural changes
   b. To inform study patients of study progress

4. Continue (modify if necessary) certification procedures for staff of participating centers

5. Update and distribute revised study handbooks and manuals of operations

6. Continue to update and distribute study address directory, mailing

labels, forms (when necessary), etc.

7. Communicate with personnel of all participating centers concerning timetable and procedures for close-out stage, especially in the use of new data collection forms or techniques

D. **Quality assurance**

1. Review and revise study quality assurance procedures as appropriate

2. Continue to prepare monitoring reports summarizing:
   a. Adherence to study protocol
   b. Adherence to data collection and examination schedule
   c. Quality of data generated
   d. Data collection activities at clinical centers
   e. Data processing activities at the data center

3. Continue periodic review of adequacy of documentation for:
   a. Reporting of primary and secondary outcomes
   b. Classification of causes of death or other major outcomes
   c. Modification of data collection forms
   d. Modification of study protocol
   e. Ongoing data management procedures

E. **Treatment monitoring**

1. Revise data analysis and reporting procedures required to monitor study results for evidence of adverse or beneficial treatment effects

2. Initiate procedures for review and implementation of protocol modifications recommended by the treatment effects monitoring committee

F. **Authorship and publications**

1. Paper writing activities:
   a. Establish and activate writing teams

b. Develop papers on study findings

c. Develop papers on natural history and ancillary studies

2. Draft paper containing main study conclusions

3. Prepare stand-by press release for use in the event study findings appear in the news media prior to publication in a scientific journal

4. Continue procedures for distribution of published papers to study investigators

5. Update and distribute listing of study publications to study investigators

G. Management

1. Review and, if necessary, revise study guidelines concerning:

a. Patient care

b. Inquiries from outside the study regarding study design or study results

c. Rights of access to study data

d. Informed consent procedures

e. Information sources to be used in classification of major events

2. In the event of a major protocol change or in preparation for close-out discuss and establish procedures for:

a. Informing patients of close-out

b. Informing referring physicians of close-out

c. Developing special data collection forms for close-out

d. Developing special patient consent forms for post-trial follow-up (if planned)

3. Develop detailed patient close-out procedures

4. Establish timetable for close-out activities, including timetable for termination of funding for data collection at participating clinical centers

5. Recommend procedures to be followed at clinical centers in termination of patient follow-up

6. Prepare special informational material to be dispensed to patients at the close-out examination

7. Develop plan to monitor for possible adverse effects associated with treatment in the close-out stage

8. Review data storage, backup, security, and integrity procedures

9. Review and revise organizational structure of the trial

10. Continue making priority assignments for data analysis activities

H. Other activities

1. Continue procedures for distribution of study drugs during the follow-up phase

2. Continue FDA reporting procedures (if trial involves INDA)

3. Reproduce and distribute data collection forms to be used during close-out stage

4. Review timetable for remainder of study and prepare request for additional funding (if necessary)

5. Update central repository of data slides for use by study investigators in making study presentations

V. PATIENT CLOSE-OUT STAGE

A. Treatment and patient care

1. Initiate procedures for unmasking treatment assignments, when masking is involved

2. Monitor for adverse effects due to treatment termination (if appropriate)

3. Inform the study investigators of study results and their implications for patient care

4. Formulate treatment recommendations to be made to patients on close-out

5. Inform patients of study results and recommended future treatment

6. Inform patients' primary care physicians of study results

7. Update patient identifying information to facilitate post-trial follow-up

8. Inform patients of plans for post-trial follow-up (if any) and of methods to be used to maintain contact with them after termination of regular follow-up

9. Request data center to prepare summaries of accumulated follow-up data needed by clinic personnel when reviewing care needs of individual patients and for facilitating transfer of pertinent data to primary care physicians

10. Effect transfer of patient care responsibilities to appropriate sources

11. Document that all active patients have been informed of study results

B. Data processing and analysis

1. Perform final edit of accumulated study data. Identify items that need review or corrections

2. Initiate special search procedures to locate patients classified as lost to follow-up for final data analysis

3. Develop and carry out data analyses that summarize study findings, including results from the close-out process

C. Quality assurance

1. Prepare final reports summarizing:
   a. Adherence to study protocol
   b. Adherence to data collection and examination schedule
   c. Quality of data generated
   d. Performance of all participating

D. Treatment monitoring

1. Prepare final report on treatment effects

2. Hold final meeting of treatment effects monitoring committee

3. Monitor close-out process to ensure adherence to indicated procedures for separation of patients from the trial

E. Authorship and publications

1. Write and submit for publication paper(s) summarizing study results

2. Supply advance copy of paper(s) on results to participating clinics for distribution to staff and referring physicians

3. Establish coordinated approach to dissemination of information to the medical public in conjunction with publication of study results, including press releases, if needed

4. Develop paper writing and analysis plans for termination stage of study, including procedures for review of papers prepared in that stage

5. Develop mechanism for support of travel and work of writing teams and leadership committees during termination stage

6. Develop mechanism for distribution of papers published during termination stage

7. Update and distribute list of publications to study investigators

F. Management

1. Develop plans and policies for:
   a. Disposition of equipment purchased with study funds
   b. Disposition of unused study drugs and other supplies
   c. Disposition of centrally stored study materials, such as frozen serum specimens, ECGs, fundus photographs
   d. Disposition of patient medical records and materials accumulated at clinical centers in a manner consistent with local statutes

e. Final disposition of study data on completion of the termination stage

2. Review study organizational structure and propose revisions for termination stage

3. Review timetable for termination stage and develop plans for additional funding (if necessary)

4. Develop plans for disengaging study investigators and related staff from the trial

G. Other activities

1. Update central repository of data slides for use by study investigators in making presentations of study findings

2. Update and distribute address directory

VI. TERMINATION STAGE

A. Treatment and patient care

1. Verify that all clinics have complied with close-out procedures (e.g., verify that all patients have been informed of study results, have been taken off their assigned treatment, and have had care responsibilities transferred)

2. Review and revise, if necessary, conclusions of the study after completion of final data analysis

B. Data processing and analysis

1. Complete final edit procedures and create final data file

2. Prepare data listings or data tapes (disks) needed by writing teams

3. Update backup tapes and repository listings of data files

C. Authorship and publications

1. Implement plans for support of travel and work of writing teams and leadership committees remaining in operation in termination stage

2. Implement plan for authorship and review of manuscripts prepared during termination stage

3. Distribute copies of finished papers to study investigators

4. Distribute updated list of study publications to participating investigators

D. Management

1. Establish policy on type and amount of data to be made available outside the study structure during and after the termination stage

2. Establish approach for dealing with inquiries regarding the study and the study results

3. Establish study stewardship body after termination of the trial

E. Repository

1. Establish a suitable repository for all study materials to be retained beyond the termination stage, such as:

   a. Patient medical records
   b. Completed data forms
   c. Associated records, such as ECGs and fundus photographs
   d. Serum samples, biopsy slides, etc.

2. Establish a central repository for patient identifying and locator information

3. Store computer data files and backup copies

F. Other activities

1. Dispose of unused study drugs (if any)

2. Complete phase-out of study personnel

3. Dissolve all remaining study committees, except for stewardship committee

4. Submit final report to FDA (if trial involved INDA)

5. Inform IRB of completion of study

6. Prepare final version of data slides for use by study investigators in presenting results of the trial

7. Maintain communications with participating investigators

VII. POST-TRIAL FOLLOW-UP STAGE (optional)

A. Preparatory steps

1. Re-establish contact with clinics to:
   a. Inform them of the proposed follow-up
   b. Update address directory
   c. Address special procedural and ethical questions posed by the follow-up

2. Assemble roster of patients to be followed

3. Outline approach to be used in the follow-up and the amount of data to be collected

4. Obtain IRB approval for the proposed follow-up study

B. Follow-up

1. Initiate mechanisms to establish patient contact

2. Implement special procedures to locate patients who do not respond to initial contact or who cannot be located

3. Update patient identifying and locator information

4. Assemble data collected from the post-trial follow-up

C. Data analysis and publication

1. Link added follow-up data with existing patient files

2. Carry out analyses to summarize post-trial follow-up results

3. Prepare manuscript summarizing results

D. Other activities

1. Store updated patient identifying and location information for future follow-up

2. Distribute a copy of any manuscript(s) produced to study investigators

E. Sample consent statements

E.1 Consent statement for the Macular Photocoagulation Study (MPS): Senile Macular Degeneration Study

E.2 Consent statement for the Persantine Aspirin Reinfarction Study (PARIS)

E.3 Consent statement for the Hypertension
Prevention Trial (HPT)

Table E-1 Content checklist for sample consent statements

This appendix contains consent statements from
three of the multicenter trials sketched in Appendix B:

- Macular Photocoagulation Study (MPS): Se-
nile Macular Degeneration Study
- Persantine Aspirin Reinfarction Study
(PARIS)
- Hypertension Prevention Trial (HPT)

The statements used by the individual clinics may
have differed. All clinics could expand on information contained in the prototype statements,
but could not delete or abridge information.

Table E-1 provides a content analysis of the
three statements. The checklist is based on Table
14-4. None of the statements covered all of the
items in the checklist. The MPS statement had
the largest number of content deficiencies—16.
There were 9 noted for the PARIS and 7 for the
HPT statements.

The last line in Table E-1 gives the reading
grade level of the text, derived using a scoring
system developed by McLaughlin (1969). The
PARIS statement had the highest reading level.
It also contained language designed to speak for
the patient (e.g., as in use of the phrase *I understand*)—a defect largely avoided in the other two
statements.

E.1 CONSENT STATEMENT FOR THE
MACULAR PHOTOCOAGULATION
STUDY (MPS): SENILE MACULAR
DEGENERATION STUDY

Macular degeneration is a major cause of visual
loss in the U.S. It results from aging changes
that affect the pigment cells and small blood
vessels behind the retina. There is a familial
tendency. No form of treatment is known to be
effective.

Sometimes, a progressive deterioration of the
pigment cells results in a slow reduction in vision. At other times, a break in the membrane
behind the retina permits a blood vessel to grow
through and leak fluid and/or blood beneath the
retina and into the retina causing a rather sudden loss of vision.

Photographs taken after fluorescein dye injection locate the position of the leaking blood
vessel. The closer this vessel is to the center of
the retina, the greater the threat to vision. If the
vessel is somewhat removed from the center, it
may be possible to close the vessel with the laser
and prevent further growth and further bleeding.
If the vessel is directly central, laser treatment is
not recommended.

Prior to laser treatment, numbing medication
is given to prevent discomfort and motion of the
eye. Rarely, this injection may cause some swelling behind the eye and some visual loss.

Possible complications of laser treatment include bleeding, retinal wrinkling, pigment loss,
and damage to the center of the retina which
may cause vision to be worse than before treatment. It is important to recognize, however, that
each of these problems can occur without the use
of the laser.

At present, it is not known whether your
chances of maintaining good central vision are
better with or without laser treatment, and your
doctor has agreed to participate in a randomized
trial to find an answer to this question. If your
eye is eligible and if you agree to participate, you
will be assigned in random fashion to a treatment group or to a non-treatment group. Randomization is similar to flipping a coin so that
there is one chance in two of being treated or not
treated with the laser. This provides an opportunity to balance the risks and benefits of laser
treatment.

There is another important benefit. Patients
with a second eye at risk have much to gain from
participation since we anticipate the results of
this study may provide information that will
help the ophthalmologist with the management
of the second eye.

Table E-1 Content checklist* for sample consent statements

Topic	MPS	PARIS	HPT
General descriptive and design information			
• Disease or condition to be studied	✓	✓	✓
• Type of people to be studied	✓	✓	✓
• Length of follow-up	—	—	✓
• Method of follow-up	—	—	✓
• Description of data collection procedures and schedule	—	—	✓
Treatment procedures described			
• Test treatment	✓	✓	✓
• Control treatment	—	✓	✓
• Method of treatment administration	✓	✓	✓
• Method of treatment assignment	✓	✓	✓
• Treatment masking	NA	✓	NA
• Rationale for choice of treatment	—	✓	✓
• Alternative treatments	—	✓	NA
Risk-benefit information detailed			
• Nature of treatment side effects	✓	✓	—
• Risk-benefit of test treatment	✓	✓	—
• Risk-benefit of control treatment	—	—	NA
• Potential side effects of test treatment	✓	✓	—
• Potential side effects of control treatment	✓	NA	NA
• Risk-benefit of special procedures to be performed	✓	NA	NA
Patient responsibilities and safeguards			
• Patient follow-up responsibilities detailed	—	✓	✓
• Provisions for protecting patient from prolonged denial of a beneficial treatment or exposure to a harmful treatment detailed	—	✓	—
• Safeguards for protecting patient's right to privacy detailed	—	—	✓
• Patient's right to withdraw from trial stated	✓	✓	✓
• Statement of right to have questions answered before enrollment provided	—	✓	✓
• Types of information that will not be disclosed during trial detailed	—	—	—
• Policy on care and payment for study related injuries detailed	—	—	✓
• Statement of where and how personal identifiers will be used	—	—	✓
• Amount and type of information provided to patient during trial indicated	—	✓	—
• Amount and type of information provided to patient at end of trial indicated	—	—	—
SMOG grade	12	14	12

*A checkmark indicates the item was covered. A dash indicates it was not. NA indicates not applicable.

Results of the study will be analyzed regularly; and any significant findings will be made known to the patient, especially findings which would alter the management of either eye.

To be certain that the physician will be able to locate all patients in case there are important study findings, we ask you for the names of relatives and others who may be contacted in case the patient cannot be located at some future date.

My signature below indicates that I understand all of the above and agree to participate in this program. I recognize that I am under no obligation to join this study, that I am free to withdraw at any time, and that neither failure to join nor withdrawal will prejudice the medical care which I receive at the Johns Hopkins Medical Institutions.

Patient's Signature   _____

Doctor's Signature   _____

Witness   _____

Date   _____

E.2　CONSENT STATEMENT FOR THE PERSANTINE ASPIRIN REINFARCTION STUDY (PARIS)

I agree to permit Dr. _____ and the study physician to treat me, _____, with Persantine (dipyridamole) and/or aspirin (acetylsalicylic acid) or placebo (inactive substance) for coronary heart disease. It has been explained to me that some studies have shown that aspirin may produce favorable results in the treatment of heart attacks and blood clot disorders by affecting the function of the blood platelets (the small cells in the blood that are necessary to keep blood from clotting [sic]). There is also some indication that the addition of Persantine may enhance these effects. However, at present there are no clear-cut data showing that people having one heart attack will not have another heart attack if they are given drugs which change platelet function. This study is designed to test the possibility that these drugs may help to prevent a recurrent heart attack.

It has been further explained to me that all of the persons participating in this study will be assigned at random to one of the following three groups. Neither I nor my physician will know to which group I belong.

1. One group will be given aspirin. Along with aspirin this group will receive a placebo pill (inactive substance) resembling the second drug, Persantine. Persons in this group will take 325 mg of aspirin three times a day.

2. A second group in this study will take aspirin and Persantine. Persons in this group will take 325 mg of aspirin and 75 mg of Persantine three times a day.

3. The third group will be what is called the control group. Those selected at random for this group will be given two placebos, that is, pills appearing like the other drugs in the study but with no active medication in them. This group will be compared with the other groups to see if there is a difference between the groups taking medication and the group taking placebos.

I understand that aspirin may cause stomach irritation or a bleeding tendency. No one who has had a personal sensitivity or history of significant problems taking aspirin will be asked to participate. I also understand that Persantine may cause lightheadedness or dizziness as a result of lowered blood pressure. I understand that there are no data in humans to suggest that its long-term use will lead to the development of any serious illness. Studies are in progress to determine whether or not this drug has any potential to cause tumors in animals. Should information become available suggesting any adverse effects, I understand that I would immediately be notified by the study physicians and that any such measures deemed necessary for the protection of my health would be carried out promptly. I also understand that if I should have any reactions to the medication during the study, I should notify the study physician so that appropriate treatment could be carried out promptly.

I understand that the reason for the placebo group is that there is always a chance, in fact a reasonable possibility, that the drugs may be ineffective and may cause some side effects which outweigh any beneficial effects. It has been explained to me that if at any point during this study it becomes evident that patients on one treatment are not doing as well as the patients on the other treatments, they will be switched to one of the superior treatments.

It has also been explained to me that there are other methods of possible prevention of recurrent heart attack including diet, weight reduction, exercise programs, drug control of high blood pressure, cessation of smoking, various types of heart surgery, or use of anticoagulants which reduce the clotting ability of blood without affecting blood platelets. I understand that all of these forms of treatment, with the exception of anticoagulant drugs which cannot be given together with PARIS medications, are available to me with the advice of my personal physician. I also understand that I must avoid taking aspirin and aspirin-containing drugs during my participation in this study.

I have read and have understood the foregoing explanation and I fully understand the program of study. I also understand that my participation in this study is of great value to me and to others like myself who have coronary disease and have survived a heart attack. I have had an adequate chance to ask questions and I may ask questions at any time while the study is in progress. I voluntarily consent to participate, or to continue my participation, in this study and to treatment with these drugs or placebo. I understand that I may withdraw my consent and discontinue my participation in the study at any time.

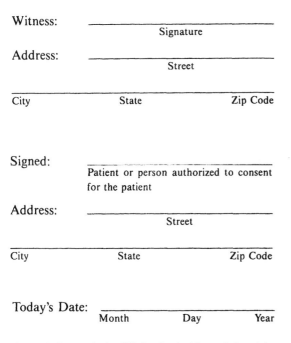

Witness: _____
　　　　　　　　　　Signature

Address: _____
　　　　　　　　　　Street

_____
City　　　　　State　　　　　Zip Code

Signed: _____
　　　　　Patient or person authorized to consent
　　　　　for the patient

Address: _____
　　　　　　　　　　Street

_____
City　　　　　State　　　　　Zip Code

Today's Date: _____
　　　　　　　Month　　　Day　　　Year

Source: Reference citation 375. Reprinted with permission of the American Heart Association, Inc., Dallas, Texas.

E.3 CONSENT STATEMENT FOR THE HYPERTENSION PREVENTION TRIAL (HPT)

The Hypertension Prevention Trial (HPT) is designed to help us determine whether or not people can avoid high blood pressure through a change in diet. Only volunteers who are not being treated for hypertension and who do not now have elevated blood pressure are eligible for the study. The main aim is to determine if people can make, and then maintain, the diet changes proposed. Each person will be studied for at least two years. The amount of change in blood pressure will be observed over that time period. The specific diets to be studied are:

- *Low-sodium diet*—participants assigned to this diet will be asked to reduce the amount of foods they eat which contain high levels of sodium. Sodium is a mineral required by the human body in small amounts. The most common source of sodium is table salt (sodium chloride).
- *Low-sodium and high potassium diet*—participants assigned to this diet will be asked to reduce the amount of high-sodium foods in their diet and also increase their use of foods which are high in potassium. Potassium is also a mineral required by the human body. The most common sources of potassium are fresh fruits and vegetables.
- *Weight loss diet*—participants assigned to this diet will be asked to reduce body weight by eating less and through increased exercise.
- *Weight loss and low-sodium diet*—participants assigned to this diet will be asked to lose weight by eating less, increasing exercise, and to reduce consumption of high-sodium foods.

People entering the study will be placed in one of two weight groups. Approximately half the people enrolled are expected to fall into each of the two groups. People in the higher weight group will be assigned to one of the above diets, or to no diet change. Those in the lower weight group will be assigned to one of the two diets above that do not involve a weight loss, or to no diet change.

The specific diet you will be asked to follow depends on an assignment made by the Data Coordinating Center located in Baltimore, Maryland. The assignment is made using a chance procedure, like rolling dice, but carried out with a computer. Hence, neither we nor you know in advance the group to which you will be assigned.

Everyone taking part in the study will need to return to the clinic for blood pressure measurement, every six months after enrollment. A 24-hour food record and overnight urine collection will be required prior to each of these visits. An electrocardiogram and a blood sample will be drawn once a year.

Participants assigned to a diet group will need to make more frequent visits to the clinic to receive instructions on how to make necessary diet changes. As a rule, these visits will be organized as group instruction sessions. Each session will last about one and one-half hours. The schedule will be:

• One session a week for the first ten weeks after enrollment
• Six additional sessions during the rest of the first year
• A minimum of four sessions in the second year, and in each year thereafter so long as the study continues

Entry into the study is voluntary. If you do decide to enroll we will keep in contact with you for the duration of the study. We may even wish to maintain written or telephone contact with you after the study is finished.

You are not obligated to continue in the study if you change your mind about participating later on. Withdrawal from the study will in no way affect any care or treatment you are receiving from other clinics in the University. However, anyone who drops out after enrollment reduces the scientific value of the study. Hence, you should not enroll if you are uncertain about the value of the study or if you know now that you cannot fulfill the study requirements. If you do decide to drop out, we will contact you by telephone or letter about once a year.

Data, including peronal information such as name and address, will be stored in a computer at the Clinic and at the Data Coordinating Center in Baltimore. All personal information is confidential and available only to study personnel. No reports will be presented or published which reveal your identity.

There will be no charge to you for any of the study procedures or clinic visits. The examination procedures used in this study are not intended for individual medical diagnosis or care. If you have any medical problems that come to our attention, we will refer you to proper sources of care.

The University has no general provision for compensation in the event of physical injury resulting from research studies. In the unlikely event that injury should occur, medical treatment is available, but may not be provided free of charge.

We believe the risks associated with participation in this trial are small. The diets being studied are consistent with general nutritional recommendations. The tests and procedures are standard and in common use.

If you are satisfied with the explanation of the Hypertension Prevention Trial and wish to take part in it, please sign below. Please do not sign until you have had all questions concerning the study and your participation in it answered to your satisfaction.

Participant
Name (print) _____

Signature _____ _____
Date

Witness
Name (print) _____

Signature _____ _____
Date

Should you have any complaint after enrollment, you may contact the HPT Clinic Director, or the University Human Volunteers Office. The Human Volunteers Office should be contacted if you desire to make the complaint without knowledge of the clinic staff.

Clinic Director:	Harry J. Jones, M.D. 684 North Fox Street Any Town, MD 47150 Phone: 872-8420
Human Volunteers Office:	Jane V. Moore, M.D. 7844 East 5th Street Any Town, MD 47150 Phone: 962-7741

CLINIC STAFF: *Please make a copy of the signed consent form for the participant*

F. Data items and forms illustrations

This appendix contains illustrations referenced in Chapter 12. Many of the items are taken from study forms as used in a clinical trial or an epidemiological study and are exact photo reproductions of the items except for the reductions necessary to fit the format of this book. Others have been retyped as they appeared except for minor differences in type style and spacing (these are labeled as facsimiles). Some of the items have been contrived (labeled as such) to illustrate specific points not covered by actual examples.

The categorization of an illustration as satisfactory or unsatisfactory relates to the point considered. A satisfactory classification in one context may be unsatisfactory in another.

F.1 ITEM NUMBERING

F.1.1 Unnumbered items (Unsatisfactory; photo reproduction)

```
                                              Study No.:_____

Date of                        Name of
Record Rev.:____/____/____      Reviewer:_____
           (mo.) (day) (yr.)

Name of Hospital:_____

Name of Patient:_____

Address:_____
                               Name in
Telephone No.:_____  Which listed:_____

History          Soc. Sec.          Medicare          Insurance
No.:_____   Number:_____   Number:_____   Number:_____

Date of Birth:____/____/____      Age:_____
             (mo.) (day) (yr.)
```

F.1.2   Numbered items (satisfactory; photo reproduction)

2. LAST NAME		3. OPD NO.	4. HOSPITAL NO.	5. SPECIAL NO.
6. FIRST NAME	7. MIDDLE	8. MAIDEN		COMPLETE ONLY IF NEEDED BY HOSPITAL
9. ADDRESS (Street and Number) (City, Zone and State)		10. TELEPHONE NO.	11. EDC	

12. DATE REGISTERED	13. DATE FORM INITIATED	14. FIRST DAY LMP	15. DATE OF BIRTH	16. AGE
Mo. Day Year	Mo. Day Year	Mo. Day Year	Mo. Day Year	

17. MARITAL STATUS	18. RACE	19. WEEKS OF GESTATION
☐S 1 ☐M 2 ☐CL 3 ☐W 4 ☐D 5 ☐SEP. 6	☐W 1 ☐N 2 ☐OR 3 ☐PR 4 ☐Other 5	

20. PATIENT STATUS	21. SAMPLING FRAME PATIENT
☐Clinic 1 ☐Private 2	SELECTED FOR STUDY ☐Based on 1 Systematic Sampling. ☐Based on 2 Special Sampling (Specify) NOT SELECTED FOR STUDY ☐Based on 7 Sampling Design ☐For Other Reasons 8 (Specify below)

F.1.3   Comment

Item numbering is mandatory if the respondent is required to skip certain items. However, it is useful even when skips are not required. The numbers serve as convenient references for data editing and processing.

F.2   ITEMS THAT INDICATE PRESENCE OR ABSENCE OF A FINDING OR CONDITION

F.2.1   (Unsatisfactory; photo reproduction)

15.   **GENERAL MEDICAL HISTORY:** Have you ever had any of the following conditions?
   For each <u>yes</u> in column 1, please fill in columns 2 to 7.

Condition	(1) Check if yes	(2) First occurrence (Yr.)	(3) First seen by physician (Yr.)	(4) Treated currently (yes or no)	(5) Current or most recent physician and/or clinic (Name & address)	
Cataracts						
Any other eye problems (specify)						
Heart trouble of any kind						
Stroke						

F.2.2 (Unsatisfactory; photo reproduction)

15. Could you list all the pets (types of animals) you/_____ had?

Index Subject

A. Pet	B. Did you have close contact with this pet? e.g., did he sit on your lap, sleep on your bed?	If YES, Ask D - G / C. Was this pet ever sick prior to your/ Index Subject's hospitalization/ physician visit in ___ - ___ ? Month Year YES | NO | UNK			D. Could you tell me the name of the disease?	E. What year was this pet sick?	F. Could you tell me the name and location of the veterinarian who treated this pet?

F.2.3 (Satisfactory; photo reproduction)

13. Has a doctor ever told you that you had ASK (a-c) FOR EACH OF THE FOLLOWING:	(A) IF YES ASK (B-C) YES | NO | UNK			(B) IF YES At what age?	(C) IF YES TO (A): Were you hospitalized? YES | NO | UNK		
Varicose veins							
Phlebitis (Inflammation of veins usually in arms or legs)							
Repeated Vaginal Infec- tions (more than 3/year)							
Repeated Pelvic and/or Uterine (female) Infections							
Venereal Disease							
Stroke							
High Blood Pressure							
Heart Disease (Specify:)							
Anemia (poor blood)							

F.2.4   (Satisfactory; photo reproduction)

a.   **Have you ever been pregnant? NO ☐ YES ☐**   b. **How many times?** _____
(If yes, please complete table below listing all pregnancies, beginning with the first pregnancy. Include miscarri
(If no, go to page 18)

Pregnancy order: No.	Child's first name	Date pregnancy ended or date of birth	Residence during pregnancy, list all if more than one (No. of mos, in each)	Physician and/or hospital (Name & address)	Pregnancy outcome and no. of months pregnant*
1.					
2.					
3.					
4.					

F.2.5   Comment

F.2.1 is deficient in that it allows the respondent to skip conditions that are absent. This design can lead to ambiguous results, especially when none of the conditons are checked. There is no way in such cases to know if the entire item was overlooked or if it was left unanswered because none of the conditions were present.

F.2.2 is defective in that it provides no indication of what the index subject is to do when the answer to the lead question is "No." Taken literally, a "No" reply means the respondent is unable to list *all* his pets. Further, the time period to which the question refers is unclear. Is the intent to list all pets the index subject has ever had or only those for some specified time period? Presumably the entire set of questions is to be skipped for an index subject reporting no pets, creating the same ambiguity as cited for F.2.1.

The items shown in F.2.3 and F.2.4 avoid this problem by requiring an answer even if the condition is absent. Example F.2.3 requires a "Yes," "No," or "Unknown" answer for each disease condition listed; example F.2.4 has a lead question that, if checked "No," allows the respondent to skip the rest of the item.

F.3   UNNECESSARY WORDS

F.3.1   (Unsatisfactory; facsimile)

Would you please tell me about how much income you and your family will get during 1971, January through December? I mean your total family income - before taxes from all sources.

1. Under $3,999
2. $4,000 - $7,999
3. $8,000 - $11,999
4. $12,000 - $15,999
5. $16,000 - $24,999
6. Over $25,000

F.3.2   (Satisfactory; contrived from F.3.1)

Please indicate your total, before tax, family income for 1971.

1. Under $3,999
2. $4,000 - $7,999
3. $8,000 - $11,999
4. $12,000 - $15,999
5. $16,000 - $24,999
6. Over $25,000

F.3.3   Comment

F.3.1 contains unnecessary words that are not helpful, and perhaps even confusing, particularly since the question simply refers to income and the "clarifying" remark following the question refers to total family income. F.3.2 conveys the same meaning as F.3.1, but with fewer words.

It is easy to find examples of items with unnecessary words. An economy of words cannot be achieved without a considerable investment of time and effort in the development, review, and testing processes involved in constructing forms.

F.4   DOUBLE NEGATIVES

F.4.1   (Unsatisfactory; facsimile)

05:38. In the past week, did you have any injuries or accidents that didn't cause you to cut down on your normal activities?

    0 NO   1 YES

F.4.2   (Unsatisfactory; contrived)

The answers to items 28 thru 32 have been reviewed by a nutritionist and they do not disqualify the candidate from enrollment.

    ( )   ( )
    Yes   No

F.4.3   (Unsatisfactory; contrived)

Since your stroke are you (check one)

( ) Unable to walk
( ) Barely unable to walk
( ) Able to walk fairly well
( ) Able to walk normally

F.4.4   (Satisfactory; contrived from F.4.1)

In the past week did you have any accidents or injuries?

    0 NO   1 YES

If yes,

Did they cause you to cut down on your normal activities?

    0 NO   1 YES

F.4.5   (Satisfactory; contrived from F.4.2)

Were items 28 through 32 reviewed by a nutritionist?

    ( ) ( )
    Yes   No

If Yes,

Do the answers qualify the candidate for enrollment in the study?

    ( ) ( )
    Yes   No

F.4.6   (Satisfactory; contrived from F.4.3)

Since your stroke are you (check one)

( ) Unable to walk
( ) Barely able to walk
( ) Able to walk fairly well
( ) Able to walk normally

F.4.7   Comment

F.4.1 is almost impossible to comprehend in this form. Compare it with the reworded version in F.4.4.

    F.4.2 is difficult to understand because it consists of two parts and a double negative phrase, "do not disqualify." The reworded version in F.4.5 divides the question into two parts and eliminates the use of the double negative.

    Example F.4.3 uses two negative terms, "barely" and "unable." F.4.6 avoids the confusion created by their use.

F.5   COMPOUND QUESTIONS

F.5.1   (Unsatisfactory; contrived)

The answers to items 28 thru 32 have been reviewed by a nutritionist and they qualify the participant for enrollment.

    ( ) ( )
    Yes   No

F.5.2   (Unsatisfactory; facsimile)

_____MONTH   _____YEAR

Why did you see a doctor? I mean, what was wrong with you?

```
00   ROUTINE CHECK-UP (GENERAL HEALTH)
01   ROUTINE CHECK-UP FOR PREGNANCY
02   JUST DIDN'T FEEL GOOD
03   RECEIVING TREATMENT FOR ILLNESS, SPECIFY ILLNESS:
```
_____

_____

```
04   RECEIVING TREATMENT FOR INJURY OR ACCIDENT?
     SPECIFY WHAT WAS WRONG. _____
```
_____

```
05   RECEIVING TREATMENT BECAUSE RESPONDENT WAS A VICTIM
     OF CRIME.  SPECIFY. _____
```
_____

```
06   OTHER, SPECIFY _____
```
_____

F.5.3   (Satisfactory; contrived from F.5.1)

Were items 28 thru 32 reviewed by a
nutritionist?

(   ) (   )
Yes   No

If <u>Yes</u>,

Do the answers qualify the candidate for
enrollment in the study?

(   ) (   )
Yes   No

F.5.4   (Satisfactory; contrived from F.5.2)

Why did you see a doctor?

```
00   ROUTINE CHECK-UP (GENERAL HEALTH)
01   ROUTINE CHECK-UP FOR PREGNANCY
02   JUST DIDN'T FEEL GOOD
03   RECEIVING TREATMENT FOR ILLNESS, SPECIFY ILLNESS:
```
_____

F.5.5   Comment

The question in F.5.1 requires two conditions to be met in order to check "Yes." Technically, a "No" could mean either that the list of questions was not reviewed by a nutritionist or that one or more of the answers disqualified the candidate from enrollment. The confusion is eliminated in F.5.3 by first asking if a nutritionist reviewed the listed items and then making the second question conditional on a "Yes" reply to the first question.

F.5.2 is unsatisfactory because the two questions require different responses. The reasons for going to a doctor may not relate to what is actually wrong. The confusion is avoided by deleting the second "clarifying" question, as in example F.5.4.

F.6 COMPARATIVE EVALUATIONS

F.6.1 Unstated standard

F.6.1.1 (Unsatisfactory; contrived)

Do you get more exercise now?

( ) ( )
Yes   No

F.6.1.2 (Satisfactory; contrived from F.6.1.1)

Do you get more exercise now than you did before your illness?

( ) ( )
Yes   No

F.6.2 Undefined standard

F.6.2.1 (Unsatisfactory; contrived)

Do you have any major diseases?

( ) ( )
Yes   No

F.6.2.2 (Better; contrived from F.6.2.1)

Do you have any major diseases, such as cancer or heart disease?

( ) ( )
Yes   No

F.6.2.3 (Satisfactory; contrived from F.6.2.2)

Do you have any of the following diseases? (Check as many as apply):

( ) Cancer
( ) Heart disease
( ) Diabetes
( ) Arthritis
( ) Other (specify)

˙.6.3 Positive versus negative standards

F.6.3.1 (Unsatisfactory; contrived)

Are you shorter than your mother?

( ) ( )
Yes   No

F.6.3.2 (Satisfactory; contrived from F.6.3.1)

Are you taller than your mother?

( ) ( )
Yes   No

F.6.3.3 (Unsatisfactory; contrived)

Would you say you are in worse health than you were a year ago?

( ) ( )
Yes   No

F.6.3.4 (Satisfactory; contrived from F.6.3.3)

Would you say you are in better health than you were a year ago?

( ) ( )
Yes   No

F.6.4 Comment

Items requiring a comparative assessment should indicate the standard for the comparison. Question F.6.1.1 is confusing because there is no specification of the time period over which the comparison is to be made. F.6.1.2 specifies a reference point for the assessment.

Care should be taken to avoid the ambiguity of an undefined term, such as in F.6.2.1. F.6.2.2 provides a general indication of what is meant by "major" disease. F.6.2.3 is even more explicit in this regard.

Comparative statements should be cast in positive terms, since they are generally easier to understand than corresponding statements cast in negative terms (e.g., F.6.3.2 and F.6.3.4 versus F.6.3.1 and F.6.3.3).

F.7 INVERTED MEANING OF A YES REPLY

F.7.1 (Unsatisfactory; contrived)

Patient does not use (answer a through c):

		Yes	No
a.	Insulin	( )	( )
b.	Oral hypoglycemic agents	( )	( )
c.	Digitalis	( )	( )

F.7.2 (Satisfactory; contrived from F.7.1)

Patient uses (answer a through c):

		Yes	No
a.	Insulin	( )	( )
b.	Oral hypoglycemic agents	( )	( )
c.	Digitalis	( )	( )

F.7.3 Comment

F.7.1 requires the respondent to check "Yes" if the patient does not use an indicated drug. The question is less confusing if the use of a drug requires a "Yes" reply, as in F.7.2.

F.8 PRESENCE VERSUS ABSENCE OF A CONDITION

F.8.1 (Unsatisfactory; contrived)

Are you free of heart disease?

( ) ( )
Yes   No

F.8.2 (Satisfactory; contrived from F.8.1)

Has a doctor ever told you that you have heart disease?

( ) ( )
Yes   No

F.8.3 Comment

F.8.1 requires an affirmative response to indicate the absence of a condition. In a sense, the question is impossible to answer since there is no way to know if one is free of heart disease.

Item F.8.2 is stated in positive terms and avoids the problem of F.8.1 by relying on an operational definition of heart disease.

F.9 TIME REFERENCES

F.9.1 Time point references

F.9.1.1 Present time point (Satisfactory; facsimile)

9. (AAW) Are you presently taking any drugs prescribed by a physician?

$(\quad)_1 \quad (\quad)_2$
Yes   No

F.9.1.2 Time frame defined in terms of a specified calendar date (Satisfactory; photo reproduction)

9. Approximately what was your weight in _____? _____ POUNDS (_____ KG)   UNKNOWN ☐
(2 YEARS PRIOR TO REF. DATE)

10. Approximately what was your weight in _____? _____ POUNDS (_____ KG)   UNKNOWN ☐
REFERENCE DATE

F.9.1.3 Time frame specified in terms of a defined event (Satisfactory; contrived)

```
Were you taking any prescription drugs
when you had your last MI?
```

( ) $_1$ ( ) $_2$
  Yes   No

F.9.2 Time interval references

F.9.2.1 Time interval defined by two events (Satisfactory; facsimile)

110. Did your doctor advise you <u>not</u> to take the pill or IUD
      between the start of your periods and your first pregnancy?

YES, IUD ☐

YES, PILL ☐   ASK: What were the reasons? _____

NO ☐   UNKNOWN ☐

F.9.2.2 Time interval defined as period from last study examination to present (Satisfactory; photo reproduction)

8) Since the patient's last completed
   follow-up visit, has he had any of the
   following (answer each question):

                                        Yes   No
A) Cardiac asthma? .... ( ) ( ) [45]

B) An obvious stroke? .... ( ) ( ) [46]

C) Weakness or paralysis of any part
   of his body? .... ( ) ( ) [47]

F.9.2.3 Time interval defined as entire "study period" (Satisfactory; facsimile)

ist all in-patient admissions during study period (for any diagnosis, to this hospital only).

Identify with a check the admission selected for review sample	Date of					
	Admission			Discharge		
	Month	Day	Year	Month	Day	Year
1st						
2nd						
3rd						
4th						
5th						
6th						

` Study Admission is the First in the Study Period, give most Recent Date of Hospitalization
:his hospital only) before Study Period:_____ None ☐

F.9.2.4   Time interval defined from some calendar time to present (Satisfactory; photo reproduction)

18.   PHYSICIAN OR CLINIC VISITS SINCE 1950

Please list all physician and/or clinic visits since 1950 <u>other than routine employment exams.</u>

Physician and/or clinic (Name & address)	Date (Mo. & yr.)	Specialty

F.9.2.5   Time interval from present to recall limit (Satisfactory; photo reproduction)

16.   Could you please tell me a few things about each time you were x-rayed? Start with the first x-ray you remember, and then tell me about later ones.   (ASK A-F)

(A) What part of the head was x-rayed? skull, tonsils, sinuses, etc.)	(B) In what year was this done?	(C) In what hospital or doctor's office was this done? NAME ADDRESS	(D) Why was the x-ray taken?	(E) About how many films were taken?

F.9.3   Comment

The examples in F.9.1 all refer to some point in time—the present, a calendar date, or the date on which a defined event occurred. The examples in F.9.2 are for defined time intervals. The interval in F.9.2.1 is defined by two events—the start of menstruation and first pregnancy. A common frame of reference for follow-up studies is illustrated in F.9.2.2 where the respondent is required to cover the time period from the last follow-up visit to the present visit. The time frame in F.9.2.3 is the entire "study period." This mode of reference is useful only when it is clear what is meant by the phrase. Example F.9.2.4 covers a time interval from 1950 to the time of the interview. The interval in F.9.2.5 is defined by the limits of a respondent's recall.

F.10   DIRECTION OF RESPONSE

F.10.1   Mixed disease categorization (Unsatisfactory; contrived)

Is the patient (answer each question):

	Yes	No
Hypertensive?	( )	( )
Euglycemic?	( )	( )
Obese?	( )	( )
Hyperlipidemic?	( )	( )

F.10.2 Mixed attitude expression (Unsatisfactory; facsimile)

How often did you feel _____ (READ CHOICES)

		NOT AT ALL (0)	ONCE (1 TIME)	SEVERAL TIMES (2-3 TIMES)	OFTEN (3+ TIMES)
03:43	Pleased about having accomplished something?	0	1	2	3
44.	Proud because someone complimented you on something you had done?	0	1	2	3
45.	Depressed or very unhappy?	0	1	2	3
46.	Bored?	0	1	2	3
47.	Particularly excited or interested in something?	0	1	2	3
48.	Downcast and dejected?	0	1	2	3

F.10.3 Comment

The difficulty with F.10.1 arises from the mixture of disease and nondisease states. This problem could be corrected by replacing "euglycemic" with "diabetic" in the check list.

F.10.2 includes a mix of positive and negative states of mind. The first two items are phrased in positive terms. The next two are stated in negative terms. Intermixing of this sort is ill-advised unless there are good reasons for doing so (e.g., to keep a respondent from automatically checking the same category for all items without thinking).

F.11 LEADING QUESTIONS

F.11.1 (Leading; contrived)

Do you still have allergies to ragweed?

( ) ( )
Yes No

F.11.2 (Not leading; contrived)

Have you ever had allergies to ragweed?

( ) ( )
Yes No

If <u>Yes,</u>

Do you still have them?

( ) ( )
Yes No

F.11.3 Comment

F.11.1 not only leads the patient but assumes he has had an allergy to ragweed in the past. As written, there is no way to answer the question if the patient has never had ragweed allergies. F.11.2 avoids the problem by beginning with a general question that determines whether the patient has ever had ragweed allergies before inquiring about current allergies.

F.12   VERTICAL VERSUS HORIZONTAL RESPONSE LISTS

F.12.1   Horizontal lists

F.12.1.1   (Unsatisfactory; photo reproduction)

Sex and Race: (check) ☐ WM; ☐ WF; ☐ NWM; ☐ NWF; ☐ OM; ☐ OF

F.12.1.2   (Unsatisfactory; photo reproduction)

11. How many times a week do you eat each of the following foods?
Fish _____; Meat _____; Poultry _____; Eggs _____; Cheese _____; Butter or margarine _____;
Breads & cereals _____; Potatoes _____; Rice _____; Vegetables _____; Green salads _____;
Fruits and fruit juices _____; Sweet desserts _____; Candy _____

F.12.1.3   (Unsatisfactory; photo reproduction)

16. Check the reactions at test sight 7-14 days after application.
☐ 0. None   ☐ 1. Erythema   ☐ 2. Edema   ☐ 3. Vesicles/oozing
☐ 4. Bulla/denudation   ☐ 5. Delayed flare

F.12.1.4   (Unsatisfactory; photo reproduction)

22. **RADIATION THERAPY**: Have you ever had any treatments with radium, cobalt 60, cobalt bomb radic ⎰
☐ NO ☐ YES ☐ DON'T KNOW   If <u>yes</u>, please complete the table below: (Start with most re ⎰

F.12.1.5   (Satisfactory; contrived from F.12.1.4)

RADIATION THERAPY: Have you ever had any treatments with radium, cobalt 60, cobalt bomb radio is ⎰
☐ NO   ☐ YES   ☐ DON'T KNOW   If yes, please complete the table below: (Start wi ⎰

F.12.1.6   (Satisfactory; contrived)

Are you taller than your mother?

(   ) (   )
Yes   No

F.12.1.7   (Unsatisfactory; photo reproduction)

14. How often do you use the following types of medicine?
Aspirin, Bufferin ....Never ☐ Occasionally ☐ Frequently ☐
Vitamin pills ....Never ☐ Occasionally ☐ Frequently ☐
Sleeping pills ....Never ☐ Occasionally ☐ Frequently ☐
Tranquilizers ....Never ☐ Occasionally ☐ Frequently ☐
Laxatives ....Never ☐ Occasionally ☐ Frequently ☐
Anti-acid medicine ....Never ☐ Occasionally ☐ Frequently ☐

F.12.1.8   (Satisfactory; photo reproduction)

16. How often do you
experience:

	Never	Occasionally	Frequently
Sensation of heart beating (except after exercise)	☐	☐	☐
Insomnia...	☐	☐	☐
Sense of exhaustion (except after exercise)..........	☐	☐	☐
Periods of alternating gloom and cheerfulness........	☐	☐	☐
Periods of being particularly self-conscious	☐	☐	☐

F.12.2 Vertical lists

F.12.2.1 (*Satisfactory; facsimile*)

(AAW) How would you characterize your ethnic
origin? (Use HPT flashcard 01)

( )1 White
( )2 Black
( )3 Hispanic
( )4 Oriental
( )5 Other (Specify)

F.12.2.2 (*Satisfactory; facsimile*)

(AAW) What is the combined income of all members of
your household? (Use list below to categorize
candidates response). (Use HPT flashcard 03)

( )0 < $5,000
( )1   5 thru 10,999
( )2 11 thru 15,999

( )3 16 thru 20,999
( )4 21 thru 25,999
( )5 26 thru 35,999

( )6 36 thru 45,999
( )7 46 thru 55,999
( )8 55,000 and over
( )9 declines to answer

F.12.2.3 (*Satisfactory; contrived from F.12.1.3*)

Check the reactions at test sight 7-14 days after application.

|☐| 0. None

|☐| 1. Erythema

|☐| 2. Edema

|☐| 3. Vesicles/oozing

|☐| 4. Bulla/denudation

|☐| 5. Delayed flare

F.12.2.4 (*Satisfactory; contrived*)

Does the patient have any of the following diseases?
(Check all that apply.)

( )1 Diabetes
( )2 Cancer
( )3 Hypertension
( )4 Heart disease
( )0 None of the above

F.12.3   Comment

A list that is horizontally arrayed requires less space than one that is vertically arrayed (e.g., compare F.12.1.3 and F.12.2.3). However, vertical layouts are generally less confusing than horizontal layouts to use (compare items in F.12.2 with those in F.12.1). The main difficulty with the examples in F.12.1 stems from the confusion the respondent is likely to have in locating the proper check space. Items F.12.1.2 and F.12.1.4 are especially defective in this regard. The uniformity of spacing makes it difficult for the respondent to decide whether the check space for the response is in front of or behind the designated reply.

A horizontal layout is acceptable for short lists. However, even in such instances it is important to use a layout, as in F.12.1.5 and F.12.1.6, that makes it easy to associate a response with the appropriate check space. The association is not obvious for F.12.1.1 and F.12.1.4 and only moderately so for F.12.1.7.

The amount of space provided for making a check in a vertical list should be adequate to avoid the confusion that can result if the check is not registered squarely in the center of the check space. For example, the vertical separations in F.12.2.3 are better than those in F.12.1.7 and F.12.1.8.

F.13   UNIT SPECIFICATIONS

F.13.1   Time units

F.13.1.1   (Unsatisfactory; contrived)

a. Date of patient's next appointment?

‾‾ ‾ ‾‾ ‾ ‾‾
Mo   Day   Yr

b. Time of patient's next appointment?

F.13.1.2   (Satisfactory; facsimile)

Time and date of BP measurement

a. Time of day   ‾ ‾ : ‾ ‾   AM
                                 PM

b. Date: ‾ ‾ ‾ ‾ ‾ ‾
                Mo   Day   Yr

F.13.2   Laboratory units

F.13.2.1   (Unsatisfactory; photo reproduction)

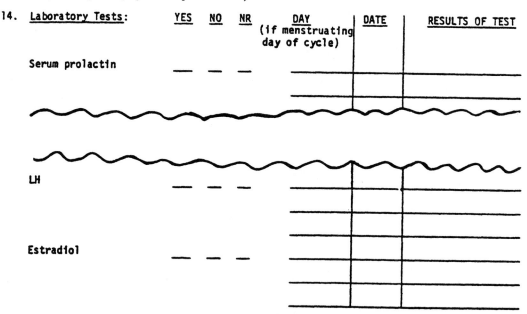

F.13.2.2 (*Fair; photo reproduction*)

If a check mark was placed after item 20-R, answer items A through E below relative to the episode which resulted in a diagnosis of myocardial infarction:

A) Highest SGOT recorded (state units): .. _____[55]
If not done, check here: .... (STOP)

B) Highest LDH recorded (state units): .... _____[56]
If not done, check here: .... ( )

C) Highest sedimentation rate recorded (min/hr): .... _____[57]

If not done, check here: .... ( )

F.13.2.3 (*Satisfactory; contrived from F.13.2.1*)

Laboratory Tests:	YES	NO	NR	DAY (if menstruating day of cycle)	DATE	RESULTS OF TEST	UNITS
Serum prolactin	—	—	—				
LH	—	—	—				
Estradiol	—	—	—				

F.13.3 Height-weight units

F.13.3.1 (*Unsatisfactory; photo reproduction*)

Height: _____ NR ☐

Weight: _____ NR ☐

F.13.3.2 (*Satisfactory; facsimile*)

13. Ht (shoes off):

inches

14. Wt (outdoor garments and shoes off):

lbs.

F.13.4   Unconventional units (Unsatisfactory; photo reproduction)

1) Results for the FIRST 90 minute collection period.

a) Serum creatinine determination. The blood sample for this determination should be taken at the start of the FIRST 90 minute collection period. Record the results in mg./ml. Carry the accuracy of the determinations four (4) places beyond the decimal point, e.g., 0.0185 mg./ml. Record the readings from both aliquots.

SERUM A

Aliquot 1 _____ mg./ml

Aliquot 2 _____ mg./ml

b) Urine creatinine concentration for the FIRST collection period. Record results in mg./ml. Carry the accuracy of the determinations three (3) places beyond the decimal point, e.g., 0.155 mg/ml. Record the readings from both aliquots.

URINE A

Aliquot 1 _____ mg./ml

Aliquot 2 _____ mg./ml

F.13.5   Comment

F.13.1.1 does not specify how time is to be recorded—on a 24-hour basis or on a 12-hour basis. If the latter, there will be ambiguity in the information supplied unless the respondent indicates AM or PM. F.13.1.2 avoids this difficulty by requiring the respondent to indicate AM or PM.

The unit of measurement should be part of the item, as in F.13.3.2 and F.13.4, when measurements are to be made using a specified unit. The item should provide space for recording the unit of measurement when it is not specified (e.g., as in F.13.2.3). The format for F.13.2.3 is better in this regard than for F.13.2.2. Items F.13.2.1 and F.13.3.1 are defective because they do not provide an indication of the unit of measurement.

The illustration in F.13.4 is taken from a form used in the University Group Diabetes Program (UGDP). Creatinine determinations are typically recorded in 100mg/ml. The UGDP form required recordings in mg/ml. The requirement resulted in a large number of recording errors.

F.14   PRECISION SPECIFICATIONS

F.14.1   Dashed lines with decimal points (Satisfactory; facsimile)

Height: _ _ . _ _   inches

Weight: _ _ _ . _   pounds

F.14.2   Boxes with decimal points (Satisfactory; contrived)

Height: ☐☐ . ☐   inches

Weight: ☐☐☐ . ☐   pounds

F.14.3   Hatched line with indication of required precision (Satisfactory; contrived)

Systolic blood pressure |_|_|_| mmHg

F.14.4   Solid line with written indication of required precision (Satisfactory; facsimile)

Blood pressure (record to nearest even number)

Diastolic   _____ mmHg

Systolic   _____ mmHg

F.14.5 Solid line with no indication of required precision (Unsatisfactory; facsimile)

```
Height        _____   inches

Weight        _____   lbs.
```

F.14.6 Comment

F.14.1 indicates the required precision through use of a series of dashed lines and decimal points. This format is preferred to those illustrated in F.14.2 and F.14.3 for reasons indicated in Section 12.6.8.2. The main problem with F.14.1 is that it requires more precision than is attainable with ordinary body height and weight measurements.

A format involving use of a solid line with no indication of required precision, such as illustrated in F.14.5, should be avoided if possible. The instructions for the item should indicate the desired precision if this format is used, as in F.14.4.

F.15   CALCULATION ITEMS

F.15.1   Bad examples

F.15.1.1   Blood pressure measurement (Facsimile)

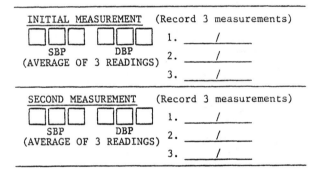

F.15.1.2   Blood pressure measurement (Photo reproduction)

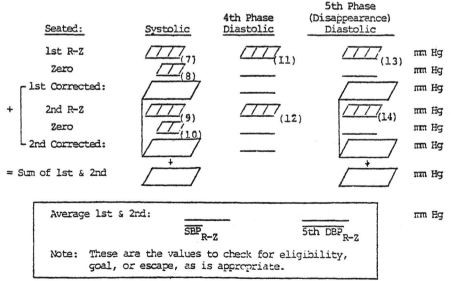

F.15.1.3   Cholesterol readings (Photo reproduction)

5) Serum cholesterol (recorded in mg. per cent). Determination made at the University of Minnesota on the basis of two .1 mL aliquots taken at both the initial and final examinations. When aliquots have been taken place a check in the appropriate parentheses at the right and record the date taken below.

Both "I" aliquots taken ( )   Both "F" aliquots taken ( )

Initial taken .... _____ _____ _____
                              Mo.   Day   Yr.

Final taken .... _____ _____ _____
                              Mo.   Day   Yr.

→		← Avg. →		←
I - F →		← Diff.
Overall →		← Avg.

Reserved for Recording Reading

F.15.1.4   Oscillometric readings (Photo reproduction)

1) Record the oscillometric readings for the RIGHT leg, for the two sites indicated.

   a) Two inches below the lower margin of the patella .... _____mm.

   b) Two inches above the apex of the internal malleolus .... _____mm.

2) Record the oscillometric readings for the LEFT leg, for the two sites indicated.

   a) Two inches below the lower margin of the patella .... _____mm.

   b) Two inches above the apex of the internal malleolus .... _____mm.

---

3) Total of all four readings on PRESENT examination (1a+1b+2a+2b) .... _____mm.

4) Total of all four readings on PREVIOUS examination (1a+1b+2a+2b) .... _____mm.

5) Item 4 — Item 3 .... _____mm.

6) Item 5 ÷ Item 4 ....

F.15.1.5   Activity assessment (Photo reproduction)

ACTIVITY (1)	Did you perform this activity? No (2)	Did you perform this activity? Yes (3)	For Clinic Personnel Use Only — Month of Activity Jan	Feb	Mar	Apr	May	June	July	Aug	Sept	Oct	Nov	Dec	Average number of times per month
SECTION A: Walking and Miscellaneous															
Walking for Pleasure and/or to Work															
Using Stairs When Elevator is Available															
Cross Country Hiking															
Back Packing															
Mountain Climbing															

F.15.2 Good examples

F.15.2.1 Blood pressure measurement (*Facsimile*)

```
RZ BP measurements
_____

                     BP in mmHg
  Reading          SBP       DBP
  _____

  1st RZ

   a. Reading      __ __     __ __

   b. Zero value   __ __     __ __

   c. a-b          __ __     __ __

  2nd RZ

    d. Reading     __ __     __ __

    e. Zero value  __ __     __ __

    f. d-e         __ __     __ __

  Avg RZ

    g. Sum (c + f) __ __ __   __ __ __

    h. Avg (g ÷ 2) __ __ __   __ __ __
```

F.15.2.2 Blood pressure measurement (*Photo reproduction*)

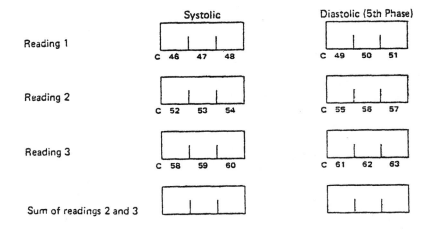

F.15.2.3 Blood pressure measurement (*Photo reproduction*)

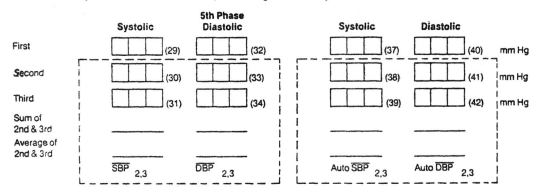

F.15.2.4   Pulse (Photo reproduction)

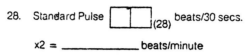

28.   Standard Pulse [| |] (28)   beats/30 secs.

x2 = _____ beats/minute

F.15.3   Comment

F.15.1.1 is bad because there is no space for calculating the average systolic and diastolic blood pressures. F.15.1.2 has a confusing layout as well as a shortage of work space. The three blood pressure examples in Section F.15.2 avoid the problems of F.15.1.1 and F.15.1.2.

F.15.1.3 is defective because of the absence of any work space for performing the additions, subtractions, and divisions required for the item. As written, the operation must be done on scratch paper. A vertical layout, such as displayed in F.15.2.1, would be required to enable the respondent to use the form to make and record intermediate calculations needed to complete the item.

The layout in F.15.1.4 could be improved by providing work space for the required additions and by having item 4 appear above item 3 to facilitate the subtraction required in item 5.

The layout of F.15.1.5 is not well suited for the averaging process, since users would almost certainly have to copy the data from the item onto a separate worksheet to perform the required additions and divisions.

F.16   INSTRUCTION ITEMS

F.16.1   STOP items

F.16.1.1   Eligibility STOP item (Satisfactory; facsimile)

13. Ht (shoes off):
                          inches

14. Wt (outdoor garments and
         shoes off):
                       — lbs. —

15. Q.I. = Wt/Ht^2 (use HPT Chart 11)

         0. __ __ __ __ lbs/in^2

16. Q.I. <0.0500 lbs/in^2
                    ( )   (stop)*
                 Yes 1   No 2

F.16.1.2   Temporary STOP item (Satisfactory; facsimile)

24. Serum specimen for central labor-
         atory determinations collected?

                    ( )   (stop)*
                 Yes 1   No 2

* Remove by drawing required blood.

F.16.2   SKIP item (Satisfactory; facsimile)

6. (AAW) Have you ever had your blood
        pressure measured before your
        first visit here?
                    ( ) ( )
                 Yes 1   No 2

If No, go to item 7.

If Yes, answer a and b

F.16.3 Comment

See Section 12.5.8 for discussion of STOP and SKIP items.

F.17 AGE AND BIRTHDATE ITEMS

F.17.1 (Satisfactory; facsimile)

> 9. (AAW) What is the month, day
>   and year of your birth?
>
> $$\overline{\text{Mo}} - \overline{\text{Day}} - \overline{\text{Yr}}$$
>
> 10. (AAW) What was your age at your
>   last birthday?
>
> — —
>
> 11. (DA) Does the birthdate fall within
>   the interval defined below?
>
> $\binom{}{\text{Yes}}_1 \binom{(\text{stop})}{\text{No}}_2$

> Candidate must be 25 or older but
> 49 or less at the time of registration
> to be eligible for enrollment into the
> HPT. Permissible birthdates for visits
> completed in 1982 are (use month and
> day recorded in item 8):
>
> $$\overline{\text{Mo}} - \overline{\text{Day}} - \overline{\text{Yr}}\ 3\ 2$$
>
> thru
>
> $$\overline{\text{Mo}} - \overline{\text{Day}} - \overline{\text{Yr}}\ 5\ 7$$

F.17.2 Comment

See Section 12.5.10.

F.18   REMINDER AND DOCUMENTATION ITEMS

F.18.1   Reminder items

F.18.1.1   Time window check (Facsimile)

5. Time window check

    a. Date of BL 1 (item 20b, Form 01CP)

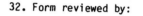

        $\overline{\text{Mo}}$ - $\overline{\text{Day}}$ - $\overline{\text{Yr}}$

    b. Is this visit at least 7 days after the date in item a.

        (   )$_1$ (stop)$^*_2$
        Yes   No

* Candidate should be rescheduled to remove this stop condition.

F.18.1.2   Procedure reminder (Facsimile)

24. Serum specimen for central laboratory determinations collected?

        (   )$_1$ (stop)$^*_2$
        Yes   No

* Remove by drawing required blood.

F.18.2   Documentation items (Facsimile)

32. Form reviewed by:

    a. Name: _____

    b. HPT Cer. No.   __ __ - __ __

    c. Date: $\overline{\text{Mo}}$ - $\overline{\text{Day}}$ - $\overline{\text{Yr}}$

33. Data entered by:

    a. Name: _____

    b. HPT Cer. No.   __ __ - __ __

    c. Date: $\overline{\text{Mo}}$ - $\overline{\text{Day}}$ - $\overline{\text{Yr}}$

F.18.3   Comment

See Section 12.5.13.

F.19 FULL-PAGE VERSUS TWO-COLUMN LAYOUT

F.19.1 Full-page layout

F.19.1.1 (Unsatisfactory; photo reproduction)

1. When were you born? _____/_____/_____
   <small>MONTH   DAY   YEAR</small>

2. Were you born in the U.S.? ☐ No   ☐ Yes
   IF YES, in what state? _____

3. Sex: ☐ Male   ☐ Female

4. Race: ☐ White   ☐ Black   ☐ Hispanic   ☐ Asian
   ☐ American Indian   ☐ Other_____

5. Please circle the highest grade in school you have completed:

   0   1   2   3   4   5   6   7   8   9   10   11   12   13   14   15   16   16+

6. Have you smoked at least 100 cigarettes (five packs) in your entire life?   ☐ No   ☐ Yes   IF YES ➤

   > a) How old were you when you first started regular smoking?_____years old
   > b) On the average of the entire time you smoked, how many cigarettes did you smoke per day?_____cigarettes per day
   > c) Did you ever stop smoking cigarettes for a year or more, and then start again?   ☐ No   ☐ Yes, stopped for____years
   > d) Do you smoke cigarettes now?
   >   ☐ No   IF NO, how old were you when you stopped? _____years old
   >   ☐ Yes   IF YES, how many cigarettes a day do you smoke now?_____cigarettes
   > e) Do you (or did you) inhale?   ☐ No, rarely   ☐ Yes, usually
   > f) Do you (or did you) smoke filter cigarettes   ☐ No, rarely   ☐ Yes, usually
   > g) Did you ever smoke cigarettes which you rolled yourself?   ☐No   ☐ Yes, for_____years

7. Have you ever smoked a pipe regularly?   ☐ No   ☐ Yes   IF YES ➤

   > a) How old were you when you started regular pipe smoking?_____years old
   > b) On the average of the entire time you smoked, how much pipe tobacco did you smoke? _____pipefuls per_____
   >   <small>(day or week)</small>
   > c) Did you ever stop smoking a pipe for a year or more and then start again?   ☐ No   ☐ Yes, stopped for_____years
   > d) Do you smoke a pipe now?
   >   ☐ No   IF NO, how old were you when you stopped?_____years old
   >   ☐ Yes   IF YES, how much tobacco do you smoke now?_____pipefuls per_____
   >   <small>(day or week)</small>

8. Have you ever smoked cigars regularly?   ☐ No   ☐ Yes   IF YES ➤

   > a) How old were you when you started regular cigar smoking?_____years old
   > b) On the average of the entire time you smoked, how many cigars did you smoke?_____cigars per_____
   >   <small>(day or week)</small>
   > c) Did you ever stop smoking cigars for a year or more, and then start again?   ☐ No   ☐ Yes, stopped for_____years
   > d) Do you smoke cigars now?
   >   ☐ No   IF NO, how old were you when you stopped?_____years old
   >   ☐ Yes   IF YES, how many cigars do you smoke per day or per week? _____cigars per_____
   >   <small>(day or week)</small>

F.19.1.2   (Satisfactory; photo reproduction)

PART III: Clinical Findings.

		Yes	No	Not possible to test
1) Is the femoralis artery palpable?	Right leg	( )	( )	( )
	Left leg	( )	( )	( )

		Yes	No	Not possible to test
2) Is the dorsalis pedis artery palpable?	Right foot	( )	( )	( )
	Left foot	( )	( )	( )

PART IV: Oscillometric Examination. The upper margin of the cuff for the knee measurement should be placed two (2) inches below the lower margin of the patella. The lower margin of the cuff for the ankle reading should be placed two (2) inches above the apex of the internal malleolus. The patient should be reclining and the knee unflexed with the ankle in a neutral position. If a particular reading cannot be taken because the site is missing or the patient has a lesion in the area of the site of the measurement, please indicate this by writing "Not Possible" in the space reserved for recording the measurement. Record the results in mm.

1) Record the oscillometric readings for the RIGHT leg, for the two sites indicated.

   a) Two inches below the lower margin of the patella _____ _____mm.

   b) Two inches above the apex of the internal malleolus _____ _____mm.

2) Record the oscillometric readings for the LEFT leg, for the two sites indicated.

   a) Two inches below the lower margin of the patella _____ _____mm.

   b) Two inches above the apex of the internal malleolus _____ _____mm.

F.19.2 Two-column layout

F.19.2.1 Right-hand justification for response boxes (Satisfactory; photo reproduction)

Item 6 continued:

C) How much exertion would it typically take to precipitate such an episode (check only one)?

Walking at less than ordinary pace ...... (1)[25]
Walking at an ordinary pace .... (2)
Walking hurriedly or up hill, or climbing stairs .... (3)
Not related to exertion .... (4)

D) Can excitement, emotion, or meals precipitate such an episode? .... ( )Yes ( )No [26]

E) Does rest typically relieve such an episode?

Not at all .... (1)[27]
After more than 10 minutes .... (2)
In less than 10 minutes .... (3)
Rest not used .... (4)

F) Does nitroglycerin typically relieve such an episode?

Not at all .... (1)[28]
After more than 10 minutes .... (2)
In less than 10 minutes .... (3)
Nitroglycerin not used .... (4)

G) What has been the longest duration of such an episode?

Less than 10 minutes .... (1)[29]
10 to 30 minutes .... (2)
More than 30 minutes .... (3)

H) Have any of the episodes been such that rest or nitroglycerin did *NOT* bring relief in the typical manner? ( )Yes ( )No [30]

I) Did the patient get medical attention in connection with any episode of pain, aching, etc., during this period? .... ( )Yes ( )No [31]

If *NO*, proceed to item 6-J.

If *YES*, please give the place where such medical information may be found:

Then avail yourself of this information and answer items i through viii below. (If medical attention was obtained on more than one occasion, answer the questions in connection with the most serious of the episodes.)

Item 6-I continued:

ii) Any evidence of shock? .... ( )Yes ( )No [33]

iii) Arrhythmia? .... ( )Yes ( )No [34]

iv) Leucocytosis? .... (3)Not Done (1)Yes (2)No [35]

If *YES*, what was the highest recorded value (cells/mm^3)? ....

v) Elevated sedimentation rate? .... (3)Not Done (1)Yes (2)No [36]

If *YES*, what was the highest recorded value (mm/hr)? ....

vi) Abnormal SGOT? .... (3)Not Done (1)Yes (2)No [37]

If *YES*, what was the highest recorded value (state units)? ....

vii) Abnormal LDH? .... (3)Not Done (1)Yes (2)No [38]

If *YES*, what was the highest recorded value (state units)? ....

viii) ECG evidence of a new myocardial infarction?

ECG not done .... (1)[39]
Negative .... (2)
Suggestive .... (3)
Definite .... (4)

J) Did any of the episodes since the last completed follow-up visit result in a diagnosis of:

	Suspect	Yes	No
i) Myocardial infarction?	(3)	(1)	(2)[40]
ii) Acute coronary insufficiency?	(3)	(1)	(2)[41]
iii) Angina pectoris?	(3)	(1)	(2)[42]

7) Has the patient required nitroglycerin since his last completed follow-up visit? ( )Yes ( )No [43]

F.19.2.2   *Left-hand justification for response boxes (Satisfactory; photo reproduction)*

12. If death was not witnessed, what is the estimated time between when the patient was last known to be alive and the death?

[1] ≤ 1 minute   47

[2] 1–4 minutes

[3] 5–29 minutes

[4] 30–59 minutes

[5] 1–24 hours

[6] > 24 hours

[7] Unknown

[8] Death witnessed

PART V: Pathology Noted on Autopsy

13. Was an autopsy performed?

[1] Yes   48

[2] No

Were there findings of the following? (Check each item)

		Inadequate	
Yes	No	Information	
[1]	[2]	[3]	A. Esophagitis	49
[1]	[2]	[3]	B. Gastritis	50
[1]	[2]	[3]	C. Superficial gastric erosion(s)	51

13. (Continued)

		Inadequate	
Yes	No	Information	
[1]	[2]	[3]	M. Other non-neoplastic renal pathology
[1]	[2]	[3]	N. Malignant neoplasm
[1]	[2]	[3]	O. Benign neoplasm
[1]	[2]	[3]	P. Recent acute myocardial infarction
[1]	[2]	[3]	Q. Old myocardial infarction or scar
[1]	[2]	[3]	R. Rupture of myocardium
[1]	[2]	[3]	S. Myocardial aneurysm
[1]	[2]	[3]	T. Recent coronary occlusion by thrombosis or embolism
[1]	[2]	[3]	U. Recent coronary occlusion by hemorrhage into plaque
[1]	[2]	[3]	V. Pulmonary embolism

F.19.3   Comment

The layout for F.19.1.1 is confusing and cluttered. The lack of a standard location for check spaces adds to the confusion. The layout in F.19.1.2 is cleaner. It requires more page space but makes the response positions of the items easier to locate than in F.19.1.1.

The two-column layout in the examples shown in F.19.2 makes more efficient use of page space than is the case in F.19.1.2. The examples in F.19.2 differ with regard to location of check positions; either arrangement is acceptable.

F.20 LAYOUT FOR SKIP ITEMS

F.20.1 Arrows and pointers

F.20.1.1 (Unsatisfactory; photo reproduction)

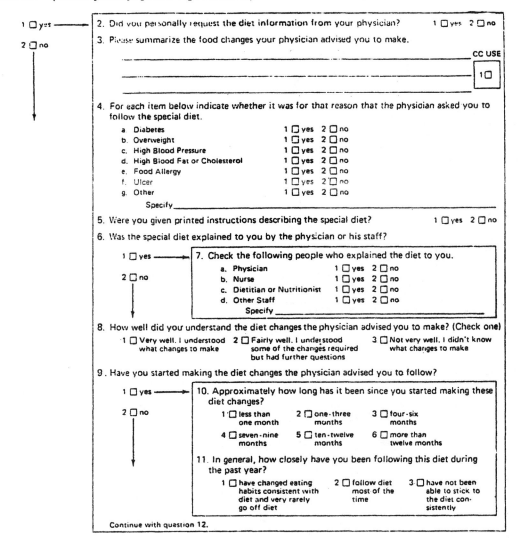

F.20.1.2   (Unsatisfactory; photo reproduction)

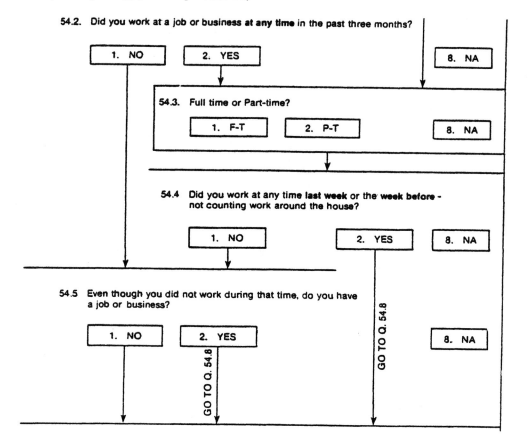

54.2. Did you work at a job or business at **any time** in the past three months?

| 1. NO | 2. YES | 8. NA |

54.3. Full time or Part-time?

| 1. F-T | 2. P-T | 8. NA |

54.4 Did you work at any time **last week** or the week before - not counting work around the house?

| 1. NO | 2. YES | 8. NA |

54.5 Even though you did not work during that time, do you have a job or business?

| 1. NO | 2. YES | 8. NA |

GO TO Q. 54.8

F.20.1.3   (Satisfactory; photo reproduction)

7. Have you ever smoked a pipe regularly?   ☐ No   ☐ Yes   **IF YES** ☛

> a) How old were you when you started regular pipe smoking?_____years old
> b) On the average of the entire time you smoked, how much pipe tobacco did you smoke?_____pipefuls per_____
> (day or week)
> c) Did you ever stop smoking a pipe for a year or more and then start again?   ☐ No   ☐ Yes, stopped for_____years
> d) Do you smoke a pipe now?
> ☐ No   IF NO, how old were you when you stopped?_____years old
> ☐ Yes   IF YES, how much tobacco do you smoke now?_____pipefuls per_____
> (day or week)

8. Have you ever smoked cigars regularly?   ☐ No   ☐ Yes   **IF YES** ☛

> a) How old were you when you started regular cigar smoking?_____years old

F.20.1.4 *(Satisfactory; photo reproduction)*

If the shipyard worker is DECEASED

a. Date of Death: _____
   Mo.   Day   Year

b. Place of Death: _____
   City   State

c. Cemetery: _____
   Name   City   State

d. Cause of Death: _____

Please **GO TO PAGE 3** (YELLOW FORM) and answer the questions ABOUT THE DECEASED.

F.20.2 SKIP or GO TO items

F.20.2.1 *(Satisfactory; facsimile)*

9. (AAW) Are you presently taking any
   drugs prescribed by a physician?

   ( )₁ (stop)₂
   Yes   No

   If No, go to Item 10, Page 4

   If Yes, answer items a thru d

F.20.2.2 *(Satisfactory; photo reproduction)*

11. Have you ever had any surgery or operations, even minor ones such as tonsillectomy?

    YES ☐ ASK Q. 12   NO ☐ SKIP TO Q. 13   UNKNOWN ☐ SKIP TO Q. 13

    IF YES, ASK:

12. Could you tell me:

(A) What type of surgery?				IF YES, ASK B, C: (B) How old were you at the time?	(C) Were you hospitalized?		
	YES	NO	UNK		YES	NO	UNK
Tonsillectomy							
Appendectomy							
*Hysterectomy (removal of uterus)							
*Removal of ovaries							

F.20.3 Comment

The layouts for F.20.1.1 and F.20.1.2 are cluttered. Those for F.20.1.3 and F.20.1.4 are better.

The illustrations in F.20.2.1 and F.20.2.2 involve use of GO TO or SKIP instructions in place of arrows or pointers. Arrows and pointers have more visual impact than GO TO or SKIP instructions, but they add to the clutter of the form, as seen in F.20.1.1 and F.20.1.2. GO TO or SKIP instructions are preferable to arrows or pointers when the form involves a lot of skips on the same page or when the skips are to other pages of the form.

F.21   INSTRUCTIONAL INFORMATION

F.21.1   Shading or highlighting (Photo reproduction)

PLEASE COMPLETE THE <u>ONE</u> SECTION BELOW WHICH APPLIES TO YOU.

If you ARE the person named above ▶

> **Did you ever work in a shipyard?**
>
> 1 ☐ YES Please **GO TO PAGE 3** and complete the yellow form. Skip page 2.
>
> 0 ☐ NO Please **RETURN THIS QUESTIONNAIRE** in the enclosed envelope so we can correct our records and prevent another mailing to you. Do not complete the remainder of this questionnaire.

If you ARE NOT the person named above ▶

> ☐ Please check box and **COMPLETE PAGE 2** of the white form.

THIS SURVEY IS AUTHORIZED UNDER THE DOE ORGANIZATION ACT PL 95-91. OMB NO. 1901-0250 EXP. DATE 9/30/84

F.21.2   Boxes

F.21.2.1   *Boxed instructions for entire form (Photo reproduction)*

> Complete this form for all candidates who remain eligible after BL 1. Proceed immediately to Form 04CP once this form is completed.
>
> Answers to questions with boxed ☐ item numbers must be reviewed by an HPT physician. Questions preceded by (AAW) are to be asked as written; those preceded by (SAW) are to be shown as written using HPT flashcards. Questions preceded by (DA) are to be answered using information from previous items.

F.21.2.2   *Boxed instructions for specific item (Photo reproduction)*

14. BL 2 Appointment:

                                   AM

    a. Time of day: __ __ : __ __ PM

    b. Day of week: _____

    c. Date: __ __ - __ __ - __ __
                 Mo   Day   Yr

> NOTE: Date in item 14 must be at least 7 days after date in item 20b on Form 01CP

15. Candidate given:

    ( )1 Appointment card
    ( )1 Participant reminder form
    ( )1 Informed consent material
    ( )1 Material introducing HPT
    ( )1 Other (specify):

F.21.3   Comment

Instructional information contained on a form should be identified. This is done via reverse image printing, pointers, and use of a different print font in F.21.1. Boxes are used to set off instructional material in F.21.2.

F.22 UNFORMATTED RESPONSES

F.22.1 (Unsatisfactory; photo reproduction)

34	IS THERE A PREVIOUS HISTORY OF STROKE? 1. _____YES 2. _____NO 3. _____ UNKNOWN
35	IF YES, MONTH_____ DAY_____ YEAR _____ UNKNOWN .
36	IF THERE WAS A CEREBROVASCULAR DISEASE DIAGNOSIS: APPROXIMATE DATE OF ONSET: MONTH_____ DAY_____YR. _____ DATE UNKNOWN _____NO STROKE ___
37	ACTIVITY AT ONSET OF STROKE _____ UNKNOWN _____ NO STROKE ___
38	PLACE AT ONSET OF STROKE _____ UNKNOWN _____NO STROKE ___
39	APPROXIMATE HOUR OF ONSET OF STROKE _____ UNKNOWN_____ NO STROKE ___

F.22.2 (Satisfactory; photo reproduction)

2) Has the patient been hospitalized at any time since his last quarterly examination? . . . ( ) ( )
                                                                                           Yes   No

If YES, give the date, duration and reason for each hospitalization in the space below.

DATE	DURATION (Days)	REASON
....	....
....	....
....	....

F.22.3 (Satisfactory; facsimile)

7. Did the participant die in a
   hospital?

   ( )   ( )   ( )
   Yes 1 No 2 Unk 3

   If Yes, give the name and address
   of the hospital and attending
   physician.

   a. Name and address of hospital.

   ┌─────────────────────────┐
   │   │
   │   │
   │   │
   │   │
   └─────────────────────────┘

   b. Name and address of attending
      physician.

   ┌─────────────────────────┐
   │   │
   │   │
   │   │
   └─────────────────────────┘

F.22.4 Comment

There is not enough vertical space between lines in F.22.1. There should be at least ¼″ of separation between lines, as in F.22.2, or the form should provide a boxed space of adequate size, as in F.22.3, when handwritten responses are required.

F.23 FORMATTED RESPONSES

F.23.1 Boxes (Photo reproduction)

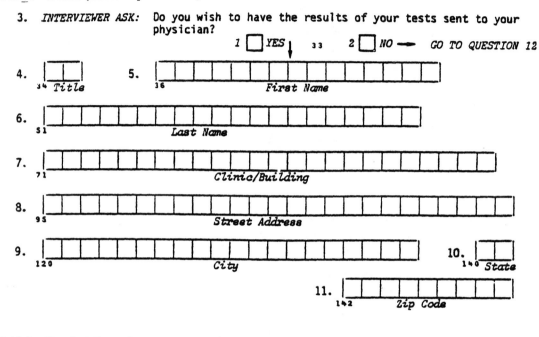

F.23.2 Hatched lines (Photo reproduction)

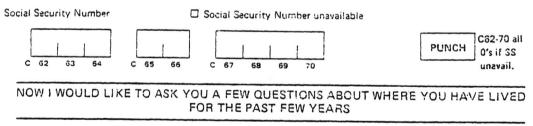

F.23.3 Comment

See Section 12.6.8.

F.24 LAYOUT FOR CHECK POSITIONS

F.24.1 Varied order for yes-no responses (Unsatisfactory; photo reproduction)

7. At least once a week, do you engage in any regular activity akin to brisk walking, jogging, bicycling, etc. long enough to work up a sweat?

  □ No
  □ Yes ——— How many times per week?_____ Activity _____

SOCIAL AND DIETARY HABITS

9. Do you smoke CIGARETTES now?   □ No □ Yes How many CIGARETTES per day? _____
   Do you drink COFFEE now?   □ No □ Yes How many CUPS per day?   _____
   Do you drink TEA now?   □ No □ Yes How many CUPS per day?   _____
   Do you drink MILK now?   □ No □ Yes How many GLASSES per day?   _____ *(1 glass = 8 oz.)*

---

12. When eating meat, do you avoid eating the fat? Yes □ No □

13. Do you often add salt to your food? Yes □ No □ Pepper? Yes □ No □
    Catsup, mustard, or spices? Yes □ No □   Mayonnaise or salad oil? Yes □ No □

F.24.2 Scattered check positions (Unsatisfactory; photo reproduction)

```
3.  Long leg sitting (knees <90° flex) with arm support R/L
                  (I) without arms support ___ time
        weight distribution —symmetrical —more on L/R
        hips abd —neutral; pelvis:thigh ⚡ ___ | pelvis:thigh ⚡ ___
        hip rotation ___ neutral            | w/knees pass. ext. to ___
        trunk ___ erect ___ kyphosis ___ lateral flexion R/L
        shoulders ___ elevated ___ retracted ___ protracted
        head ___ erect ___ cradled ___ lateral flexion R/L
        LE's ___ relaxed ___ fixing in flexion ___ tonic extension knees
        UE support ___ forward R/L ___ lateral R/L ___ posterior R/L
        shifts weight to ___ L ___ recovers ___ R ___ recovers
                      ___ ant ___ recovers ___ post ___ recovers
                      ___ diag back L ___ recovers
                      ___ diag back R ___ recovers
```

F.24.3 Scattered check positions (Photo reproduction)

25. When was the last time you smoked that much? ____/____   UNKNOWN □
                                                  MONTH YEAR

26. About how many cigarettes per day did you smoke 2 years ago? _____ UNKNOWN □

27. Did you smoke cigarettes a year ago? YES □ ASK Q. 28 NO □ SKIP TO Q. 32 UNKNOWN □ SKIP TO Q. 29

IF YES, ASK:

28. About how many cigarettes did you smoke a year ago? _____ UNKNOWN □

29. Was there ever any period of time when you stopped smoking?

    YES □ ASK Q. 30-31   NO □ SKIP TO Q. 34   UNKNOWN □ SKIP TO Q. 34

F.24.4   Inadequate check space (Photo reproduction)

SCHOLARLY QUALITY OF PROGRAM FACULTY

1. ( ) DISTINGUISHED
2. ( ) STRONG
3. ( ) GOOD
4. ( ) ADEQUATE
5. ( ) MARGINAL
6. ( ) NOT SUFFICIENT FOR DOCTORAL EDUCATION

0. ( ) DON'T KNOW WELL ENOUGH TO EVALUATE

FAMILIARITY WITH WORK OF PROGRAM FACULTY

1. ( ) CONSIDERABLE FAMILIARITY
2. ( ) SOME FAMILIARITY
3. ( ) LITTLE OR NO FAMILIARITY

EFFECTIVENESS OF PROGRAM IN EDUCATING RESEARCH
      SCHOLARS/SCIENTISTS

1. ( ) EXTREMELY EFFECTIVE
2. ( ) REASONABLY EFFECTIVE
3. ( ) MINIMALLY EFFECTIVE
4. ( ) NOT EFFECTIVE

0. ( ) DON'T KNOW WELL ENOUGH TO EVALUATE

CHANGE IN PROGRAM QUALITY IN LAST FIVE YEARS

1. ( ) BETTER THAN FIVE YEARS AGO
2. ( ) LITTLE OR NO CHANGE IN LAST FIVE YEAR
3. ( ) POORER THAN FIVE YEARS AGO

0. ( ) DON'T KNOW WELL ENOUGH TO EVALUATE

F.24.5   Unsatisfactory list layout (Photo reproduction)

18. Please check Marital Status: NEVER
                                         MARRIED ☐1   MARRIED ☐2   SEPARATED ☐3   (55)
                                         DIVORCED ☐4   WIDOWED ☐5

19. How many GRADES of school, including College, did you complete? .... _____ grades(56-57)

20. Are you under treatment for high blood pressure? .... YES ☐1   NO ☐2   (58)

21. How many hours has it been since your last meal?   .... _____ hours   (59)

F.24.6   Satisfactory list layout (Contrived from F.24.5)

Please check marital status:

(   )1 Never married
(   )2 Married
(   )3 Separated
(   )4 Divorced
(   )5 Widowed

F.24.7   Excessive white space (Contrived from F.24.8)

Hepatobiliary Pathology on Autopsy (check one or more)

1. No autopsy   ( )
2. Normal liver   ( )
3. Hepatitis   ( )
4. Fatty metamorphosis   ( )
5. Cirrhosis   ( )
6. Congestion   ( )
7. Nonspecific changes   ( )
8. Gall stones   ( )
9. Other findings (please specify):   ( )

F.24.8   Eye lines (Photo reproduction)

Hepatobiliary Pathology on Autopsy (check one or more)

1. No autopsy .... ( )
2. Normal liver .... ( )
3. Hepatitis .... ( )

4. Fatty metamorphosis .... ( )
5. Cirrhosis .... ( )
6. Congestion .... ( )

7. Nonspecific changes .... ( )
8. Gall stones .... ( )
9. Other findings (please specify): .... ( )

F.24.9 Eye lines and blocking (Contrived from F.24.8)

Hepatobiliary Pathology on Autopsy (check one or more)

```
1. No autopsy ....................................................  (   )
2. Normal liver .................................................  (   )
3. Hepatitis ....................................................  (   )

4. Fatty metamorphosis ..........................................  (   )
5. Cirrhosis ....................................................  (   )
6. Congestion ...................................................  (   )

7. Nonspecific changes ..........................................  (   )
8. Gall stones ..................................................  (   )
9. Other findings (please specify) ..............................  (   )
```

F.24.10 Blocked list (Facsimile)

```
10. (AAW) Have you taken any of these
    caffeine containing, non-prescription
    drugs in the last month?  (Use HPT
    Chart 13 as a flash card if you wish)

       (   )ı  Anacin
       (   )ı  Appedrine
       (   )ı  Bromoquinine

       (   )ı  Coryban D
       (   )ı  Dexatrim
       (   )ı  Dristan

       (   )ı  Excedrin
       (   )ı  Midol
       (   )ı  Nodoz

       (   )ı  Permathene - 12
       (   )ı  Prolamine
       (   )ı  Triaminicin
       (   )ı  Vanquish
```

F.24.11 Comment

The layout in F.24.1 is confusing because of the variation in the position of the Yes-No check spaces. In question 7 the No is above the Yes. In question 9 Yes follows No. The order is reversed in questions 12 and 13.

Items F.24.2 and F.24.3 are both examples of layouts with scattered locations for check positions. Contrast these layouts with those shown for illustrations F.24.6 through F.24.10.

The parentheses for recording checks are too small and there is not enough separation between the lines in F.24.4. The lack of line separation can cause confusion when data from completed forms are keyed. A slight error in placement of a check can cause the item to be keyed incorrectly.

F.24.5 is included to illustrate the importance of layout in a list of items. The format in the example can be expected (as was the actual case) to result in an understatement of the number of people married. Unless one is careful, the first space will be used to denote a married individual because of where the word *Never* appears. The problem could be avoided with a single-column vertical layout as shown in F.24.6, or with better spacing or different placement of the check boxes.

F.24.6 through F.24.10 involve lists with vertical layouts. The layout in F.24.7 requires the respondent to identify the item to be checked on the left hand side of the page and then locate the check space on the right hand side of the page without any lines to aid the eye. Eye lines should be used, as in F.24.8 and F.24.9, when the list and check spaces are separated. Blocking, as illustrated in F.24.9, also helps to avoid confusion in locating the proper check space. Placement of the check space to the left of the item, as shown in F.24.10, avoids the need for eye lines.

F.25　FIELD DESIGNATIONS AND PRECODED RESPONSES

F.25.1　Field designations (Satisfactory; photo reproduction)

III.　FAMILY HISTORY

	Age if Living	Age at Death	Cause of* Death
20. Father	⌐45-46⌐	⌐47-48⌐	⌐49
21. Mother	⌐50-51⌐	⌐52-53⌐	⌐54
22. Brother(s) .... A	⌐55-56⌐	⌐57-58⌐	⌐59
B	⌐60-161⌐	⌐62-63⌐	⌐64
C	⌐65-66⌐	⌐67-68⌐	⌐69
D	⌐70-71⌐	⌐72-73⌐	⌐74
E	⌐75-76⌐	⌐77-78⌐	⌐79
23. Sister(s) .... A	⌐80-81⌐	⌐82-83⌐	⌐84
B	⌐85-86⌐	⌐87-88⌐	⌐89
C	⌐90-91⌐	⌐92-93⌐	⌐94
D	⌐95--96⌐	⌐97-98⌐	⌐99
E	⌐200-01⌐	⌐202-03⌐	⌐204

24. Comments: _____

_____

*Causes of Death:

    1 - Coronary Heart Disease (Heart Attack)
    2 - Stroke
    3 - Hypertensive Heart Disease
    4 - Cancer
    5 - Other Heart Disease (specify) _____
    6 - Other Disease (specify)

        _____
    7 - Accident or trauma
    8 - Unknown
    9 - Old Age

F.25.2   Precoded responses

F.25.2.1   (*Satisfactory; photo reproduction*)

10.   Which choice below would help you lose the most weight?

(Circle one.)

Jogging 1 mile. 01
Walking 3 miles. .02
Refusing one piece of cherry pie. 03
Refusing one 12-ounce soda 04

11.   Read each statement below and then circle the number to the right of the statement that best describes how
YOU feel. If you STRONGLY AGREE with a statement, circle number 1. If you STRONGLY DISAGREE,
circle number 5. Try not to circle 3 unless you are really unsure of how you feel.

(Circle one number on each line.)

	Strongly Agree	Agree	Unsure	Disagree	Strongly Disagree
a. My health is directly affected by the actions I take every day	01	02	03	04	05
b. I am doing all I can to keep myself healthy	01	02	03	04	05
c. People can't do anything to reduce their chances of having a heart attack	01	02	03	04	05
d. I am not concerned about preventive health measures	01	02	03	04	05
e. I just go on doing the things that make me less healthy even when I know I shouldn't	01	02	03	04	05

F.25.2.2   (*Photo reproduction*)

8) In your best judgment (based on a capsule
count and/or any other information or impressions obtained from the patient at this
visit), what percentage of the capsules of AL-
LOCATED medication (i.e., from bottles 1-30)
prescribed since Initial Visit 3 has the patient
actually taken?

At least 80% --- (1)[15]
At least 60% but less than 80% ----------------- (2)
At least 40% but less than 60% ----------------- (3)
At least 20% but less than 40% ----------------- (4)
Less than 20% --- (5)

F.25.2.3   (*Facsimile*)

29. (AAW) Who usually prepares the
meals you eat at home? (Use
list below to categorize response)

( )[1]   Candidate alone
( )[2]   Spouse or partner, alone
( )[3]   Someone else, alone

( )[4]   Candidate and spouse or
partner
( )[5]   Candidate and someone else
( )[6]   Other (specify)

_____

F.25.3   Comment

The numbers appearing in items 20 through 23 in F.25.1 correspond to field designations for the data entry process. The numbers appearing in F.25.2.1, in the parentheses in F.25.2.2, and next to the parentheses in F.25.2.3, correspond to defined codes for designated fields.

G. Sample manual of operations, handbook, and monitoring report

G.1 INTRODUCTION

The sample documents contained herein were provided by the Hypertension Prevention Trial (HPT), Macular Photocoagulation Study (MPS), National Cooperative Gallstone Study (NCGS), and Persantine Aspirin Reinfarction Trial (PARIS). All four trials are sketched in Appendix B.

G.2 TABLE OF CONTENTS OF THE NATIONAL COOPERATIVE GALLSTONE STUDY CLINIC MANUAL OF OPERATIONS (July 1975 Version)

G.3 LISTING OF PAGES IN THE HYPERTENSION PREVENTION TRIAL HANDBOOK (April 7, 1983 Version)[1]

1. Background

- Abbreviations
- Definitions (3 pages)
- Proposed time schedule
- HPT objectives
- Specific aims and operational tasks of Stage 1
- HPT landmark dates
- Design and operating synopsis for Stage 1
- Projected distribution of participants for Cohorts 1, 2, and 3 combined
- Minimal detectable treatment-control difference
- Test cohort distribution of participants by treatment assignment
- Anticipated distribution of participants by treatment group for Cohorts 1, 2, and 3 combined (2 pages)

1. Each line in the listing represents a page in the Handbook, except where indicated.

- Identification numbers
- Document numbering scheme (3 pages)
- HPT numbered documents (2 pages)

2. Organization

- HPT centers
- HPT bodies
- Investigative Group specifications (IG)
- Steering Committee specifications (SC)
- Executive Committee specifications (EC)
- Quality Assurance Committee specifications (QAC)
- Intervention Methods Committee specifications (IMC)
- Laboratory Committee specifications (LC)
- Treatment Effects Monitoring and Analysis Committee specifications (TEMAC)
- Policy Advisory Board specifications (PAB)
- HPT participating centers
- HPT functions by centers
- Steering Committee and Executive Committee composition
- Policy Advisory Board composition
- HPT meetings
- Steering Committee rules
- HPT Committee structure

3. Enrollment

- Major HPT inclusion and exclusion criteria
- HPT Chart 05: Exclusion conditions by form and item number (2 pages)
- HPT Chart 06: Baseline Visit 1 exclusion drugs (2 pages)
- HPT recruitment approaches
- Number of persons to be covered in recruitment mailing
- Randomization features
- HPT consent and enrollment procedures (2 pages)

4. Weight strata

- HPT weight strata
- HPT Chart 07: Minimal BL 1 body weight required for classification in the high (H) weight stratum
- HPT Chart 15: BL 1 body weight exclusion limit for a Quetelet's Index ≥ 0.0500
- HPT Chart 11: Quetelet's index by height and weight

5. Intervention

- HPT Stage 1 study treatments
- HPT Chart 13: Time schedule for intervention contacts
- Required forms and procedures for intervention contacts
- HPT Chart 16: Intervention documents list

6. Data schedule

- Forms list
- Charts list
- Flashcards list
- Required forms and related documents for data collection visits (2 pages)
- HPT Chart 18: HPT data collection examination schedule (2 pages)
- HPT procedures by data collection visit
- Blood pressure measurement
- Height measurement
- Weight measurement
- Blood collection
- Blood processing for serum collection
- Upper right arm girth measurement
- Skinfold thickness measurement
- Electrocardiogram (ECG)
- 24-hour food record collection
- 24-hour food record processing
- 24-hour food record review and mailing
- Urine collection
- Urine processing

7. Time constraints

- Cohort specifications
- Time window specifications for baseline visits
- Time window specifications for follow-up visits
- HPT Chart 13: Time schedule for intervention contacts

8. Assurance procedures

- Quality assurance procedures
- Certification and recertification schedule
- Equipment inspection and maintenance schedule
- Clinic certification and recertification
- Personnel certification and recertification

- BP observer certification and recertification specifications
- Center director certification and recertification specifications
- Clinic coordinator certification and recertification specifications
- Data entry operator certification and recertification specifications
- Dietary interventionist certification and recertification specifications
- Food record documentor certification and recertification specifications
- Laboratory technician certification and recertification specifications
- ECG technician certification and recertification specifications
- Skinfold observer certification and recertification specifications
- Study physician certification and recertification specifications
- Wt-Ht observer certification and recertification specifications
- General inspection and maintenance procedures
- Standard BP manometer inspection procedure
- Standard BP manometer maintenance procedure
- Random zero BP manometer inspection procedure
- Random zero blood pressure manometer maintenance procedures (2 pages)
- Scale inspection procedure
- Scale maintenance procedure
- Skinfold caliper inspection procedure
- Room thermometer inspection procedure

9. Policy matters

- Design and data separation principles
- HPT policy prohibitions
- HPT document access policy
- HPT publicity policy
- HPT authorship policy
- HPT presentation and publication policy
- HPT ancillary study policy
- HPT abstract submission clearance policy (2 pages)
- HPT external presentation clearance procedure
- HPT manuscript clearance procedure
- HPT distributed data analysis policy

10. Miscellaneous

- Medical management principles
- Clinic supply procedures
- Document storage and distribution
- Center to center communications ground rules (2 pages)

- Exercise and diet preparation for BL 1, 2, 3, IE and all FUs
- Data rounding rules
- Data entry and correction procedures
- Data documentation assurance

G.4 SAMPLE TABLES FROM MACULAR PHOTOCOAGULATION STUDY TREATMENT MONITORING REPORT (January 31, 1982 Report)

Full report available via the National Technical Information Service, Springfield, VA, accession no. PB83-168-179.

Available information* by assignment, SMD study, 01-31-82

	Untreated			Treated		
Visit	Completed	Missed	Delinquent†	Completed	Missed	Delinquent†
Initial visit	111	—	—	113	—	—
Treatment visit	—	—	—	113	—	—
Post-treatment (6–weeks)	—	—	—	106	—	—
Follow-up 01 (3 months)	97	1	3	100	0	1
Follow-up 02 (6 months)	81	3	0	81	1	2
Follow-up 03 (12 months)	52	0	1	53	0	0
Follow-up 04 (18 months)	23	0	0	18	2	0
Follow-up 05 (24 months)	10	0	1	10	0	1
Follow-up 06 (30 months)	0	0	0	2	0	0
All follow-up visits	263	4	5	264	3	4
All visits	374	4	5	596	5	5

*The numbers in this table reflect clinic forms received and entered at the coordinating center.

†Delinquent visits (visits for which the time window has expired, but no form has been received in the coordinating center).

Change in visual acuity from initial visit (IV) to specified follow-up visits (FV), SMD study

	Untreated	*Treated*	
Distribution of change from IV to FV01:			
> 1.5 lines better	4 (4.1)	16 (16.0)	
< 1.5 lines change	45 (46.4)	57 (57.0)	
1.5–3.5 lines worse	23 (23.7)	9 (9.0)	
3.5–5.5 lines worse	15 (15.5)	4 (4.0)	
5.5–7.5 lines worse	8 (8.2)	6 (6.0)	
> 7.5 lines worse	2 (2.1)	8 (8.0)	
Total eyes	97	100	
Distribution of change from IV to FV02:			
> 1.5 lines better	4 (4.9)	16 (19.8)	
< 1.5 lines change	22 (27.2)	38 (46.9)	
1.5–3.5 lines worse	18 (22.2)	13 (16.0)	
3.5–5.5 lines worse	13 (16.0)	1 (1.2)	$p = 0.06$
5.5–7.5 lines worse	8 (9.9)	6 (7.4)	
> 7.5 lines worse	16 (19.8)	7 (8.6)	
Total eyes	81	81	
Distribution of change from IV to FV04:			
> 1.5 lines better	2 (8.7)	0 (0.0)	
< 1.5 lines change	5 (21.7)	11 (61.1)	
1.5–3.5 lines worse	2 (8.7)	1 (5.6)	
3.5–5.5 lines worse	1 (4.3)	2 (11.1)	$p = 0.06$
5.5–7.5 lines worse	5 (21.7)	0 (0.0)	
> 7.5 lines worse	8 (34.6)	4 (22.2)	
Total eyes	23	18	
Distribution of change from IV to LAST FV after FV01:			
> 1.5 lines better	7 (8.3)	14 (17.1)	
< 1.5 lines change	16 (19.0)	33 (40.2)	
1.5–3.5 lines worse	14 (16.7)	8 (9.8)	
3.5–5.5 lines worse	9 (10.7)	15 (18.3)	$p = 0.00003$
5.5–7.5 lines worse	13 (15.5)	3 (3.7)	
> 7.5 lines worse	25 (29.8)	9 (11.0)	
Total eyes	84	82	

Number of patients with selected baseline characteristics, SMD study

	Untreated	*Treated*		*Untreated*	*Treated*
Study Eye			**Diabetes**		
Right	66 (59.5)	60 (53.1)	No	105 (94.6)	109 (96.5)
Left	45 (40.5)	53 (46.9)	Yes or ?	6 (5.4)	4 (3.5)
Sex			**Hypertension**		
Male	63 (56.8)	46 (40.7)	None	23 (20.7)	16 (14.2)
Female	48 (43.2)	67 (59.3)	BP > 140/80 or on	88 (79.3)	95 (84.1)
Race			medication		
Caucasian	111 (100.0)	113 (100.0)	**Cigarette use**		
Black	0 (0.0)	0 (0.0)	Little or none	84 (75.7)	86 (76.1)
Other	0 (0.0)	0 (0.0)	> 10 per day	27 (24.3)	27 (23.9)
Histo belt resident			**Aspirin use**		
Never	54 (48.6)	57 (50.4)	< 4 per week	87 (78.4)	79 (69.9)
Ever	57 (51.4)	56 (49.6)	4–28 per week	22 (19.8)	27 (23.9)
Presently	38 (34.2)	38 (33.6)	> 28 per week	2 (1.8)	7 (6.2)

G.5 LISTING OF TABLES IN THE FINAL TREATMENT EFFECTS MONITORING REPORT[2] OF THE PERSANTINE ASPIRIN REINFARCTION STUDY (October 15, 1979 Database)

Section 1. Patient follow-up

- Status of patients by treatment group
- Number and percentage missed visits by treatment group and follow-up visit

Section 2. Fatal and nonfatal events

- Number and percentage dead by treatment group and cause of death (15 pages)
- Percentage dead by selected baseline characteristics and treatment group (4 pages)
- Percentage of patients with specified nonfatal events as reported on follow-up visit forms by treatment group (3 pages)
- Number and percentage of patients with specified nonfatal events as classified by the Mortality and Morbidity Committee by treatment group
- Percentage of patients with de novo and recurrent angina by specified baseline characteristics and treatment group (2 pages)
- Percentage of fatal and nonfatal events by treatment group (6 pages)
- Number and percentage fatal and nonfatal events as classified by the Mortality and Morbidity Committee by treatment group
- Plot of Z-values for observed differences in proportion of deaths and critical boundaries for $\alpha = 0.05$ (2 pages)
- Plot of Z-values for observed differences in proportion of coronary deaths or definite MIs and critical boundaries
- Plot of Z-values for observed differences in proportion of deaths or definite MIs and critical boundaries for $\alpha = 0.05$ (2 pages)
- Percentage of selected fatal and nonfatal events by clinic and treatment group (7 pages)
- Cumulative fatal and nonfatal event rates and number of patient intervals by treatment group and months of follow-up (5 pages)
- Lifetable plots by treatment groups of:
  - Death—all causes
  - Coronary death

2. Supplied by Persantine Aspirin Reinfarction Study Coordinating Center, April 1983.

- Sudden coronary death
- Definite nonfatal MIs
- Fatal or nonfatal pulmonary coronary death or definite MI
- Fatal or nonfatal pulmonary embolism or thrombophlebitis
- Death—all causes or definite MI
- Cardiovascular (CV) death or any CV event, new angina excluded
- Death—all causes or any CV event, new angina excluded
- New angina
- CV death or any CV event
- Death—all causes or any CV event
- Percentage of patients hospitalized by reason and treatment group, all follow-up visits combined
- Percentage of patients hospitalized for specified symptoms by treatment group, all follow-up visits combined

Section 3. Adherence and side effects

- Percentage distribution of patients by adherence level and follow-up visits (2 pages)
- Percentage distribution of patients by number of tablets prescribed and follow-up visits
- Percentage of patients with non-compliance as defined by the urine salicylate and urine dipyridamole tests by follow-up visit and treatment group (3 pages)
- Percentage of patients with non-compliance as defined by the urine salicylate and urine dipyridamole tests by follow-up visit and treatment group, excluding patients on zero prescription (3 pages)
- Percentage of patients with non-compliance as defined by the urine salicylate and urine dipyridamole tests by clinic, follow-up visit and treatment group (10 pages)
- Percentage of all possible tablets taken, by clinic and treatment group, all follow-up visits combined
- Percentage of all possible tablets taken, by follow-up visit and treatment group, all clinics combined
- Percentage of patients with reduced level of adherence by reason and treatment group, all follow-up visits combined (2 pages)

- Percentage of patients complaining of specific types of problems by treatment group, all follow-up visits combined
- Percentage of patients with reduced prescription by reason and treatment group, all follow-up visits combined
- Number of side effects forms submitted, by clinic and treatment group
- Percentage of patients with side effects forms by reason and by treatment group, all follow-up visits combined (2 pages)
- Mean urine salicylate and percent of patients with urine salicylate level above 10 mg/100 ml by visit and treatment group
- Percentage of patients with positive dipyridamole test for specified visits by treatment group
- Percentage of patients using or prescribed specific types of medication since entry, by follow-up visit and treatment group (2 pages)

Section 4. Laboratory and clinical findings

- Percentage of patients reporting specified symptoms by treatment group, all follow-up visits combined
- Percentage of patients with one or more laboratory or clinical measurements outside given limits by treatment group, all follow-up visits combined (2 pages)

- Percentage of patients with one or more laboratory or clinical measurements outside given limits by treatment group, all follow-up visits combined excluding patients outside the limits at baseline (2 pages)
- Distribution of changes from baseline to first annual visit of laboratory measurements by treatment group (5 pages)
- Distribution of changes from baseline to second annual visit of laboratory measurements by treatment group (5 pages)
- Distribution of changes from baseline to third annual visit of laboratory measurements by treatment group (5 pages)
- Distribution of changes from baseline to fourth annual visit of laboratory measurements by treatment group (5 pages)
- Percentage of patients with changes from baseline to third anual visit in systolic blood pressure and fasting glucose by selected baseline characteristics and treatment group (4 pages)

Section 5. Non-study drug usage

- Percentage of patients using non-study medications by treatment group, all follow-up visits combined (2 pages)
- Percentage of patients using acetaminophen or dextropropoxyhene hydrochloride, by follow-up visit

H. Budget summary for Hypertension Prevention Trial Data Coordinating Center

The tables in this Appendix are from documents prepared by the Hypertension Prevention Trial (HPT) Data Coordinating Center (DCC). See Sketch 13, Appendix B, for design details. The ceiling support levels reported in Table H-1 correspond to actual values recorded in the Notice of Grant Award from the National Heart, Lung, and Blood Institute (August 17, 1981). The total direct cost figures in Table H-2 are from tables prepared by the DCC in a rebudgeting process, prior to the award. Final negotiations led to a modest reduction in the funds awarded for each of the five years, thereby accounting for small discrepancies in the total direct costs in Table H-2 compared to Table H-1.

Table H-1 DCC ceiling support levels as specified in NHLBI Notice of Grant Award

| Study year | Time period covered | | Ceiling DCC support level |
	Start	End	
01	Sept. 1, 1981	Aug. 31, 1982	$ 297,120
02	Sept. 1, 1982	Aug. 31, 1983	$ 524,963
03	Sept. 1, 1983	Aug. 31, 1984	$ 590,080
04	Sept. 1, 1984	Aug. 31, 1985	$ 636,524
05	Sept. 1, 1985	Aug. 31, 1986	$ 551,670
Total			2,600,357

Table H-2 Projected allocation of funds by budget category and year of study

| Category | Year of study | | | | |
	01	02	03	04	05
1. Personnel*	$136,224	$198,441	$224,148	$237,596	$251,851
2. Consultant	5,750	5,750	5,750	5,750	5,750
3. Equipment	8,660	500	550	605	731
4. Supplies	4,250	4,800	5,450	6,200	6,750
5. Travel (Table H-4)	34,000	35,750	41,140	45,258	32,252
a. DCC-related	17,000	17,050	16,940	18,618	11,728
b. NonDCC-related	17,000	18,700	24,200	26,640	20,524
6. Other expenses (Table H-5)	112,610	284,136	317,920	346,029	258,648
a. DCC-related	49,666	72,182	98,003	118,884	121,775
b. NonDCC-related	62,944	211,954	219,917	227,145	136,873
7. Total direct costs	301,494	529,377	594,958	641,438	555,982

*Includes salaries as well as cost of fringe benefits.

Table H-3   Projected staffing patterns by year of study, in fulltime equivalents (FTEs)*

Study position†	Year of study				
	01	02	03	04	05
A. Professional					
✓ DCC director	0.20	0.20	0.20	0.20	0.20
✓ DCC deputy director	0.20	0.20	0.20	0.20	0.20
✓ Senior statistician	0.20	0.20	0.20	0.20	0.20
✓ Junior statistician	0.15	0.40	0.40	0.40	0.20
✓ Physician coinvestigator	0.05	0.10	0.10	0.10	0.10
✓ Nutritionist	0.10	0.10	0.10	0.10	0.10
✓ Research associate	0.50	0.50	0.50	0.50	0.50
✓ Research associate	0.10	0.20	0.20	0.20	0.20
✓ DCC coordinator	1.00	1.00	1.00	1.00	1.00
Senior programmer	1.00	1.00	1.00	1.00	1.00
Junior programmer	—	0.50	0.50	0.50	0.50
Assistant programmer	0.20	0.50	0.75	0.75	0.75
Total professional FTEs	3.70	4.90	5.15	5.15	4.95
B. Support					
Secretary	0.50	1.00	1.00	1.00	1.00
Secretary	0.20	0.50	0.75	0.75	0.75
Clerk-typist	0.65	0.65	0.65	0.65	0.65
Administrator	0.15	0.15	0.15	0.15	0.15
Administrator	0.10	0.10	0.10	0.10	0.10
Total support FTEs	1.60	2.40	2.65	2.65	2.65
C. Total FTEs	5.30	7.30	7.80	7.80	7.60

*The corresponding table submitted to the NHLBI contained actual projected salaries for each person or position listed.

†Positions preceded by the symbol ✓ had a named individual listed in the application. Those not so identified were designated in the proposal as TBA (to be appointed).

Table H-4 Projected travel expenses by year of study*

	Study year				
Type of travel	01	02	03	04	05
A. Travel for DCC staff					
1. Advisory-Review Committee:					
Person meetings/year	2	2	2	2	2
Cost	$ 1,000	$ 1,100	$ 1,210	$ 1,332	$ 1,466
2. Steering Committee:					
Person meetings/year	6	6	6	4	4
Cost	$ 3,000	$ 3,300	$ 2,420	$ 2,664	$ 1,466
3. Executive Committee:					
Person meetings/year	2	2	2	2	2
Cost	$ 1,000	$ 1,100	$ 1,210	$ 1,332	$ 1,466
4. Standing subcommittees:					
Person meetings/year	2	2	2	2	2
Cost	$ 1,000	$ 1,100	$ 1,210	$ 1,332	$ 1,466
5. Treatment Effects Monitoring Committee:					
Person meetings/year	3	3	6	6	3
Cost	$ 1,500	$ 1,650	$ 3,630	$ 3,996	$ 2,199
6. Training sessions for clinic personnel:					
Person sessions/year	3	3	3	3	0
Cost	$ 1,500	$ 1,650	$ 1,815	$ 1,998	0
7. Clinic site visits:					
Person site visits/year	12	8	4	4	0
Cost	$ 6,000	$ 4,400	$ 2,420	$ 2,664	0
8. Professional meetings:					
Person meetings/year	4	5	5	5	5
Cost	$ 2,000	$ 2,750	$ 3,025	$ 3,300	$ 3,665
Total DCC travel	$17,000	$17,050	$16,940	$18,618	$11,728
B. Travel for non-DCC staff					
1. Executive Committee:					
Person meetings/year	4	6	6	6	6
Cost	$ 2,000	$ 3,300	$ 3,630	$ 3,996	$ 4,398
2. Standing subcommittees:					
Person meetings/year	6	6	6	6	6
Cost	$ 3,000	$ 3,300	$ 3,630	$ 3,996	$ 4,398
3. Treatment Effects Monitoring Committee:					
Person meetings/year	6	6	12	12	6
Cost	$ 3,000	$ 3,300	$ 7,260	$ 7,992	$ 4,398
4. Food Record Coding Center personnel:					
Person trips/year	4	4	4	4	2
Cost	$ 2,000	$ 2,200	$ 2,420	$ 2,664	$ 1,466
5. Study consultants:					
Person trips/year	14	12	12	12	8
Cost	$ 7,000	$ 6,600	$ 7,260	$ 7,992	$ 5,864
Total other travel	$17,000	$18,700	$24,200	$26,640	$20,524
C. Total travel (Sum of parts A and B)	$34,000	$35,750	$41,140	$45,258	$32,252

*Costs calculated assuming $500 per person trip in year 01 and increased by 10% each year thereafter.

Table H-5 Other DCC expenses by year of study

Item	01	02	03	04	05
A. Johns Hopkins (JHU)					
1. Computing time	$ 11,000	$ 19,500	$ 30,000	$ 41,000	$ 41,000
2. Intelligent terminals					
a. JHU central terminal	7,212	7,933	8,726	9,599	10,559
b. Satellite terminals (8)	27,072	59,560	65,520	72,072	44,592
3. CRT workstation terminals (2)	3,000	3,300	3,630	3,992	4,392
4. Word processor	7,200	7,920	8,712	9,588	10,548
5. Telecopier	840	924	1,016	1,118	1,230
6. Telephone line charges	1,000	1,200	1,400	1,550	1,000
7. Photocopying	3,800	4,400	4,820	5,162	5,636
8. Data entry services	1,500	2,500	4,500	4,500	4,000
9. Forms printing	3,500	2,000	2,000	1,000	0
10. Manuscript page charges	0	0	1,000	4,000	6,000
11. Postage	750	900	1,100	1,200	600
12. Microfilming	0	250	400	550	700
13. Bank vault rental	300	400	475	550	625
14. Books and journals	150	200	250	300	300
15. Equipment maintenance	400	500	550	600	650
16. Central Laboratory	3,869	48,265	48,463	49,958	13,739
17. Food Record Coding Center	2,340	63,577	54,789	49,342	13,563
18. Study insurance	19,490	21,439	23,583	25,941	28,536
Total JHU	93,423	44,768	260,934	282,022	187,670
B. Maryland Medical Research Institute (MMRI)					
19. Computing time	1,500	5,000	10,000	12,500	15,000
20. Word processor	1,080	3,960	6,534	7,191	7,911
21. Telephone line charges	400	600	800	900	800
22. Photocopying	800	1,000	1,200	1,400	1,600
23. Postage	200	300	400	500	600
24. Microfilming	0	0	100	200	300
25. Bank vault rental	0	100	150	175	200
26. Books and journals	150	200	250	300	350
27. Space rental	1,500	1,650	1,800	2,000	2,200
28. MMRI overhead	13,557	26,558	35,752	38,841	42,017
Total MMRI	19,187	39,368	56,986	64,007	70,978
C. Total (Sum of parts A and B)	112,610	284,136	317,920	346,029	258,648

Table H-6 DCC percent allocation of funds, excluding nonDCC related costs*

Category	Study year				
	01	*02*	*03*	*04*	*05*
Personnel	63.1	67.7	65.0	62.2	64.1
Equipment	4.0	0.2	0.2	0.2	0.2
Supplies	2.0	1.6	1.6	1.6	1.7
Travel	7.9	5.8	4.9	4.9	3.0
Other expenses	23.0	24.6	28.4	31.1	31.0
Total	100.0	100.0	100.0	100.0	100.0
Total cost after exclusions	$215,800	$292,973	$345,091	$381,903	$392,835

*Excluding costs for consultants (line 2, Table H-2), nonDCC travel (Part B of Table H-4), Central Laboratory, Food Record Coding Center, and study insurance (lines 16–18, Table H-5). Also excluded are costs for seven of the eight terminals (line 2b, Table H-5) and overhead payments to MMRI (line 28, Table H-5).

Table H-7 Cost of the DCC relative to total projected HPT cost

	Study year					Total 5-year cost
	01	*02*	*03*	*04*	*05*	
a. Projected dollar cost, all HPT centers combined*	879,966	2,054,880	1,597,509	1,671,896	1,541,713	7,745,964
b. DCC dollar cost (from Table H-6)	215,800	292,973	345,091	381,903	392,835	1,628,602
c. DCC cost as percentage of line a	24.5%	14.3%	21.6%	22.8%	25.5%	21.0%

*Based on totals derived from summary prepared prior to actual award. Funded totals differ only slightly from those cited above.

I. Combined bibliography

This appendix contains a listing of all citations appearing in this book, except those in Appendixes B and C. The citations are arranged in chronologic order by first author. Journal abbreviations correspond to those used by the National Library of Medicine in *Index Medicus* and MEDLINE. The numbers and letters appearing in the right-hand margin correspond to chapters and appendixes in which the citations appear.

A

1. **Abt K:** Problems of repeated significance testing. *Controlled Clin Trials* 1:377–381, **1981**.   20

2. **Alamercery Y, Lo Presti F, Karisson T, Bowden G, and IMPACT Research Group:** Functional equality of coordinating centers in a multicenter clinical trial: Experience of the International Mexiletine and Placebo Antiarrhythmic Coronary Trial: IMPACT (abstract). *Controlled Clin Trials* 3:149, **1982**.   5

3. **Amberson JB Jr, McMahon BT, Pinner M:** A clinical trial of sanocrysin in pulmonary tuberculosis. *Am Rev Tuberc* 24:401–435, **1931**.   1

4. **American Bible Society:** *The Holy Bible: Old and New Testaments.* King James Version (1611), New York, **1816**.   1

5. **Anderson LK, Hendershot RA, Schoolmaker RC:** Self-checking digit concepts. *J Systems Management* 25:36–42, **1974**.   A

6. **Anscombe FJ:** Sequential estimation. *JRSS* 40(series B):1–21, **1953**.   20

7. **Anscombe FJ:** Fixed-sample size analysis of sequential observations. *Biometrics* 10:89–100, **1954**.   20

8. **Anscombe FJ:** Sequential medical trials. *JASA* 58:365–383, **1963**.   9

9. **Anturane Reinfarction Trial Research Group:** Sulfinpyrazone in the prevention of cardiac death after myocardial infarction: The Anturane Reinfarction Trial. *N Engl J Med* 298:289–295, **1978**.   9, 18

10. **Anturane Reinfarction Trial Research Group:** Sulfinpyrazone in the prevention of sudden death after myocardial infarction. *N Engl J Med* 302:250–256, **1980**.   9, 22

11. **Armitage P:** Restricted sequential procedures. *Biometrika* 44:9–26, **1957**.   9

12. **Armitage P:** Sequential medical trials: Some comments on FJ Anscombe's paper. *JASA* 58:384–387, **1963**.   9

13. **Armitage P, McPherson CK, Rowe BC:** Repeated significance tests on accumulating data. *JRSS* 132(series A):235–244, **1969**.   9, 20

14. **Armitage P:** *Statistical Methods in Medical Research.* John Wiley and Sons, New York, **1971**.   18

15. **Armitage P:** *Sequential Medical Trials* (2nd ed.). John Wiley and Sons, New York, **1975**.   9

16. **Aspirin Myocardial Infarction Study Research Group:** *Aspirin Myocardial Infarction Study: Design, Methods, and Baseline Results.* Publ. no. 80-2106, National Heart, Lung, and Blood Institute, Bethesda, MD, **1980a**.   6

17. **Aspirin Myocardial Infarction Study Research Group:** A randomized, controlled trial of aspirin in persons recovered from myocardial infarction. *JAMA* 243:661–669, **1980b**.   16, 18

B

18. **Backstrom CH, Hursh-Cesar G:** *Survey Research* (2nd ed). John Wiley and Sons, New York, **1981**.   12

19. **Bailey NTJ:** *The Mathematical Approach to Biology and Medicine.* John Wiley and Sons, New York, **1967**.   20

20. **Barker KN:** Data collection techniques: Observation. *Am J Hosp Pharm* 37:1235-1243, **1980.**   12

21. **Barnard PJ, Wright P, Wilcox P:** Effects of response instructions and question style on the   12
ease of completing forms. *J Occup Psychol* 52:209-226, **1979.**

22. **Baron J:** The life of Edward Jenner: With illustrations of his doctrines and selections from his   1
correspondence (book review). *Br Foreign Med Rev* 6:477-497, **1838.**

23. **Bayes T:** An essay towards solving a problem in the doctrine of chances (reproduced in   1
Biometrika 45:296-315, 1958). *Philos Trans Roy Soc Lond* 53:370-418, **1763.**

24. **Beatty WK:** Searching the literature and computerized services in medicine: Guides and   2
methods for the clinician. *Ann Intern Med* 91:326-332, **1979.**

25. **Beeson PB, McDermott W, Wyndgaarden JB** (editors): *Cecil's Textbook of Medicine* (15th   7
ed). WB Saunders Co, Philadelphia, **1979.**

26. **Begg CB, Iglewicz B:** A treatment allocation procedure for sequential clinical trials. *Biometrics*   10
36:81-90, **1980.**

27. **Bégin G, Boivin M, Bellerose J:** Sensitive data collection through the random response   12
technique: Some improvements. *J Psychol* 101:53-65, **1979.**

28. **Bégin G, Boivin M:** Comparison of data gathered on sensitive questions via direct question-   12
naire, randomized response technique, and a project method. *Psychol Rep* 47:743-750, **1980.**

29. **Bégun JM, Gabriel KR:** Closure of the Newman-Keuls multiple comparisons procedure.   20
JASA 76:241-245, **1981.**

30. **Beta Blocker Heart Attack Trial Research Group:** Beta Blocker Heart Attack Trial: Design   8
features. *Controlled Clin Trials* 2:275-285, **1981.**

31. **Bishop GF, Oldendick RW, Tuchfarber AJ:** Effects of presenting one versus two sides of an   12
issue in survey questions. *Public Opinion Quart* 46:69-85, **1982.**

32. *Boston Globe (The):* Data changed to put patients in cancer test. June 30, **1980a.**   19

33. *Boston Globe (The):* Research staff feared for patient's welfare. July 1, **1980b.**   19

34. *Boston Globe (The):* Passing the buck. July 2, **1980c.**   19

35. *Boston Globe (The):* MD under fire gets new grant. July 3, **1980d.**   19

36. *Boston Sunday Globe:* Cancer research data falsified; Boston project collapses. June 29, **1980.**   19

37. **Box JF:** R. A. Fisher and the design of experiments, 1922-1926. *Am Statistician* 34:1-7, **1980.**   1

38. **Brandt AM:** Racism and research: The case of the Tuskegee Syphilis Study. *Hastings Center*   14
Report 8:21-29, Dec, **1978.**

39. **Braunwald E:** Coronary-artery surgery at the crossroads. *N Engl J Med* 297:661-663, **1977.**   2

40. **Breslow NE, Day NE:** *Statistical Methods in Cancer Research* (vol 1, pg 93). International   A
Agency for Research on Cancer, Lyon, **1980.**

41. **Bross I:** Sequential medical plans. *Biometrics* 8:188-205, **1952.**   9

42. **Bross IDJ:** Laetrile. *N Engl J Med* 307:118, **1982.**   2

43. **Brown BW Jr, Hollander M:** *Statistics: A Biomedical Introduction.* John Wiley and Sons,   18
New York, **1977.**

44. **Brown BW Jr:** Designing for cancer clinical trials: Selection of prognostic factors. *Cancer*   10
Treat Rep 64:499-502, **1980.**

45. **Brown BW Jr:** Comments on the Dupont manuscript. *Controlled Clin Trials* 4:13-17, **1983.**   20

46. **Bryan LS Jr:** Blood-letting in American medicine, 1830-1892. *Bull Hist Med* 38:516-529, **1964.**   2

47. **Bull JP:** The historical development of clinical therapeutic trials. *J Chronic Dis* 10:218-248,   1
1959.

48. **Bulpitt CJ:** *Randomised Controlled Clinical Trials.* Martinus Nijhoff Publishers, London,   18
1983.

49. **Burton BT, Hirschman GH:** Demographic analysis: End-stage renal disease and its treatment   7
in the United States. *Clin Nephrol* 11:47-51, **1979a.**

50. **Burton BT, Hirschman GH:** Treatment trends of end stage renal disease in the United States.   7
Artif Organs 3(suppl):29-33, **1979b.**

51. **Buyse ME, Staquet MJ, Sylvester RJ** (editors): *Cancer Clinical Trials: Methods and Practices.*   18
Oxford University Press, Oxford, **1984**.

C

52. **Canner PL:** Monitoring clinical trials data for evidence of adverse or beneficial treatment   20
effects (in *Essais Controles Multicentres: Principles et Problemes,* edited by JP Boissel, CR
Klimt). *Institut National de la Santé et de la Recherche Medicale* (INSERM) 76:131–149,
1977a.

53. **Canner PL:** Monitoring treatment differences in long-term clinical trials. *Biometrics* 33:603–   20
615, **1977b**.

54. **Canner PL:** Comment on "Statistical inference from clinical trials: Choosing the right p   20
value." *Controlled Clin Trials* 4:13–17, **1983a**.

55. **Canner PL:** Further comment on "Statistical inference from clinical trials: Choosing the right   20
p value." *Controlled Clin Trials* 4:35, **1983b**.

56. **Canner PL, Krol WF, Forman SA:** External quality control programs. *Controlled Clin Trials*   16
4:441–466, **1983c**.

57. **Carleton RA, Sanders CA, Burack WR:** Heparin administration after acute myocardial   8
infarction. *N Engl J Med* 263:1002–1005, **1960**.

58. **Casagrande JT, Pike MC, Smith PG:** The power function of the "exact" test for comparing   9
two binomial distributions. *Appl Statist* 27:176–180, **1978**.

59. **Cascinelli N, Davis HL Jr, Flamant R, Kenis Y, Lalanne CM, Muggia FM, Rozencweig M,**   7
Staquet MJ, Veronesi U: *Methods and Impact of Controlled Therapeutic Trials in Cancer*
(part II). Union Internationale Contre le Cancer Report Series (vol 59), Geneva, **1981**.

60. **Cassel GH, Ferris FL III:** Site visits in a multi-center ophthalmic clinical trial. *Controlled Clin*   14, 16
Trials 5:251–262, **1984**.

61. **Chalmers TC, Block JB, Lee S:** Controlled studies in clinical cancer research. *N Engl J Med*   4, 7
287:75–78, **1972**.

62. **Chalmers TC:** The impact of controlled trials on the practice of medicine. *Mt Sinai J Med*   7
41:753–759, **1974**.

63. **Chalmers TC:** Randomization of the first patient. *Med Clin North Am* 59:1035–1038, **1975**.   8

64. **Chalmers TC, Matta RJ, Smith H Jr, Kunzler A:** Evidence favoring the use of anticoagulants   7
in the hospital phase of acute myocardial infarction. *N Engl J Med* 297:1091–1096, **1977**.

65. **Chalmers TC, Silverman B, Shareck EP, Ambroz A, Schroeder B, Smith H Jr:** Randomized   2
control trials in gastroenterology with particular attention to duodenal ulcer (in *Report to the
Congress of the United States of the National Commission on Digestive Diseases,* Vol IV:
*Reports of the Workgroups: Part 2B: Subcommittee on Research—Targeted and Non-
Directed,* pp. 223–255). Publ no. NIH 79-1885, National Institute of Arthritis, Metabolism,
and Digestive Diseases, Bethesda, Md, **1978**.

66. **Chalmers TC, Smith H Jr, Blackburn B, Silverman B, Schroeder B, Reitman D, Ambroz A:** A   A
method for assessing the quality of a randomized control trial. *Controlled Clin Trials* 2:31–49,
1981.

67. **Chalmers TC:** Informed consent, clinical research and the practice of medicine. *Trans Am Clin*   7, 14
Climatol Assoc 94:204–212, **1982a**.

68. **Chalmers TC:** A potpourri of RCT topics. *Controlled Clin Trials* 3:285–298, **1982b**.   8

69. **Chandor A:** *The Facts on File Dictionary of Microcomputers.* Facts on File, Inc, New York,   A
1981.

70. **Charen T:** *MEDLARS Indexing Manual.* No. PB 271-306, National Technical Information   2
Service, Springfield, Va. **1977**.

71. **Chlebowski RT, Weiner JM, Ryden VMJ, Bateman JR:** Factors influencing the interim   19, 20
interpretation of a breast cancer trial: Danger of achieving the "expected" result. *Controlled
Clin Trials* 2:123–132, **1981**.

72. **Christiansen I, Iverson K, Skouby AP:** Benefits obtained by the introduction of a coronary   2
care unit: A comparative study. *Acta Med Scand* 189:285–291, **1971**.

73. **Cobb LA, Thomas GI, Dillard DH, Merendino KA, Bruce RA:** An evaluation of internal-mammary-artery ligation by a double-blind technic. *N Engl J Med* 260:1115–1118, **1959**. 8

74. **Cocco AE, Cocco DV:** A survey of cimetidine prescribing. *N Engl J Med* 304:1281, **1981**. 6

75. **Cochran WG:** Some methods of strengthening the common X^2 tests. *Biometrics* 10:417–451, **1954**. 9, 18

76. **Cochran WG, Cox GM:** *Experimental Designs* (2nd ed). John Wiley and Sons, Inc, New York, **1957**. 9, 10

77. **Collen MF, Cutler JL, Siegelaub AB, Cella RL:** Reliability of a self-administered medical questionnaire. *Arch Intern Med* 123:664–681, **1969**. 12

78. **Collins JF, Bingham SF, Weiss DG, Williford WO, Kuhn RM:** Some adaptive strategies for inadequate sample acquisition in Veterans Administration Cooperative Clinical Trials. *Controlled Clin Trials* 1:227–248, **1980**. 6, 14

79. **Colsky J:** Clinical investigator: The clinical investigator and evaluaion of new drugs. *Am J Hosp Pharm* 20:517–519, **1963**. 1

80. **Colton T:** A model for selecting one of two medical treatments. *JASA* 58:388–400, **1963**. 9

81. **Commission on Professional and Hospital Activities:** Diabetes mellitus: Use of oral antidiabetics. *PAS Reporter* 10:263, Nov 24, **1972**. 7

82. **Commission on Professional and Hospital Activities:** *Hospital Record Study: 1969–1975.* Joint publications of CPHA and IMS America, Ltd, Ann Arbor, Mich, **1976**. 7

83. **Committee for the Assessment of Biometric Aspects of Controlled Trials of Hypoglycemic Agents:** Report of the Committee for the Assessment of Biometric Aspects of Controlled Trials of Hypoglycemic Agents. *JAMA* 231:583–608, **1975**. 7, 10, 16, 19, 24

84. **Committee on Drugs:** Unapproved use of approved drugs: The physician, the package insert, and the FDA. *Pediatrics* 62:262–264, **1978**. 6

85. **Committee on Lipoproteins and Atherosclerosis Technical Group and the Committee on Lipoproteins and Atherosclerosis of the National Advisory Heart Council:** Evaluation of serum lipoprotein and cholesterol measurements as predictors of clinical complications of atherosclerosis: Report of a cooperative study of lipoproteins and atherosclerosis. *Circulation* 14:691–741, **1956**. 1

86. **Coordinating Center Models Project Research Group:** *Coordinating Center Models Project: A Study of Coordinating Centers in Multicenter Clinical Trials: I. Design and Methods* (in two parts). Division of Heart and Vascular Diseases, National Heart, Lung, and Blood Institute, Bethesda, Md, March, **1979a**. 5, A

87. **Coordinating Center Models Project Research Group:** *Coordinating Center Models Project: A Study of Coordinating Centers in Multicenter Clinical Trials: II. RFPs for Coordinating Centers: A Content Evaluation.* Division of Heart and Vascular Diseases, National Heart, Lung, and Blood Institute, Bethesda, Md, March, **1979b**. 3, 21

88. **Coordinating Center Models Project Research Group:** *Coordinating Center Models Project: A Study of Coordinating Centers in Multicenter Clinical Trials: IV. Terminology.* Division of Heart and Vascular Diseases, National Heart, Lung, and Blood Institute, Bethesda, Md, Aug, **1979c**. A

89. **Coordinating Center Models Project Research Group:** *Coordinating Center Models Project: A Study of Coordinating Centers in Multicenter Clinical Trials: VI. Phases of a Multicenter Trial.* Division of Heart and Vascular Diseases, National Heart, Lung, and Blood Institute, Bethesda, Md, Sept, **1979d**. 3, 5

90. **Coordinating Center Models Project Research Group:** *Coordinating Center Models Project: A Study of Coordinating Centers in Multicenter Clinical Trials: XIV. Enhancement of Methodological Research in the Field of Clinical Trials.* Division of Heart and Vascular Diseases, National Heart, Lung, and Blood Institute, Bethesda, Md, Sept, **1979e**. 1

91. **Cornfield J:** Principles of research. *Am J Ment Defic* 64:240–252, **1959**. 8

92. **Cornfield J:** A Bayesian test of some classical hypotheses—With applications to sequential clinical trials. *JASA* 61:577–594, **1966a**. 9, 20

93. **Cornfield J:** Sequential trials, sequential analysis and the likelihood principle. *Am Statistician* 20:18–23, **1966b**. 20, A

94. **Cornfield J:** The Bayesian outlook and its application (including discussion by S Geisser, HO Hartley, O Kempthorne, H Rubin). *Biometrics* 25:617–657, **1969**. 1, 20, A

95. **Cornfield J:** The University Group Diabetes Program: A further statistical analysis of the mortality findings. *JAMA* 217:1676–1687, **1971**. 7, 19

96. **Cornfield J:** Design of clinical trials (pp 303–306 in *Research Status of Spinal Manipulative Therapy*, M Goldstein, editor). Monograph no. 15, National Institute of Neurological and Communicative Disorders and Stroke, Bethesda, Md. **1975**. 20

97. **Cornfield J:** Recent methodological contributions to clinical trials. *Am J Epidemiol* 104:408–421, **1976**. 20

98. **Coronary Artery Surgery Study Research Group:** National Heart, Lung, and Blood Institute Coronary Artery Surgery Study: A multicenter comparison of the effects of randomized medical and surgical treatment of mildly symptomatic patients with coronary artery disease, and a registry of consecutive patients undergoing coronary angiography (edited by T Killip, LD Fisher, MB Mock). *Circulation* 63(suppl I):I-1—I-81, **1981**. 2, 6, 10, 11, 12, 19, 24

99. **Coronary Artery Surgery Study Research Group:** Coronary Artery Surgery Study (CASS): A randomized trial of coronary artery bypass surgery: Survival data. *Circulation* 68:939–950, **1983**. 2

100. **Coronary Artery Surgery Study Research Group:** Coronary Artery Surgery Study (CASS): A randomized trial of coronary artery bypass surgery. Comparability of entry characteristics and survival in randomized patients and nonrandomized patients meeting randomization criteria. *J Am Coll Cardiol* 3:114–128, **1984**. 14

101. **Coronary Drug Project Research Group:** *Coronary Drug Project Data and Safety Monitoring Report*. PL Canner, University of Maryland School of Medicine, Baltimore, Feb 1, **1970a**. 8

102. **Coronary Drug Project Research Group:** The Coronary Drug Project: Initial findings leading to modification of its research protocol. *JAMA* 214:1303–1313, **1970b**. 20, 24

103. **Coronary Drug Project Research Group:** The Coronary Drug Project: Findings leading to further modifications of its protocol with respect to dextrothyroxine. *JAMA* 220:996–1008, **1972**. 4, 18, 19, 20, 24

104. **Coronary Drug Project Research Group:** The Coronary Drug Project: Design, methods, and baseline results. *Circulation* 47(suppl I):I-1—I-50, **1973a**. 1, 3, 6, 8–12, 14–16, 19, 21, 23–25

105. **Coronary Drug Project Research Group:** The Coronary Drug Project: Findings leading to discontinuation of the 2.5 mg/day estrogen group. *JAMA* 226:652–657, **1973b**. 18, 20, 24

106. **Coronary Drug Project Research Group:** Factors influencing long-term prognosis after recovery from myocardial infarction—Three year findings of the Coronary Drug Project. *J Chronic Dis* 27:267–285, **1974**. 10, 18, 24

107. **Coronary Drug Project Research Group:** Clofibrate and niacin in coronary heart disease. *JAMA* 231:360–381, **1975**. 9, 11, 15, 18, 24

108. **Coronary Drug Project Research Group:** Aspirin in coronary heart disease. *J Chronic Dis* 29:625–642, **1976**. 3, 10, 19, 24

109. **Coronary Drug Project Research Group:** Practical aspects of decision making in clinical trials: The Coronary Drug Project as a case study. *Controlled Clin Trials* 1:363–376, **1981**. 19, 20, 24

110. **Cox DR:** The regression analysis of binary sequences. *JRSS* 20(series B): 215–242, **1958**. 18

111. **Cox DR:** Regression models and life tables (including discussion). *JRSS* 34(series B):187–220, **1972**. 18, A

112. **Cox DR, Hinkley DV:** *Theoretical Statistics*. Chapman and Hall, London, **1974**. 9

113. **Creighton C:** *A History of Epidemics in Britain: From the Extinction of Plague to the Present Time (vol II)*. The University Press, Cambridge, **1894**. 1

114. **Crombie AC:** Avicenna's influence on the medieval scientific tradition (pp 84–107) in *Avicenna: Scientist and Philosopher*, edited by GM Wickens). Luzac and Co, Ltd, London, **1952**. 1

115. **Crout JR:** Controlled trials: Requirements in the Food, Drug and Cosmetic Act of 1938. National Institutes of Health, Bethesda, MD. Presented at the Society for Clinical Trials Annual Meeting, Pittsburgh, May 3, **1982**. 1

116. **Cupples LA, Heeren T, Schatzkin A, Colton T:** Multiple testing of hypotheses in comparing two groups (review). *Ann Intern Med* 100:122–129, **1984**. 20

117. **Curran WJ, Shapiro ED:** *Law, Medicine, and Forensic Science* (2nd ed). Little, Brown and Co, Boston, **1970**. 1

118. **Cutler SJ, Ederer F:** Maximum utilization of the life table method in analyzing survival. *J Chronic Dis* 8:699–712, **1958**. 18

D

119. **Dawkins HC:** Multiple comparisons misused: Why so frequently used in response-curve studies (commentary)? *Biometrics* 39:789–790. **1983**. 20

120. **Day HW:** Effectiveness of an intensive coronary care area. *Am J Cardiol* 15:51–54, **1965**. 2

121. **deAlmeida DJW, Cameron WR, Condie R, Deering RB, Fitzgerald RB, Joannou P, Johnston EM, Munro DF, Smith AGL, Valle-Jones JC:** The treatment of dyspepsia in general practice: A multicenter trial. *Practitioner* 224:105–107, **1980**. 8

122. **DeBakey ME, Lawrie GM:** Aortocoronary-artery bypass: Assessment after 13 years. *JAMA* 239:837–859, **1978**. 2

123. **DeMets DL, Ware JH:** Group sequential methods for clinical trials with a one-sided hypothesis. *Biometrika* 67:651–660, **1980**. A

124. **Department of Health, Education and Welfare:** *General Provisions for Negotiated Cost-Reimbursement Type Contract with Educational Institutions.* HEW-315 (rev 7/76), Washington, **1976**. 17

125. **Department of Health, Education and Welfare:** *The Negotiated Contracting Process: A Guide for Project Officers.* Washington, Oct, **1977**. A

126. **Department of Health and Human Services:** *Administration of Grants: Federal Regulations, Title 45, Part 74.* Washington, June 9, **1981**. 17

127. **Department of Health and Human Services:** *Health Care Financing Program Statistics: The Medicare and Medicaid Data Book, 1981.* Publ no. 03128, Health Care Financing Administration, Office of Research and Demonstrations, Baltimore, April, **1982a**. 6

128. **Department of Health and Human Services:** *Public Health Service Grants Policy Statement.* Publ no. (OASH) 82-50,000 (rev), Washington, Dec 1, **1982b**. 17, A

129. **Devan WJ, Brown MB** (editors): *Biomedical Computer Programs, P-Series.* University of California Press, Los Angeles, Calif, **1979**. 17

130. **Diabetic Retinopathy Study Research Group:** Preliminary report on effects of photocoagulation therapy. *Am J Ophthalmol* 81:383–396, **1976**. 19, 20

131. **Diabetic Retinopathy Study Research Group:** Photocoagulation treatment of proliferative diabetic retinopathy: The second report of diabetic retinopathy study findings. *Ophthalmology* 85:82–106, **1978**. 19

132. **Diabetic Retinopathy Study Research Group:** Diabetic Retinopathy Study: Report 6. Design, methods, and baseline results. *Invest Ophthalmol Vis Sci* 21:149–209, **1981**. 13

133. **Diehl HS, Baker AB, Cowan DW:** Cold vaccines: An evaluation based on a controlled study. *JAMA* 111:1168–1173, **1938**. 1

134. **Dimond EG, Kittle CF, Crockett JE:** Comparison of internal mammary artery ligation and sham operation for angina pectoris. *Am J Cardiol* 5:483–486, **1960**. 8

135. **Dixon WJ** (editor): *BMDP Statistical Software* (1981 ed). University of California Press, Los Angeles, **1981**. 17

136. **Donaldson N, Donaldson B:** *How Did They Die?* St. Martins Press, Inc, New York, **1980**. 2

137. **Draper N, Smith H:** *Applied Regression Analysis* (2nd ed). John Wiley and Sons, New York, **1966**. 18

138. **Drummond JC, Wilbraham A:** *The Englishman's Food: A History of Five Centuries of English Diet.* Jonathan Cape, London, **1940**. 1

139. **Duncan DB:** Multiple range and multiple F tests. *Biometrics* 11:1–42, **1955**. 20

140. **Duncan DB:** t tests and intervals for comparisons suggested by the data. *Biometrics* 31:339–359, **1975**. 20

141. **Duncan DB, Godbold JH:** Approximate k-ratio t tests for differences between unequally   20
replicated treatments. *Biometrics* 35:749–756, **1979.**

142. **Duncan DB, Brandt L:** Adaptive t tests for multiple comparisons. *Biometrics* 39:787–794,   20
1983a.

143. **Duncan DB, Dixon DO:** k-ratio t tests, t intervals, and point estimates for multiple compari-   20
sons. *Encyclopedia of Statistical Sciences* (S Kotz, NL Johnson, CB Read, editors, vol 4, pp
403–410). John Wiley and Sons, New York, **1983b.**

144. **Duncan WJ:** Mail questionnaires in survey research: A review of response inducement tech-   12
niques. *J Management* 5:39–55, **1979.**

145. **Duncum BM:** *The Development of Inhalation Anaesthesia—With Special Reference to the*   1
Years 1846–1900. Oxford University Press, London, **1947.**

146. **Dunnett CW:** A multiple comparison procedure for comparing several treatments with a   9, 20
control. *JASA* 50:1096–1121, **1955.**

147. **Dunnett CW:** New tables for multiple comparisons with a control. *Biometrics* 20:482–491,   20
1964.

148. **Dupont WD:** Sequential stopping rules and sequential adjusted p values: Does one require the   9, 20, A
other? *Controlled Clin Trials* 4:3–10, **1983a.**

149. **Dupont WD:** Rejoinder: Statistical inference from trials with sequential stopping rules.   20
Controlled Clin Trials 4:27–33, **1983b.**

E

150. **Early Treatment of Diabetic Retinopathy Study Research Group:** *Manual of Operations.*   3
National Eye Institute, Bethesda, Md, **1982.**

151. **Edvardsson B:** Effect of reversal of response scales in a questionnaire. *Percept Mot Skills*   12
50:1125–1126, **1980.**

152. **Efron B:** Forcing a sequential experiment to be balanced. *Biometrika* 58:403–417, **1971.**   10

153. **Elandt-Johnson RC, Johnson NL:** *Survival Models and Data Analysis.* John Wiley and Sons,   18
New York, **1980.**

154. **Elliott J:** A medical pioneer: John Haygarth of Chester. *Br Med J* 1:235–242, **1913.**   2

155. **Erickson SH, Bergman JJ, Schneeweiss R, Cherkin DC:** The use of drugs for unlabeled   6
indications. *JAMA* 243:1543–1546, **1980.**

156. **Ethics Advisory Board of the Department of Health and Human Services:** *The Request of the*   24
National Institutes of Health for a Limited Exemption from the Freedom of Information Act.
Department of Health and Human Services, Washington, **1980.**

157. **European Coronary Surgery Study Group:** Coronary bypass surgery in stable angina pectoris: 24
Survival at two years. *Lancet* 1:889–893, **1979.**

158. **European Coronary Surgery Study Group:** Prospective randomised study of coronary artery   24
bypass surgery in stable angina pectoris: Second interim report. *Lancet* 2:491–495, **1980.**

159. **European Coronary Surgery Study Group:** Prospective randomized study of coronary artery   24
bypass surgery in stable angina pectoris: A progress report on survival. *Circulation* 65(suppl
II):II–67—II–71, **1982a.**

160. **European Coronary Surgery Study Group:** Long-term results of prospective randomised study   2, 24
of coronary artery bypass surgery in stable angina pectoris. *Lancet* 2:1173–1180, **1982b.**

F

161. **Feinstein AR:** Clinical biostatistics: VII. An analytic appraisal of the University Group   7, 19, 26
Diabetes Program (UGDP) study. *Clin Pharmacol Ther* 12:167–191, **1971.**

162. **Fellegi IP, Sunter A:** A theory for record linkage. *JASA* 64:1183–1210, **1969.**   A

163. **Feller W:** *An Introduction to Probability Theory and Its Applications* (vol 1, 3rd ed). John   20, A
Wiley and Sons, New York, **1968.**

164. **Fibiger J:** Om serumbehandlung af difteri. *Hospitalstidende* 6:309–325, **1898.** 1

165. **Finkel MJ:** The development of orphan products. *N Engl J Med* 307:963–964, **1982.** 6

166. **Finney HC:** Improving the reliability of retrospective survey measures: Results of a longitudinal field survey. *Evaluation Rev* 5:207–229, **1981.** 12

167. **Fisher RA, MacKenzie WA:** Studies in crop variation: II. The manurial response of different potato varieties. *J Agric Sci* 13:311–320, **1923.** 1

168. **Fisher RA:** The arrangements of field experiments. *J Ministry Agric Great Britain* 33:503–513, **1926.** 1

169. **Fisher RA:** *Statistical Methods for Research Workers* (10th ed). Oliver and Boyd, Edinburgh, **1946.** 18

170. **Fisher RA, Yates F:** *Statistical Tables for Biological, Agricultural and Medical Research* (6th ed). Hafner Publishing Company, Inc, New York, **1963.** 10

171. **Fisher RA:** *Statistical Methods and Scientific Inference* (3rd ed). Hafner Press, Macmillan Publishing Co, Inc, New York, **1973.** 1

172. **Fleiss JL:** *Statistical Methods for Rates and Proportions* (2nd ed). John Wiley and Sons, New York, **1981.** 9, 18

173. **Fletcher RH, Fletcher SW, Wagner EH:** *Clinical Epidemiology: The Essentials.* Williams and Wilkins, Baltimore, **1982.** 7

174. **Food and Drug Administration:** Procedural and interpretative regulations: Investigational use. *Federal Register* 28:179–182, Jan 8, **1963.** 1

175. **Food and Drug Administration:** Hearing procedure for refusal or withdrawal of approval of New Drug Applications and for issuance, amendment, or repeal of Antibiotic Drug Regulations: Interpretative description of adequate and well controlled clinical investigations. *Federal Register* 34:14596–14598, Sept 19, **1969a.** 1

176. **Food and Drug Administration:** Novobiocin-tetracycline combination drugs: Calcium novobiocin-sulfamethizole tablets. Final order repealing regulations and working certificates. *Federal Register* 34:14598–14599, Sept 19, **1969b.** 1

177. **Food and Drug Administration:** Hearing requests on refusal or withdrawal of New Drug Applications and issuance, amendment or repeal of Antibiotic Drug Regulations and describing scientific content of adequate and well-controlled clinical investigations. *Federal Register* 35:3073–3074, Feb 17, **1970a.** 1

178. **Food and Drug Administration:** Hearing regulations and regulations describing scientific content of adequate and well-controlled clinical investigations. *Federal Register* 35:7250–7253, May 8, **1970b.** 1

179. **Food and Drug Administration:** Oral hypoglycemic agents: Diabetes prescribing information. *FDA Current Drug Information,* Oct, **1970c.** 7

180. **Food and Drug Administration:** Oral hypoglycemic agents. *FDA Drug Bull,* June 23, **1971.** 7

181. **Food and Drug Administration:** Oral hypoglycemic drug labeling. *FDA Drug Bull,* May, **1972a.** 7

182. **Food and Drug Administration:** DESI Who? *FDA Consumer,* Oct, **1972b.** 2

183. **Food and Drug Administration:** Drug labeling: Failure to reveal material facts; labeling of oral hypoglycemic drugs. *Federal Register* 40:28582–28595, July 7, **1975.** 7

184. **Food and Drug Administration:** Phenformin: New labeling and possible removal from the market. *FDA Drug Bull* 7:6–7, May–July, **1977a.** 7

185. **Food and Drug Administration:** HEW Secretary suspends general marketing of phenformin. *FDA Drug Bull* 7:14–16, Aug, **1977b.** 7

186. **Food and Drug Administration:** *General Considerations for the Clinical Evaluation of Drugs.* Publ no. HEW (FDA) 77-3040, Rockville, Md, Sept, **1977c.** 7, A

187. **Food and Drug Administration:** Status of withdrawal of phenformin. *FDA Drug Bull* 7:19–20, Sept–Oct, **1977d.** 7

188. **Food and Drug Administration:** Oral hypoglycemic drugs: Availability of agency analysis and reopening of comment period on proposed labeling requirements. *Federal Register* 43:52732–52734, Nov 14, **1978.** 7, 16, 24

189. **Food and Drug Administration:** Medical devices: Procedures for Investigational Device   13
Exemptions. *Federal Register* 45:3732–3759, Jan 18, **1980**.

190. **Food and Drug Administration:** *Clinical Testing for Safe and Effective Drugs. Investigational*   13
Drug Procedures. HHS publ no. (FDA) 74–3015, Rockville, MD, **1981**.

191. **Food and Drug Administration:** *Regulatory Requirements for Medical Devices: A Workshop*   13, A
Manual. HHS publ no. (FDA) 83–4165, Rockville, Md, June, **1983**.

192. **Food and Drug Administration:** *Guideline Labeling for Oral Hypoglycemic Drugs of the*   7
Sulfonylurea Class. Docket no. 83D-0304, Rockville, Md, March 16, **1984a**.

193. **Food and Drug Administration:** Labeling of oral hypoglycemic drugs of the sulfonylurea class.   7
Federal Register 49:14303–14331, April 11, **1984b**.

194. **Food and Drug Administration:** Oral hypoglycemic drug products: Availability of guideline   7
labeling. *Federal Register* 49:14441–14442, April 11, **1984c**.

195. **Food and Nutrition Board:** *Toward Healthful Diets.* National Academy of Science, Washing-   22
ton, May 28, **1980**.

196. **Francis T, Korns RF, Voight RB, Boisen M, Hemphill FM, Napier JA, Tolchinsky E:** An   1
evaluation of the 1954 poliomyelitis vaccine trial: Summary report. *Am J Public Health*
45(part II, May suppl): 1–51, **1955**.

197. **Fredrickson DS:** The field trial: Some thoughts on the indispensable ordeal. *Bull NY Acad*   2, 3
Med 44:985–993, **1968**.

198. **Freedman LS, White SJ:** On the use of Pocock and Simon's method for balancing treatment   10
numbers and prognostic factors in the controlled clinical trial. *Biometrics* 32:691–694, **1976**.

199. **Freiman JA, Chalmers TC, Smith H Jr, Kuebler RR:** The importance of beta, the type II error   2, 9
and sample size in the design and interpretation of the randomized control trial: Survey of 71
"negative" trials. *N Engl J Med* 299:690–694, **1978**.

200. **Frenette C, Begin G:** Sensitive data gathering through the random response technique: A   12
validity study. *Psychol Rep* 45:1001–1002, **1979**.

201. **Friedman LM, Furberg CD, DeMets DL:** *Fundamentals of Clinical Trials.* John Wright, PSG   10
Inc, Boston, **1982**.

G

202. **Gail M, Gart JJ:** The determination of sample sizes for use with the exact conditional test in   9
2x2 comparative trials. *Biometrics* 29:441–448, **1973**.

203. **Gail M:** Power computations for designing comparative Poisson trials. *Biometrics* 30:231–237,   9
1974.

204. **Gail M:** Applicability of sample size calculations based on a comparison of proportions for use   9
with the logrank test. *Controlled Clin Trials* 6:112–119, **1985**.

205. **Galton F:** Regression towards mediocrity in hereditary stature. *Anthropological Institute*   A
15:246–263, **1886**.

206. **Garrett HE, Dennis EW, DeBakey ME:** Aortocoronary bypass with saphenous vein graft: 2
Seven-year follow-up. *JAMA* 223:792–794, **1973**.

207. **Gart JJ:** The comparison of proportions: A review of significance tests, confidence intervals   9
and adjustments for stratification. *Review Internat Stat Inst* 39:148–169, **1971**.

208. **Gordis L, Naggan L, Tonascia J:** Pitfalls in evaluating the impact of coronary care units on   2
mortality from myocardial infarctions. *Johns Hopkins Med J* 141:287–295, **1977**.

209. **Grant AP:** Sequential trial of isocarboxazid in angina pectoris. *Br Med J* 1:513–515, **1962**.   9

210. **Greenberg BG** (chairman): *A Report from the Heart Special Project Committee to the*   1
National Advisory Heart Council: Organization, Reviews and Administration of Cooperative
Studies, May, 1967. Controlled Clin Trials 9:137–148, 1988.

211. **Greenhouse SW, Halperin M:** Jerome Cornfield: 1912–1979. *Controlled Clin Trials* 1:75–80,   1
1980.

212. **Greenhouse SW:** Discussion on early stopping. *Controlled Clin Trials* 4:23–25, **1983**.   20

213. **Grizzle JE:** A note on stratifying versus complete random assignment in clinical trials.   10
Controlled Clin Trials 3:365–368, **1982**.

H

214. **Hagans J:** The design and methodology of cooperative drug trials. *Drug Intell Clin Pharm* 8:531–534, **1974**. 5, 10

215. **Haggard HW:** *The Lame, the Halt, and the Blind: The Vital Role of Medicine in the History of Civilization.* Harper and Brothers, New York, **1932**. 2

216. **Hainline A Jr, Miller DT, Mather A:** Role and methods of the central laboratory. *Controlled Clin Trials* 4:377–387, **1983**. 16

217. **Halperin M, Rogot E, Gurian J, Ederer F:** Sample sizes for medical trials with special reference to long-term therapy. *J Chronic Dis* 21:13–24, **1968**. 9

218. **Hamilton MP:** Role of an ethicist in the conduct of clinical trials in the United States. *Controlled Clin Trials* 1:411–420, **1981**. 23

219. **Harville DA:** Experimental randomization: Who needs it? *Am Statistician* 29:27–31, **1975**. 19

220. **Haseman JK:** Exact sample sizes for use with the Fisher-Irwin test for 2x2 tables. *Biometrics* 34:106–109, **1978**. 9

221. **Hauck WW:** Letter to the editor concerning random number generators. *Controlled Clin Trials* 3:73, **1982**. 10

222. **Haupt BJ:** Deliveries in short-stay hospitals: United States, 1980. *Vital and Health Statistics of the National Center for Health Statistics*, no. 83, Hyattsville, Md, Oct 8, **1982**. 2

223. **Haverkamp AD, Thompson HE, McFee JG, Cetrulo C:** The evaluation of continuous fetal heart rate monitoring in high-risk pregnancy. *Am J Obstet Gynecol* 125:310–320, **1976**. 2

224. **Haverkamp AD, Orleans M, Langendoerfer S, McFee J, Murphy J, Thompson HE:** A controlled trial of the differential effects of intrapartum fetal monitoring. *Am J Obstet Gynecol* 134:399–412, **1979**. 2

225. **Hawkins BS, Canner PL:** Impact of closeout on operations at two coordinating centers. The Johns Hopkins University, Baltimore. Presented at the 4th Annual Symposium on Coordinating Clinical Trials, Arlington, Va, May 25–26, **1978**. 15

226. **Hawkins BS:** Staffing the coordinating center: Who is minding the data? (in *Coordinating Center Models Project: A Study of Coordinating Centers in Multicenter Clinical Trials: XVI. CCMP Manuscripts Presented at the Annual Symposia on Coordinating Clinical Trials*, pp. 155–187). Division of Heart and Vascular Diseases, National Heart, Lung, and Blood Institute, Bethesda, Md, June, **1979**. 5

227. **Hawkins BS:** Perusing the literature. *Controlled Clin Trials* 1:71–74, 181–185, 269–274, **1980**. 26

228. **Hawkins BS:** Perusing the literature. *Controlled Clin Trials* 2:51–57, 257–265, 327–333, **1981**. 26

229. **Hawkins BS:** Perusing the literature. *Controlled Clin Trials* 3:371–383, **1982**. 26

230. **Hawkins BS:** Perusing the literature. *Controlled Clin Trials* 4:75–86, 239–253, **1983**. 26

231. **Haygarth J:** *Of the Imagination, as a Cause and as a Cure of Disorders of the Body: Exemplified by Fictitious Tractors, and Epidemical Convulsions.* R Cruttwell, Bath, **1800**. 1, 2

232. **Helsing KJ, Comstock GW:** Response variation and location of questions within a questionnaire. *Internat J Epidemiol* 5:125–130, **1976**. 12

233. **Hill AB:** *Statistical Methods in Clinical and Preventive Medicine.* Oxford University Press, New York, **1962**. 1

234. **Hill AB:** *Principles of Medical Statistics* (9th ed). Oxford University Press, New York, **1971**. 5

235. **Hill JD, Holdstock G, Hampton JR:** Comparison of mortality of patients with heart attacks admitted to a coronary care unit and an ordinary medical ward. *Br Med J* 2:81–83, **1977**. 2

236. **Hill JD, Hampton JR, Mitchell JRA:** A randomised trial of home-versus-hospital management for patients with suspected myocardial infarction. *Lancet* 1:837–841, **1978**. 2

237. **Himmelfarb S, Edgell SE:** Additive constants model: A randomized response technique for eliminating evasiveness to quantitative response questions. *Psychol Bull* 87:525–530, **1980**. 12

238. **Hochstim JR, Renne KS:** Reliability of response in a sociomedical population study. *Public Opinion Quart* 35:69–79, **1971**. 12

239. **Holland WW, Ashford JR, Colley JRT, Morgan DC, Pearson NJ:** A comparison of two respiratory symptoms questionnaires: I. Methodology and observer variation. *Br J Prev Soc Med* 20:76–96, **1966**. 12

240. **Holman DV:** Venesection before Harvey and after. *Bull NY Acad Med* 31:661–670, **1955**.   2

241. **Howard JM, DeMets D, and the BHAT Research Group:** How informed is informed consent?   8, 14
The BHAT experience. *Controlled Clin Trials* 2:287–303, **1981**.

242. **Hypertension Detection and Follow-Up Program Cooperative Group:** Five-year findings of   1, 11, 14
the Hypertension Detection and Follow-Up Program: I. Reduction in mortality of persons
with high blood pressure, including mild hypertension. *JAMA* 242:2562–2571, **1979a**.

243. **Hypertension Detection and Follow-Up Program Cooperative Group:** Therapeutic control of   8
blood pressure in the Hypertension Detection and Follow-Up Program. *Prev Med* 8:2–13,
1979b.

I

244. **IMS America, Ltd** (Ambler, Pa): Diabetic therapy. *National Disease Therapeutic Review* 8:7,   7
June, **1977**.

245. **Ingelfinger JA, Mosteller F, Thibodeau LA, Ware JH:** *Biostatistics in Clinical Medicine*.   18
Macmillan Publishing Co, New York, **1983**.

246. **International Committee of Medical Journal Editors:** Uniform requirements for manuscripts   25
submitted to biomedical journals. *Br Med J* 284:1766–1770, **1982**.

J

247. **James G, James RC** (editors): *Mathematics Dictionary* (multilingual ed). D Van Nostrand   A
Company, Inc, Princeton, NJ, **1959**.

248. **Jenner E:** *An Inquiry into the Causes and Effects of the Variolae Vaccinae*. Sampson Low,   1
London, **1798**.

249. **Jones JH:** *Bad Blood: The Tuskegee Syphilis Experiment*. The Free Press, New York, **1981**.   14

250. **Juhl E, Christensen E, Tygstrup N:** The epidemiology of the gastriontestinal randomized   4
clinical trial. *N Engl J Med* 296:20–22, **1977**.

K

251. **Kalbfieisch JD, Prentice RL:** *The Statistical Analysis of Failure Time Data*. John Wiley and   18
Sons, New York, **1980**.

252. **Kaplan EL, Meier P:** Nonparametric estimation from incomplete observations. *JASA* 53:457–   18, A
481, **1958**.

253. **Keefer CS, Blake FG, Marshall EK Jr, Lockwood JS, Wood WB Jr:** Penicillin in the treatment   1
of infections: A report of 500 cases. *JAMA* 122:1217–1224, **1943**.

254. **Keen H, Jarrett RJ:** The effect of carbohydrate tolerance on plasma lipids and atherosclerosis   7
in man (pp 435–444, 446–449 in *Atherosclerosis*, RJ Jones, editor). Springer-Verlay, New
York, **1970**.

255. **Keen H:** Factors influencing the progress of atherosclerosis in the diabetic. *Acta Diabet Lat*   7
8(suppl 1):444–456, **1971**.

256. **Kelsey FO:** Government: The Kefauver-Harris Amendments and investigational drugs. *Am J*   1
Hosp Pharm 20:515–517, **1963**.

257. **Kelso IM, Parsons RJ, Lawrence GF, Arora SS, Edmonds DK, Cooke ID:** An assessment of   2
continuous fetal heart rate monitoring in labor: A randomized trial. *Am J Obstet Gynecol*
131:526–532, **1978**.

258. **Kendall MG, Buckland WR:** *A Dictionary of Statistical Terms* (2nd ed). Hafner Publishing   A
Company, New York, **1960**.

259. **Kenton C, Scott YB:** MEDLINE searching and retrieval. *Med Inf* 3:225–235, **1978**.   2

260. **Kidder LH:** *Selltiz, Wrightsman and Cook's Research Methods in Social Relations* (4th ed).   12
Holt, Rinehart and Winston, New York, **1981**.

261. **Kilo C, Miller JP, Williamson JR:** The achilles heel of the University Group Diabetes   7, 26
Program. *JAMA* 243:450–457, **1980**.

262. **King LS:** The blood-letting controversy: A study in the scientific method. *Bull Hist Med* 35:1–13, **1961.** 2

263. **Klein E:** *A Comprehensive Etymological Dictionary of the English Language.* Elsevier Scientific Publishing Co, Amsterdam, **1971.** 1, A

264. **Kleinbaum DG, Kupper LL, Chambless LE:** Logistic regression analysis of epidemiologic data: Theory and practice. *Commun Statist-Theor Meth* 11:485–547, **1982.** 18

265. **Klimt CR, Canner PL:** Terminating a long term clinical trial. *Clin Pharmacol Ther* 25:641–646, **1979.** 15

266. **Klimt CR:** Terminating a long-term clinical trial. *Controlled Clin Trials* 1:319–325, **1981.** 15

267. **Knatterud GL:** Lessons learned in monitoring for treatment effects in the Diabetic Retinopathy Study (abstract). *Am J Epidemiol* 106:247, **1977.** 8

268. **Knatterud GL:** Methods of quality control and of continuous audit procedures for controlled clinical trials. *Controlled Clin Trials* 1:327–332, **1981.** 3

269. **Knatterud GL, Forman SA, Canner PL:** Design of data forms. *Controlled Clin Trials* 4:429–440, **1983.** 12

270. **Knox JHM Jr:** The medical history of George Washington, his physicians, friends and advisers. *Bull Inst Hist Med* 1:174–191, **1933.** 2

271. **Knox RA:** The pill for diabetics. *Boston Sunday Globe*, Nov 7, **1971.** 7

272. **Knuth DE:** *Seminumerical Algorithms* (vol 2 of *The Art of Computer Programming*). Addison-Wesley Publishing Co, Reading, Mass, **1969.** A

273. **Kolata GB:** Controversy over study of diabetes drugs continues for nearly a decade. *Science* 203:986–990, **1979.** 7

274. **Kotz S, Johnson NL, Read CB** (editors): *Encyclopedia of Statistical Sciences.* John Wiley and Sons, New York, **1982.** A

275. **Krol WF:** Closing down the study. *Controlled Clin Trials* 4:505–412, **1983.** 15

276. **Kruskal WH, Tanur JM** (editors): *International Encyclopedia of Statistics* (in 2 vols). The Free Press, Macmillan Publishing Co, Inc, New York, **1978.** A

L

277. **Lachin JM:** Introduction to sample size determination and power analysis for clinical trials. *Controlled Clin Trials* 2:93–113, **1981.** 9

278. **Last JM** (editor): *A Dictionary of Epidemiology.* Oxford University Press, New York, **1983.** A

279. **Layne BH, Thompson DN:** Questionnaire page length and return rate. *J Soc Psychol* 113:291–292, **1981.** 12

280. **Ledger RR:** Safety of Upjohn's oral antidiabetic drug doubted in study: Firm disputes findings. *Wall Street Journal*, May 21, **1970.** 7

281. **Lee ET:** *Statistical Methods for Survival Data Analysis.* Lifetime Learning Publications, Wadsworth Inc, Belmont, Calif, **1980.** 18

282. **Levine J, Guy W, Cleary PA:** Therapeutic trials of psychopharmacologic agents: 1968–1972 (in *Principles and Techniques of Human Research*, vol VIII, *Psychopharmacological Agents*, edited by FG McMahon). Futura Publishing Co, Mt. Kisco, NY, **1974.** 2

283. **Levine MM:** Informed consent (abstract). *Am J Epidemiol* 104:350, **1976.** 14

284. **Levine RJ, Lebacqz K:** Some ethical considerations in clinical trials. *Clin Pharmacol Ther* 25:728–741, **1979.** 14

285. **Levine RJ:** *Ethics and Regulations of Clinical Research.* Urban and Schwarzenberg, Baltimore, **1981.** 1, 14

286. **Lieberman GJ, Owen DB:** *Tables of the Hypergeometric Probability Distribution.* Stanford University Press, Stanford, Calif, **1961.** 18

287. **Lilienfeld AM:** Ceteris paribus: The evolution of the clinical trial. *Bull Hist Med* 56:1–18, **1982.** 1

288. **Lind J:** *A Treatise of the Scurvy* (reprinted in *Lind's Treatise on Scurvy*, edited by CP Stewart,   1, 8
D Guthrie, Edinburgh University Press, Edinburgh, 1953). Sands, Murray, Cochran, Edin-
burgh, **1753**.

289. **Lindley DV:** *The Role of Randomization in Inference.* Report no. M 627, Department of   19
Statistics, Florida State University, Tallahassee, **1982**.

290. **Lipid Research Clinics Program:** Recruitment for clinical trials: The Lipid Research Clinics   14
Coronary Primary Prevention Trial experience: Its implication for future trials (WS Agras,
RH Bradford, GD Marshall, editors). *Circulation* 66 (suppl IV):IV-1—IV-78, **1982**.

M

291. **Macular Photocoagulation Study Group:** Argon laser photocoagulation for senile macular   7, 18
degeneration: Results of a randomized clinical trial. *Arch Ophthalmol* 100:912-918, **1982**.   20, 24

292. **Macular Photocoagulation Study Group:** Argon laser photocoagulation for ocular histoplas-   18, 20,
mosis: Results of a randomized clinical trial. *Arch Ophthalmol* 101:1347-1357, **1983a**.   24

293. **Macular Photocoagulation Study Group:** Argon laser photocoagulation for ideopathic   18, 24
neovascularization. Results of a randomized clinical trial. *Arch Ophthalmol* 101:1358-1361,
1983b.

294. **Macular Photocoagulation Study Group:** Changing the protocol: A case report from the   7
Macular Photocoagulation Study. *Controlled Clin Trials* 5:203-216, **1984**.

295. **Management Committee of the Australian Therapeutic Trial in Mild Hypertension:** The   24
Australian Therapeutic Trial in Mild Hypertension. *Lancet* 1:1261-1267, **1980**.

296. **Mantel N, Haenszel W:** Statistical aspects of the analysis of data from retrospective studies of   18, A
disease. *J Natl Cancer Inst* 22:719-748, **1959**.

297. **Mantel N:** Evaluation of survival data and two new rank order statistics arising in its   18
consideration. *Cancer Chemother Reports* 50:163-170, **1966**.

298. **Market Facts, Inc:** *The Impact of Two Clinical Trials on Physician Knowledge and Practice.*   7
Final Report. Division of Heart and Vascular Diseases, National Heart, Lung, and Blood
Institute, Bethesda, Md, March, **1982**.

299. **Marks IN, Wright JP, Denyer M, Garisch JAM, Lucke W:** Comparison of sucralfate with   8
cimetidine in the short-term treatment of chronic peptic ulcers. *S Afr Med J* 57:567-573, **1980**.

300. **Marks RG:** *Designing a Research Project: The Basics of Biomedical Research Methodology.*   12
Lifetime Learning Publications, Wadsworth Inc, Belmont, Calif, **1982**.

301. **Martin GL, Newman IM:** Randomized response: A technique for improving the validity of   12
self-reported health behaviors. *J Sch Health* 52:222-226, **1982**.

302. **Mather HG, Pearson NG, Read KLQ, Steed GR, Thorne MG, Jones S, Guerrier CJ, Eraut**   2
CD, McHugh PM, Chowdhury NR, Jafary MH, Wallace TJ: Acute myocardial infarction:
Home and hospital treatment. *Br Med J* 3:334-338, **1971**.

303. **Mather HG, Morgan DC, Pearson NG, Read KLQ, Shaw DB, Steed GR, Thorne MG,**   2
Lawrence CJ, Riley IS: Myocardial infarction: A comparison between home and hospital care
for patients. *Br Med J* 1:925-929, **1976**.

304. **Matts JP, Long JM, and POSCH Group:** Modeling recruitment from the population to the   14
randomized patient (abstract). *Controlled Clin Trials* 1:169, **1980**.

305. **McCarn DB:** MEDLINE: An introduction to on-line searching. *J Am Soc Inf Sci* 31:181-192,   2
1980.

306. **McDill M:** Activity analysis of data coordinating centers (in *Coordinating Center Models*   3, 5
Project: A Study of Coordinating Centers in Multicenter Clinical Trials: XVI. CCMP Manus-
cripts Presented at the Annual Symposia on Coordinating Clinical Trials, pp 105-125).
Division of Heart and Vascular Diseases, National Heart, Lung, and Blood Institute, Bethesda,
Md, June, **1979**.

307. **McFarland SG:** Effects of question order on survey responses. *Public Opinion Quart* 45:208-   12
215, **1981**.

308. **McLaughlin GH:** SMOG grading—a new readability formula. *J Reading* 12:639-646, **1969**.   E

309. **Meadows AJ:** *Dictionary of New Information Technology.* Nichols Publishing Co, New York,   A
1982.

310. **Medical Research Council:** Clinical trials of new remedies (annotations). *Lancet* 2:304, **1931.** 1

311. **Medical Research Council:** Streptomycin treatment of pulmonary tuberculosis: A Medical Research Council investigation. *Br Med J* 2:769–782, **1948.** 1

312. **Meier P:** Stratification in the design of a clinical trial. *Controlled Clin Trials* 1:355–361, **1981.** 10

313. **Meinert CL:** Quality assurance in clinical trials. *Institut National de la Santé et de la Recherche Medicale* (INSERM) 76:123–130, **1977.** 6

314. **Meinert CL:** Cost profiles of data coordinating centers (in *Coordinating Center Models Project: A study of Coordinating Centers in Multicenter Clinical Trials: XVI. CCMP Manuscripts Presented at the Annual Symposia on Coordinating Clinical Trials*, pp. 127–153). Division of Heart and Vascular Diseases, National Heart, Lung, and Blood Institute, Bethesda, Md, June **1979a.** 5, 6

315. **Meinert CL:** Recommendations and comments on the organization of multicenter trials (in *Coordinating Centers Models Project: A Study of Coordinating Centers in Multicenter Clinical Trials: XVI. CCMP Manuscripts Presented at the Annual Symposia on Coordinating Clinical Trials*, pp 257–284). Division of Heart and Vascular Diseases, National Heart, Lung, and Blood Institute, Bethesda, Md, June **1979b.** 23

316. **Meinert CL:** Terminology—A plea for standardization (editorial). *Controlled Clin Trials* 1:97–99, **1980a.** 1, A

317. **Meinert CL:** Clinical trials and data integrity (editorial). *Controlled Clin Trials* 1:189–192, **1980b.** 16

318. **Meinert CL:** Organization of multicenter clinical trials. *Controlled Clin Trials* 1:305–312, **1981.** 1, 4, 23

319. **Meinert CL:** Funding for clinical trials. *Controlled Clin Trials* 3:165–171, **1982.** 6

320. **Meinert CL, Heinz EC, Forman SA:** Role and methods of the coordinating center. *Controlled Clin Trials* 4:355–375, **1983.** 5, 17

321. **Meinert CL, Tonascia S, Higgins K:** Content of reports on clinical trials: A critical review. *Controlled Clin Trials* 5:328–347, **1984.** 2, 25

322. **Miller RG Jr:** *Simultaneous Statistical Inference.* McGraw-Hill Book Company, New York, **1966.** 20

323. **Miller RG Jr:** Developments in multiple comparisons: 1966–1976. *JASA* 72:779–788, **1977.** 20

324. **Milman N, Scheibel J, Jessen O:** Lysine prophylaxis in recurrent herpes simplex labialis: A double-blind, controlled crossover study. *Acta Derm Venereol* 60:85–87, **1980.** 8

325. **Milne JS, Williamson J:** Comparison of teaching machine with an observer in detection of angina pectoris by questionnaire. *Br J Prev Soc Med* 25:105–108, **1971.** 12

326. **Mintz M:** Antidiabetes pill held causing early death. *The Washington Post*, May 22, **1970a.** 7

327. **Mintz M:** Discovery of diabetes drug's perils stirs doubts over short-term tests. *The Washington Post*, June 8, **1970b.** 7

328. **Moertel CG, Fleming TR, Rubin J, Kvols LK, Sarna G, Koch R, Currie VE, Young CW, Jones SE, Davignon JP:** A clinical trial of amygdalin (Laetrile) in the treatment of human cancer. *N Engl J Med* 306:201–206, **1982.** 2

329. **Montgomery B:** Abuses of Freedom of Information Act. *JAMA* 242:1007–1009, **1979.** 24

330. **Morgenstern H, Bursic ES:** A method for using epidemiologic data to estimate the potential impact of an intervention on the health status of a target population. *J Community Health* 7:292–309, **1982.** A

331. **Morris RA, Sales BD, Berman JJ:** Research and the Freedom of Information Act. *American Psychol* 36:819–826, **1981.** 7

332. **Morris W** (editor): *The American Heritage Dictionary of the English Language.* American Heritage Publishing Co, Inc and Houghton Mifflin Co, New York, **1973.** A

333. **Moses LE, Oakford RY:** *Tables of Random Permutations.* Stanford University Press, Stanford, Calif, **1963.** 10

334. **Mosteller F, Gilbert JP, McPeek B:** Reporting standards and research strategies for controlled trials: Agenda for the editor. *Controlled Clin Trials* 1:37–58, **1980.** 2, 9

335. **Mount FW, Ferebee SH:** Control study of comparative efficacy of isoniazid, streptomycin-isoniazid, and streptomycin-para-aminosalicylic acid in pulmonary tuberculosis therapy: I. Report on twelve-week observations on 526 patients. *Am Rev Tuberc* 66:632–635, **1952.** 1

336. **Mount FW, Ferebee SH:** Control study of comparative efficacy of isoniazid, streptomycin-isoniazid, and streptomycin-para-aminosalicylic acid in pulmonary tuberculosis therapy: II. Report on twenty-week observations on 390 patients with streptomycin-susceptible infections. *Am Rev Tuberc* 67:108–113, **1953a.** 1

337. **Mount FW, Ferebee SH:** Control study of comparative efficacy of isoniazid, streptomycin-isoniazid, and streptomycin-para-aminosalicylic acid in pulmonary tuberculosis therapy: III. Report on twenty-eight-week observations on 649 patients with streptomycin-susceptible infections. *Am Rev Tuberc* 67:539–543, **1953b.** 1

338. **Multicenter Investigation of the Limitation of Infarct Size Research Group:** *Organization and Bylaws.* Division of Heart and Vascular Diseases, National Heart, Lung, and Blood Institute, Bethesda, Md, **1983.** 22

339. **Multiple Risk Factor Intervention Trial Research Group:** Statistical design considerations in the NHLI Multiple Risk Factor Intervention Trial (MRFIT). *J Chronic Dis* 30:261–275, **1977.** 1

340. **Multiple Risk Factor Intervention Trial Research Group:** Multiple Risk Factor Intervention Trial: Risk factor changes and mortality results. *JAMA* 248:1465–1477, **1982.** 4, 14, 16, 19, 20, 22

341. **Mundy GR, Fleckenstein L, Mazzullo JM, Sundaresan PR, Weintraub M, Lasagna L:** Current medical practice and the Food and Drug Administration: Some evidence for the existing gap. *JAMA* 229:1744–1748, **1974.** 6

342. **Murphy ML, Hultgren HN, Detre K, Thomsen J, Takaro T, and participants of the Veterans Administration Cooperative Study:** Treatment of chronic stable angina: A preliminary report of survival data of the randomized Veterans Administration Cooperative Study. *N Engl J Med* 297:621–627, **1977.** 2

343. **Murray JAH, Bradley H, Craigie WA, Onions CT** (editors): *The Oxford English Dictionary: A New English Dictionary on Historical Principles* (in 13 vols). Clarendon Press, Oxford, **1970.** A

N

344. **National Cancer Institute:** *Compilation of Experimental Cancer Therapy Protocol Summaries* (7th ed). Bethesda, Md, **1983.** 2

345. **National Center for Health Statistics:** *National Death Index: User's Manual.* HHS publ no. (PHS) 81–1148, Hyattsville, Md, **1981.** 6, 15, A

346. **National Cooperative Gallstone Study Group:** Design and methodological considerations in the National Cooperative Gallstone Study: A multicenter clinical trial. *Controlled Clin Trials* 2:177–299, **1981a.** 5, 11, 12–14, 16, 18, 19, 20, 23, 24

347. **National Cooperative Gallstone Study Group:** Chenodiol (chenodeoxycholic acid) for dissolution of gallstones: The National Cooperative Gallstone Study: A controlled trial of efficacy and safety. *Ann Intern Med* 95:257–282, **1981b.** 11, 13, 22, 24

348. **National Cooperative Gallstone Study Group:** Major issues in the organization and implementation of the National Cooperative Gallstone Study (NCGS). *Controlled Clin Trials* 5:1–12, **1984.** 13

349. **National Diet-Heart Study Research Group:** The National Diet-Heart Study: Final report. *Circulation* 37(suppl I):I–1—I–428, **1968.** 19

350. **National Heart, Lung, and Blood Institute:** *National Conference on High Blood Pressure Education: Report of Proceedings.* Publ no. (NIH) 73–486, Bethesda, Md, **1973.** 7

351. **National Institute of Arthritis, Metabolism, and Digestive Diseases:** *Request for Research Cooperative Agreement Application: Clinical Centers for a Collaborative Clinical Trial on the Relationship Between Blood Glucose Control and Vascular Complications of Insulin-Dependent Diabetes Mellitus.* RFA NIAMDD 81–01, Bethesda, Md, **1981a.** 21

352. **National Institute of Arthritis, Metabolism, and Digestive Diseases:** *Request for Proposal: Data Coordinating Center for a Collaborative Clinical Trial on the Relationship Between Blood Glucose Control and Early Vascular Complications of Insulin-Dependent Diabetes Mellitus.* RFP NH-NIAMDD 81-9, Bethesda, Md, **1981b.** 21

353. **National Institutes of Health:** *NIH Inventory of Clinical Trials: Fiscal Year 1975* (in two vols). Division of Research Grants, Research Analysis and Evaluation Branch, Bethesda, Md, **1975.** 2, 4, 6

354. **National Institutes of Health:** *NIH Inventory of Clinical Trials: Fiscal Years 1976 through 1979* (unpublished). Data tapes obtained from the Division of Research Grants, Research Analysis and Evaluation Branch, Bethesda, Md, **1980**. 2, 4, 6, 21

355. **National Institutes of Health:** *Basic Data Relating to the National Institutes of Health.* Office of Program Planning and Evaluation, and the Division of Research Grants, Bethesda, Md, May **1981a**. 6

356. **National Institutes of Health:** *NIH Almanac.* Publ no. 81-5, Division of Public Information, Bethesda, Md, **1981b**. 1

357. **National Institutes of Health Clinical Trials Committee** (RS Gordon Jr, chairman): Clinical trial activity. *NIH Guide for Grants and Contracts* 8:29, June 5, **1979**. 20

358. **National Library of Medicine:** *Medical Subject Headings: Index Medicus.* NIH publ no. 81-259, Bethesda, Md, **1980**. 2

359. **National Library of Medicine:** *List of Journals Indexed in Index Medicus.* NIH publ no. 83-267, Bethesda, Md, **1983**. 25

360. **National Research Council:** *Report of Ad Hoc Committee on Dimethyl Sulfoxide.* Division of Medical Sciences, National Academy of Sciences, Washington, **1973**. 2

361. **Neyman J, Pearson ES:** *Joint Statistical Papers.* University of California Press, Berkeley, Calif, **1966**. 9

362. **Norusis Mj:** *SPSS^X Introductory Statistics Guide.* McGraw-Hill Book Co, New York, **1983**. 17

O

363. **O'Brien PC, Fleming TR:** A multiple testing procedure for clinical trials. *Biometrics* 35:549-556, **1979**. 20

364. **O'Brien PC:** The appropriateness of analysis of variance and multiple-comparison procedures. *Biometrics* 39:787-788, **1983**. 20

365. **Office for Protection from Research Risks:** *Code of Federal Regulations: Title 45: Public Welfare, Part 46: Protection of Human Subjects.* National Institutes of Health, Bethesda, Md, **1983**. 13, 14

366. **Office of Technology Assessment:** *The Impact of Randomized Clinical Trials on Health Policy and Medical Practice: Background Paper.* OTA-BP-H-22, United States Congress, Washington, Aug, **1983**. 7

367. **Ott WJ:** Primary cesarean section: A critical analysis. *Obstet Gynecol* 58:691-695, **1981**. 2

368. **Overton HH:** Perceptions of the coordinating center—As viewed by a clinical coordinator. *Controlled Clin Trials* 1:131-136, **1980**. 23

P

369. **Paasikivi J:** Long-term tolbutamide treatment after myocardial infarction. *Acta Med Scand* suppl 507:1-82, **1970**. 7

370. **Packard FR:** *Life and Times of Ambroise Parè, 1510-1590.* Paul B Hoeber, New York, **1921**. 1

371. **Park WH, Bullowa JGM, Rosenbluth MB:** The treatment of lobar pneumonia with refined specific antibacterial serum. *JAMA* 91:1503-1508, **1928**. 1

372. **Patulin Clinical Trials Committee** (of the Medical Research Council): Clinical trial of Patulin in the common cold. *Lancet* 2:373-375, **1944**. 1

373. **Payne SL:** *The Art of Asking Questions.* Princeton University Press, Princeton, NJ, **1951**. 12

374. **Perry GT, Dunphy JV, Fruin RC, Littman A:** Gastric freezing for duodenal ulcer: A double blind study. *Gastroenterology* 47:6-9, **1964**. 8

375. **Persantine Aspirin Reinfarction Study Research Group:** Persantine Aspirin Reinfarction Study: Design, methods and baseline results. *Circulation* 62(suppl II): II-1—II-42, **1980a**. 5, 6, 10, 16, 21-23, 25, E

376. **Persantine Aspirin Reinfarction Study Research Group:** Persantine and aspirin in coronary heart disease. *Circulation* 62:449-461, **1980b**. 9, 11, 18, 24, 25

377. **Peto R, Pike MC, Armitage P, Breslow NE, Cox DR, Howard SV, Mantel N, McPherson K,**   10, 18
     Peto J, Smith PG: Design and analysis of randomized clinical trials requiring prolonged
     observation of each patient: I. Introduction and design. *Br J Cancer* 34:585–612, **1976.**

378. **Peto R, Pike MC, Armitage P, Breslow NE, Cox DR, Howard SV, Mantel N, McPherson K,**   18
     Peto J, Smith PG: Design and analysis of randomized clinical trials requiring prolonged
     observation of each patient: II. Analysis and examples. *Br J Cancer* 35:1–39, **1977.**

379. **Pines WL:** *A Primer on New Drug Development.* Publ no. 1980–311–254/83, Food and Drug   A
     Administration, Rockville, Md, **1980.**

380. **Pitman EJG:** Significance tests which may be applied to samples from any populations: III.   8
     The analysis of variance test. *Biometrika* 29:322–335, **1937.**

381. **Plackett RL:** Current trends in statistical inference. *JRSS* 129 (series A):249–267, **1966.**   9

382. **Pocock SJ, Simon R:** Sequential treatment assignment with balancing for prognostic factors in   10
     the controlled clinical trial. *Biometrics* 31:103–115, **1975.**

383. **Pocock SJ:** Group sequential methods in the design and analysis of clinical trials. *Biometrika*   A
     64:191–199, **1977.**

384. **Pocock SJ:** *Clinical Trials: A Practical Approach.* John Wiley and Sons, Chichester, **1983.**   10, 18

385. **Presberg J, Timnick L:** Federal investigation into heart research project here. *St. Louis Globe-*   19
     Democrat, May 3, **1976.**

386. **Prout TE, Knatterud GL, Meinert CL:** Diabetes drugs: Clinical trial (letter). *Science* 204:362–   7
     363, **1979.**

R

387. **Rand Corporation** (The): *A Million Random Digits with 100,000 Normal Deviates.* The Free   10
     Press, Glencoe, Ill, **1955.**

388. **Rand LI, Knatterud GL:** Certification of clinics and staff in a multicenter clinical trial.   3
     University of Maryland, Baltimore. Presented at the Combined Annual Scientific Sessions of
     the Society for Clinical Trials and the 7th Annual Symposium for Coordinating Clinical Trials,
     Philadelphia, May 6–8, **1980.**

389. **Ray AA** (editor): *SAS User's Guide: Statistics* (1982 ed). SAS Institute Inc, Cary, NC, **1982.**   17

390. **Relman AS:** Publications and promotions for the clinical investigator. *Clin Pharmacol Ther*   24
     25:673–676, **1979.**

391. **Relman AS:** Closing the books on Laetrile. *N Engl J Med* 306:236, **1982.**   2

392. **Remington RD:** Problems of university-based scientists associated with clinical trials. *Clin*   4, 24
     Pharmacol Ther 25:662–665, **1979.**

393. **Renou P, Chang A, Anderson I, Wood C:** Controlled trial of fetal intensive care. *Am J Obstet*   2
     Gynecol 126:470–476, **1976.**

394. **Research Development Committee, Society for Research and Education in Primary Care**   26
     Internal Medicine (RH Fletcher, chairman): Clinical research methods: An annotated bibliog-
     raphy. *Ann Intern Med* 99:419–424, **1983.**

395. **Rheumatic Fever Working Party of the Medical Research Council of Great Britain and the**   1
     Subcommittee of Principal Investigators of the American Council of Rheumatic Fever and
     Congenital Heart Disease, American Heart Association: The evolution of rheumatic heart
     disease in children: Five year report of a cooperative clinical trial of ACTH, cortisone and
     aspirin. *Circulation* 22:503–515, **1960.**

396. **Robbins H:** Some aspects of the sequential design of experiments. *Bull Am Mathematics Soc*   A
     58:527–535, **1952.**

397. **Robbins H:** A sequential decision problem with finite memory. *Proc Natl Acad Sci* 42:920–   A
     923, **1956.**

398. **Romm FJ, Hulka BS:** Developing criteria for quality of care assessment: Effect of the Delphi   12
     technique. *Health Serv Res* 14:309–312, **1979.**

399. **Roper FW, Boorkman J:** *Introduction to Reference Sources in the Health Sciences.* Medical   26
     Library Association, Inc, Chicago, Ill, **1980.**

400. **Roth A, Klassen D, Lubin B:** Effects of follow-up procedures on survey results. *Psychol Rep* 47:275–278, **1980**.   12

401. **Rothman DJ:** Were Tuskegee and Willowbrook "Studies in Nature"? *Hastings Center Report* 12:5–7, April **1982**.   14

402. **Royall RM:** Discussion of Dupont's "Statistical inference from clinical trials: Choosing the right p value." *Controlled Clin Trials* 4:23–25, **1983**.   20

S

403. **Sackett DL, Gent M:** Controversy in counting and attributing events in clinical trials. *N Engl J Med* 301:1410–1412, **1979**.   A

404. **Sackett DL:** The competing objectives of clinical trials. *N Engl J Med* 303:1059–1060, **1980**.   A

405. **Schade RR, Donaldson RM:** How physicians use cimetidine: A survey of hospitalized patients and published cases. *N Engl J Med* 304:1281–1284, **1981**.   6

406. **Scheffé H:** A method for judging all contrasts in the analysis of variance. *Biometrika* 40:87–104, **1953**.   20

407. **Schlesselman JJ:** *Case-Control Studies: Design, Conduct, Analysis.* Oxford University Press, New York, **1982**.   9, A

408. **Schmeck HM Jr:** Scientists wary of diabetic pill: FDA study indicates oral drug may be ineffective. *New York Times*, May 22, **1970**.   7

409. **Schor S:** The University Group Diabetes Program: A statistician looks at the mortality results. *JAMA* 217:1671–1675, **1971**.   7, 19, 26

410. **Schriesheim CA:** The effect of grouping or randomizing items on leniency response bias. *Educat Psychol Measurement* 41:401–411, **1981**.   12

411. **Schuman SH, Olansky S, Rivers E, Smith CA, Rambo DS:** Untreated syphilis in the male Negro: Background and current status of patients in the Tuskegee Study. *J Chronic Dis* 2:543–558, **1955**.   14

412. **Schwartz D, Lellouch J:** Explanatory and pragmatic attitudes in therapeutic trials. *J Chronic Dis* 20:637–648, **1967**.   A

413. **Schwartz TB:** The tolbutamide controversy: A personal perspective. *Ann Intern Med* 75:303–306, **1971**.   7

414. **Sciotti H, Sciotti S, Zogbi M** (editors): *Ubrich's International Periodicals Directory* (21st ed, in 2 vols). RR Bowker Co, New York, **1982**.   26

415. **Scott DHT, Arthur GR, Scott DB:** Haemodynamic changes following buprenorphine, and morphine. *Anaesthesia* 35:957–961, **1980**.   8

416. **Seigel D** (chairman, editorial committee): *A Memorial Symposium in Honor of Jerome Cornfield. Biometrics* 38(suppl):1–165, **1982**.   1

417. **Seigel D, Milton RC:** Further results on a multiple-testing procedure for clinical trials. *Biometrics* 39:921–928, **1983**.   20

418. **Selmer ES:** Registration numbers in Norway: Some applied number theory and psychology. *JRSS* 130(series A):225–231, **1967**.   A

419. **Seltzer HS:** A summary of critcisms of the findings and conclusions of the University Group Diabetes Program (UGDP). *Diabetes* 21:976–979, **1972**.   7, 19, 26

420. **Shapiro SH, Louis TA** (editors): *Clinical Trials: Issues and Approaches.* Marcel Dekker, Inc, New York, **1983**.   18

421. **Sherwin R, Kaelber CT, Kezdi P, Kjelsberg MO, Thomas HE Jr:** The Multiple Risk Factor Intervention Trial (MRFIT): II. The development of the protocol. *Prev Med* 10:402–425, **1981**.   3, 13

422. **Simon R:** Adaptive treatment assignment methods and clinical trials. *Biometrics* 33:743–749, **1977**.   10, A

423. **Smith CV, Pyke R:** The Robbins-Isbell two-armed-bandit problem with finite memory. *Ann Math Statistics* 36:1375–1386, **1965**.   A

424. **Smith TW:** Qualifications to generalized absolutes: "Approval of hitting" questions on the GSS. *Public Opinion Quart* 45:224–230, **1981**.   12

425. **Smith WM:** Problems in long-term trials. Merck, Sharp and Dohme, West Point, Pa. Presented at the Joint WHO/ISH Meeting on Mild Hypertension, Susona, Japan, Sept, **1978.**   3

426. **Smythe M:** Record numbering (pp 179–187 in *Record Linkage in Medicine*, HD Achison, editor). The Williams and Wilkins Co, Baltimore, **1968.**   A

427. **Snedecor GW, Cochran WG:** *Statistical Methods* (6th ed). The Iowa State University Press, Ames, Iowa, **1967.**   9

428. **Snell, ES, Armitage P:** Clinical comparisons of diamorphine and pholcodine as cough suppressants: By a new method of sequential analysis. *Lancet* 1:860–862, **1957.**   9

429. **Society for Clinical Trials, Inc:** By Laws. *Controlled Clin Trials* 1:83–89, **1980.**   1

430. **Stallones RA:** The effects of the Freedom of Information Act on research. *Am J Public Health* 72:335–337, **1982.**   7

431. **Stokes J, Noren J, Shindell S:** Definition of terms and concepts applicable to clinical preventive medicine. *J Community Health* 8:33–41, **1982.**   A

432. **Strauss MB** (editor): *Familiar Medical Quotations*. Little, Brown and Company, Boston, **1968.**   2

433. **Stross JK, Harlan WR:** The dissemination of new medical information. *JAMA* 241:2622–2624, **1979.**   7

434. **Stross JK, Harlan WR:** Dissemination of relevant information on hypertention. *JAMA* 246:360–362, **1981.**   7

435. **Sudman S, Bradburn NM:** *Asking Questions: A Practical Guide to Questionnaire Design*. Jossey-Bass Inc, Publishers, San Francisco, **1983.**   12

436. **Sutton HG:** Cases of rheumatic fever. *Guy's Hosp Rep* 11:392–428, **1865.**   1

437. **Szklo M:** The epidemiologic basis for hypertension control. *J Pub Hlth Policy* 1:312–327, **1980.**   7

T

438. **Taylor SH, Silke B, Ebbutt A, Sutton GC, Prout BJ, Burley DM:** A long-term prevention study with oxprenolol in coronary heart disease. *N Engl J Med* 307:1293–1301, **1982.**   A

439. **Temple R, Pledger GW:** Special report: The FDA's critique of the Anturane Reinfarction Trial. *N Engl J Med* 302:1488–1492, **1980.**   9, 18

440. **Thorndike EL, Lorge I:** *The Teacher's Word Book of 30,000 Words*. Columbia University, New York, **1944.**   12

441. **Tonascia J:** Lecture notes from Epidemiology 2. The Johns Hopkins School of Hygiene and Public Health, Baltimore, **1983.**   18

442. **Tucker WB:** The evolution of the cooperative studies in the chemotherapy of tuberculosis of the Veterans Administration and Armed Forces of the USA: An account of the evolving education of the physician in clinical pharmacology. *Adv Tuberc Res* 10:1–68, **1960.**   1

443. **Tukey JW:** "Quick and dirty methods in statistics." Part II: A simple analysis for standard designs. *Proceedings of the 5th Annual Convention of the American Society for Quality Control*, pp 189–197, **1951.**   20

444. **Tukey JW:** Some thoughts on clinical trials, especially problems of multiplicity. *Science* 198:679–684, **1977.**   20

445. **Tuskegee Syphilis Study Ad Hoc Advisory Panel:** *Final Report of the Tuskegee Syphilis Study Ad Hoc Advisory Panel* (47 pages). United States Department of Health, Education, and Welfare, Washington, **1973.**   14

446. **Tygstrup N, Lachin JM, Juhl E** (editors): *The Randomized Clinical Trial and Therapeutic Decisions*. Marcel Dekker, Inc, New York, **1982.**   18

U

447. **United States Congress** (87th): *Drug Amendments of 1962*, Public Law 87-781, S 1522. Washington, Oct 10, **1962.**   1

448. **United States Congress** (94th): *Medical Device Amendments of 1976*, Public Law 94-295, S 510. Washington, May 28, **1976.**   1

449. **United States Congress** (97th): *Small Business Innovation Research Act of 1981* (S 881). 5
Washington, Dec 8, **1981**.

450. **United States Court of Appeals for the District of Columbia Circuit:** Peter H Forsham et al, 7
versus Joseph A Califano, Jr, et al. No. 76–1308, July 11, **1978**.

451. **United States Court of Appeals for the First Circuit:** Robert F Bradley, et al, versus Caspar W 7
Weinberger, Secretary of Health, Education, and Welfare et al. No. 73–1014, July 31, **1973**.

452. **United States District Court for the District of Columbia:** Forsham et al, versus Mathews, 7
et al. No. 75–1608, Sept 30, **1975**.

453. **United States District Court for the District of Columbia:** Peter H Forsham et al, versus David 7
Mathews, et al. No. 75–1608, Feb 5, **1976**.

454. **United States District Court for the District of Delaware:** Pharmaceutical Manufacturers 1
Association versus Robert H Finch, Secretary of Health, Education, and Welfare and Herbert
L Ley, Jr, Commissioner of Food and Drugs. Affidavit of William Thomas Beaver, MD. Civil
action no. 3797, **1969**.

455. **United States District Court for the District of Delaware:** Pharmaceutical Manufacturers 1
Association versus Elliot Richardson, Secretary of Health, Education, and Welfare and
Charles C Edwards, Commissioner of Food and Drugs. Order denying preliminary injunction
and granting summary judgment of dismissal. Civil action no. 3946, Oct 20, **1970**.

456. **United States District Court for the District of Maryland:** Shirley Bailey et al. versus Robert J 14
Lally, etc., et al. Civ nos. K-74-1102, K-75-1370, K-75-1371 and K-75-1372, July 21, **1979**.

457. **United States District Court for the Southern District of New York:** Ciba-Geigy Corporation 7
versus David Mathews, et al. No. 75 Civ 5049, Oct 14, **1975**.

458. **United States District Court for the Southern District of New York:** Ciba-Geigy Corporation 7
versus David Mathews, et al. No. 75 Civ 5049 (CHT), March 8, **1977**.

459. **United States Senate Select Committee on Small Business:** *Oral Hypoglycemic Drugs: Hearing* 7
before the Subcommittee on Monopoly, Sept 18, 19, and 20, 1974. Part 25, U.S. Government
Printing Office, Washington, **1974**.

460. **United States Senate Select Committee on Small Business:** *Oral Hypoglycemic Drugs: Hearing* 7
before the Subcommittee on Monopoly, Jan 31, July 9-10, 1975. Part 28, U.S. Government
Printing Office, Washington, **1975**.

461. **United States Supreme Court:** Peter H Forsham, et al, versus Joseph A Califano, et al. 7
Petition for a writ of certiorari to the United States Court of Appeals for the District of
Columbia Circuit, Oct term, **1978**.

462. **United States Supreme Court:** Forsham, et al, versus Harris, Secretary of Health, Education 7, 24
and Welfare, et al. Certiorari to the United States Court of Appeals for the District of
Columbia Circuit. No. 78–1118, argued Oct 31, 1979, decided March 3, **1980**.

463. **University of Chicago Press:** *The Chicago Manual of Style* (13th ed). Chicago, **1982**. 25

464. **University Group Diabetes Program Research Group:** The effects of hypoglycemic agents on 7
vascular complications in patients with adult-onset diabetes: 1. Design and methods (abstract).
Diabetes 19 (suppl 1):387, **1970a**.

465. **University Group Diabetes Program Research Group:** The effects of hypoglycemic agents on 7
vascular complications in patients with adult-onset diabetes: 2. Findings at baseline (abstract).
Diabetes 19 (suppl 1):374, **1970b**.

466. **University Group Diabetes Program Research Group:** The effects of hypoglycemic agents on 7
vascular complications in patients with adult-onset diabetes: 3. Course and mortality (abstract). *Diabetes* 19 (suppl 1):375, **1970c**.

467. **University Group Diabetes Program Research Group:** A study of the effects of hypoglycemic 3, 6, 7,
agents on vascular complications in patients with adult-onset diabetes: I. Design, methods, and 8, 10, 11,
baseline characteristics. *Diabetes* 19 (suppl 2):747–783, **1970d**. 19, 24,
25

468. **University Group Diabetes Program Research Group:** A study of the effects of hypoglycemic 1, 4, 7,
agents on vascular complications in patients with adult-onset diabetes: II. Mortality results. 8, 10, 11,
Diabetes 19 (suppl 2):785–830, **1970e**. 15, 17–
20, 24, 25

469. **University Group Diabetes Program Research Group:** Effects of hypoglycemic agents on vascular complications in patients with adult-onset diabetes: III. Clinical implications of UGDP results. *JAMA* 218:1400–1410, **1971a.** — 7

470. **University Group Diabetes Program Research Group:** Effects of hypoglycemic agents on vascular complications in patients with adult-onset diabetes: IV. A preliminary report on phenformin results. *JAMA* 217:777–784, **1971b.** — 7, 8, 20, 24

471. **University Group Diabetes Program Research Group:** The UGDP controversy: Clinical trials versus clinical impressions. *Diabetes* 21:1035–1040, **1972.** — 7

472. **University Group Diabetes Program Research Group:** A study of the effects of hypoglycemic agents on vascular complications in patients with adult-onset diabetes: V. Evaluation of phenformin therapy. *Diabetes* 24(suppl 1): 65–184, **1975.** — 7, 17, 19, 20, 24, 25

473. **University Group Diabetes Program Research Group:** Effects of hypoglycemic agents on vascular complications in patients with adult-onset diabetes: VI. Supplementary report on nonfatal events in patients treated with tolbutamide. *Diabetes* 25:1129–1153, **1976.** — 7

474. **University Group Diabetes Program Research Group:** University Group Diabetes Program releases data on 1,027 patients. *Diabetes* 26:1195, **1977.** — 7, 17, 24

475. **University Group Diabetes Program Research Group:** Effects of hypoglycemic agents on vascular complications in patients with adult-onset diabetes: VII. Mortality and selected nonfatal events with insulin treatment. *JAMA* 240:37–42, **1978.** — 1, 7, 8

476. **University Group Diabetes Program Research Group:** Effects of hypoglycemic agents on vascular complications in patients with adult-onset diabetes: VIII. Evaluation of insulin therapy: Final report. *Diabetes* 31(suppl 5):1–81, **1982.** — 7, 8, 15, 17, 23, 24, 25

477. **University Group Diabetes Program Research Group:** Paper listing of baseline and follow-up data on UGDP patients (one volume per treatment group). No. PB 83-136-325, *National Technical Information Service* (NTIS), Springfield, VA, **1983a.** — 7

478. **University Group Diabetes Program Research Group:** Magnetic tape of baseline and follow-up data on UGDP patients. No. PB 83-129-122, *National Technical Information Service* (NTIS), Springfield, VA, **1983b.** — 7

V

479. **Veterans Administration Cooperative Studies Program:** *Guidelines for VA Cooperative Studies* (5th ed). Washington, April, **1982.** — 5, 23

480. **Veterans Administration Cooperative Study Group on Antihypertensive Agents:** Effects of treatment on morbidity in hypertension: Results in patients with diastolic blood pressure averaging 115 through 129 mm Hg. *JAMA* 202:1028–1034, **1967.** — 7, 16

481. **Veterans Administration Cooperative Study Group on Antihypertensive Agents:** Effects of treatment on morbidity in hypertension: II. Results in patients with diastolic blood pressure averaging 90 through 114 mm Hg. *JAMA* 213:1143–1152, **1970.** — 7, 16

482. **Vonderlehr RA, Clark T, Wenger OC, Heller JR Jr:** Untreated syphilis in the male Negro: A comparative study of treated and untreated cases. *J Vener Dis Inform* 17:260–265, **1936.** — 14

W

483. **Wade N:** Food Board's fat report hits fire: Academy discovers Cassandra's problem: What good is the truth if its not spreadable? *Science* 209:248–250, **1980.** — 22

484. **Wald A:** *Sequential Analysis.* John Wiley and Sons, New York, **1947.** — 9

485. **Warner R, Wolfe SM, Rich R:** *Off Diabetes Pills: A Diabetic's Guide to Longer Life.* Public Citizen's Health Research Group, Washington, **1978.** — 7

486. **Waterhouse B:** *A Prospect of Exterminating the Small Pox.* Cambridge Press, Cambridge, **1800.** — 1

487. **Waterhouse B:** *A Prospect of Exterminating the Small Pox.* (part II). University Press, Cambridge, **1802.** — 1

488. **Watson BL:** Disclosure of computerized health care information. *Am J Law Medicine* 7:265–300, **1981.** — 7

489. **Wei LJ, Durham S:** The randomized play-the-winner rule in medical trials. *JASA* 73:840–843,   10
1978.

490. **Weichert BG:** Health care expenditures (in *Health—United States 1981*, pp 81–85). Publ no.   6
(PHS) 82-1232, Department of Health and Human Services, Washington, **1981**.

491. **Weik MH:** *Standard Dictionary of Computers and Information Processing*. Hayden Book   A
Company, Inc, New York, **1970**.

492. **West KM:** Recent trends in dietary management (pp 67–89 in *Clinical Diabetes: Modern*   7
Management, edited by S Podolsky). Appleton-Century-Crofts, New York, **1980**.

493. **Williams ME, Lannon L, O'Donnell R, Barth SN** (editors): *Computer-Readable Data Bases:*   1, 2
A Directory and Data Sourcebook. American Society for Information Science, Washington,
1979.

494. **Woodward, WE:** Informed consent of volunteers: A direct measurement of comprehension   14
and retention of information. *Clinical Research* 27:248–252, **1979**.

495. **Woolf HB** (editor in chief): *Webster's New Collegiate Dictionary*. G and C Merriam Co,   A
Springfield, Mass, **1981**.

496. **Working Group on Arteriosclerosis:** Decline in coronary heart disease mortality, 1968–78 (in   7
Arteriosclerosis 1981, vol 2, pp 159–263). Publ no.82-2035, National Heart, Lung, and Blood
Institute, Bethesda, Md, Sept, **1981**.

497. **Wright IS, Marple CD, Beck DF:** *Myocardial Infarction: Its Clinical Manifestations and*   8
Treatment with Anticoagulants: A Study of 1,031 Cases (Report of the Committee on Anticoagulants). Grune and Stratton, New York, **1954**.

498. **Wright P, Haybittle J:** Design of forms for clinical trials (1) *Br Med J* 2:529–530, **1979a**.   12

499. **Wright P, Haybittle J:** Design of forms for clinical trials (2) *Br Med J* 2:590–592, **1979b**.   12

500. **Wright P, Haybittle J:** Design of forms for clinical trials (3) *Br Med J* 2:650–651, **1979c**.   12

Z

501. **Zdep SM, Rhodes IN, Schwarz RM, Kilkenny MJ:** The validity of the randomized response   12
technique. *Public Opinion Quart* 43:544–549, **1979**.

502. **Zelen M:** Play the winner rule and the controlled clinical trial. *JASA* 64:131–146, **1969**.   10, A

503. **Zelen M.** A new design for randomized clinical trials. *N Engl J Med* 300:1242–1245, **1979**.   14

504. **Zelnio RN:** Data collection techniques: Mail questionnaires. *Am J Hosp Pharm* 37:1113–1119,   12
1980.

505. **Zukel WJ:** Evolution and funding of the Coronary Drug Project. *Controlled Clin Trials* 4:281–   13, 21
312, **1983**.

Index

This index consists of 613 author headings and 975 subject headings. The author portion of the index covers the 505 references listed in the Combined Bibliography (Appendix I), but does not include authors represented in the 130 references in Table B-3 of Appendix B or those in the 180 references listed in Appendix C.

The index contains an entry for each person or corporate entity represented in a bibliographic citation, even if that author's name does not appear on the page cited (e.g., when the number of the reference is cited or the author is not the first author on papers involving three or more authors). A superscript asterisk next to the page cited in the index is used to denote citations of the latter type. All author listings have a minimum of two page listings, at least one of which refers to a page in the Combined Bibliography (pages 430 through 451). Names of persons that appear in the text only as authors are listed as they appear in the Combined Bibliography (i.e., last name followed by initials). The person's first (or second) name is used if the heading contains citations related to the person in a context other than as an author.

Sixty-six of the authors represented are corporate entities. Corporate names related to bibliographic citations from multicenter trials contain the name of the study and end with the term *group* or *research group*. Listings with these terms in parentheses—for example, as in Coronary Drug Project (CDP) (Research Group)—include references to the study itself as well as to papers produced on its behalf.

The terminology conventions discussed in Chapter 1 (pages 8 and 9) and reflected in comments throughout the Glossary (Appendix A) have been followed in constructing this index. Page designations for definitions appear in italics, the majority of which refer to pages in the Glossary (pages 281 to 308).

A

Abt, K: 212, 214, 430
acts: *see* legislative acts and regulations
adherence: *see* treatment, adherence
adverse side effect, adverse drug reaction: *see* side effect, adverse
Alamercery, Y: 31, 430
Albert Einstein College of Medicine: 354
Albrink, Margaret J: 349
allocated (assigned) treatment: 199–200, *282*
allocation: 6, 12, 16, *282*, *305*, *see also* randomization
  adaptive: *281*
    baseline: *282*
    number: *295*
    outcome: *296*
    play the winner: *298*
    two-armed bandit: *307*
  design: *281*, *290*, *305*
  dynamic: *see* allocation, adaptive
  equal: *see* allocation, uniform
  fixed: *289–90*
  methods: 12, 16, 25–26, 67–68
  probability: 91, *305*
  ratio: 78 (choice of), 92–93, 196, 199–200, *289–90*, *295*, *303*, *305*
  restricted: *301*
  schedule: *282*, *290*, *301*, *305*, *307*
  strata: 93, *305*
  stratified: *303*
  systematic: 6, 68, 198
  uniform: 78, 92, *289*, *295*, *307*
  unit: 10, *305*
  unrestricted: *307*
Amberson, JB Jr: 4, 6, 430

Ambroz, A: 15*, 300*, 432
American Bible Society: 3, 430
American Diabetes Association: 51, 53, 263
American Heart Association: 7, 102, 123
American Medical Association (Journal of): 59, 257
analysis: 8, 72–74, 80, 96, 173, 175–95, 201–2, 204–6, 208–16, 269, 275, *282–83*, *286*, *288–92*, *294*, *301–2*, *304*, 363–64, 367
  adjustment procedures: 193–95, *286*, *294*, *304*
    multiple regression: 194–95, *286*, *294*
    subgrouping: 193–94, *304*, *see also* stratification
  Bayesian: 8, *283*
  (by) intention to treat: 186, 204, *282*
  (by) treatment administered: 186, *282*
  cohort analysis: 192–93
  database: 179–84, *282*
  fixed sample size: 72–74, 185–95
  groundrules: 80, 185–87, 201–2, 204–5
  group sequential: *290*
  interim: 96, 173, 206, 208–16, *291*, *see also* interim result
  lifetable: 188–92, *292*
  procedures: 185–95, 204–6, 208–15, 269, 275, 363–64, 367, *see also* analysis, adjustment procedures; analysis, lifetable; chi-square test (of significance); Fisher's exact test (of significance); Mantel-Haenszel test statistic; inverse sine transform test (of significance); log rank test statistic; mutiple, comparisons; multiple, looks; Poisson test (of significance); *t*-test (of significance)
  regression procedures: *see* analysis, adjustment procedures
  risk factor: *301*
  sequential: 72–73, *302*
  subgroup analysis: 204, 213–15, *see also* analysis, adjustment procedures

453